CRANIAL COMPUTED TOMOGRAPHY

CRANIAL COMPUTED TOMOGRAPHY

Seungho Howard Lee, M.D.

Professor of Radiology
Chief of Neuroradiology
Department of Radiology
State University of New York
Upstate Medical Center
Syracuse, New York

Krishna C.V.G. Rao, M.D.

Associate Professor of Radiology
  and Clinical Neurosurgery
Chief of Neuroradiology
Department of Radiology
University of Maryland School of Medicine and Hospital
Baltimore, Maryland

McGraw-Hill Book Company

New York   St. Louis   San Francisco   Auckland   Bogotá   Guatemala   Hamburg   Johannesburg
Lisbon   London   Madrid   Mexico   Montreal   New Delhi   Panama   Paris
San Juan   São Paulo   Singapore   Sydney   Tokyo   Toronto

NOTICE

Medicine is an ever-changing science. As new research and clinical experience broaden our knowledge, changes in treatment and drug therapy are required. The editors and the publisher of this work have made every effort to ensure that the drug dosage schedules herein are accurate and in accord with the standards accepted at the time of publication. Readers are advised, however, to check the product information sheet included in the package of each drug they plan to administer to be certain that changes have not been made in the recommended dose or in the contraindications for administration. This recommendation is of particular importance in regard to new or infrequently used drugs.

CRANIAL COMPUTED TOMOGRAPHY

Copyright © 1983 by McGraw-Hill, Inc. All rights reserved. Printed in the United States of America. Except as permitted under the United States Copyright Act of 1976, no part of this publication may be reproduced or distributed in any form or by any means, or stored in a data base or retrieval system, without the prior written permission of the publisher.

1234567890 HDHD 898765432

ISBN 0-07-037399-X

This book was set in Palatino by Ruttle, Shaw & Wetherill, Inc.; the editors were Robert P. McGraw, Stuart D. Boynton, and Mark W. Cowell; the production supervisor was Jeanne Skahan; the designer was Murray Fleminger.
Halliday Lithograph Corporation was printer and binder.

Library of Congress Cataloging in Publication Data
Main entry under title:

Cranial computed tomography.

  Bibliography: p
  Includes index.
  1. Cranium—Radiography. 2. Head—Diseases—
Diagnosis. 3. Tomography. I. Lee, Seungho H.
(Seungho Howard) II. Rao, Krishna C.V.G.
RC936.C717 1983   617'.4107572   82-14009
ISBN 0-07-037399-X

*To our wives, Taeja Kim and Kusuma, and
to our children, Michele, Jennifer, Anil, and Sudhir*

Contents

List of Contributors

Larissa T. Bilaniuk, M.D.
Associate Professor of Radiology
University of Pennsylvania School of Medicine and
  Hospital
Philadelphia, Pennsylvania

Norman E. Chase, M.D.
Professor and Chairman
Department of Radiology
New York University School of Medicine and Hospital
New York, New York

Richard E. Fernandez, M.D.
Instructor in Radiology
Medical College of Virginia and Hospital
Richmond, Virginia

Charles R. Fitz, M.D.
Associate Professor of Radiology
Sick Children's Hospital
University of Toronto College of Medicine
Toronto, Canada

Mokhtar H. Gado, M.D.
Professor of Radiology
Mallinckrodt Institute of Radiology and
Washington University School of Medicine
St. Louis, Missouri

Herbert I. Goldberg, M.D.
Professor of Radiology
University of Pennsylvania School of Medicine and
  Hospital
Philadelphia, Pennsylvania

Kalyanmay Ghoshhajra, M.D.
Clinical Associate Professor of Radiology
University of Pittsburgh
Pittsburgh, Pennsylvania

Derek C. Harwood-Nash, M.D.
Professor and Chairman
Department of Radiology
Sick Children's Hospital
University of Toronto College of Medicine
Toronto, Canada

Stephen A. Kieffer, M.D.
Professor and Chairman
Department of Radiology
State University of New York
Upstate Medical Center
Syracuse, New York

Pulla R.S. Kishore, M.D.
Professor of Radiology
Medical College of Virginia and Hospital
Richmond, Virginia

Jonathan Kleefield, M.D.
Assistant Professor of Radiology
Tuft Medical School and Boston Veterans Hospital
Boston, Massachusetts

Irvin I. Kricheff, M.D.
Professor of Radiology
New York University School of Medicine and Hospital
New York, New York

Seungho Howard Lee, M.D.
Professor of Radiology
State University of New York
Upstate Medical Center
Syracuse, New York

Harvey L. Levine, M.D.
Associate Professor of Radiology
Tufts Medical School and Boston Veterans Hospital
Boston, Massachusetts

Maurice H. Lipper, M.B., Ch.B.
Associate Professor of Radiology
Medical College of Virginia and Hospital
Richmond, Virginia

Jaime H. Montoya, M.D.
Assistant Professor of Radiology
Temple University School of Medicine and Hospital
Philadelphia, Pennsylvania

Krishna C.V.G. Rao, M.D.
Associate Professor of Radiology and Clincial
   Neurosurgery
Department of Radiology
University of Maryland Medical School and Hospital
Baltimore, Maryland

Karel G. TerBrugge, M.D.
Assistant Professor of Radiology
University of Toronto College of Medicine
Toronto Western Hospital
Toronto, Canada

Theodore Villafana, Ph.D.
Professor of Radiology
Temple University School of Medicine and Hospital
Philadelphia, Pennsylvania

J. Powell Williams, M.D.
Professor of Radiology
University of Southern Alabama School of Medicine
Mobile, Alabama

Robert A. Zimmerman, M.D.
Professor of Radiology
University of Pennsylvania School of Medicine and
   Hospital
Philadelphia, Pennsylvania

Preface

The introduction of computed tomography (CT) has been one of the most significant advances among the imaging modalities. CT plays such a vital role today that good practice in clinical neurosciences is not conceivable without its utilization. Since its introduction in 1973, technical improvements have been made at a rapid pace, resulting in significantly better image resolution and extensive utilization for parts of the body other than the cranium. Indeed, this one modality has created an impact not only in its clinical utilization but also in bringing about bureaucratic controls, because of the cost of CT equipment.

Vast amounts of information on both technical and clinical application of cranial CT has accumulated in the last several years. This book is intended to summarize and consolidate information relating to the clinical aspect of cranial computed tomography. Although we do not intend this book to be an encyclopedia of cranial CT, we have attempted to depict the state of the art in clinical cranial CT in the early 1980s, aiming to place it in a clinical perspective for the students, the trainees, and the practitioners of neurosciences; radiologists, neurologists, and neurosurgeons.

Preparing this book was made especially difficult because CT technology has evolved so rapidly, which is amply exhibited by the varying quality of the CT images in the text, representing a few generations of CT scanners. Futhermore, all of the contributing authors had to adhere to rigid deadlines to insure that the chapters were written and published within a short period of time. We are extremely grateful to the contributing authors for undertaking such an admittedly difficult task.

The editors are deeply indebted to our colleagues who have contributed many of the interesting cases. Indeed, they are in a true sense coauthors of the present work. We are extremely thankful to the editors of McGraw-Hill, Robert McGraw, Mark Cowell, Stuart Boynton and Edward Schultheis; our secretaries, especially Tricia Mead and Suellen Molloy; and the photographers, especially David Crandall and John G. Hodgson, for their help in preparation of this book.

We also wish to express our sincere gratitude to Drs. Marc S. Lapayowker and William A. Buchheit at Temple University, Philadelphia; John Murray Dennis, Joseph E. Whitely and Thomas B. Ducker at the University of Maryland, Baltimore; and E. Robert Heitzman, Stephen A. Kieffer and Robert B. King at Upstate Medical Center, Syracuse, New York, for their understanding, encouragement, and assistance in our undertaking of this project.

Seungho Howard Lee
Krishna C.V.G. Rao

1

PHYSICS AND INSTRUMENTATION

Theodore Villafana

INTRODUCTION

Few innovations in radiology have fomented as much excitement and fundamental change as has computed, or computerized, tomography (CT). It turns out that a wealth of radiological information had been overlooked in classical radiology and tomography (Ter-Pogossian 1974). In fact, even now, computed tomography as we know it is probably just the beginning of what may come. Radiologists, of course, have been caught up in this imaging revolution. They must become increasingly familiar with the physical principles, instrumentation, and technical limitations of computed tomography in order to make accurate and precise diagnostic interpretations. The purpose of this chapter is to provide a fuller understanding of the basic CT scanning principles of direct importance to the clinician. The presentation here consists, first, of a brief review of the basis and the limitations of classical radiographic imaging. Second, classical tomography, as an attempt to overcome some of the problems of classical radiography, is also briefly discussed. Finally, computed tomography and its limitations are discussed fully.

Basic X-Ray Image Formation

The basic aim of diagnostic radiology is to record on a film (or display on a monitor) a pattern of densities (or illumination levels on a monitor) which corresponds to and conveys diagnostic information on

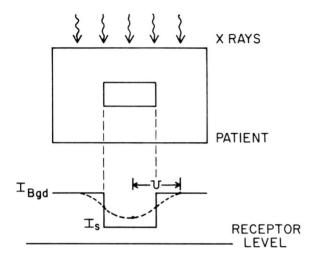

Figure 1-1 An intensity profile of the x-ray beam as it emerges from the patient. Here a hypothetical square anatomical structure ideally casts a shadow (I_s) relative to the adjoining background tissue (I_{Bgd}). The depth of the shadow or subject contrast, C_s, depends on the difference in attenuation between the two areas. Factors such as scatter, motion, and focal spot size tend to degrade both subject contrast and the edge character of the pattern (dashed curve) U as the resulting unsharpness or distance edge is blurred over.

the size, shape, and distribution of the anatomic tissues within a patient. For instance, in Figure 1-1, we see a beam of x-rays penetrating a "simplified patient" consisting of simply a square block of tissue surrounded by a different but uniform tissue background. As the x-rays pass through the patient they are attenuated, that is, they are both absorbed and scattered within the patient. Attenuation, however, will depend on the type of tissues present and on the x-ray beam energy. Finally, the x-rays emerge from the patient and arrive at the image receptor level, where they are recorded.

Figure 1-1 depicts one particular x-ray intensity profile. It is important to realize that this x-ray intensity profile is the sum total of the transmitted primary beam and the scattered radiation reaching the receptor level. Each point along the final profile thus depends on the x-ray attenuation which occurred along each ray-path within the patient, as well as the scatter generated. Note also that the final two-dimensional image is composed of the col-

lection of all such intensity profiles within the patient for the entire exposed field.

Let us study further the representation of radiographic images by intensity profiles, as this is the key to understanding CT technology. Referring again to Figure 1-1, we see that if x-rays penetrate a square object, a square x-ray profile is expected. This profile exhibits a certain depth (object shadow) as well as a certain edge character. It should be clear that if the anatomic square structure under study had been more similar in atomic number and density to the background medium, the pattern depth or shadow would have been diminished and visualization would have been poorer. The relative x-ray intensity difference between the background and the anatomic structure of interest is referred to as the *relative subject contrast* (C_s).

$$C_s = \frac{I_{Bgd} - I_s}{I_{Bgd}} \qquad (1)$$

Subject contrast depends on a number of factors, of which the beam energy is one of the two most important. Beam energy in turn is governed by the operating kilovoltage and the beam filtration present in the beam. The second factor is the atomic number difference between the background and the anatomic structure in question. Figure 1-2 plots subject contrast as a function of beam energy for various combinations of anatomic tissues. Note that subject contrast diminishes as beam energy increases and as tissues become more similar. The practical importance of the C_s measure and how it limits routine radiography can be illustrated by the case of blood vessels within soft-tissue surrounds. Visualization of brain or renal vasculature, for instance, is extremely poor even under the most advantageous circumstance. However, introduction of contrast media into the blood vessel drastically increases its attenuation properties as compared to the surrounding tissues, and the blood vessels "light up." Introducing contrast media greatly increases subject contrast, and visualization is markedly improved.

In addition to subject contrast, a second important aspect of the x-ray image is its edge character. Figure 1-1 shows the ideal case, in which the x-ray image has exactly the same well-defined edges as the structure itself. In general, this is not the case; unsharp edges usually appear. Deviation from a well-defined edge is quantitated with the concept of *unsharpness* (or *blur*). Unsharpness represents the smear around the edge and is simply expressed as the distance from the point of maximum intensity to the point of minimum intensity. A number of factors affect unsharpness in the x-ray image. The most important of these are anatomic and patient motion, scatter, focal-spot size, relative geometry of the patient, and the x-ray source. The concept of unsharpness can be applied not only to the x-ray image but also to the final recorded and visible image by incorporating the recording-system image-degrading effects.

In addition to subject contrast and unsharpness, a third aspect of the x-ray image is *quantum mottle* (or *x-ray image noise*). Quantum mottle can be simply defined as the relative fluctuation in photon number arriving at the image plane. Figure 1-3 illustrates how quantum mottle can seriously obscure both the edge character and the depth character of a given

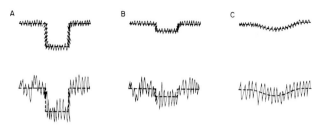

Figure 1-3 The effects of x-ray noise (quantum mottle) on x-ray intensity profiles. **A.** Ideal intensity profile with relatively high subject contrast (depth of shadow). Increasing amounts of noise mask the x-ray image but it may still be detected. **B.** Ideal profile with relatively low subject contrast. Increasing amounts of noise readily obscure pattern. **C.** Unsharp and low subject contrast pattern is also readily obscured by noise.

image, especially for low subject contrast and small object sizes. Quantum mottle arises from the fact that there are random fluctuations in the x-ray emission spectrum of the x-ray source as well as in the interactions the x-rays undergo within the patient.

To minimize the effect of quantum mottle in the x-ray image, the overall photon levels at the image plane must be increased. This can be accomplished by increases in x-ray tube current, or kilovoltage, or by a decrease in distance from the x-ray source to the image receptor. Attempts to decrease quantum mottle in such a manner, however, usually result in increased radiation dose to the patient.

CLASSICAL RADIOGRAPHY

In classical radiography, one attempts to record directly the x-ray intensity profiles in the form of a density distribution on a film. This process, though simple and direct, forms the major limitation for classical radiography. The reason for this limitation is clear when one considers the fact that the patient is made up of a complex distribution of different tissues and structures. Any particular x-ray intensity profile emerging from the patient is thus the compounded sum of the attenuation which occurred in the patient along a particular ray-path.

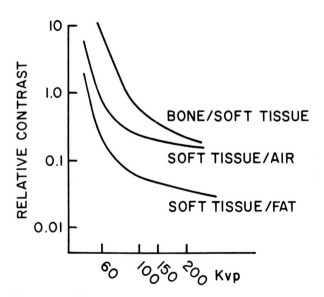

Figure 1-2 Plot of subject contrast between typical tissues as a function of energy. Note how subject contrast diminishes with increasing energy and with increasing similarity in tissue densities. (Adapted from Meredith and Massey, 1972.)

Under these conditions contour can interfere with contour and shadow with shadow. What will finally be most prominent in the recorded image is that anatomic structure with the greatest absorption. Thus lesions can be "lost" behind the ribs or the heart shadow or, in the skull, behind the fossa as well as along the base of the calvarium. In practice, this information loss is compensated for in part by obtaining two views perpendicular to each other, such as anterior-posterior and lateral views, as well as other views such as obliques.

Other limitations in classical radiography include the presence of scatter and the use of nonlinear receptors. Scatter is a major source of image degradation, hence scatter-eliminating grids are generally used. It is true that the use of high-ratio grids reduces scatter as much as 95 to 98 percent, depending on patient thickness and grid ratio. However, it is also true that the difference in subject contrast between such structures as gray matter and white matter is less than 1 percent. As a result, even a small percentage of scatter can obscure visualization.

In the case of nonlinear receptors, the basic problem is the fact that at low subject- or tissue-contrast different structures may have densities falling in the nonlinear response region of the receptor. These nonlinear regions yield less film contrast. This can be seen in the H&D response curve and the corresponding film contrast curve illustrated in Figure 1-4. Here, film contrast is merely the slope of the H&D response curve and determines the actual density differences seen on the film. Note that the point of maximum film contrast occurs at about the middle of the linear region. This means that slight exposure or x-ray intensity differences at this level of the H&D curve result in the greatest displayed density differences. Film contrast progressively falls toward both the high-density and low-density sides of the linear region. Final displayed density difference is referred to as *image, radiographic,* or *broad-area contrast.*

Figure 1-4 illustrates these ideas graphically. Here a given slight exposure difference along *B* is finally displayed with a density difference of Δ*B*. If exposures had been such that tissue structures of

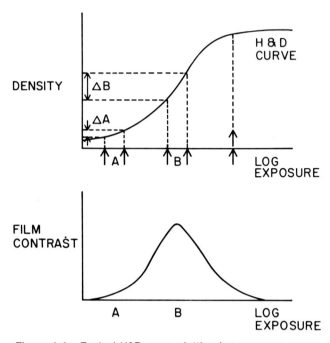

Figure 1-4 Typical H&D curve plotting log exposure versus resulting optical density. Nonlinearity of this curve results in a variable film contrast as seen in the lower figure where the film contrast at any point of the curve is plotted as merely the slope of the H&D curve at each point. Slight differences in exposure along *B* lying on the linear portion of the H&D curve are displayed with the greatest difference in densities or image contrast (Δ*B*) and thus are better visualized. Exposures at the lower densities (*A*) or at higher densities are visualized at lower image contrast (Δ*A*).

interest were in the low-density region, i.e., along *A*, then final displayed contrast would be Δ*A*, and the observed density difference would be less than that obtained along the center of the H&D curve. Radiographically, this can be seen in Figure 1-5A, where a bullet is not visible in an approximately correctly exposed chest film, which usually leaves the mediastinum area at very low densities and thus low display contrast. Figure 1-5B shows the same patient but with exposures sufficiently high so that structures of interest are displayed at higher densities and thus higher display contrast; presence of the bullet then becomes obvious.

One last observation should be made here, that even if the exposure factors (kilovoltage and milliamperage) are selected optimally for a given tissue

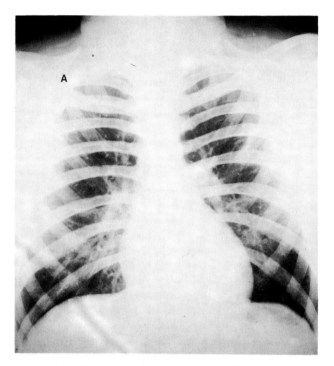 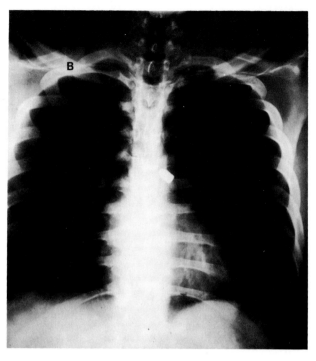

Figure 1-5 Example of loss of important image details in classical radiography as a function of density on the film. **A.** Correctly exposed chest film leaving heart shadow at low density and thus low image contrast. **B.** Bullet obviously present when film is exposed to higher density levels where image contrast is higher.

or subject contrast, one may still be limited by a relatively small final display contrast. In CT scanning, under computer control one can increase and optimize the display contrast, utilizing the full black-and-white capability of modern cathode ray tube (CRT) monitors. This is referred to as *windowing*. For instance, exposures along *B* in Figure 1-4, rather than being displayed with display contrast ΔB, can be windowed in such a way that one can arbitrarily assign them any desired gray-scale values, including the full range of white to black. This important feature is discussed further in a subsequent section.

The following limiting factors of classical radiography as seen in this section can then be summarized:

1. Superimposition of three-dimensional information onto two dimensions causes the loss of low-tissue-contrast anatomic structures.
2. Presence of scatter obscures low-tissue-contrast anatomic structures.
3. Presence of nonlinear film receptors limits display contrast at high and low densities, as well as the fact that display contrast is not adjustable on film.

CLASSICAL TOMOGRAPHY

Classical tomography was formulated in an attempt to minimize the problem of the superimposition of three-dimensional information onto two dimensions. It is based on moving the x-ray source and film cassette relative to each other in such a way that the recorded images of anatomic structures within the patient are blurred. However, one anatomic layer (referred to as the *focal, fulcrum,* or *pivot plane*) within the patient remains stationary relative to the film and is recorded unblurred. Thus the third dimension (patient thickness, or depth) is removed, and presumably only the specified or pivot layer is recorded at full contrast and sharpness. It is clear, however, that the scatter problem is still present, as well as the limitations of nonlinear film and screen systems.

Classical tomography has been reviewed in depth (Littleton 1976), and the reader is referred to a wealth of literature already available. What must be emphasized here is that tomography has certain inherent limitations which result in less than optimal information acquisition. These limitations can be summarized as follows:

1. There is incomplete tomographic blurring of the nonfocused planes. This means that obscuring anatomy is never completely and totally removed. The degree of blurring depends on distance from the focal plane. Therefore structures near the focal plane affect the image to a greater extent than structures far from the focal plane.
2. Some blur occurs within the focal plane itself, obscuring the anatomy one desires to visualize, since theoretically only an infinitesimally thin plane is truly in focus. This may be overcome in part by scanning over wide-arc angles (thin-section tomography). Finally, some blur also may occur within the focal plane because of mechanical vibration of the moving apparatus.
3. Tomographic blur is dependent on the direction of motion relative to the shape of the anatomy to be blurred. For example, linear tomography does not blur structures whose boundaries are parallel to the direction of arc motion; rather, only structures whose margins are at an angle to the arc motion are blurred.
4. Even though unwanted structures are blurred, they contribute fog background density to the film, which lowers the relative contrast of the structures within the pivot plane.

COMPUTED TOMOGRAPHY

We now come to computed tomography (CT). CT has in great measure overcome the various limitations of both classical radiography and classical tomography. This has been accomplished by

1. Scanning only a thin, well-defined volume of interest, which serves to minimize the superimposition effect
2. Minimizing scatter by collimating down to relatively thin volumes
3. Using linear detectors with computerized windowing functions

The final success of the diagnostic task hinges on how well the image displays or conveys diagnostic information on the distribution of anatomic structures within the patient. In classical radiography the emerging x-ray beam is recorded directly, with an intensifying screen/film combination. The emerging beam, however, represents the total attenuation which occurred within the patient cross section, and as discussed previously the superimposition effect is present. Ideally, one would like to have displayed a point-by-point characterization of the anatomical cross section under study. The characterization presently most useful is that of x-ray attenuation in tissue. Recently a host of other characterizations and different radiation types have been proposed and studied with varying degrees of success. These include the atomic number and electron density (Phelps 1975; Rutherford 1976; Latchaw 1978), nuclear magnetic resonance properties (Hinshaw 1979; Moore 1980; Holland 1980; Partain 1980), ultrasound acoustic impedance (Carson 1977; Kak 1979), microwaves (Kak 1979; Maini 1980), neutrons (Koeppe 1981), protons (Cormack 1976) and isotopic emission (Emission Computed Tomography I, 1980; Emission Computed Tomography II, 1981). CT reconstructions based on fluoroscopic techniques have also been developed (Baily, 1976; Kak, 1977).

The computed tomography approach consists in isolating a specific planar volume within the patient. This plane, or slice, has a thickness z as seen in

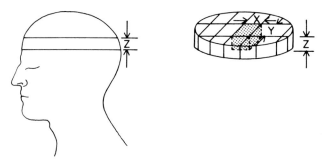

Figure 1-6 Cross-sectional slice across patient—the expanded view showing arrangement of pixels (or picture elements) of dimensions *x* by *y* in a grid array. Volume element (or voxel) is formed in a third dimension due to the finite slice thickness.

Figure 1-6. The x-ray beam to be utilized passes through only this volume, thus superimposition and scatter effects are greatly minimized but not totally eliminated. Final characterization of tissues within the scanned volume will be expressed and displayed for each element area given by *x* and *y* as seen in Figure 1-6. This element area is referred to as a *pixel* (*pic*ture *el*ement). The volume formed by virtue of the slice having some thickness *z* is referred to as a *voxel* (*vo*lume *el*ement). In practice, the whole patient part is arbitrarily broken down into a matrix array of such pixels. The pioneer EMI Mark I unit consisted of an 80 × 80 array in which each pixel corresponded to a 3 mm × 3 mm area within the patient and had a slice thickness of 13 mm. Matrix sizes of modern units are 256 × 256, 512 × 512, or even higher. Pixel sizes now correspond to 1 mm by 1 mm or an even smaller area within the patient. Different CT units have different pixel configurations. In most cases, however, the critical parameter is not the number of pixels but rather the area they correspond to within the patient.

Attenuation Coefficients and Algorithms

The tissue type within each pixel is characterized by the tissue's property of x-ray attenuation, which is defined simply as the removal of x-ray photons from the beam. This removal can be accomplished either by absorption (energy deposited at or near the site of photon interaction) or scatter events (energy removed from the site of photon interaction). Tissues in general have different attenuation properties, depending on their atomic number and physical density and the incident photon energy. One can describe the attenuation of a material in terms of the *attenuation coefficient,* usually symbolized by the Greek letter μ and having units of cm^{-1}. The attenuation coefficient is quite familiar to radiological scientists and with the advent of CT scanning has taken on special importance to the clinical radiologist. Table 1-1 lists typical biological tissues of interest and their corresponding attenuation coefficients. Also shown is their representation on an arbitrary scale on which bone is specified as $+1000$, air as -1000, and water as zero. This scale is now usually referred to as the Hounsfield scale in honor of the inventor of computed tomography, Godfrey N. Hounsfield (1972). Formerly these numbers were referred to as EMI and delta numbers by the CT manufacturers. More commonly they are simply referred to as *CT numbers.* (For extensive tabulation of attenuation coefficients and CT numbers, see Phelps 1975b, Rao 1975, and McCullough 1975.)

The decision to characterize tissue types by Hounsfield numbers and to specify an array of pixels within the patient still leaves the problem of actually determining the value of the CT number

Table 1-1   Attenuation Coefficient and CT No. for Biological Tissues at 60 keV

Tissue	*Attenuation coefficient* μ *(cm^{-1})*	*CT number*
Bone	0.400	+1000
Blood	0.215	+100 (approx.)
Brain Matter	0.210	+30 (approx.)
CSF	0.207	+5 (approx.)
Water	0.203	0
Fat	0.185	−100 (approx.)
Air	0.0002	−1000

Source: Adapted from Phelps et al. 1975b.

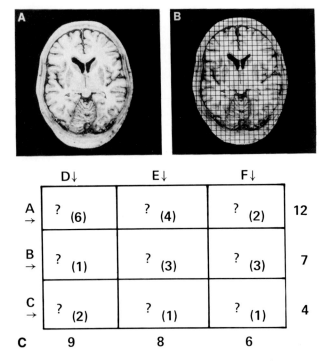

Figure 1-7 A Cross sectional slice of brain showing structures to be imaged. **B.** Grid array of pixels superimposed over brain slice. The task in CT scanning is to determine tissue type within each pixel. **C.** As an example of how pixel values are determined, here is an unknown 3 × 3 array of pixels. Each pixel has some number value. Even though the interior values are unknown, the total exterior sums along the horizontal paths A, B, and C and vertical paths D, E, and F can be determined (transmission values when using x-rays). Mathematical techniques (algorithms) are available to reconstruct the true interior values from this type of exterior data even for a very large number of pixels.

for each pixel within that patient. Figure 1-7 shows a simplified 3 × 3 matrix array containing nine pixels, each having specific but unknown values of attenuation. The task is to determine the attenuation for each pixel. If x-rays are passed through ray-path *A*, an attenuation corresponding to, for instance, 12 units is determined. This value is referred to as a *ray sum* and represents the total attenuation occurring from the sum of the attenuation in all the pixels along that ray. Likewise, ray-paths *B* and *C* yield totals of 7 and 4, respectively. The process is repeated from another angle perpendicular to the first (ray-paths *D*, *E*, and *F*), and ray sums of 9, 8,

and 6 are found. Now the task is to assign or reconstruct values for each pixel which will conform with ray sums experimentally found from the two angles used. One may, in fact, "play" with the numbers and finally arrive at the correct distribution, such as that indicated in Figure 1-6.

In the case of matrix arrays which are, for instance, 512 × 512 in extent, one must determine ray scans over many different angles (from 180° to 360°), and the amount of data to be collected is formidable—so much so that a computer is necessary to keep track of the data and to perform the actual calculations necessary for a successful reconstruction. The model, or calculation scheme used for reconstruction, is referred to as an *algorithm*. The most popular algorithm for commercial scanners is the back-projection algorithm. In this algorithm the ray sum for each row of pixels, for a first approximation, is assigned to each pixel along that·row (this is called *back projection*). As each new set of data corresponding to a new angle of scan is determined, it is also back-projected and averaged into each pixel. Such a procedure, though not directly intuitive, does in fact, as seen in Figure 1-8, result in a successful image reconstruction. Note in Figure 1-8 that back projection is accomplished by linearly

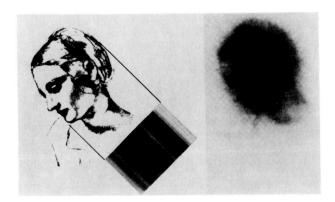

Figure 1-8 Example of back-projection technique using a pictorial view of a face. The value of the density along each line is given by the average along each line. In this particular case the average is obtained via a smearing motion (equivalent to back projection). When all such projections are summed, the original face is, surprisingly enough, reconstructed. (After Gordon 1975.)

smearing (back-projecting) the image for a number of different angles, and the sum, or superimposition, of all the views represents a reconstruction of the original image.

For CT images it is the computer which processes the ray sums and accomplishes the necessary back projections. In practice, before back projection is implemented, each intensity profile is modified or filtered to minimize starlike artifacts caused by use of a finite set of angular images made to correspond to a square pixel. A number of *filter functions* are incorporated in the algorithms which have been used or proposed, and the reader is referred to various reviews (Gordon 1974; Brooks 1975). These filter functions, which are sometimes called *kernels*, can also incorporate varying degrees of *smoothing*. Smoothing may sometimes be of value when noise limits the detail visible in the image (Joseph 1978a). Many CT units have a number of filter functions available, and the user should be aware of possible improvements in the images and the possibility of decreasing patient dose with their use. It should, however, also be realized that the smoothing operation degrades image resolution and thus limits the smallest sizes that can be displayed. It should be considered only as a noise suppressant in imaging relatively large structures.

Data Collection Geometry

It is worth repeating that the reconstruction process involves the collection of x-ray transmission values outside the patient. These transmission values are an index of how much the radiation was attenuated in passage through the patient. The collection of such data from a number of different angles around the patient is used to calculate the attenuation occurring at each picture element within the patient. Various data-collection schemes have been employed for the acquisition of x-ray transmission data. All schemes involve some geometrical pattern of scanning around the patient coupled with use of a suitable radiation detector. The signal from the radiation detector is digitized by the use of an analog-to-digital (A/D) converter and passed onto the computer for processing. After the reconstruction is completed, the results are displayed on a video monitor. The images can be preserved for long-term storage either on discs or on magnetic tape. The overall layout is illustrated in Figure 1-9.

Translate/Rotate Geometry

The first successful clinical CT scanner was based on a translate/rotate gantry geometry. In this type of system the x-ray beam is collimated down to the desired slice thickness and to a narrow slit, typically 3 mm in width. The resulting x-ray pattern is referred to as a *pencil beam.* The pencil beam is then passed through the patient and is incident on a radiation detector, as seen in Figure 1-10. The quantity of radiation arriving at the detector for each ray-path will depend on the total attenuation which

Figure 1-9 Block diagram of a typical CT system. After x-rays emerge from the patient they are detected, amplified, and digitized with an analog-to-digital (A/D) converter. After computer processing, the reconstruction results are assigned a gray scale and displayed on a CRT video monitor from which hard-copy views may be obtained. Alternatively, CT number data can be outputted to a line printer for quantitative analysis. Normally a tape or disc system is also used for storage of data for later redisplay and/or image manipulation.

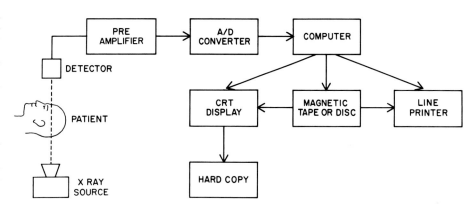

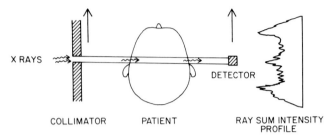

X RAYS

COLLIMATOR   PATIENT   RAY SUM INTENSITY
                                  PROFILE

DETECTOR

Figure 1-10 First-generation type CT configuration. A pencil beam is formed with a collimator and passed through the patient at a particular angle onto a detector traversing the patient along with the x-ray pencil beam. A ray sum intensity profile is thus detected and channeled to the computer for processing. The process is repeated at 1° intervals for 180°.

occurred along the ray-path for each volume element (voxel) traversed.

In order to determine the ray-attenuation sums for each row of voxels, the pencil beam is made to linearly scan, or translate, across the patient. During the translate motion the detector, being rigidly connected to the x-ray tube, moves in such a manner that it always intercepts the x-ray pencil beam. The signals detected during the translation motion form a profile representing the ray sums along all voxel rows.

To determine the ray-sum profiles at different angles, the unit must sequentially rotate and perform a translation movement across the patient for each angle of rotation. The original EMI Mark I system rotated a total of 180° one degree at a time (the configuration usually referred to as *first-generation geometry*). These movements required a total of 5½ to 6 minutes to complete. Unfortunately, patient motion and resulting mismatch between patient position and pixel position resulted in severe image streaks. To reduce overall patient examination time, two detectors were placed side by side in the *Z* (or slice thickness) directions and the x-ray beam made wide enough to include both these detectors. This had the effect of providing two image slices simultaneously and shortening the overall time needed to obtain all the slices desired, as well as minimizing patient motion between slices.

Individual slice scan times may be reduced sig-

nificantly by providing for multiple pencil beams, with each beam directed at its own detector. This has the effect of obtaining ray sums from different angles on one translation (the configuration referred to as *second-generation geometry*). This is illustrated in Figure 1-11 for a three-pencil-beam system. Here the pencil beams are configured to be at a 1° angle to one another. Consequently, during one translation data are collected for three different angles, and the unit can be rotated 3° instead of 1° as for a single-pencil-beam configuration. Scan times can thus be reduced approximately three times, since the unit need complete only one-third the number of rotations and translations. (Sixty rotations at 3° increments will still provide for 180° around the patient and 180 ray-sum profiles.) Additionally, one may provide for a second bank of detectors identical to the first, to detect and process two slices simultaneously. To further reduce scan times one may incorporate even more pencil beams, each with its own detector. Thus 10 beams will require 10 detectors and only 18 rotations, 20 beams will require 9 rotations, etc. In fact, given sufficient beams and detectors, scan times can be effectively reduced to a few seconds. In this latter case, since scan times are relatively short, the second bank of detectors may be eliminated, for a considerable cost saving.

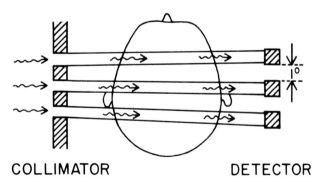

COLLIMATOR   DETECTOR

Figure 1-11 Configuration for second-generation gantry systems. A series of pencil beams pass through the patient at an angle of 1° to one another. To obtain 180° of information the number of translations across the patient is then reduced to 180/*N* where *N* is the number of detectors. When possible another row of detectors is added to obtain a second slice simultaneously with the first slice.

Rotate-Only Geometry

The logical extension of using more and more pencil beams is to open up the x-ray beam in the transverse plane to produce a fan beam large enough to encompass the entire patient. This is the so-called *third-generation geometry*. This fan beam is incident on a whole array of detectors, which move along with the fan, as in Figure 1-12. In this process one eliminates entirely the time-consuming translation motion. Note that not only must detectors number at least 180 (one for each of the 180° of view), but actually one needs even more detectors, since the array must be large enough to include a wide range of patient diameters. It is also necessary to include additional detectors to serve as monitoring chambers to correct for any variations in x-ray output. Modern third-generation units use from 300 to over 600 detectors, with scan times of 5 to 10 seconds. At these scanning times it is not necessary to have a second array of detectors for simultaneous two-plane scanning, as was common with single-pencil and some multiple-pencil systems. This reduces the cost and complexity of the equipment considerably.

One problem, however, with third-generation configuration is related to the detector calibration problem. The reconstruction process requires extremely high precision, and slight variations (even less than 1 percent) in x-ray output or in detector electronics must be corrected for. Each individual detector must then be calibrated to assure constancy and uniformity of response as compared to adjacent detectors. In first- and second-generation systems, because of the translation motion, the detectors were out from behind the patient and were directly

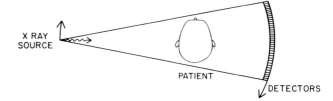

Figure 1-12   Configuration for a third-generation gantry system. Here an entire fan of x-rays is passed through the patient onto the array of detectors. Since all portions of the patient are viewed, translation motion across the patient is entirely eliminated.

exposed through air to the x-ray beam at the extreme ends of their travel during each scan motion. They could thus be easily calibrated in air before traversing the patient. Third-generation systems preclude the possibility of frequent calibrations, in that detectors are always behind the patient and cannot be calibrated between individual scans. The result is the formation of artifactual ring structures, each ring corresponding to a drift in one or more detectors, as seen in Figure 1-13. Ring artifacts can be minimized with certain algorithm corrections; however, stability of detector system as well as uniformity of detector response are crucial. In fact, detector drifts of less than 1 percent can cause visible artifacts (Shepp 1977).

One possible method of avoiding detector-calibration problems, as found in third-generation configurations, is to use a ring of detectors fixed around the entire periphery of the gantry (*fourth-generation geometry*). This configuration is seen in Figures 1-14 and 1-15. In such an arrangement the x-ray beam rotates around the patient and always radiates a

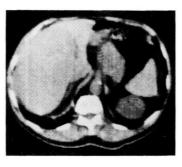
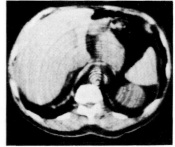

Figure 1-13   Demonstration of typical third-generation ring artifacts (on right). These ring structures are caused by slight detector calibration drifts (typically less than 1 percent). View on left shows the same scan without ring artifacts.

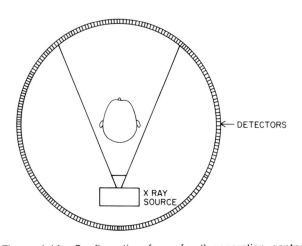

Figure 1-14 Configuration for a fourth-generation gantry system. Here detectors are fixed around the entire gantry and the x-ray tube rotates around the patient.

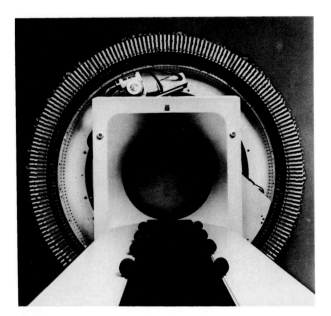

Figure 1-15 Photograph of detector configuration for a fourth-generation gantry system.

freshly calibrated detector. The added complexity and cost of fixing detectors around the entire gantry periphery and the associated electronics are obvious. Recently, some modern CT designs have reverted back to third-generation configurations, especially in view of the fact that algorithms to

minimize ring-artifact formation have been greatly improved. Variations on the fourth-generation configuration include putting the x-ray tube outside the detector array. This allows the use of a smaller detector ring as well as more closely packed detectors. In this configuration (which was pioneered by the EMI Corporation), provision is made for moving the detector ring out of the direct x-ray beam path—a motion called by the manufacturer *nutation*. Another variation, put forward by the Artronics Corporation (no longer in business), is the so-called "hula hoop" gantry. Here tube and detectors move around the patient in hula hoop fashion so that the x-ray beam is effectively parallel through the patient, allowing for more effective collimation. The reader is referred to a number of review papers for further discussion on geometries and CT scanning in general (Gordon 1975; Ter-Pogossian 1977; Brooks 1976*b*; Kak 1979).

Detectors

Let us now look at the various radiation detector types commonly used in CT scanning. Three general types of detection system have emerged: the scintillation detector/photomultiplier, the scintillation detector/photodiode multiplier, and the pressurized ionization chamber. Each of these is briefly discussed in turn.

Scintillation Detector/Photomultiplier

This type of detector package is most familiar to the clinician in that it is the type commonly used for nuclear medicine scans. It consists of a solid scintillation crystal such as NaI (Tl), which has the property of emitting light when x-ray or gamma photons are incident upon it. This emitted light falls upon a photocathode surface which converts the light to an electronic signal, which in turn is amplified within a photomultiplier. In CT scanning the signal is then digitized and transmitted to the computer for processing. Examples of typical scintillation crystals used in such configurations are seen in Table 1-2. Scintillation crystal/photomultiplier technology is

Table 1-2 CT Detectors

Detector types	Chemical form
Scintillation crystals + photomultiplier	Sodium iodide NaI (TI)
	Calcium fluoride CaF$_2$
	Bismuth germanate Bi$_4$Ge$_3$O$_{12}$ (BGO)
Scintillation crystals + photodiode	Cadmium tungstate CdWO$_4$
	Cesium iodide CsI (Na)
Ionization chamber	Xenon (under pressure)

well established and is used extensively in first- and second-generation CT units.

The photomultiplier itself is a configuration of surfaces called *dynodes,* arranged so that each electron emitted from the photocathode falling on such a surface knocks out three to ten electrons. These in turn are accelerated to another dynode surface, where each knocks out another three to ten electrons. This multiplication process continues for nine to ten dynode stages, and electron multiplication by millions is possible. Photomultiplier drift, a function of applied voltage and electronic stability, critically affects the multiplication process. In spite of this, systems of this type are very efficient and have made CT scanning possible.

Scintillation Crystal/Photodiode Multiplier

There is at present a definite trend toward the use of solid-state photodiode-multiplier scintillation-crystal systems. Here, instead of coupling the emitted scintillation light to a photomultiplier, it is coupled to a silicon photodiode. Advantages include high stability, small size, and possible cost saving.

One solid-state variation on detector packages which is under development is the use of a semiconductor photoconductive crystal which produces an electric current directly when irradiated, without the intermediate step of light production. As for any other CT detector, sensitivity and stability as well as size must be evaluated.

Pressurized Ionization Chambers

One of the requirements for CT detectors is that they be small and capable of being configured very close to one another to provide for full capture of the incident radiation. The ionization chamber approach comes closest to providing these features. Such a chamber consists of one large assembly having very thin walls defining each small collection region as in Figure 1-16. This configuration yields a very high packing density of these small detectors. Additionally, xenon gas is perfused evenly throughout the assembly to assure uniformity of response. Some disadvantages include the fact that xenon gas does not provide for as much absorption efficiency as solid state detectors. To compensate for these losses, ionization chambers are pressurized at 10 to 30 atm (providing more gas molecules for absorbing the x-ray beam) and are constructed with relatively great depths (providing greater path length for x-ray photons to be absorbed). Some attenuation loss is experienced within the relatively thick face plate needed to withstand the relatively high xenon gas pressure, and this serves to attenuate the x-ray beam.

Detector Requirements

Detectors, to be effective in CT scanning applications, should have the characteristics listed in Table 1-3. The need for *high absorption efficiency* is self-

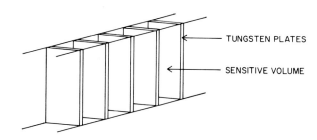

Figure 1-16 Close-up view of adjacent plates within a pressurized xenon gas detector. The small size of these detectors allows for very small data sampling distances; also, there is minimal information loss between detector cells (high capture ratio).

Table 1-3 Favorable Detector Characteristics

High absorption efficiency
High conversion efficiency
High capture efficiency
Good temporal response (little afterglow)
Wide dynamic range
High reproducibility and stability

evident. This provides for maximum utilization of the photons incident on the face of the detector. Here the important factors are the physical density, atomic number, size, and thickness of the detector. *Conversion efficiency* relates to the ability of the detector to convert the absorbed x-ray energy to a usable electronic signal. *Capture efficiency* means that the size of the detector and the distance to adjacent detectors should be such that as many as possible of the photons passing through the patient are incident on (or captured by) the detector face. The *temporal response* of a detector should be as fast as possible in that in a scanning configuration each detector sees the radiation for a relatively short time measured in milliseconds. Within this time, the signal must be processed and the detector be ready for the next measurement. It is clear that the performance of a unit would be severely degraded if the detector had a significantly delayed response, sometimes referred to as *phosphorescence* or *afterglow*. With significant afterglow, correlation between the specific voxel the x-ray beam is traversing and the signal received by the computer would be lost. Afterglow would be especially limiting for fast, dynamic scanning. *Wide dynamic range* refers to the ability of the detector to respond linearly to a wide range of x-ray intensities. When scanning patients the x-ray beam is sometimes passing through air having negligible attenuation and consequently forming a very intense signal at the detector and may then traverse a thick patient or body part having a high beam attenuation. The x-ray signal formed at the detector would then be relatively low. Ideally a detector should respond linearly between these two extremes; a dynamic range of 10,000 to 1 should be minimal. Finally, *high reproducibility and stability* are

required to avoid drift and the resultant detector fluctuation or noise.

CT Image Display and Recording

What the computer understands to be an image consists merely of an array of CT numbers, one number corresponding to each pixel. In order for the viewer to see a "real" image, this array of numbers must be displayed on a suitable medium such as a video monitor. Three considerations must be taken into account for the proper display and storage of CT images:

1. Adjustment of the video monitor display characteristics of brightness and display contrast, i.e., the video gray scale
2. Selection of settings (center and window) to optimize the display of anatomic tissues of interest within the given video gray scale
3. Recording of the image for long-term storage

Video Gray Scale

Every video device has its own gray scale. The gray scale refers to the manner in which the device goes from its darkest to its brightest illumination. The gray scale usually is displayed as a graded series of steps, that at one end representing the darkest and that at the other end the brightest illumination. Steps in between, therefore, have intermediate values of gray, and the rapidity with which they go from light to dark is the video monitor contrast. Rather than steps, some units have a continuous illumination strip. In any case the result is the same, namely, that one can observe the actual display brightness and contrast of the monitor. Adjustments can be made exactly as one controls monitor display characteristics during image-intensified fluoroscopy, ultrasound video, or home video viewing. These settings are usually chosen initially and remain fixed thereafter. The basis for actual settings varies for each individual viewer. Usually, however, the final gray scale should display both the very darkest and the very brightest that the monitor can display, as well as a relatively uniform gradation of gray between these two extremes. Most installations have a monitor for direct viewing and a monitor to obtain hard-copy films. In the latter case, the gray scale should be adjusted to match the needs of the film which will be used to record the image. Selection of film, as well as the monitor brightness and contrast used to record the film, are not trivial matters, and care must be taken to assure the best possible film image (Schwenker 1979).

Variations in window and center settings reported between CT sites are usually due in part to differences in initial gray-scale settings and differences in video monitor display characteristics.

Center and Window Settings

One of the biggest differences between radiographic film viewing and CT viewing is the ability in the latter to *window* the anatomic tissues of interest. By this is meant that one can optimize the viewing of particular tissues of interest by assigning to them the full range of blacks and whites available on the CRT monitor. For example, the center setting assigns the video mid-gray value to the CT number (or tissue) desired; the window setting defines the CT number range which will occupy the scale from black to white. To illustrate, consider a head CT scan viewed at a center of +50 and a window of

200 CT units. The +50 corresponds to the approximate CT number of gray and white matter, and it is these tissues that will be displayed with the mid-gray illumination. A window of 200 CT units implies that the range will be from +150 (100 above 50) to −50 (100 below 50). Consequently all tissues having CT numbers of 150 or above will be displayed as white, while all tissues at −50 and below will be displayed as black. On these settings, bone calcifications and blood pools will appear light and ventricular volumes will appear darker. The above settings may be ideal for a head scan, but different settings are needed for body scanning, since body scanning involves a greater range of tissue types, and a greater window must be selected.

The power of the windowing function will be appreciated when it is recalled that in film radiography one must accept whatever exposure was made and is limited to what is seen on the film. Film, however, is nonlinear and thus results in different image contrast, depending on the density. Additionally, films may be underexposed or overexposed. In either case, as discussed previously, information is lost at both the low- and high-density regions of the film. Figure 1-17 illustrates the role of windowing using linear detectors. If the full tissue range of −1000 to +1000 is displayed, note that the particular tissues of interest in the previous example (−50 to +150) would be limited to a relatively small range of grays, and visualization would

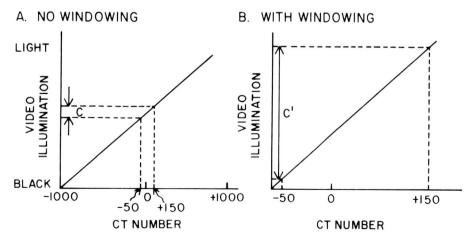

Figure 1-17 On a scale of −1000 to +1000, if no windowing is available, a given CT number difference such as −50 to +150 is displayed with only a limited range of gray values (low image contrast *C*). With windowing invoked, the same CT number range can be displayed with up to the maximum video range from white to black (high image contrast *C*); thus, −50 can be assigned full dark and +150 is assigned full light.

be poor. However, with windowing as in Figure 1-17, the full black-and-white range is assigned between the -50 and $+150$ CT values, and visualization of these particular tissues is optimum in that the greatest illumination difference results.

Long-term Storage Media

It has always been necessary to record the final image for patient records and subsequent comparisons and for referring physicians. Such recording can be done on film as for classical radiography. However, it is advantageous to record the actual computer image, consisting of all the pixel values, since pixel values, if available, can allow for subsequent windowing and redisplay and for computer manipulations such as magnification, CT number, or tissue identification and various image-enhancement routines. Thus magnetic tape and magnetic disc systems are usually incorporated into the basic CT instrumentation. In fact, the basic image-recording configuration of a clinical scanner may consist of some or all of the items listed in Table 1-4.

FILM Film continues to be the most popular and economical long-term storage medium. It should be realized that the films used in CT imaging are quite different from the films used in radiography, inas-

much as one is recording an image off a video monitor. Consequently, the film usually consists of a single emulsion sensitive to the light-emission spectrum of the video-screen phosphor. Additionally, these nonscreen films tend to be linear. To facilitate film recording, multi-image-format cameras have been developed, consisting of a self-enclosed video monitor with independent access to the computer pixel image information. The arrangement is such that the camera exposes the film to the particular size format desired. For instance, both four views (or image slices) on an 8×10 film and nine views on a 14×17 film are quite popular.

Polaroid film originally had three drawbacks: limited film contrast range, expense, and the need for mounting for permanent records. To a lesser extent there was also the nuisance of paper wrappers, the wait for development, and the need for coating. Newer Polaroid film emulsions available have extended film contrast range and do not need coating. This form of image recording, however, will probably still remain limited to relatively low patient-volume sites where the capital cost of multi-image cameras or tape recorders is a factor and sites where rapid film processing equipment is not available.

MAGNETIC TAPE Magnetic tape recording of computer outputs is a well-established technology. Pixel values, as well as patient identification data, can be readily recorded in relatively short times (a few seconds). This means that images can be redisplayed at any subsequent time, and different computer manipulations of the images, including windowing, are possible. Additionally, the fidelity of the images is excellent. A number of drawbacks exist, however. For example, storage space is limited to between 100 and 300 images per tape, depending on the number of pixels in the image. Thus a 256×256 pixel array demands less tape space than a 512×512 pixel array. A few hundred images, in the case of a busy site, means that only one or two days' worth of patient images may be stored on one tape. In practice, this is a severe limitation, since accessing patient images on different tapes requires an inordinate amount of time, because of the need for

Table 1-4 Storage Media

Medium	Pixels recoverable?	Comments
Polaroid film	No	Relatively expensive; relatively poor contrast scale
Film	No	Convenient, various sizes available
Magnetic tape	Yes	Access time long, good for long-term storage
Floppy disc	Yes	Convenient size and format; relatively expensive
Magnetic discs	Yes	Expensive but fast

loading and reloading tapes, as well as the relatively slow search times characteristic of magnetic tape systems. Finally, the number of tapes accumulated and the required floor storage space have dictated the recycling of tapes. Thus it is not uncommon to find tapes covering only 6 to 12 months, or even less, at a particular site.

DISC-BASED SYSTEMS Two basic approaches to disc imaging have evolved. One approach uses so-called "floppy" discs. These discs are relatively small and are flexible. In many cases a full patient examination or more can be recorded on one disc and can be conveniently transported to another room or site for image review at an independent viewing station. Disc search time is essentially negligible. However, the cost of each disc is such that many sites rely on magnetic tape recording for long-term storage and use floppy discs only for recent patients or for particularly interesting cases.

Another disc-based system consists of a bank of large discs capable of storing thousands of images. These are random-access devices, so that stepping through every image in the file to find the required one is not necessary and search and access times are minimal. Viewing at remote consoles is possible, however, only via direct data-link connection to the computer. The overall costs of such a system are relatively high.

Artifacts in CT Scanning

CT scanning artifacts are currently the subject of active research. Many artifacts have multiple causes, and their description requires rigorous mathematical techniques. Here we present a number of the more significant artifacts that the clinician should be aware of. Artifacts can manifest themselves either visibly in the form of streaks or quantitatively in the form of inaccurate CT numbers.

Streaks arise in general because there is an inconsistency in a particular ray-path through the patient. This inconsistency can be due either to an error along the ray or to inconsistencies between rays. Table 1-5 summarizes the various sources of

Table 1-5 Sources of CT Artifacts

Source area	Cause
Data formation	Patient motion
	Polychromatic effects
	Equipment misalignment
	Faulty x-ray source
Data acquisition	Slice geometry
	Profile sampling
	Angular sampling
Data measurement	Detector imbalance
	Detector nonlinearity
	Scatter collimation
Data processing	Algorithm effects

artifacts. Classification of artifacts has been troublesome (Joseph 1981). For our purposes here we have classified artifacts according to what is happening to the data. Each of the artifacts listed in Table 1-5 is discussed in turn.

Data Formation

In this section we are concerned with how data are formed as the x-rays pass through the patient. As previously discussed, the transmitted x-ray beam detected in CT scanning is an index of the degree of attenuation which has occurred as the beam passed through the patient. Reference to Figure 1-6 shows that the patient contour is arbitrarily divided up into pixels. To accomplish the CT scan process, ray-paths along different angles around the patient are obtained. Thus data are collected for the attenuation at each point in the field from different angles. If such ray-path data are inconsistent—that is, if the pixel does not contribute the same attenuation regardless of the particular angle of view—then streaks result. The most familiar example of data inconsistency is that casued by patient motion.

PATIENT MOTION Motion has plagued CT scanning from the beginning (Alfidi 1976). The original CT scan units took up to 6 minutes of scan time. The inordinate amount of time allowed for considerable patient motion during the course of the examination. When such motion occurs during the scanning process, the computer has no means of keeping track of where the pixels are in space and which ray-path sums belong to which row and column. This inconsistency results in severe streaking and is especially aggravated by the presence of high-density structures. In early CT units, the relatively long scanning time necessary was so limiting that it provided the impetus to develop faster and faster scanners. Presently, modern scanners can routinely perform scans in less than 5 to 10 seconds.

It should be clear that motion not only introduces artifactual streaks but, as in classical radiography, may cause both a loss of *spatial resolution* (the ability to visualize fine spatial detail) and a loss of *tissue resolution* (the ability to visualize small differences in tissue densities), also called *density resolution* and referring to the subject contrast measure. These latter losses are usually minimal as compared to the presence of streaks. To minimize motion artifacts one may, in addition to scanning faster, provide for immobilization of the patient. Another possibility involves overscanning. Here the patient is typically scanned 40° to 60° beyond the normal 180° or 360°, the rationale being that one is then collecting repeat, or redundant, views. For instance, if the patient has moved between the beginning of the scan and the end, there will be a discrepancy between the data collected on the 0° pass and the 180° pass. If the patient has not moved during the scan, these two views should be identical; any difference detected is entirely due to patient motion. Under computer control these differences can be averaged (or feathered) out. One obvious drawback to overscanning is the fact that scan times are longer, introducing the possibility of further motion artifacts. In spite of this, however, overscanning has been shown to be useful.

POLYCHROMATIC EFFECTS Probably the best-known polychromatic artifact referred to in clinical practice is the beam-hardening artifact. The basis for this artifact is the fact that in the reconstruction process one attempts to assign an attenuation coefficient value to each volume element (voxel) within the patient. However, attenuation coefficients are highly dependent on x-ray beam energy. Photons in x-ray beams do not have a unique energy but rather are polychromatic, that is, they are made up of photons having a wide distribution of energy. As the beam passes through the patient, the lower-energy photons are preferentially absorbed, and we say that the beam becomes harder. (This is similar to the rationale for the use of filters in diagnostic radiology to reduce the patient dose.) Any given voxel within the patient is, however, viewed along different ray-paths for each different angular projection. Consequently, the x-ray beam, having experienced different degrees of beam hardening, will have a different energy as it passes any particular voxel along these different ray-paths (see Fig 1-18). The overall result will be a general decrease in the CT numbers, since higher energies imply lower attenuation coefficients. This effect is most notable along ray-paths containing thicker and denser bony structures, as along the orbit-base views. The visual result is dark streaks, since higher energies result in the display of CT numbers denoting less dense tissues. The best example of this effect is the interpetrous bone hypodensity streaks seen in Figure 1-19. This particular artifact is also caused in part by the nonlinear partial volume effect (Glover 1980).

Beam hardening also leads to a spillover effect near the interface of bony structures with adjoining softer tissues. This is evident at the edge of the skull and was originally interpreted as the cerebral cortex (Ambrose 1973). Its artifactual nature was demonstrated by Gado and Phelps (1975), and it is now referred to as the *pseudocortex*. The basis for this effect, which is also referred to as *cupping*, is illustrated in Figure 1-18: rays passing through the periphery of a structure suffer less hardening than rays passing through the center of that structure. The central regions thus are displayed as having lower CT numbers and appear darker. The original water-bag systems circumvented many of these problems by providing for an essentially equal path length for all rays in all projections. Another approach to minimize beam hardening effects is to add filtration to the beam or to add specially shaped compensating attenuators to the beam. These ap-

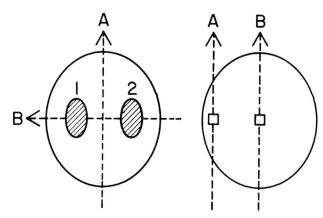

Figure 1-18 Demonstration of beam hardening in CT scanning. *Left:* Interpetrous bone hypodensity artifact. Ray *A* suffers a different degree of beam hardening from Ray *B*, which travels through bony structures 1 and 2. The result is an inconsistency in the CT numbers calculated, and streaks result between the bony structures. *Right:* Cupping artifact. Rays such as *A*, passing through the periphery of a uniform structure, suffer less attenuation than rays such as *B*, passing through the center of that structure. Result is an apparent cupping, or increase in tissue density toward the periphery.

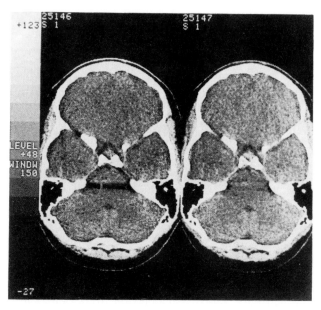

Figure 1-19 *Left:* Interpetrous bone artifact. *Right:* Same view after bone corrections are performed.

proaches will be discussed further under the section on CT number variations.

Beam hardening has been discussed at length and a number of algorithms have been proposed to correct for the beam-hardening artifact (Brooks 1976*a*; Duerinckx 1978; McDavid 1977*a*; Joseph 1978*b*). Typical CT scanners include within their reconstruction algorithm a so-called water correction based on the linearization of the data collected. However, a more complete correction usually involves off-line processing which may take from seconds to minutes per image to perform. Algorithms of this kind are referred to as *bone* or *calcium correction algorithms* and, because of the necessity of off-line processing, are often implemented only for specially selected cases.

EQUIPMENT MISALIGNMENT Mechanical misalignment of the x-ray source and radiation detectors may lead to artifactual streak formation. The basic problem is that of isocenter location (Shepp 1977). If an aluminum pin is placed at the isocenter and scanned, its position will be isocentric for all views

and projections. If a misalignment is present, an inconsistency results between angular views, and streaks sometimes referred to as "tuning fork" streaks result.

Another misalignment problem may occur for 180° dual-slice scanners. Hounsfield (1977) has described what happens when the central ray of the x-ray beam is not aligned perpendicular to the axis of the patient's head. Under these conditions a bony structure may be included within the collimated x-ray field in the Z direction for the 0° view but excluded from the 180° view. The result is a vertical streak along the edges of the bony object. One practical lesson from this is that when possible one should align the patient in such a way that bony structures fall along the 90° views and not along the 0° and 180° views. The petrous bones, for instance, satisfy this for scanners rotating 180° from the posterior to the anterior hemispheres. However, the eye lens is then exposed to the primary beam, and relatively high radiation dose results (McCullough 1980). Since the appearance of this artifact depends mainly on the 0° and 180° views, overscanning will serve to minimize it.

FAULTY X-RAY SOURCE   If the x-ray output varies during the scan process, an obvious inconsistency in data immediately arises, since detectors cannot distinguish between increases or decreases in radiation level due to increases or decreases in x-ray output and those due to increased or decreased absorption along the ray-path. All CT units include reference detectors to detect output variations for the purpose of correcting for such changes. These corrections, however, are for data from a single angular view. If variations are present between angular views, streaks crisscrossing the image field and forming moiré patterns result (Joseph 1981; Stockham 1979). These are assumed to be most likely related to the speed of anode rotation, which is also called *anode wobble*. Other possible x-ray source problems include momentary high-voltage arcing and fluctuations, which may reduce or increase instantaneous x-ray output. Again, such changes, though detected by reference chambers, still result in inconsistencies between angular views, and streaks result.

Data Acquisition

In this section, artifactual effects resulting from the manner in which the data are collected are studied.

SLICE GEOMETRY   The thickness of the slice scanned determines a very significant though nonvisible artifact: the partial volume effect. To understand this effect and its significance in practice, remember that the pixel displayed represents a volume in the patient given by both the area size and the slice thickness (the voxel). The voxel representing some finite patient volume may contain more than one tissue type. What happens is that the total contents of the voxel are averaged, and it is this average CT number which is assigned to the voxel. Figure 1-20 illustrates this effect. For instance, if half of the pixel is filled with a tissue having a CT number of 100 and the other half with a tissue having a CT number of 200, the average of the two is 150, and this voxel will be displayed as if it were filled with a tissue type of CT number 150 which, in fact, is not present within the voxel.

This effect is significant for relatively small ana-tomic structure sizes or for tissue volumes which are rapidly changing in size. Examples are the orbital base level and regions near the calvarium. Additionally, vascular structures, blood clots (Lim 1977), and thin flat structures, as well as optic nerve visualization (Salvolini 1978), are subject to the partial volume effect. The result of the partial volume effect is the loss of tissue and spatial resolution and not necessarily streaks. In many instances, however, volume averaging is nonlinear in that tissue types within the voxel have widely different CT numbers. This, in turn, results in wide exponential and nonlinear absorption differences. An example of this, would be the bony structures of the petrous ridges and the adjacent brain matter. The result is the interpetrous ridge lucency artifact which has been discussed previously. At first this artifact was thought to be entirely due to beam-hardening effects. However, these artifacts were subsequently shown to be partly due to the nonlinear partial volume effect, which in turn is related to the sampling slice thickness (Glover 1980). Thus this artifact can be minimized by diminishing the slice thickness, although it cannot be eliminated entirely unless beam hardness is also corrected for.

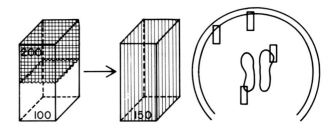

Figure 1-20   *Left:* Example of the partial volume artifact. Here, if a particular voxel contains different tissues, the final computed value will be characterized by some weighted average CT number. If the CT numbers are very different from each other, the summing average process is exponential and therefore nonlinear, and streaks may result.   *Right:* Cross-sectional view of voxel positions at various levels within the skull, showing a varying degree of partial-volume averaging for different tissue-structure boundaries.

The basis for the nonlinear partial volume effect is that the detector response varies nonlinearly with the degree of bony intrusion into any given volume element; that is, the net signal at the detectors depends on the relative amount of soft tissue and bony tissue within the voxel. However, this dependence does not vary linearly, since attenuation in each material is an exponential function. These nonlinearities result in an inconsistency in the data collected as the volume element is viewed from various angles around the patient, and it is this inconsistency that creates the streaks observed. These streaks appear not only across the petrous bones but also from the occipital protuberance and wherever there are relatively large, abrupt variations in tissue or structure densities. To minimize this artifact, one merely reduces the slice thickness, in which case one must contend with more image noise because of less photons being detected. Alternatively, x-ray tube factors may be adjusted upward, resulting in a greater patient dose for the thinner slices.

Another slice-geometry artifact is that associated with the fact that the x-ray beam is diverging as it passes through the patient. This causes some interesting effects. For instance, where is the slice thickness indicated? Figure 1-21 shows that there is no unique slice thickness; thickness varies throughout the scanned volume! By convention, we specify the thickness at the center of rotation (isocenter) of the CT unit. If the scan is completely around the patient (360°) the volume actually being imaged is symmetrically depressed in the center. The consequences of this effect are:

1. Partial volume effects are then a function of position in the field, as well as whether 180° or 360° scans are obtained. As a result, greater spatial and tissue resolution will be found in the center than at the periphery.
2. A missed volume may occur between slices, as with the EMI Mark I unit, where as much as 10 percent of the total scan volume could be missed (Goodenough 1975). These effects are minimized when patient scan volumes are relatively far from the x-ray source (less beam divergence) and the x-ray source (less beam divergence) and

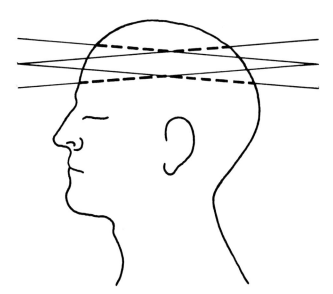

Figure 1-21 Beam diverges as it passes through patient. As beam rotates around patient it forms, not a parallel-sided slice, but rather a concave slice with center thinner than the periphery.

when slices are exactly juxtaposed (or overlapped) at the center. Overlapping, of course, results in an increase in patient dose.

PROFILE SAMPLING Figure 1-22 shows an intensity profile of the x-ray beam after it has emerged from the patient. This profile, together with all the other profiles taken at different angles or views around the patient, represents the total ray-sum information necessary for the reconstruction process. In third- and fourth-generation systems, this intensity profile is sampled by the detector array. Each detector intercepts and averages that portion of the profile which is incident over its face. This constitutes a sampling process. The sampled profile as it is transmitted to the computer is then seen to be not the exact replica of the incident profile but only a representation of it, and in fact generally is degraded. This degradation takes the final form of decreased tissue and spatial resolution (note that valleys and peaks tend to flatten or smooth out). Additionally, information is lost between detectors. These effects are a function of how large the detec-

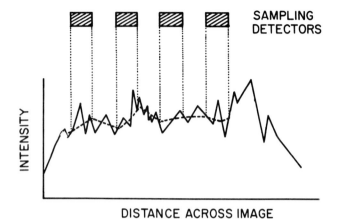

SAMPLING
DETECTORS

INTENSITY

DISTANCE ACROSS IMAGE

Figure 1-22   Demonstration of how a series of finite-size detectors sample an x-ray intensity profile as it emerges from the patient. Each detector responds in proportion to the average intensity sampled. The discrete distribution processed by the computer is then given by the dashed curve. Note the loss of information at the peaks and valleys as well as in the voids between the detectors.

tors are as well as the space between them. As either of these dimensions increases, progressive degradation occurs.

First- and second-generation systems provide for continuous sampling along the scans, and no inter-detector dead spaces exist. From Figure 1-22 it can be seen that the sampled image has features in it that are not present in the original profile. These bogus features consist of valleys and peaks that do not match the original profiles. In general, low-frequency details* not present in the original image are introduced into the resulting data. This effect is referred to as *aliasing* and is characteristic of all digitizing and sampling systems. The aliasing effect is further illustrated in Figure 1-23. Here we have an elementary sinusoidal-type profile having some particular frequency. It is seen that if the profile is sampled over very short intervals (Fig. 1-23A), that profile is completely and accurately determined both in frequency and in amplitude. However, if sampling distances are relatively long, as in Figure

* By frequency is meant the rapidity with which profiles change; thus high frequency implies sharp edges or relatively small structures.

1-23D, the pattern resulting has totally different amplitudes and has a lower frequency than the original pattern. Thus a poorly sampled profile introduces patterns in the final result not present in the original.

If the pattern is sampled only once within each cycle, the response is flat, as in Figure 1-23C. Figure 1-23B shows that when the pattern is sampled at least twice in a cycle, the frequency recorded is

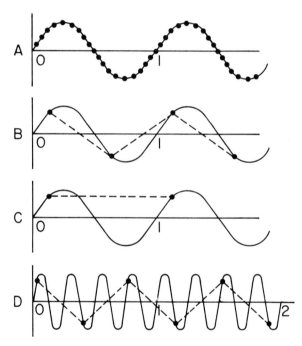

Figure 1-23   Demonstration of the aliasing effect with a pure sinusoidal profile distribution.   *Curve A:* If samples are taken at rates much greater than the frequency of the information distribution being sampled, all the frequency as well as all the amplitude information is saved.   *Curve B:* If samples are taken at twice the frequency of the distribution, as shown here, all the frequency information is saved (this is the Nyquist frequency). Note, however, that some amplitude information is still lost.   *Curve C:* If samples are taken at a rate equal to the frequency of the information distribution, all the frequency and amplitude information will be lost, that is, a flat response results.   *Curve D:* Aliasing occurs if sampling rate is less than twice the frequency of the information distribution. Information *not* present in the original is then produced. For example, if time distribution is 4 cycles per millimeter and a sample is obtained every 1½ cycles, as shown here, then the apparent frequency detected is approximately ¾ cycle per millimeter. In general, aliasing results in lower frequencies appearing. The result is streaks in the image.

identical to that of the original pattern. We refer to this sampling frequency as the *Nyquist frequency* (f_n). The Nyquist frequency is seen to be merely twice the maximum frequency (f_m) present in the x-ray profile:

$$f_n = 2f_m \qquad (2)$$

The maximum frequency associated with a structure of dimension *d* is $1/d$. Thus to sample at the Nyquist frequency the profile must be sampled at

$$f_n = \frac{2}{d} \qquad (3)$$

When sharp discontinuities are present in the scanned image, Equation (3) does not hold and aliasing artifacts appear in the reconstructed image.

Visually, aliasing artifacts for a complete reconstruction appear as shown for a computer simulation in Figure 1-24. Aliasing patterns serve to mask details in the clinical reconstruction. However, in practice their visibility may at times be suppressed by noise present in the image (Stockham 1979). Aliasing streaks can be serious. Examples are clip or star artifacts, which usually consist of streaks emanating from small high-density structures within the patient such as a surgical clip or any metallic object. Similar artifacts can also be seen coming from tooth fillings, gas/liquid interfaces in the stomach, and bony protuberances in skull. It should also be noted that these streaks are partly due to nonlinear partial volume effects, detector nonlinearity, and angular undersampling. One final artifact related to the presence of small or sharp high-contrast structure is that related to the presence of markers on the surface of patients to correlate anatomic level with radiographic views. It has been shown that the use of opaque catheters for this purpose does indeed generate artifacts (Villafana 1978*b*).

Since aliasing is due to insufficient sampling, an obvious solution is to sample at higher rates, taking readings closer together or using smaller detectors packed closer. The minimum rate to avoid aliasing effects as discussed above, is the Nyquist rate, which is a function of the anatomic structure sizes and the presence of sharp discontinuities. Another method which can be used to minimize aliasing is

to purposely smooth or eliminate sharp discontinuities in the profiles before they are sampled. This is accomplished by having a relatively wide sampling aperture. One drawback of this approach is that spatial and tissue resolution are sacrificed as well.

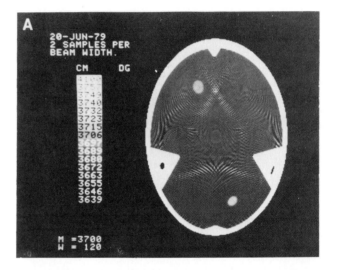

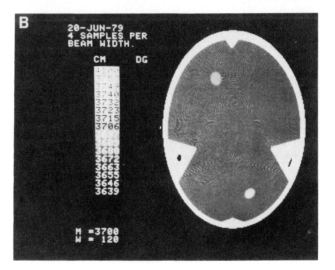

Figure 1-24 Aliasing streaks due to undersampling. Overlapping streaks emanating over the periphery of the skull result in a moiré pattern. The lower figure shows a phantom simulation sampled at a rate twice that of the upper figure: 0.96 mm sample spacing versus 0.48 mm (After Stockham 1979 and Joseph 1981).

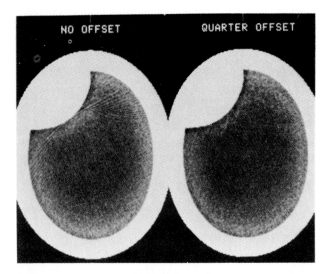

Figure 1-25 Verification of the removal of aliasing streaks seen on the left by quarter offset or shift of the central detector in a third-generation geometry detector array. (After Brooks 1979.)

A third method to suppress aliasing, which has the advantage of not degrading resolution, is the one-quarter detector shift technique. This technique, which has been successfully applied to fan-beam third-generation geometry (Peters 1977; Brooks 1979), consists of offsetting the central detector by one-fourth of the detector dimensions. As a result, as the scanner obtains views around the patient, all the views from 180° to 360° are exactly interleaved with the views from 0° to 179°—that is, the view at 180° is interleaved with that from 0°, and the 360° view is interleaved with that from 180°. The result is that each view is offset by one-half of the detector dimensions. The significance of this is that the highest frequency available at the detector is determined by the detector dimensions, and we thus need, according to Equation (3), to obtain two samples per detector width d (a frequency of 2/d); the quarter offset provides exactly this sampling interval, and aliasing streaks are markedly reduced, as seen in Figure 1-25.

ANGULAR SAMPLING Just as a particular profile can be undersampled as discussed above, the number of profiles or angular view samples around the pa-

tient can be deficient. Such angular undersampling also leads to the formation of streak artifacts. However, these streaks, although radiating from small, dense objects, always occur at some distance from the object. It has been shown that undersampling along the profile is more important and leads to more severe aliasing streaks as compared to undersampling the number of angular views around the patient (Brooks 1979; Schulz 1977). Streaks due to view undersampling usually lead to artifacts in the image emanating from the undersampled structure but first appear at some distance from that structure.

To summarize this section: Data acquisition or sampling schemes play a key role in the quality and accuracy of the final image. Sampling includes the thickness of the slice, the sampling along each profile, and the number of views around the patient. Effects can range from simple inaccuracies in the CT number to severe streaks obliterating the desired diagnostic information. Some of the ways to minimize aliasing streaks include thinner slices, closely packed small detectors, and quarter-shifted detector geometry.

Data Measurement

DETECTOR IMBALANCE we have already emphasized that detectors should have high efficiency and high reproducibility. Of importance also is that each detector in an array of detectors be matched in response as compared to the other detectors in the array. When an imbalance occurs, ring artifacts such as those in Figure 1-13 result. Imbalance may result from individual detector gain shifts. Shepp (1977) has shown that shifts as low as 0.1 percent can result in visible streaks. Furthermore, the appearance of streaks is more severe if detector error affects only one ray-path or a small group of ray-paths, as in first-, second-, and third-generation systems. Fourth-generation system detector errors affect the whole view (each detector sees the whole patient), and as a result, inconsistency is smoothed over the whole image.

When shifts occur they can be calibrated out. This calibration is performed whenever the detector is out from behind the patient. Calibration is automatic for first-, second-, and fourth-generation systems. Third-generation systems, however, present a problem in that the detectors are behind the patient throughout the examination. The resulting ring artifacts (Fig. 1-13) are particularly troublesome.

DETECTOR NONLINEARITIES   Ideally, the response of a detector should be directly proportional to the quantity of radiation incident on it. In CT scanning, the range of x-ray intensities may be as high as 10,000 to 1 or even higher. The detector should have a dynamic range at least this high. Some factors contributing to detector nonlinearity (Joseph 1981) are dark current or leakage (current flow in the absence of radiation), saturation (detector output is at its maximum and higher intensities do not evoke higher output), and hysteresis (detector continues to respond after irradiation ends). One form of hysteresis is the afterglow of scintillation detectors. All these may lead to inconsistency in data and can result in streaks. The severity of these streaks is related to the contrast of the structure as well as the presence of abrupt discontinuities in its shape. One way to minimize the detector nonlinearity problem is to reduce the range of intensities arriving at the detector. This can be accomplished by placing the patient within a water box or by the use of a compensating wedge filter (see Fig. 1-27).

SCATTER COLLIMATION   Scatter present at the detector plane is similar to that from leakage in the detector. This can be appreciated by considering a very dense object. The primary x-ray intensity behind this object is expected to be low; however, small amounts of scatter at the detector will indicate a higher than actual transmission. The resulting data are inconsistent with data from ray-paths not traversing the high-contrast object, and streaks can result. Scatter is less of a problem in first-, second-, and third-generation systems, where scatter-rejecting collimation can be incorporated into detectors. In fourth-generation systems, unlike the others, stationary detectors must accept radiation from a wide range of angles, and collimation cannot be used.

Consequently these latter systems are more susceptible to scatter effects.

Data Processing

The final step to be considered here is how the data are processed within the computer. The specific algorithm used may introduce artifacts into the final image which are not due to sampling or measurement factors. Examples of this are the use of an edge-enhancement algorithm, which can result in a false subarachnoid space. Another example is that described by Hounsfield (1977), Stockham (1979), and Joseph (1981), involving scanning long, straight-edged, bony, or high-contrast structures. Approximations normally used in algorithms lead to the formation of streaks along the edge of such structures. These streaks can be minimized by using narrower collimators for first- and second-generation units and smaller detectors for third- and fourth-generation units. The use of hardened (filtered) x-ray beams also helps. Needless to say, algorithm-induced artifacts are mathematically complex, and further discussion is beyond our scope here.

CT Number Accuracy

In the previous section the factors resulting in mainly visible streak artifacts were studied. In this section the factors affecting actual accuracy of the CT numbers are considered.

A number of factors limiting the absolute accuracy of CT numbers are listed in Table 1-6. As discussed in an earlier section, the CT reconstruction process computes a value for the linear attenuation coefficient of each volume element within the patient scanned. In most CT designs, the computer then assigns to the attenuation coefficient a value based on the arbitrary -1000 for air to $+1000$ for bone scale. (Additionally, some units are capable of accurately computing and displaying values up to $+3000$.) These values (CT numbers or Hounsfield numbers) represent quantitative data from which tissue identification can be attempted. In general, they are related to the attenuation coefficient of water (μ_w) as follows:

$$\text{CT no.} = \frac{\mu - \mu_w}{\mu_w} \times 100 \qquad (4)$$

where μ = the attenuation coefficient of the material the CT number is specified for. Table 1-1 gives a short list of CT numbers for typical tissues. All CT scanners have provision for determining the CT number for any specified point or region of points in the image field, either by direct interaction with the video display, using a region-of-interest (ROI) indicator, or by direct printout on a line printer.

Since CT numbers characterize the tissue or its chemical composition, it is no wonder that considerable effort has been expended to use these quantitative data. This involves not only identifying gross tissue type but, among other more sophisticated applications, the determination of bone mineral content (Weissberger 1978; Exner 1979; Revak 1980) and the identification of calcified versus noncalcified pulmonary nodules (Siegelman 1980). In fact, CT scanning can be configured to determine directly the effective atomic numbers or electron densities (tomochemistry) instead of the attenuation coefficients (McDavid 1977b; Latchaw 1978).

The question of validity must be posed before undue reliance is placed on CT numbers. A number of factors affect the validity of correlating directly the CT number obtained from a particular CT machine and the tissue it is supposed to characterize (McCullough 1977). Specific factors to be considered are given in Table 1-6, from which it is easy to see that one cannot in fact expect the CT numbers from one machine to match those from another exactly. One reason is that CT numbers are dependent on

Table 1-6   Factors Affecting CT Number Accuracy

X-ray beam kilovoltage and filtration
Patient thickness and shape
Tissue type and location
Partial volume effect
Algorithm and calibration shifts

x-ray beam energy. Thus correlation cannot be expected between units operated at different kilovoltage (Ruegsegger 1978) or even between similar units operated at the same nominal kilovoltage, because of kilovoltage calibration inaccuracies. CT number anomalies can also occur for the same unit whenever the kilovoltage shifts. In general, the CT number of any material will shift as a function of the difference between the atomic number of that material and the atomic number of water: it will increase for materials with an atomic number less than water and decrease for materials with an atomic number greater than water (Zatz 1976). A tight quality-assurance program monitoring the constancy of CT numbers for a given unit is necessary.

Beam filtration also affects the energy distribution of the x-ray beam. In general, the greater the filtration the harder the beam (or the greater the effective beam energy), and also the beam becomes more monochromatic and therefore less subject to further hardening. This means that CT numbers are subject to variation between units depending on the degree of beam filtration incorporated in each unit as well as the calibration and shift effects discussed above. It is also interesting to note that some CT units provide for two filtration modes, one for head scans and a relatively thicker filtration for body scans, the rationale being that the greater tissue-path lengths in bodies would produce greater beam hardening. Greater initial filtration would then reduce this effect, in that the beam is prehardened via the additional filter and closer to a monochromatic beam before it enters the patient. Patient thickness is crucial in determining the CT numbers finally computed. Again, beam hardening is involved, in that different patient thicknesses yield different beam paths and different degrees of beam hardening. This is illustrated in Figure 1-26. It can also be seen that results will depend on the shape of the body parts. Figure 1-26 also illustrates the so-called apical artifact (DiChiro 1978), in which CT number variations occur between the slice levels scanned, owing to varying head thickness and thus different degrees of beam hardening.

It should be noted that the original EMI Mark I

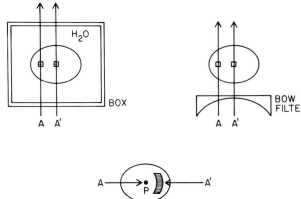

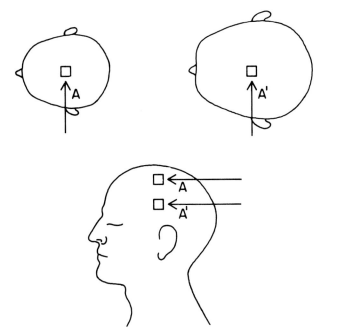

Figure 1-26 Different degrees of beam hardening yielded by different patient thicknesses and the effect on CT number accuracy. Ray-path *A* to any particular pixel is shorter in the smaller patient on the left than ray-path *A'* in the larger patient on the right. As shown in the lower figure, even in the same patient path length to any given pixel can differ depending on slice level (apical artifact). All these effects are further compounded when the beam rotates around the patient and path length is a function of ray angle.

Figure 1-27 *Left:* In original CT units a water bath providing a fixed path length for any and all ray-paths, such as *A* and *A'*, resulted in minimal beam-hardening effects on CT numbers. *Right:* In an attempt to equalize ray-paths *A* and *A'* without a water bath one can provide for a "bow tie" filter arrangement. Here varying filter thickness results in attenuation matching the curvature of the patient. *Bottom:* Presence of dense structures (shaded region) aggravates the beam-hardening problem between ray-paths *A* and *A'*, since the beam through a point such as *P* suffers different beam hardening along the two paths indicated. This is particularly severe for ray-paths falling along the edges of the structures, and image streaks are usually formed.

unit provided a water box surrounding the patient's head. This meant that all ray-paths were more nearly equal, as seen in Figure 1-27, for any orientation around the head. With such a configuration beam hardening is minimal. Figure 1-27 also shows one attempt to provide for a fixed path length by providing for a "bow tie" compensating filter. Here added filter thickness toward the periphery of the bow tie presumably compensates for decreased peripheral patient thickness. Patient centering here will obviously be important, and the configuration will not be as effective as a water box. Figure 1-27 also shows how the presence of dense structures adds to the beam-hardening problem. Discrepancies for ray-paths tangent to the edges of the structure in fact result in severe image streaking.

The partial volume effect also strongly influences

CT number accuracy. This was discussed in the previous section and will not be discussed further here.

Finally, the question of algorithms must be addressed. Each CT manufacturer attempts to minimize the beam-hardening problem and to calibrate its CT number scale to maximize accuracy. Such algorithms vary between manufacturers, and the actual field calibrations on any given unit and at any given time will vary.

This section can be summarized simply by stating that great caution must be exercised in using CT numbers, not only between and within different manufacturers' models but also for one's own unit, as a function of the factors listed in Table 1-6.

CT Reconstruction Performance

As already seen, CT performance is a somewhat complex area of study. A number of different aspects of it require discussion, as seen in Table 1-7.

Table 1-7   Aspects of CT Reconstruction Performance

CT number performance
    CT number accuracy
    CT number linearity
    Spatial independance of CT numbers
    Sensitivity to artifactual effects
    Contrast scale

Geometrical and mechanical factors
    Divergence of beam
    Focal-spot penumbra
    Source and detector collimation and alignment
    Dual-slice effects
    Slice location and table incrementation
    Mechanical vibration

Imaging performance
    Spatial resolution
    Tissue resolution
    Noise characteristics

Patient dose
    Single-slice dose
    Multiple-slice dose
    Dose profile

The interested reader is also referred to a number of articles reviewing CT performance and comparisons between specific CT units (Weaver 1975; McCullough 1976; Bassano 1977; Cohen 1979*b*; McCullough 1980).

CT Number Performance

CT NUMBER ACCURACY   CT numbers have been discussed at length in previous sections, especially as related to factors causing artifactual variations in their reproducibility and accuracy. To quantitate the accuracy of CT numbers one merely scans a collection of plastics having known attenuation coefficients (or CT numbers) in a water bath. The CT numbers computed are then compared to the known values. In addition, these data when plotted should form a straight line (CT number linearity). There is no generally accepted performance standard covering day-to-day variations in CT numbers;

each site should set it own limits, taking into account the manufacturer's recommendations. It should again be noted that CT numbers vary with beam energy. Thus kilovoltage and beam filtration as well as size of the phantom used will affect the CT number. Proper calibration of the unit, however, will assure that water gives a CT number of zero for a given reconstruction scan circle or field size and that the known plastics scanned also display their correct CT numbers.

SPATIAL INDEPENDENCE OF CT NUMBERS   Clearly it is desirable for computed CT numbers to be independent of spatial position in the reconstruction field. Spatial independence or uniformity is readily measured by scanning a uniform water bath. Variations in CT numbers can be quantitated by computing the standard deviation. This computation is readily available on all commercial scanners, as is the selection of the region of interest over which such determinations are made. In general, for a water bath, the standard deviation in CT numbers in particular regions over the field should not be greater than a factor of 2 as compared to the central region (McCullough 1976).

CONTRAST SCALE   Reference is often made to the contrast scale, defined as the change in the linear attenuation coefficient per CT number (McCullough 1976). It specifies the range of attenuation coefficients which will appear as one CT number. Thus, if the manufacturer's specified performance is 0.5 percent accuracy, the contrast scale should be at least 0.5 percent per CT number. In general, the contrast scale is used to compare results between different CT units. It is necessary because different CT number normalizations may be incorporated in individual CT units. Examples of this would be, for instance, a scale of -500 to $+500$ as in early CT units as compared to the current -1000 to $+1000$ scale. Even if two units have the same nominal scale, there may still be differences. Thus, to make one's results independent of one's particular unit, one should specify the contrast scale. This would particularly apply in making statements pertaining to CT numbers and noise performance values.

It is relatively simple to determine the contrast scale (CS). IT may be done by simply scanning Plexiglas in a water bath and using the following equation:

$$CS = \frac{\mu_{plex} - \mu_{H_2O}}{(CT\ no.)_{plex} - (CT\ no.)_{H_2O}} \frac{cm^{-1}}{CT\ no.} \quad (5)$$

In this equation the average linear attenuation coefficient difference between Plexiglas and water ($\mu_{plex} - \mu_{H_2O}$) is constant and is equal to 0.001 cm^{-1} for the range of 100 to 150 kV and for moderate beam filtration (AAPM, Report Number 1). $(CT\ no.)_{plex} - (CT\ no.)_{H_2O}$ is the measured CT number difference.

Geometrical and Mechanical Factors

A number of geometric and mechanical factors affect the performance of CT scanners. It has been shown, for instance, that the slice is not necessarily uniformly thick throughout the patient volume; also, all points within the defined slice volume do not contribute equally to the image (Goodenough 1977; Brooks 1977). Six reasons for this effect are discussed in the following paragraphs.

DIVERGENCE OF BEAM   The x-ray beam is not parallel but rather diverges as it passes through the patient (see Fig. 1-21). If the beam is then made to rotate 180° or 360° around the patient, the actual volume scanned is depressed in the center. Slice width is defined at the center of rotation, therefore this results in volume elements at the center contributing more to the CT response than those off the center. This is shown in Figure 1-28 (top), where a theoretical slice is shown. When the x-ray beam is superimposed, the voxels at the periphery intercept less x-rays than those at the center.

FOCAL-SPOT PENUMBRA   As is true for classical radiography, finite size focal spots are utilized for CT scanning x-ray tubes, thus focal-spot effects are also expected. These effects take the form of the expected decrease in overall resolution. Probably more important, however, the focal spot contributes to nonuniformity of the slice along the z direction. This

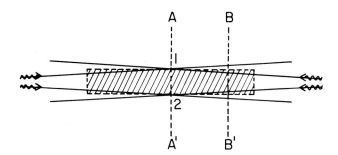

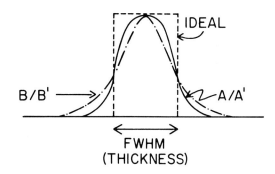

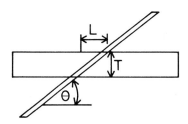

Figure 1-28   Determination of sensitivity profiles. *Top:* CT response varies along lines perpendicular to the slice plane such as *AA'* and *BB'* because of the divergent nature of beam. *Middle:* Curve *AA':* sensitivity profile along the center defines the slice thickness as the full width of half maximum (*FWHM*). Curve *BB':* sensitivity profile along a line closer to the periphery. Note the greater degree of flaring out in the tails and the decreased response within the slice thickness borders. The ideal sensitivity curve should be uniform within the confines of the slice and drop to zero response just outside the slice. *Bottom:* Slice thickness and sensitivity profiles may be determined by scanning an inclined ramp (usually made of a thin slice of aluminum). Thickness (*T*) is determined from length *L* measured on the CT scan. Slice thickness is computed from knowledge of the ramp angle (Θ) and simple trigonometry (e.g., *T* = *L* tangent Θ).

nonuniformity in turn results in a nonuniform sensitivity response of the detector. This effect is particularly true for dual-slice units utilizing relatively large focal-spot dimensions extending along the *z* direction.

SOURCE AND DETECTOR COLLIMATION Any given size focal spot will form some penumbral region at the detector. To reduce unnecessary dose to the patient, efforts at collimation or increasing detector size may be made. These efforts, however, add to the nonuniformity of the CT response, since the beam will then be even more divergent, because tighter source collimation provides for a smaller effective focal-spot size, and there is more divergence from a point source than from an extended source. Also, larger detector sizes result in larger beam diameter, which in turn results in more divergence, that is, the beam is parallel along the central ray and becomes less so for peripheral rays as the beam diameter increases.

Collimation, since it affects x-ray beam field size, obviously affects scatter degradation of the image and also contributes to the patient dose. First-, second-, and third-generation CT systems can easily incorporate collimation, but fourth-generation systems cannot, since detectors must view x-rays emerging from the patient from different angles. Self-collimation can be incorporated in xenon ionization chamber detector systems. Here the chamber walls, though thin, are made up of a highly absorbent material like tungsten arranged in relatively long channels. As a result, image scatter degradation is minimized.

Detector collimator alignment also presents a possible source of problems. This effect, as well as how to measure it on dual-slice units, has been described by Goodenough (1977).

DUAL-SLICE EFFECTS Units that scan two slices simultaneously inherently produce two partially overlapped and inclined beams, as seen in Figure 1-29. This effect may lead to asymmetric slice profiles. Hounsfield (1977) has described an additional consequence of this: the possibility of just including an object at the 0° view (clipping it) and

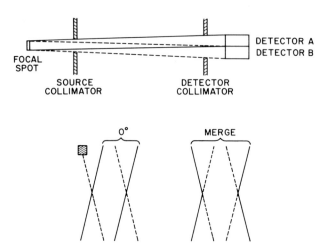

Figure 1-29 *Top:* Asymmetric sensitivity profiles result from dual slice units due to the partial overlapping and inclination (beams are not perpendicular to axis of the head) which are inherent for extended focal-spot and detector sizes. *Bottom:* Because of beam inclination relative to the axis of the head, there is a possibility of clipping a high-density object (shaded) on the 180° view and missing it on the 0° view, resulting in image streaks. If the unit rotates a full 360° or even just a few degrees beyond 180°, the data merge and the inconsistency and thus the streaking will be minimized.

missing it at the 180° view; the resulting inconsistency in the data would lead to streaking, especially if the object was very dense, like bone. If one rotates over 360°, this inconsistency is minimized as is the resulting streaking. In fact, even rotating only an extra 30° to 60° may alleviate the clipping problem. Extra rotation also provides for the possibility of motion correction, in that views beyond 180° are redundant. For example, the 185° view corresponds to the original 5° view. A comparison routine could then be invoked within the computer, with any differences between redundant views assumed to be due to patient motion and averaged (or feathered) out. In typical gantry geometries for dual-slice units, the beam inclination and overlap problems are relatively small, but the resulting artifacts may still be significant. Fortunately, petrous bone imaging is affected only slightly, since petrous bones are usually at the 90° position and not near the center of the picture.

To illustrate the consequences of having nonuniform slice thickness and resulting nonuniform response sensitivity, refer to Figure 1-28. Imagine a dense, high-contrast point placed at different levels along a line perpendicular to the slice plane at the center of the slice (along line AA' in Figure 1-28). Ideally, the response of the CT unit should be rectangular (dashed curve), in that the test point will be detected with equal response as long as it is within the slice thickness (points 1 to 2) and will not be detected at all if it falls outside the slice. In practice, the situation does not follow the ideal; rather, a loss of response occurs inside the slice width borders and some response occurs beyond the borders of the slice due to the effects discussed above and to focal-spot penumbra and collimation effects discussed earlier. The final response is as shown in Figure 1-28 (solid line). If a similar test had been conducted along a line closer to the periphery, such as BB', a broader response would have occurred (alternating dash-circle curve). These curves are termed *sensitivity profiles.* By convention the slice thickness is defined as the full width at half maximum of the sensitivity profile through the center of the slice.

A number of methods to measure the slice thickness have been proposed, including use of small beads on a 45° ramp (Goodenough 1975), inclined cylinders (Sorenson 1979) or wires, or an aluminum ramp (AAPM, Report Number I; Brooks 1977). All these methods are based on the fact that projection of the inclined objects will demonstrate different lengths, as seen in Figure 1-28 (bottom). Here, with knowledge of the angle of inclination, one can calculate the slice thickness directly from simple trigonometric considerations. Phantoms can be made up with such inclines at various positions in the field to test for variations in slice thickness. Sensitivity profiles can be approximated by plotting out the CT numbers along the inclination.

SLICE LOCATION AND TABLE INCREMENTATION   CT scanners normally have a number of light alignment devices to locate and align the patient. In addition, provision is usually made for automatic incrementation of the table to move the patient into position for consecutive scans. The most recent CT scanners, in fact, provide for both automatic incrementation

of the table and inclination of the gantry. These features are indeed convenient and time-saving and offer potentially more accuracy than manual incrementation. Their benefit, however, is clearly compromised if they themselves lack accuracy. The accuracy of all alignments and incrementation features should be verified at regular intervals.

MECHANICAL VIBRATION   Inherent to the CT scan process is mechanical motion. Such motion may and usually does create some degree of vibration, which in turn may induce image-degrading effects. The best example of this is the problem of microphonics for third-generation xenon ionization chamber systems. The term *microphonics* refers to the vibrations induced in ionization chamber walls by the various gantry motions. These vibrations induce fluctuations in output signals, which result in additive CT image noise. To minimize microphonics, thicker chamber walls with smaller overall area must be used. However, this then affects image quality since ideally walls should be as thin as possible and placed as close to each other as possible. Because of the relative inefficient quantum absorption of the gas, long chamber walls are required to maintain low patient dosage. This in turn may make the chamber susceptible to further vibration.

CT Imaging Performance

In addition to the problem of artifact sensitivity, as discussed previously, there are three basic descriptors of CT imaging performance: spatial (or high-contrast) resolution, image noise, and tissue (or low-contrast) resolution.

Spatial Resolution

Spatial resolution is the ability of a CT scanner to record fine, high-contrast detail. Various measures of spatial resolution are available (see Table 1-8). What they all have in common is essentially 100 percent contrast and noise-free conditions. These measures do not necessarily predict the actual performance of a CT unit when imaging tissues having

Table 1-8   Spatial Resolution Measures (100 Percent Contrast and Noise-Free Conditions)

Measure	Mathematical equivalent
Resolution bar and pin pattern	Zero cutoff of MTF
Sunburst pattern	Zero cutoff of MTF
Point spread function (PSF)	Basic response function
Line spread function (LSF)	Integral of PSF along line
Edge response function (ERF)	Integral of LSF along line (slope of ERF = LSF)
Modulation transfer function (MTF)	Fourier transform of LSF

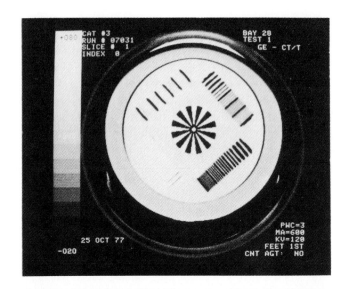

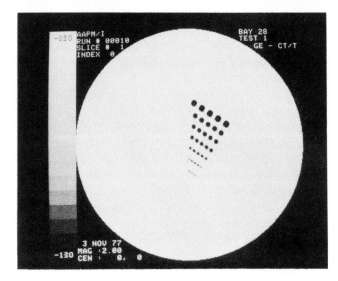

Figure 1-30   Examples of spatial resolution test-scan results for two popular phantom configurations.   *Top:* Starburst and bar pattern scans. Four different bar patterns of differing subject contrast can be displayed on the Catphan phantom (Alderson Research Laboratories; Goodenough 1977).   *Bottom:* Phantom made up of Plexiglas with different-diameter holes in each row (AAPM phantom; AAPM Report Number 1). Both these phantoms have a variety of test objects in addition to those shown here for evaluating the full range of CT system performance as well as for ongoing quality control tests.

similar attenuation coefficients. The resolution-bar pattern is probably the most familiar test object used in general radiology. It can be configured for CT scanning (Goodenough 1977; Maue-Dickson 1979), for instance with a series of Plexiglas strips (or similar material) in a water bath in such a manner that equal widths of Plexiglas alternate with equal spaces of water. These Plexiglas widths form a *line pair* with the adjoining water space, and each line pair is made progressively narrower—that is, a greater number of line pairs per millimeter, or higher line-pair frequency, is formed. The resolving power of the system is that line-pair frequency which is just barely visible on the image.

A variation of the basic resolution bar pattern is the sunburst phantom (Goodenough 1977), in which alternate radial strips and spaces are arranged in a tapered manner around a circle like wheel spokes to provide for continuously varying frequencies. Resolution is given by the distinctly visible tapered pattern closest to the center. This approach was actually used to approximate the modulation-transfer function of a CT system (MacIntyre 1976), which is another measure of resolution. Instead of repetitive bar patterns, a series of varying-diameter Plexiglas, high-contrast pins in a water bath can be used to assess spatial resolution. Alternatively, one can have holes of varying diameters in Plexiglas. Figure 1-30 shows results for two popular phantoms incorporating various spatial-resolution patterns.

A number of other spatial-resolution descriptors are shown in Table 1-8. Though each is distinct, they are all interrelated. The *point-spread function* (PSF) is the most fundamental measure and is defined as the response of a system to a point object. The PSF can be measured by scanning a high-contrast wire pin which is perpendicular to the long axis of the slice. The *line-spread function* (LSF) is the response of the system to a line object lying within or along the long axis of the slice plane. Mathematically, the LSF can be obtained from the PSF by integrating the PSF along a line. The *edge-response function* (ERF) in turn is merely the mathematical integration of the LSF along a plane. Experimentally, the ERF may be obtained directly by scanning an edge object.

Next to the resolution-bar and pin patterns, the *modulation-transfer function* (Villafana 1978a) approach is probably the most commonly cited descriptor of spatial resolution. The MTF is defined as the response of the system to a sinusoidally varying object. Because of the difficulty of constructing objects with sinusoidally varying CT numbers, usually the PSF (Weaver 1975; Goodenough 1977), LSF (Bishop 1977; Judy 1976), or ERF (Judy 1976) are measured and then mathematically converted to the MTF. For instance, the LSF may be subjected to a Fourier transform operation and converted to an MTF. For the interested reader, Jones (1954) has reviewed in depth the various mathematical relationships between these various measures.

To illustrate the use of MTFs, Figure 1-31 shows for comparison purposes the MTF for GE CT/T 7800 and 8800 systems. The 8800 system has a detector aperture nearly one-half the size of the 7800. As a result, the MTF of the 8800 system is correspondingly better (about twice as good). This can be seen from the fact that the MTF response of the 8800 system drops at higher frequencies than the drop for the 7800 system.

The ideal MTF would correspond to a unit (MTF = 1) response regardless of frequency. Such comparisons can be of great value in assessing per-

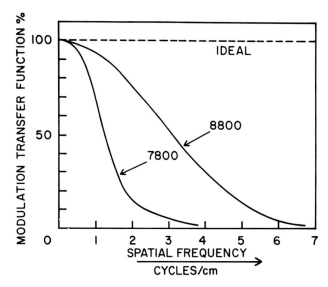

Figure 1-31 The modulation transfer functions (MTF) for the GE CT/T 7800 and 8800 systems. The GE 8800 system has a detector aperture size nearly half as large as the 7800 and the detectors are correspondingly more closely spaced. The improvement in the MTF is significant (nearly two times). The ideal curve represents the situation in which the system response is unity regardless of how high the frequency is. (Adapted from GE brochure.)

formance. Comparisons can also be made between different manufacturers' models and even between subcomponents of a given model CT. This latter application has been admirably demonstrated by Barnes (1979), as shown in Figure 1-32, where it is seen that for the particular CT unit under study, the algorithm (or filter function) represents the limiting system component, since its MTF drops to zero the most quickly, and the focal spot is the component least limiting CT performance. The overall total or composite curve is obtained from the product of the MTFs of all the system components at each frequency; that is, in the general case:

$$MTF_{TOT} = MTF_1 \times MTF_2 \times MTF_3 \times \ldots \quad (6)$$

Note that the composite MTF is in general lower than, and at most equal to, the lowest MTF response component in the system. Attempts to improve the spatial resolution of this system should be directed to improving the lowest response link in the system.

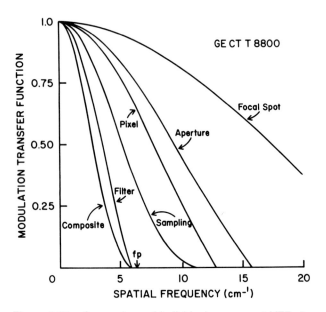

Figure 1-32 Comparison of individual-component MTFs for a given CT system. System shown is the GE CT/T8800 for a 24-cm diameter patient circle, 0.78-mm pixel size. (Adapted from Barnes et al 1979.) Here the sampling and the algorithm filter function would be the limiting component, while the focal spot would be the least limiting. Also shown is the composite or total MTF curve, which is the product of all the component curves. Note that the composite is poorer than any individual component.

In the specific case shown in Figure 1-32, the sampling MTF would be the next most advantageous component to improve.

As previously seen, insufficient sampling leads to aliasing and artifactual streak formation. Even if algorithms are available to remove such artifacts, a generalized loss of spatial resolution will still be present as predicted by the sampling MTF in Figure 1-32. The pixel MTF refers to the fact that for computer reconstruction the image must still be displayed, and choice of pixel size will affect the resolution of the final image. For instance, a smaller patient or reconstruction circle results in smaller effective pixel size and higher resolution. Finally, the aperture (or collimator) MTF in Figure 1-32 refers to the physical opening at the detector.

It should be noted that some systems having relatively large detectors provide for an absorbing pin which can be placed in front of the detector to reduce its effective size and thus improve its MTF or resolution response. Here again, component MTF curves can predict the possible success of such a maneuver. For instance, in the case of the GE CT/T, such an absorbing pin would be essentially futile, since the aperture MTF is not limiting. This is true for all third-generation xenon ionization chamber systems, since such systems can be configured with small detector face area.

Finally, we again caution that MTF data do not of themselves predict actual clinical performance, since they are defined for 100 percent contrast and for essentially noise-free conditions. Consequently they should be used for comparative purposes only.

Noise

In detecting low-contrast tissue structures (tissues of similar CT numbers), noise plays a dominant role; it is, in general, the limiting factor in CT scanning, since in many applications diagnosis hinges on the visualization of tissue structures having very similar CT numbers. For instance, gray- and white-matter tissues are separated by only 5 to 10 CT numbers. Noise can be defined as the standard deviation in CT numbers in a scanned, uniform water bath. All CT scanners provide for a region-of-interest selector where one can read out automatically the standard deviation of the CT numbers falling within the selected area (usually about 25 pixels in size). To make the noise measure independent of the particular CT unit and contrast scale (CS) (see Equation 5), the following expression is used:

$$\text{Noise} = \frac{\text{CS} \times \sigma_w}{\mu_w} \times 100 \qquad (7)$$

where μ_w = the linear attenuation coefficient of water (0.195 cm^{-1} for 70 keV) and σ_w is the observed standard deviation for a uniform water-bath region.

It is crucial to note that image noise is directly related to the number of photons received and processed at the detectors. Consequently, to decrease CT noise one must increase the number of photons passing through the patient and available at the detectors. This, of course, increases the patient dose. The statistical variation in the photon number in a uniform beam incident on the detectors is given by the standard deviation of the photon number (often called the *quantum mottle*) and is given by

$$\sigma_N = \sqrt{N} \tag{8}$$

σ_N here, as the fluctuation in the photon number N (which is related to patient dose), must be distinguished from σ_w as specified for the standard deviation in CT numbers of the final reconstructed uniform water field, the difference between these two being the contribution of algorithm noise (Joseph 1978a).

From Equation (8) emerges an underlying and crucial conclusion, namely, that *CT imaging performance depends on patient radiation dose.* This is true because the number of photons at the detector is directly related to the number of photons passing through the patient, which in turn determines patient dose. Because of the dependence of image quality on patient dose, one must specify the patient dose associated with any image performance specification. Stated another way, an image may be of very high quality but may have been obtained at the cost of an unacceptably high radiation dose to the patient. Haage et al. (1981) have recently illustrated how photon levels of different milliamperage affect actual visualization.

Brooks and DiChiro (1976c) have shown that quantum mottle σ_N, pixel size w (representing the limiting resolution measure), slice thickness h, dose D, and the fractional attenuation of the patient B are related as follows:

$$\sigma_N = \left(\frac{KB}{w^3 h D}\right)^{1/2} \tag{9}$$

where K is a proportionality constant for any given unit. Equation (9) reveals that in general, as slice thickness decreases, the noise value increases. This is evident, since less thickness h implies a narrower beam and consequently the delivery of fewer photons to the detector. A similar statement is true for the patient-dose factor D, in that a lower dose to the patient (for instance, less tube milliamperage or scan time) results in fewer photons at the detector. Both these factors vary as the square root, which

means that halving either one results in a $\sqrt{2}$ times greater noise level. The noise dependence on pixel size, on the other hand, is as the third power. Thus halving the pixel size (which may result in doubling the resolution) results in an eightfold increase in dose to maintain the same level of noise! Not only does CT image performance depend on noise, but attempts at increasing performance by reducing noise may indeed result in a very considerable dose increase to the patient.

If noise is, in fact, limiting CT performance, and not spatial resolution, one may opt, for instance, to increase pixel size. Such a move would reduce noise and might improve visualization of large but low-contrast structures; but care must be taken, since a net reduction of spatial resolution would also result. As discussed above in Equation (9), noise dependence varies with slice thickness to the 1/2 power. Thus increases in slice thickness also reduce noise, but not nearly to the same degree as increases in pixel width, which vary to the 3/2 power. The rationale for the noise dependence on pixel width and slice thickness is simply that reduction in these sizes causes a reduction in the number of photons available to make up the image for each pixel. A reduced number of photons, in turn, creates greater statistical variation, and image noise is increased.

An interesting approach to reducing final noise without increase in dose to the patient is by mathematical smoothing (Joseph 1978a). Algorithms can be configured to include various smoothing routines (referred to as *kernels* or algorithm filters). Such smoothing, however, may result in blurring and thus a loss of spatial resolution. However, if accomplishment of a particular task is indeed limited by the presence of noise, smoothing may in fact yield significant results, as reported by Joseph (1978a). This area, however, still needs considerable clinical investigation.

Finally, it should be stated that other descriptors of noise even more complete and general are available. For instance, noise power spectra can be constructed (Riederer 1978). These describe noise as a function of spatial frequency, hence they are similar to and can be combined with the MTF descriptor. For further details, the reader is referred to the literature (Barnes 1979; Riederer 1978; Rossman 1972).

Tissue Resolution

Tissue, or low-contrast, resolution may be defined as the smallest object or pin size detectable under low-contrast conditions. Low contrast is considered to exist when scanning CT number differences of less than 0.5 percent or 5 CT numbers. (For a -1000 to $+1000$ CT system, each CT number represents 0.1 percent difference.) Phantoms used are similar to the bar and pin object types already discussed. Recent CT units have a tissue resolution of 4 to 5 mm, compared to a spatial high-contrast resolution of 1 mm or less. Tissue resolution is also called *low-contrast detectivity* or *low-contrast sensitivity*.

The tissue-resolution measure is more accurate in predicting clinically expected performance, since low-contrast conditions are more clinically relevant. Also, since low-contrast conditions are specified, the influence of noise is incorporated. Because of crucial interplay among noise, performance, and patient dose, tissue-resolution specifications must be accompanied by statements of pixel size, patient dose, phantom diameter, kilovoltage or filter, and other reconstruction details (McCullough 1980).

Recently another approach describing system resolution has been introduced which uses so-called contrast-detail curves (Cohen 1979a, 1979b). In this approach both the low-contrast and the high-contrast resolution response of a system is specified. Figure 1-33 shows a contrast-detail curve for two levels of radiation dose and two different CT systems. In general, spatial resolution is relatively good for both units at high contrast and is independent of dose (noise). Note that in both cases spatial resolution still does not get better than a certain minimum detectable size (called the *resolution limit* and occurring at 100 percent contrast). As contrast decreases, resolution falls. At low-contrast levels, curves tend to flatten out (this is referred to as the *noise limit*. Note from Figure 1-33 that if noise levels are reduced (dose increased), detectable size decreases at low-contrast levels but not at high-contrast levels.

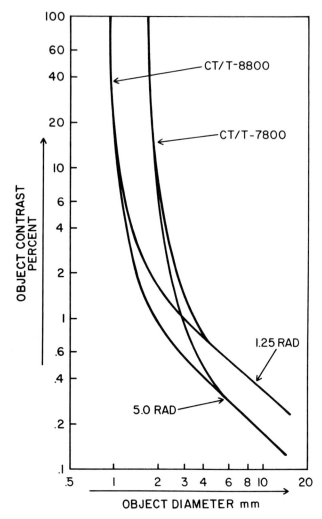

Figure 1-33 Detail-contrast curves. Plot of object diameter visible on both the GE 7800 and the GE 8800 versus object contrast for two different dose levels. At high contrast the smallest possible object diameter is visible (the resolution limit), independent of dose or noise. At low contrast, noise becomes a significant factor and results are highly dependent on dose. (Adapted from GE brochure.)

Finally, mention should be made of still another approach to quantitating the performance of CT equipment. This consists in using receiver- (or reader) operator-characteristic (ROC) curves. Here, an attempt is made to compare the number of false positive and false negative detection rates as a function of reader bias and decision criteria. The interested reader is referred elsewhere for further details (Weaver 1975; Goodenough 1974*a*, 1974*b*; Rossman 1972).

Pixel Sizes, Zoom, and CT Performance

Various aspects of pixels have been previously discussed. Since much discussion concerning CT units centers around statements of pixel sizes, we now summarize some pertinent facts. (1) Pixels are the basic building blocks of the CT image. They represent an element or area of the view over which the reconstruction process has calculated a CT number. (2) Pixels represent a weighted nonlinear average CT number of the various tissues which fall within a given volume element (voxel) within the patient (volume-averaging or partial volume effect) and as a result may be artifactual, especially in regions of the patient where tissue type and structure are rapidly changing. (3) The original EMI Mark I pixel sizes were relatively large, in that they represented a $3 \times 3 \times 13$ mm volume (80×80 array). Currently pixel sizes can be configured to less than 1 mm on a side. (4) Changing pixel sizes can indeed improve CT images, in that the partial volume effect is reduced and consequently both spatial and low-contrast tissue resolution can improve. Improvement, however, is dependent on whether there is a corresponding increase in photon levels to overcome the greater noise levels inherent with smaller pixels (that is, smaller pixel sizes imply a greater number of pixels and thus fewer photons per pixel) and whether the imaging limitation was in fact the pixel size. It is clear that other components such as motion, focal-spot size, or detector-aperture size may be limitations, in which case pixel-size reduction may only result in either image degradation due to noise or an increase in patient dose if photon levels are increased to overcome the higher noise levels for smaller pixel sizes.

Other features which affect pixel size and imaging performance are magnification and zoom. There are a variety of ways in which magnification and zoom can be accomplished. There is as yet no accepted terminology describing these, and the author proposes the terms geometric zoom, interpolated zoom, and reconstructed zoom.

GEOMETRIC ZOOM   Geometric zoom refers to image enlargement accomplished by varying geometric factors such as sampling distances, number of detectors used for the reconstruction process, or mechanical configuration of the gantry. For instance, in first- and second-generation CT systems, a particular detector scans across the total patient cross section. The resulting number of pixels may be the number of intervals over which summing and digitization take place. If a smaller reconstruction area is chosen and if the number of pixels is the same, the patient volume size corresponding to each pixel decreases, allowing for an increase in system performance. For instance, if a particular system is configured for displaying 256×256 pixels for a reconstruction circle of 400 mm, each pixel represents $400/256 = 1.56$ mm. If the reconstruction circle is reduced to 200 mm, each pixel represents $200/256 = 0.78$ mm. To exploit this, CT units have selectable lengths or reconstruction circles over which data can be collected, selection being based on the size of the patient. One must be careful to distinguish between the gantry opening (or patient window), which is the physical opening within which the patient is placed, and the reconstruction circle, which is that region within the gantry opening over which the data are collected and processed, as discussed above. For the best images, the CT operator should select the smallest possible reconstruction circle. Actually, in some applications where resolution is critical, a reconstruction circle even smaller than the patient size is selected and centered around a particular region of interest, as in scanning the cervical spine, for instance.

Sometimes this latter approach is also referred to as *region-of-interest* (ROI) scanning (still a form of geometric zoom). In ROI scanning, caution must be observed in interpreting the resulting CT numbers, since inaccuracies may be introduced by the contribution of patient volumes outside the region of interest. As already stated, the pixel size for small reconstruction circles represents a smaller volume in the patient. As a consequence of this, the actual size of the patient image on the display screen is enlarged. Furthermore, this represents a true zoom, in that enlargement of the image is accomplished with each pixel still representing actual patient data.

In third- and fourth-generation systems, the detectors see the full patient contour, and the millimeters of patient per pixel, and thus data sampling distances, are fixed, thus the use of small detectors is especially necessary. These units, however, still have a selectable reconstruction circle and different possible degrees of final display magnification, in that the smaller regions scanned can still be imaged over the full display with the total pixels available. Image quality is again usually improved, but such improvement will depend on the relative role of the sampling and pixel size MTFs.

One interesting variation of geometric zoom is referred to as *geometrical enlargement.* This configuration provides for variable magnification within the gantry. For example, the detector array, along with the x-ray source, can be moved closer to or farther away from the patient in such a manner that the full array of detectors is always used. When the x-ray source is closer to the patient (and detectors far), a smaller patient diameter is viewed. For larger patient diameter, the source is placed farther away. In either case all the detectors are utilized. With this arrangement, the sampling distances and therefore the image quality can always be optimized.

INTERPOLATED ZOOM This is quite different from geometric zoom. Interpolated zoom enlarges the image of a relatively small region of interest within an already processed image and, under computer control, expands it to fill the entire display by averaging the CT numbers in each particular pixel over the neighboring pixels. Therefore while the final pixels represent a smaller patient volume, they do not represent unique and true patient data but arithmetic averages (or interpolations) over adjacent pixels. Note that this type of zoom corresponds to the straight magnification modes made available in the early first- and second-generation units. It is always performed on a finished image without a reconstruction routine.

RECONSTRUCTED ZOOM This type of zoom depends on original data being available to allow reconstruction over a smaller area. Typically, reconstructed zoom can be performed with optimal results when scan sampling distances are smaller than the pixel display sizes. For example, if a third-generation scanner with 576 detectors is used but final reconstruction results are condensed and displayed on a 256×256 pixel array, then, if original data are still available, a reconstructed zoom of over two times ($576/256 = 2.25$) can be invoked on the original image. This is a true zoom in that original patient data are reconstructed and displayed.

In summary, then, it can be stated that pixel size is indeed an important parameter determining CT imaging performance. A statement of array size by itself is not, however, sufficient. Rather, it is important to state what size (or volume) the pixel actually represents in the patient. There are various ways to enlarge or magnify the image which correspond to decreasing the volume each pixel represents. Such zooming in may or may not lead to an increase in perceived image quality.

Patient Radiation Dose

We have already discussed the fact that CT scanning is noise-limited in that image quality increases as the number of x-ray photons utilized increases. A greater number of photons, however, results in greater patient dose. Fortunately, radiation dosimetry, in general, is an established technology. Even though there are some unique aspects to the dose problem in CT scanning, such as highly collimated scanning fields, these can be taken into account.

The radiological units of roentgens and rads are familiar to all. The *roentgen* is a measure of the ionization occurring in air. The International Commission on Radiological Units (ICRU) has recently recommended dropping this unit, and the clinician will be seeing less and less of it. The *rad* is a measure of the absorbed energy per unit mass, or absorbed dose (1 rad $= 2.58 \times 10^{-4}$ joules per kilogram). Given the roentgen exposure, the rad dose may be

Physics and Instrumentation **39**

obtained by multiplication by a suitable factor (0.91 for diagnostic x-ray energies and soft tissue). The ICRU has also recommended the use of the unit *gray* for absorbed dose (1 gray = 1 joule per kilogram) as a replacement for the rad. Presently most dose information is available in rads, but this is expected to shift toward the gray in the future (1 gray = 100 rads).

Table 1-9 summarizes the various factors affecting patient dose. The factors most familiar to the clinician are patient thickness, beam filtration, and the radiographic factors of kilovoltage and milliamperage. To these must be added a number of factors unique to CT scanning such as beam collimation.

PATIENT THICKNESS It stands to reason that as patient thickness increases, so does the attenuation of the x-ray beam and the amount of radiation which must pass through the patient to provide the required number of photons at the detector level. As a consequence, more total energy is absorbed in the patient. The fact that larger patients have their entry skin surface closer to the x-ray source also results in greater patient skin dose.

KILOVOLTAGE Kilovoltage affects the dose in two possible ways. If kilovoltage is increased because more photons are needed to form the image field, then patient dose is also increased. Dose is decreased on increasing kilovoltage only if this allows a greater proportional decrease in the milliamperage. This relative decrease comes about because the number of photons arriving at the detector is greater, owing to the higher penetrating ability of the higher-kilovoltage beam.

FILTRATION Added beam filtration always leads to lower patient doses. The reason for this is the same as in clinical radiography: filtration removes the softer, low-energy photons which are readily absorbed in the patient and have little probability of penetrating through to the detectors. Selection of filters on CT scanners, however, is not to provide for dose saving but rather to harden the beam to avoid beam-hardening effects within the patient. Typically, such added filtration is selected for scanning large body

Table 1-9 Factors Affecting Patient Dose

Patient thickness

Generator and tube factors:
  Kilovoltage and filtration
  Tube current (milliamperage) and scan on time
  Focal-spot size (penumbral spread)

Gantry factors:
  Beam collimation
  Slice width and overlap
  Scan orientation

Image quality desired

parts as compared to scanning heads. (The filtration referred to here should not be confused with the filters incorporated in an algorithm, which are part of the mathematical reconstruction process.)

TUBE CURRENT AND SCAN ON TIME Tube current represents the flow of electrons across the x-ray tube, and it controls the final quantity of x-rays emitted. By convention it is measured in milliamperes. Scan "on time" refers to the period of time milliamperes are actually flowing and x-rays are actually on or not shuttered. Pulsing units are configured to fire, or turn on for x-ray pulses or various intervals of time (pulse length). These pulses are repeated at various angles as the x-ray tube rotates around the patient. It is the product of the tube current and the "on time" (the milliamperage product) which is the important dose-determining factor. First- and second-generation units, as well as some fourth-generation units, typically do not pulse, and the x-ray beam is on during the entire scan. Many CT units offer a fast scan at low image quality and a slower scan at higher image quality (if patient motion is not limiting). Typically, the faster scans are accomplished by pulsing at fewer intervals around the patient or an overall reduction in scan times. Since the milliamperes product will be lower for such fast scans, the dose also will be lower.

BEAM COLLIMATION Typically, CT scanning involves the use of highly collimated beams.

First-generation systems used pencil beams approximately 3 mm wide by 30 mm long. Second-generation systems utilized multiple pencils, each having approximately the same dimensions as the first-generation pencil beams. Fan beams, as used in third- and fourth-generation systems are opened up along the horizontal direction. As far as dose is concerned, the important idea is that the x-ray beam should be collimated down to approximately the height dimensions of the detectors. Figure 1-34 shows examples of a poorly collimated beam and a well-collimated beam. Note that for poor collimation the region which extends beyond the dimensions of the detector unnecessarily adds to the patient dose and forms a region of overlapping dose when the adjacent slice is scanned. To study this in more detail, dose profiles are usually obtained across the patient in a direction perpendicular to the slice

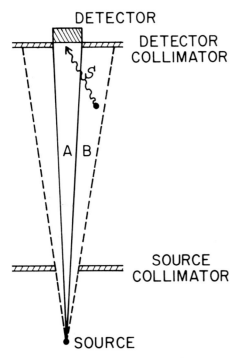

Figure 1-34   A. Well-collimated beam confined to the dimensions of the detector.   **B.** Poorly collimated beam. Radiation passing through the patient is not utilized at the detector. Additionally, scatter (*S*) may degrade image quality.

plane (along *z* axis). These can be obtained by the use of thermoluminescent dosimeters (TLD),* for instance, placed on tissue-equivalent phantoms or on patients directly. Alternatively, ionization chambers placed on phantoms can be used.

One of the prime means of evaluating the dose efficiency of a CT scanner is to compare the dose profiles with the sensitivity profiles. It will be recalled that the sensitivity profile is the response of the CT system along the perpendicular (*z* direction) to the scan plane. The dose profile is the radiation distribution along the same direction. Ideally, the dose profile should be identical to the sensitivity profile for a particular set of scan parameters when both are compared at the patient level. Thus the ratio of the two should be 1.0, or 100 percent. Dose efficiency is also referred to as *dose utilization*. The practitioner is cautioned that a particular CT unit may have a high dose efficiency yet also result in a relatively high dose to the patient, since dose efficiency indicates how efficiently the radiation was detected but does not yield the magnitude of the actual dose received.

SLICE WIDTH AND OVERLAP   As slice width decreases, the penumbral region of the field becomes relatively more important, because the tails of the dose profiles then represent a proportionately larger fraction of the dose distribution, and overlapping on multiple scans becomes correspondingly more serious. Additionally, some degree of slice overlap may be incorporated into the scan sequence. Thus a 1.3-mm slice width being scanned may be incremented, for instance, by a 1.2-mm distance. This results in a 1-mm scan overlap, which drives the patient dose even higher. Figure 1-35 shows how

* TLD detectors usually consist of a small lithium fluoride chip (typically about 1.0 mm × 3 mm × 3 mm), which has the advantage of being small and tissue-equivalent; however, it is low-energy-dependent and must be calibrated very carefully. The TLD detector is based on the principle that electrons liberated by the incident radiation are trapped at certain impurity centers, or electron traps, within the crystal. When the crystal is heated, the electron traps are emptied and light is emitted as the electrons fall back to the ground state. This emitted light is proportional to the original incident radiation.

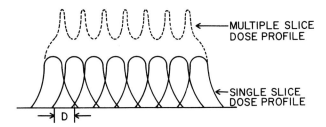

Figure 1-35 Determination of dose distribution over an extended body part when multiple scans are obtained. Appropriate summation of the dose profiles is accomplished by superimposing the dose profiles with incrementation distance *D*. Because of the tailing off of the dose profiles and the degree of overlap in incrementation, dose peaks may appear in the distribution.

total dose distribution for a series of consecutive scans can be obtained by summation of a single-scan dose profile incremented by some known amount; it also shows the case in which peaks may appear in dose distribution, depending on the extent of the tails in the dose profile and the degree of overlap incorporated in the scan sequence.

SCAN ORIENTATION A number of factors associated with scan orientation should be noted. For instance, in a 180° head scanner the x-ray tube should rotate over the posterior of the patient, sparing the eye lens a considerable dose (Villafana, 1978*c*; Batter 1977) (a factor of about 10!). Third- and fourth-generation scanners typically rotate 360° around the patient periphery. Some units incorporate an overscan feature for patient-motion and streak correction. In this case, more than 360° is scanned and the dose is greater in the region of overscan. Such a case requires particular attention to avoid having the scan both begin and end over a critical organ such as the eye lens.

Expressing Dose

There are a number of ways to express patient dose. For instance, average or maximum skin dose, or dose at the middepth of the patient, or even the dose at some critical organ such as the eye lens or gonads has been used (Villafana 1978*c*; Isherwood 1978; Shrivastava 1977; Gyldensted 1977; Mc-Cullough 1974; Perry 1973). Other measures include total integrated energy absorbed in the body (integral dose). Since image quality depends on dose and dose in turn depends on many factors (see Table 1-9), care must be exercised in interpreting dose data. For example, the average dose for a 180° scanner would be relatively low in that only half the patient is irradiated directly, but the dose may be averaged over the indirectly irradiated region. Moreover, depending on the extent of the dose profile tails, very high dose regions may exist which may be masked by the average. The simplest adequately descriptive measures of patient dose are the single-scan dose profile and the multiple-scan dose factor. These should be known to the user for the various operating modes of the equipment used. Along with the dose profiles, a plot of dose distribution along the total body part, similar to that in Figure 1-35, should be available.

The most complete description of the patient dose is that using isodose curves (Perry 1973; Agarwal 1979; Jucius 1977; Wall 1979). Figure 1-36 shows such curves. From these the relative dose at any point or level can readily be picked out, since each isodose curve represents the points having the same dose within the patient, and the points falling between the curves can easily be interpolated. If isodoses are stated in terms of percent of peak dose, the peak dose must be explicitly stated.

A way of expressing CT dose which has been recently proposed is the "computed tomography dose index" (CTDI). The CTDI is obtained at a particular measurement site by integrating the single-slice dose profile and dividing by the nominal slice thickness (Shope 1981). The volume of the CTDI turns out to be equal to the average dose at the measurement site which would result from scanning a series of contiguous slices as in a typical procedure. The CTDI is usually measured with a special long ionization chamber.

GONAD DOSE When the head or upper torso is scanned, the gonads receive a relatively low dose

A

Anterior

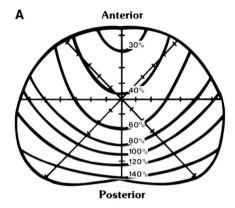

Posterior

B

Anterior

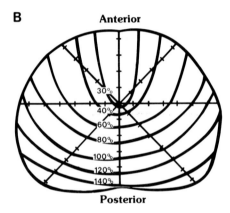

Posterior

Figure 1-36 Isodose curves in a Rando phantom for a Delta 50FS2 20-second scanner, 140 kVp, 35 mA, 42-cm scan circle, 13-mm slice thickness. **A.** Distribution for a multiple-scan examination average in which 100% = 1.1 R. **B.** Distribution for a single-scan peak exposure at 100% = 1.1 R. *(From Jucius 1977.)*

(typically 10 mrad or less). The gonads are exposed to both scattered radiation produced within the patient and leakage radiation from the x-ray tube. Scatter in general must pass through and be extensively attenuated by whatever tissue thickness exists between the region scanned and the position of the gonads. Gonad dose increases as the distance to the irradiated region decreases. Tube-leakage levels are limited by law to a maximum of 100 mR/h at 1 meter. As with any diagnostic x-ray tube, most CT tubes have leakage rates well within this maximum because of the lead lining usually placed inside the tube housing. Even for slower scanners requiring 10 to 15 minutes total examination scan time, this would amount to 10 to 15 mR even under maximum leakage levels. In addition to internally scattered and leakage radiation, there is the possibility of radiation scattering from various portions of the gantry components, which also can contribute to patient dose. Each unit should be evaluated as to gonad doses as well as radiation dosages to persons remaining in the scan room to hold or calm patients.

In summary, then, it is recognized that CT scanning-image quality is noise-limited. Noise in turn is dependent on the number of photons utilized to make up the image. Therefore patient dose, noise, and image quality are all intimately related. When evaluating the performance of a CT scanner, the dose must be explicitly stated for the conditions under which the image was obtained.

Bibliography

AAPM: *Phantoms for Performance Evaluation and Quality Assurance of CT Scanners*, Report Number 1. New York, AAPM, 1978.

AGARWAL SK, FRIESEN EJ, BHADURI D, COURLAS G: Dose distribution from a delta 25 head scanner. *Med Phys* **6**:302–304, 1979.

ALFIDI RJ, MACINTYRE WJ, HOAGAN JR: The effects of biological motion on CT resolution. *Am J Roentgenol* **127**:11–15, 1976.

AMBROSE J: Computerized transverse axial scanning (tomography): Part 2. Clinical application. *Br J Radiol* **46**:1023–1047, 1973.

BAILY NA, KELLER RA, JAKOWATZ CV, KAK AC: The capability of fluoroscopic systems for the production of computerized axial tomograms. *Invest Radiol* **11**:434–439, 1976.

BARNES G, YESTER MV, KING MA: Optimizing computed tomography (CT) scanner geometry. *Proc Soc Photo-opt Eng* **173**:(Med VII) 225–237, 1979.

BASSANO DA, CHAMBERLAIN CC, MOSLEY JM, KIEFFER SA: Physical performance and dosimetric characteristics of the delta 50 whole body/brain scanner. *Radiology* **123**:455–462, 1977.

BATTER S: A philosophy of dose specification for computed tomography. *Med Mundi* **22**:3, 11-12, 1977.

BISHOP CJ, EHRHARDT JC: Modulation transfer function of the EMI head scanner. *Med Phys* **4**:163–167, 1977.

BROOKS RA, DICHIRO G: Beam hardening in x-ray reconstructive tomography. *Phys Med Biol* **21**:390–398, 1976a.

BROOKS RA, DICHIRO G: Principles of computer assisted tomography (CAT) in radiographic and radioisotopic imaging. *Phys Med Biol* **21**:689–732, 1976b.

BROOKS RA, DICHIRO G: Slice geometry in computer assisted tomography. *J Comput Assist Tomogr* **1**:191–199, 1977.

BROOKS RA, DICHIRO G: Statistical limitations in x-ray reconstructive tomography. *Med Phys* **3**:237–240, 1976c.

BROOKS RA, DICHIRO G: Theory of image reconstruction in computed tomography. *Radiology* **117**:561–572, 1975.

BROOKS RA, GLOVER AJ, TOLBERT RL, EISNER FA, DIBIANCA FA: Aliasing, a source of streaks in computed tomograms. *J Comput Assist Tomogr* **3**:511–518, 1979.

CARSON PL, OUGHTON TV, HENDEE WR, AHIYA AS: Imaging soft tissue through bone with ultrasound transmission tomography by reconstruction. *Med Phys* **4**:302–309, 1977.

COHEN G, DIBIANCA FA: The use of contrast-detail-dose evaluation of image quality in a computed tomographic scanner. *J Comput Assist Tomogr* **3**:189–195, 1979a.

COHEN G: Contrast-detail-dose analysis of six different computed tomographic scanners. *J Comput Assist Tomogr* **3**:197–203, 1979b.

CORMACK AM, KOEHLER AM: Quantitative proton tomography: Preliminary experiments. *Phys Med Biol* **21**:560–569, 1976.

CRAWFORD CR, KAK AC: Aliasing artefacts in computerized tomography. *App Opt* **18**:3704–3711, 1979.

DICHIRO G, BROOKS RA, DUBAL L, CHEN E: The apical artifact: Elevated attenuation values toward the apex of the skull. *J Comput Assist Tomogr* **2**:65–70, 1978.

DUERINCKX AJ, MACOVSKI A: Polychromatic streak artefacts in computed tomography images. *J Comput Assist Tomogr* **2**:481–487, 1978.

Emission computed tomography I. *Semin Nucl Med* vol 10, 1980.

Emission computed tomography II. *Semin Nucl Med* vol 11, 1981.

EXNER GU, ELSASSER U, RUEGSEGGER P, ANLIKER M: Bone densimetry using computed tomography: Parts 1 and 2. *Br J Radiol* **52**:14–28, 1979.

GADO M, PHELPS M: Peripheral zone of increased density in computed tomography. *Radiology* **117**:71–74, 1975.

GLOVER GN, PELC NJ: Nonlinear partial volume artefacts in x-ray computed tomography: *Med Phys* **7**:238–248, 1980.

GOODENOUGH DJ, ROSSMAN K, LUSTED LB: Radiographic applications of receiver operating characteristic curves. *Radiology* **110**:89–95, 1974a.

GOODENOUGH DJ, ROSSMAN K, LUSTED LB: Factors affecting the detectability of a simulated radiographic signal. *Invest Radiol* **8**:339–344, 1974b.

GOODENOUGH DJ, WEAVER KE, DAVIS DO: Potential artefacts associated with the scanning pattern of the EMI scanner. *Radiology* **117**:615–619, 1975.

GOODENOUGH DJ, WEAVER KE, DAVIS DO: Development of a phantom for evaluation and assurance of image quality in CT scanning. *Opt Eng* **16**:52–65, 1977.

GORDON R, HERMAN GT: Three dimensional reconstructions from projections: A review of algorithms. *Int Rev Cytol* **38**:111–151, 1974.

GORDON R, HERMAN GT, JOHNSON SA: Image reconstruction from projections. *Sci Am* pp 56–68, October 1975.

GYLDENSTED C: Gonadal thermoluminescence dosimetry in cranial computed tomography with the EMI scanner. Neuroradiology **14**:111–112, 1977.

HAAGE J, MIRALDI F, MACINTYRE W, LIPUMA JP, BRYAN PS, WIESEN E: The effect of mAs variation upon computed tomography image quality as evaluated by invivo and invitro studies. *Radiology* **138**:449–454, 1981.

HERMON G: Demonstration of beam hardening correction in computerized tomography of the head. *J Comput Assist Tomogr* **3**:373–378, 1978.

HINSHAW WS, ANDREW ER, BOTTOMLEY PE, HOLLAND FW, MORRE WS, WORTHINGTON BS: An invivo study of the forearm and hand by thin section NMR imaging. *Br J Radiol* **52**B:6–43, 1979.

HOLLAND GN, HAWKES RC, MOORE WS: Nuclear magnetic resonance (NMR) tomography of the brain: Coronal and sagittal sections. *J Comput Assist Tomogr* **4**:429–433, 1980.

HOUNSFIELD N: A Method of and Apparatus for Examination of a Body Part by Radiation such as X-ray or Gamma Radiation. British Patent 1283915, 1972.

HOUNSFIELD N: Some practical problems in computerized tomography scanning, in Ter-Pogossian MM et al (eds): *Reconstruction Tomography in Diagnostic Radiology and Nuclear Medicine.* University Park Publ., 1977.

ISHERWOOD I, PULLON BR, RITCHINGS RT: Radiation dose in neuroradiological procedures. *Neuroradiology* **16**:477–481, 1978.

JONES RC: On the point and line spread functions of photographic images. *J Opt Soc Am* **44**:468, 1954.

JOSEPH PM: Artefacts in computed tomography, in *Radiology of the Skull and Brain: Technical Aspects of Computed Tomography.* vol 5. St. Louis, Mosby, 1981.

JOSEPH PM: Image noise and smoothing in computed tomography (CT) scanners. *Opt Eng* **17**:396–399, 1978a.

JOSEPH PM, SPITAL RD: A method for correcting bone induced artefacts in computed tomography scanners. *J Comput Assist Tomogr* **2**:100–108, 1978b.

JUCIUS RA, KAMBIC GX: Radiation dosimetry in computed tomography. *Proc Soc Photo-Opt Instrument Eng* **127**(Med IV):286–295, 1977.

JUDY PF: The line spread function and modulation transfer function of a computed tomographic scanner. *Med Phys* **3**:233, 1976.

KAK AC: Computerized tomography with x-ray emission and ultrasound sources. *Proc IEEE* **67**:1245–1272, 1979.

KAK AC, JAKOWATZ CV, BAILY NA, KELLER RA: Computerized tomography using video recorded fluoroscopic images. *IEEE Trans BioMed Eng BME* **24**:157–169, 1977.

KIJEWSKI PK, BJARNGARD B: Correction for beam hardening in computed tomography. *Med Phys* **5**:209–214, 1978.

KOEPPE RA, BRIGGER RM, SCHLAPPER GA, LARSEN GN, JOST RJ: Neutron computed tomography. *J Comput Assist Tomogr* **5**:79–88, 1981.

LATCHAW RE, PAYNE JT, GOLD LHA: Effective atomic number and electron density as measured with a computed tomography scanner: Computation and correlation with brain tumor histology. *J Comput Assist Tomogr* **2**:199–208, 1978.

LIM ST, SAGE DJ: Detection of subarachnoid blood clot and other flat thin structures by computed Tomography. *Radiology* **123**:79–84, 1977.

LITTLETON JT, DURIZCH ML, CROSBY EH, GEORY JC: Tomography: Physical principles and clinical applications, in Robbins LL (ed): *Golden's Diagnostic Radiology*, Sec. 17. Baltimore, Williams & Wilkins, 1976.

MACINTYRE WJ, ALFIDE RJ, HAAGA J, CHERNAK E, MEANY TF: Comparative modulation transfer functions of the EMI and delta scanners. *Radiology* **120**:189–191, 1976.

MAINI R, ISKANDER MF, DURNEY CH: On electro-magnetic imaging using linear reconstruction techniques. *Proc IEEE* **68**:1550–1552, 1980.

MAUE-DICKSON W, TREFLER M, DICKSON DR: Comparison of dosimetry and image quality in computed and conventional tomography. *Radiology* **131**:509–514, 1979.

MCCULLOUGH EC: Factors affecting the use of quantitative information from a CT scanner. *Radiology* **124**:99–107, 1977.

MCCULLOUGH EC: Photon attenuation in computed Tomography. *Med Phys* **2**:307–320, 1975.

MCCULLOUGH EC: Specifying and evaluating the performance of computed tomography (CT) scanners. *Med Phys* **7**:291–296, 1980.

MCCULLOUGH EC et al: On evaluation of the quantitative and radiation features of a scanning x-ray transverse axial tomograph: The EMI scanner. *Radiology* **111**:709–715, 1974.

MCCULLOUGH EC, PAYNE JT, BAKER HL, HATTERY RR, SHEEDY PF, STEPHENS DH, GEDGAUDUS E: Performance evolution and quality assurance of computed tomography scanners with illustrations from the EMI, beta and delta scanners. *Radiology* **120**:173–188, 1976.

MCDAVID WD, WAGGENER RG, PAYNE WH, DENNIS MJ: Correction for spectral artefacts in cross sectional reconstruction from x-rays. *Med Phys* **4**:54–57, 1977*a*.

MCDAVID WD, WAGGENER RG, DENNIS MJ, SANK VS, PAYNE WH: Estimation of chemical composition and density from computed tomography carried out at a number of energies. *Invest Radiol* **12**:189–194, 1977*b*.

MEREDITH WJ, MASSEY JB: The effect of x-ray absorption on the radiographic image, in *Fundamental Physics of Radiology*, 2d ed, chap 19 Baltimore, Williams & Wilkins, 1972.

MOORE WS, HOLLAND GN, KNEEL L: The NMR CAT scanner—A new look at the brain. *CT: J Comput Tomogr* **4**:1–7, 1980.

NALCIOGLU O, LOU RY: Post reconstruction method of beam hardening in computerized tomography. *Phys Med Biol* **24**:330–340, 1979.

PARTAIN CL, JAMES AE, WATSON JT, PRICE RR, COULAM CM, ROLLO FD: Nuclear magnetic resonance and computed tomography. *Radiology* **136**:767–770, 1980.

PERRY BJ, BRIDGES C: Computerized transverse and axial scanning (tomography): Part III. Radiation dose considerations. *Br J Radiol* **46**:1048–1051, 1973.

PETERS JM, LEWITT RM: Computed tomography with fan beam geometry. *J Comput Assist Tomogr* **1**:429–436, 1977.

PHELPS ME, GADO MH, HOFFMAN EJ: Correlation of effective atomic number and electron density with attenuation co-efficients. *Radiology* **117**:585–588, 1975*a*.

PHELPS ME, HOFFMAN EJ, TER-POGOSSIAN MM: Attenuation coefficients of various body tissues, fluids and lesions at photon energies 18 to 136 Kev. *Radiology* **117**:573–583, 1975*b*.

RAO PS, GREGG EC: Attenuation of monoenergic gamma rays in tissues. *Am J Roentgenol* **123**:631–637, 1975.

RAO PS, SANTOSH K, GREGG EC: Computed tomography with microwaves. *Radiology* **135**:769–770, 1980.

REVAK CS: Mineral content of cortical bone measured by computed tomography. *J Comput Assist Tomogr* **4**:342–350, 1980.

RIEDERER SJ, PELC NJ, CHESTER DA: The noise power spectrum in computed x-ray tomography. *Phys Med Biol* **23**:446–454, 1978.

ROSSMAN K: Image quality and patient exposure. *Curr Probl Radiol* **2**:2–34, 1972.

RUEGSEGGER P, HANGARTNER TH, KELLER HU, HINDERLING TH: Standardization of computed tomography images by means of a material-selective beam hardening correction. *J Comput Assist Tomogr* **2**:184–188, 1978.

RUTHERFORD RA, PULLAN BR, ISHERWOOD I: Measurement of effective atomic number and electron density using an EMI scanner. *Neuroradiology* **11**:15–21, 1976.

SALVOLINI U, CABANIS EA, RODOLLEE A, MENICHELLI F, POSQUINI FU, IBA-ZIZEN MT: Computed tomography of the optic nerve: I. Normal results. *J Comput Assist Tomogr* **2**:141–149, 1978.

SCHULZ RA, OLSON EC, HON KS: A comparison of the number of rays versus the number of views in reconstruction tomography. *Proc SPIE* **127**:25–27, 1977.

SCHWENKER RP: Film selection considerations for computed tomography and ultrasound video photography. *Proc Soc Photo-Opt Instrum Eng* **173** (Med VII): 75–80, 1979.

SHEPP LA, STEIN JA: Simulated reconstruction artifacts in computerized x-ray tomography," in Ter-Pogossian M, Phelps M, Brownell GL, Cox JR, Davis DO, Evans RG (eds): *Reconstruction Tomography in Diagnostic Radiology and Nuclear Medicine,* University Park Press, 1977.

SHOPE T, GAGNE R, JOHNSON G: A method for describing the doses delivered by transmission x-ray computed tomography. *Med Phys* **8**:488–495, 1981

SHRIVASTAVA PN, LYNN SL, TING JY: Exposures to patient and personnel in computed axial tomography. *Radiology* **125**:411–415, 1977.

SIEGELMAN SS, ZERHOUNI EA, LEO FP, KHOURI NF, STITIK FP: CT of the solitary pulmonary nodule. *Am J Radiol* **135**:1–13, 1980.

SORENSON JA: Technique for evaluating radiation beam and image slice parameters of CT scanners. *Med Phys* **6**:68–69, 1979.

STOCKHAM CD: A simulated study of aliasing in computed tomography. *Radiology* **132**:721–726, 1979.

TER-POGOSSIAN MM: Computerized cranial tomography seminars in roentgenology. **12**:13–25, 1977.

TER-POGOSSIAN MM, PHELPS ME, HOFFMAN EJ, EICHLING JO: The extraction of the yet unused wealth of information in diagnostic radiology. *Radiology* **113**:515–520, 1974.

VILLAFANA T: Advantage of limitations and significance of the modulation transfer function in radiologic practice. *Curr Probl Diagn Radiol* **7**:10, 1978a.

VILLAFANA T, LEE SH, LAPAYOWKER MS: A device to indicate anatomical level in computed tomography. *J Comput Assist Tomogr* **2**:368–371, 1978b.

VILLAFANA T, SCOURAS J, KIRKLAND L, MCELROY N, PARAS P: Health physics aspects of the EMI computerized tomography brain scanner. *Health Phys J* **34**:71–82, 1978c.

WALL BF, GREEN DAC: Radiation dose to patients from EMI brain and body scanners. *Br J Radiol* **52**:189–196, 1979.

WEAVER KE, GOODENOUGH DJ, DAVIS DO: Physical measurements of the EMI computerized axial tomographic imaging system. *Proc Soc Photo-Opt Instrum Eng* **70**:299–309, 1975.

WEISSBERGER MA, ZOMENHOF RG, ARANON S, NEER RM: Computed tomography scanning for the measurement of bone mineral in the human spine. *J Comput Assist Tomogr* **2**:253–262, 1978.

ZATZ LM: The effect of the kVp level on EMI values. *Radiology* **119**:683–688, 1976.

2

NORMAL CRANIAL CT ANATOMY

Mokhtar H. Gado

The human brain consists of well-known anatomical components. Some parts of these components have been shown to be concerned with certain functions. A complete cranial CT examination consists of a stack of several slices obtained in a sequence. The ultimate goal of this chapter is to pinpoint those slices or parts of slices that depict a given anatomical structure or several structures that deal with a given function. To achieve this goal, the discussion of CT cranial anatomy is presented in three sections.

The first section deals with description of the different components of the brain with reference to the configuration, surfaces, and borders of the brain that one has to be familiar with before addressing the CT image, with no reference to the detailed internal structure that is not visualized on the CT image.

The second section describes the appearance of the CT images of the cranium taken at different axial levels. The discussion emphasizes the features of each slice that enable one to identify the slice and therefore determine its correct position in the complete stack of cranial CT slices. These distinctive features of a given slice are largely anatomical. Familiarity with the morphologic features of the brain in the first section are therefore essential to the text of the second section.

In the third section the different components of the brain are discussed individually in the context of a CT examination. Each individual structure, such as a lobe of a cerebral hemisphere, is approached with particular emphasis on which slices may depict that particular structure. The boundaries of the structure within each of the different slices are determined whenever possible. In the same fashion, localization of a particular functional part of that structure in one or more slices is addressed. Familiarity with the terminology and text of the first and second sections is thus necessary for the discussion of the third section.

COMPONENTS OF THE BRAIN

The brain consists of three major components, each of which is composed of several parts:

Forebrain (prosencephalon):
    Telencephalon
    Diencephalon
Midbrain (mesencephalon)
Hindbrain:
    Pons and medulla
    Cerebellum

The ventricular system consists of an interconnected series of cavities lying within the three major components just mentioned. In the forebrain it includes the lateral ventricles within the telencephalon and the third ventricle surrounded by the structures of the diencephalon. In the midbrain it consists of the aqueduct of Sylvius. In the hindbrain it is the fourth ventricle.

The Forebrain or Prosencephalon

The forebrain consists of two components: the diencephalon (the "between brain") and the telencephalon (the endbrain).

The Telencephalon

The telencephalon consists of the two cerebral hemispheres that occupy most of the cranial cavity (Fig. 2-1). In the midline the interhemispheric fissure separates these two hemispheres on both sides. Ante-

riorly, the interhemispheric fissure extends down to the floor of the cranial fossa. In its middle part the interhemispheric fissure stops at the corpus callosum, which connects the two cerebral hemispheres. Posteriorly, the interhemispheric fissure stops at the upper surface of the cerebellum, which is wedged in pyramidlike fashion between the two occipital lobes.

The falx cerebri is a midline sheet of dura that lies in the interhemispheric fissure (Fig. 2-2). In the anterior part of the fissure the falx is attached to the anterior part of the bony floor of the cranial cavity. In its middle part the falx has a free edge which hangs over the corpus callosum. In its posterior part the falx cerebri is attached to the tentorium cerebelli, which is a dural partition overlying the superior surface of the cerebellum and separates it from the inferior surfaces of the cerebral hemispheres. The straight sinus lies at the meeting of the falx and the two leaflets of the tentorium cerebelli (Fig. 2-2). The superior sagittal sinus lies at the root of the falx along the inner table of the cranial vault in the midline. At its posterior end, therefore, the superior sagittal sinus meets the posterior end of the straight sinus at the torcular Herophili. From the torcular, on each side of the midline a transverse sinus extends against the inner table of the occipital bone at the line of attachment of the tentorium to this bone.

Each cerebral hemisphere consists of an outer gray substance called the cerebral cortex, an underlying white substance called the centrum semiovale, and a small group of internally located masses of central gray substance called the basal ganglia (Figs. 2-9A, 2-10A).

The *cerebral cortex* covers the surface of the cerebral hemisphere. There are three surfaces for each hemisphere, separated by three borders. The superior border separates the medial and lateral surfaces. The inferolateral border separates the lateral and inferior surfaces, and the inferomedial border separates the medial and inferior surfaces (Figs. 2-1, 2-3). The medial surface is straight and situated in the midline separated from the opposite side by the falx cerebri. The lateral surface is convex and

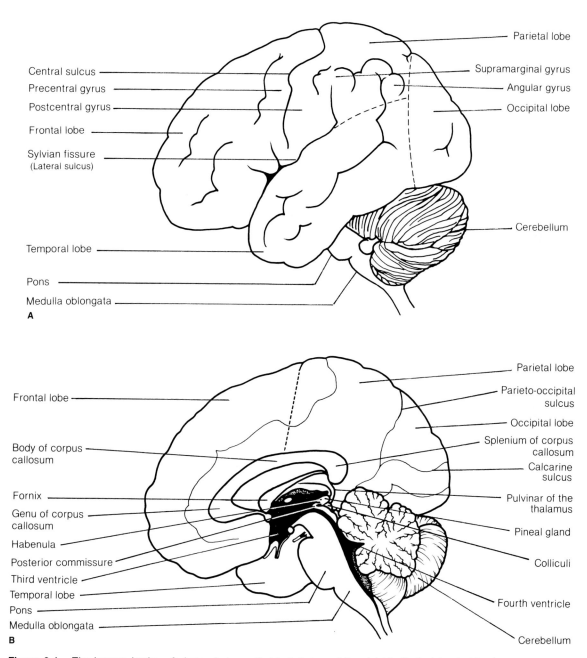

Figure 2-1 The human brain. **A.** Lateral view. **B.** Medial view of the right half of a bisected brain.

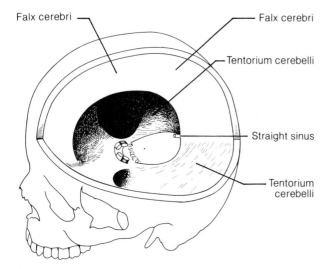

Falx cerebri

Falx cerebri

Tentorium cerebelli

Straight sinus

Tentorium cerebelli

Figure 2-2   Superior lateral view of the cranium. The left half of the vault as well as the soft tissues within the cranium have been removed with the exception of the falx cerebri and tentorium cerebelli.

lies against the inner table of the cranial vault. The inferior surface is irregular. The anterior part of the inferior surface is flat and lies against the floor of the anterior cranial fossa, which separates it from the orbits and nasal cavities. Posterior to this part, the inferior surface dips downward to occupy the hollow of the middle cranial fossa and thus lies against the inner table of the greater wings of the sphenoid bone and the anterior surfaces of the petrous bones. Farther posterior, this surface is slanted to fit the slope of the tentorium cerebelli.

The three surfaces of the cerebral hemisphere contain numerous sulci that separate the cerebral gyri. Four of these sulci or fissures are worthy of description, since they are helpful in dividing each cerebral hemisphere into its constituent lobes. The *lateral sulcus (sylvian fissure)* is identified on the lateral surface. It separates the greater part of the temporal lobe below from the frontal lobe and the anterior part of the parietal lobe above (Fig. 2-1A). The *central sulcus (rolandic fissure)* begins on the medial surface of the hemisphere at about the middle of the superior border (Fig. 2-1A, B). It runs on the lateral surface of the hemisphere downward and

forward and stops short of the lateral sulcus. The *parietooccipital sulcus* lies on the medial surface of the cerebral hemisphere (Fig. 2-1B). It starts at the superior margin at a point about 5 cm from the occipital pole and extends downward and forward, where it meets the *calcarine sulcus* near the splenium of the corpus callosum. The calcarine sulcus extends from this point backward on the medial surface of the occipital lobe and ends at the occipital pole (Fig. 2-1B).

Each cerebral hemisphere is divided into five lobes. The boundaries separating these lobes are in part formed by the sulci mentioned above and in part by imaginary lines, as will be described. The *frontal lobe* is the anterior part of the hemisphere. On the lateral surface (Fig. 2-1A) it is limited posteriorly by the central sulcus (rolandic fissure) and inferiorly by the lateral sulcus (sylvian fissure). On the medial surface (Fig. 2-1B) it is limited posteriorly by a line drawn downward and anteriorly from the end of the central sulcus to the corpus callosum. The *occipital lobe* is the small posterior part of the cerebral hemisphere. On the medial surface it is limited anteriorly by the parietooccipital sulcus (Fig. 2-1B). Its anterior border on the lateral surface (Fig. 2-1A) is an imaginary line extending from the upper end of the parietooccipital sulcus at the superior border of the hemisphere at the preoccipital notch at the inferolateral border.

The *parietal lobe* lies between the frontal lobe anteriorly and the occipital lobe posteriorly. The inferior border of the parietal lobe on the lateral surface (Fig. 2-1A) is formed by the posterior part of the lateral sulcus and an arbitrary line extending from the lateral sulcus toward the other arbitrary line which forms the anterior border of the occipital lobe described above. It will be seen, therefore, that the separation between the parietal, temporal, and occipital lobes on the lateral surface is formed by ar-

Figure 2-3   Coronal sections of the brain.   **A.** At the level of the frontal lobes anterior to the frontal horns of the lateral ventricles.   **B.** At the level of the foramina of Monro.   **C.** At the level of the occipital horns of the lateral ventricles. The falx cerebri and the tentorium cerebelli do not show.

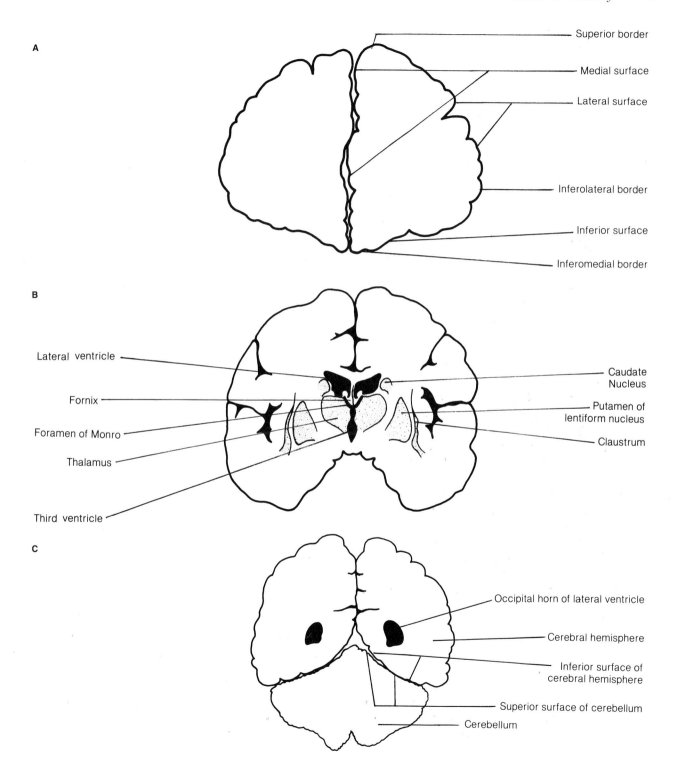

A

Superior border

Medial surface

Lateral surface

Inferolateral border

Inferior surface

Inferomedial border

B

Lateral ventricle

Fornix

Foramen of Monro

Thalamus

Third ventricle

Caudate Nucleus

Putamen of lentiform nucleus

Claustrum

C

Occipital horn of lateral ventricle

Cerebral hemisphere

Inferior surface of cerebral hemisphere

Superior surface of cerebellum

Cerebellum

bitrary lines and thus they are rather ill-defined. The area could be referred to as a zone and may be termed the *parietotemporooccipital junction.* On the medial surface (Fig. 2-1B), the posterior border of the parietal lobe is formed by the parietooccipital sulcus which separates it from the occipital lobe. The *insula (central lobe)* is hidden in the depth of the lateral sulcus and can be seen only if the lips of the sulcus are bent back or cut away. These lips are parts of the frontal, parietal, and temporal lobes. They are called the frontal, parietal, and temporal opercula, respectively.

The *centrum semiovale* constitutes the white matter of the internal portion of the cerebral hemisphere. The *corpus callosum* is a great band of central white matter that connects the two cerebral hemispheres (Fig. 2-1B). Its anterior end is bent downward and is called the *genu.* The main part of the corpus callosum is called the *body.* Its posterior end, which has a thick, rounded free edge and is called the *splenium,* overhangs the pineal body and the colliculi (see below under Midbrain).

The *basal ganglia* represent the central gray matter of the telencephalon (Figs. 2-9A, 2-10A). The *caudate nucleus* has an enlarged anterior end, the head, that indents the lateral wall of the anterior horn of the lateral ventricle. It has a narrow posterior portion, the tail, which follows the superolateral border of the thalamus. The *lentiform nucleus* has a wedge-shaped configuration in the axial cut section (Fig. 2-9A). The *internal capsule* is a thick band of white matter situated between the thalamus (see below) and the caudate and lentiform nuclei. The part of the internal capsule that lies between the caudate and lentiform nuclei is called the anterior limb. The part between the thalamus and lentiform nucleus is called the posterior limb. Both limbs meet in a right angle at the genu.

The Diencephalon

The diencephalon consists of several structures that lie around the third ventricle. It connects the midbrain on one side to the cerebral hemispheres on the other side. Its structures include the thalami, the geniculate bodies, the epithalamus, the subthalamus, and the hypothalamus.

1. The *thalami* are two large ovoid masses, small in size anteriorly and more voluminous posteriorly. Each thalamus is 4 cm long. Its medial surface forms the lateral wall of the third ventricle. It is covered with ependyma and is separated from the opposite thalamus by the third ventricle itself (Fig. 2-3B). Its superior surface forms part of the floor of the lateral ventricle on each side. The medial part of the superior surface which does not form part of the floor of the lateral ventricle is covered with the fold of pia called tela choroidea, which forms the velum interpositum in the roof of the third ventricle. The fornix lies on top of the superior surface of the thalamus, separating the lateral part from the medial part (Fig. 2-1B). The anterior end of the thalamus is small and forms the posterior boundary of the foramen of Monro, while the column of the fornix that overlies the thalamus forms at this point the anterior border of the foramen of Monro (Fig. 2-3B). Each foramen of Monro forms a communication between the lateral ventricle of that side and the third ventricle. The voluminous posterior end of the thalamus is the pulvinar. It extends farther posteriorly beyond the posterior end of the third ventricle (Fig. 2-1B), so each pulvinar overlies a superior colliculus. In the space between the two pulvinars the pineal rests in the midline just above the two superior colliculi (Figs. 2-4, 2-6). Unlike the superior and medial surfaces of the thalamus, which form part of the walls of the lateral and third ventricles, the inferior and lateral surfaces lie against other parts of the brain tissue. The inferior surface is continuous with the upper end of the tegmentum of the midbrain (see below). The lateral surface lies against the white matter that constitutes the posterior limb of the internal capsule (Fig. 2-10A). The medial surfaces of the thalami are separated by the cavity of the third ventricle, but they are connected by the massa intermedia (Fig. 2-3B).

2. The *geniculate bodies* (Fig. 2-4) are a medial and a lateral one on each side. All four structures constitute the metathalamus. The geniculate bodies

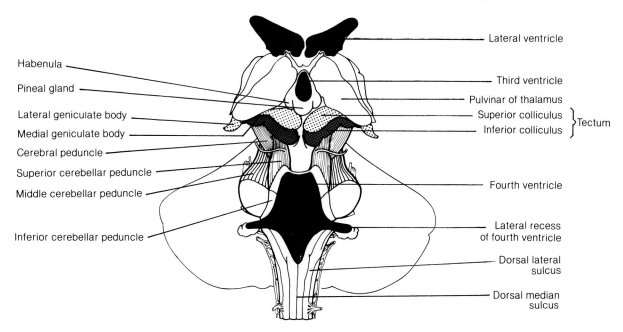

Habenula

Pineal gland

Lateral geniculate body

Medial geniculate body

Cerebral peduncle

Superior cerebellar peduncle

Middle cerebellar peduncle

Inferior cerebellar peduncle

Lateral ventricle

Third ventricle

Pulvinar of thalamus

Superior colliculus

Inferior colliculus

}Tectum

Fourth ventricle

Lateral recess
of fourth ventricle

Dorsal lateral
sulcus

Dorsal median
sulcus

Figure 2-4   Dorsal view of the diencephalon and brainstem. (*Modified from Nieuwenhuys, Vougd, Van Huijen: The Human Central Nervous System. Berlin, Heidelberg, New York, Springer-Verlag, 1979.*)

serve as relay stations. The lateral geniculate body is connected by the superior brachium to the superior colliculus and serves as part of the visual pathways that end in the visual cortex of the occipital lobe. The medial geniculate body is connected by the inferior brachium to the inferior colliculus and serves as part of the auditory pathways that end in the auditory cortex of the superior temporal gyrus.

3. The *habenula,* the *pineal body,* and the *posterior commissure* constitute the epithalamus (Figs. 2-1B, 2-6). The stalk which attaches the pineal gland consists of a superior and an inferior lamina. The superior lamina is formed by the habenula. The inferior lamina is formed by the posterior commissure. Between these two laminae is the pineal recess of the third ventricle (Fig. 2-1B).

4. The *subthalamus* is the transition zone between the thalamus and the tegmentum of the midbrain, upon which it lies and with which it is continuous.

5. The *hypothalamus* forms the wall of the anterior end of the third ventricle. It consists of several small parts: the mamillary bodies, the tuber cinereum, the infundibulum, the hypophysis, and the optic chiasm (Fig. 2-5).

The Midbrain or Mesencephalon

The midbrain (mesencephalon) is a short segment of the brainstem. It connects the pons and the cerebellum on the one hand with the forebrain on the other hand. The brainstem thus consists of the midbrain, the pons, and the medulla. The latter two are part of the hindbrain.

The midbrain consists of a smaller dorsal portion called the *tectum* (Fig. 2-4) and a larger anterior portion formed by the *cerebral peduncles* (Fig. 2-5). Between the tectum and the cerebral peduncles, the central gray substance of the midbrain surrounds the aqueduct which connects the fourth and third

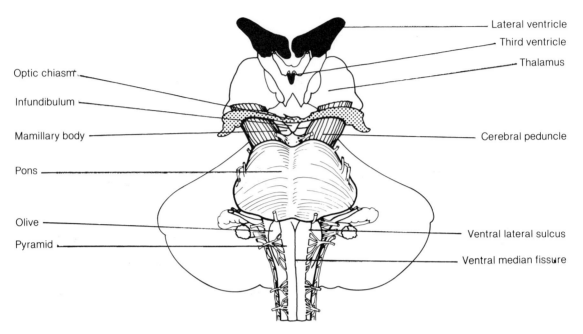

Figure 2-5   Ventral view of the diencephalon and brainstem. (*Modified from Nieuwenhuys, Vougd, Van Huijzen: The Human Central Nervous System. Berlin, Heidelberg, New York, Springer-Verlag, 1979.*)

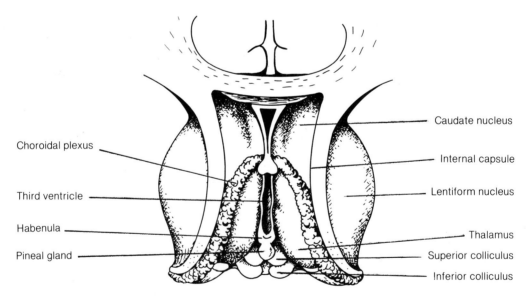

Figure 2-6   Superior view of the diencephalon. (*Modified from Carpenter MB: Human Neuroanatomy, 7th Ed. Baltimore, Williams and Wilkins, 1976.*)

ventricles. The cerebral peduncles are viewed on the ventral surface of the brain as two prominent ridges (Fig. 2-5), diverging as they approach the cerebral hemispheres. Thus a triangular area, the interpeduncular fossa, separates the two cerebral peduncles. The triangular configuration of this fossa is seen in the ventral view as well as the axial view of the midbrain. The floor of the interpeduncular fossa is the posterior perforated substance.

The tectum of the midbrain consists of four rounded prominences, the *corpora quadrigemina* or *colliculi* (Fig. 2-4). The superior colliculi are continuous on both sides with the superior brachia; each connect one superior colliculus to the ipsilateral lateral geniculate body where the ipsilateral optic tract ends. Thus the fibers of the superior brachium connect the superior colliculus and the visual cortex. Likewise, the inferior brachia extend from the inferior colliculi to the medial geniculate bodies, connecting the inferior colliculus and auditory cortex.

Each cerebral peduncle consists of a ventral part, the crus (or basis pedunculi), and a dorsal part, the tegmentum of the midbrain. The superior cerebellar peduncle (brachium conjunctivum) penetrates deeply into the tegmentum of the inferior part of the midbrain from the dorsal aspect on each side of the midline (Fig. 2-4).

The Hindbrain

The hindbrain consists of two parts. The anterior part is the *medulla oblongata* inferiorly and the *pons* superiorly. The posterior part is the *cerebellum.* Between the anterior and posterior parts of the hindbrain there is a cavity, the fourth ventricle.

The Medulla Oblongata

The medulla oblongata is continuous inferiorly with the spinal cord and superiorly with the pons. It measures 3 cm in length. Its cross-sectional dimensions are 2 cm from side to side and 1.25 cm anteroposteriorly. There are two midline grooves, a ventral and a dorsal. Anteriorly, the ventral median fissure starts below at the pyramidal decussation and ends superiorly at the inferior border of the pons (Fig. 2-5). The dorsal median sulcus is present only on the dorsal aspect of the inferior half of the medulla and stops at the superior half, where the dorsal surface of the medulla forms the floor of the fourth ventricle (Fig. 2-4). These two midline grooves thus bisect the medulla. Each half furthermore shows two longitudinal grooves, the ventral lateral sulcus and the dorsal lateral sulcus (Figs. 2-4 and 2-5).

The two lateral sulci enable several structures to be identified on the surface of each lateral half of the medulla. Anteriorly, the *pyramid* lies between the ventral median fissure and the ventral lateral sulcus (Fig. 2-5). The *olive* lies between the two lateral sulci (Fig. 2-5). Behind the dorsal lateral sulcus and lying between it and the dorsal median fissure are the cuneate and gracile tubercles (Fig. 2-4). As previously mentioned, the dorsal median sulcus is present only over the dorsal aspect of the lower half of the medulla, so these tubercles are present only on that portion of the medulla.

The upper half of the dorsal surface of the medulla shows two diverging prominences forming the lateral boundaries of the floor of the fourth ventricle (Fig. 2-4). These prominences contain the *inferior cerebellar peduncles* (restiform bodies), which connect the spinal cord and medulla with the cerebellum.

The Pons

The pons connects the medulla below with the midbrain above. It forms a massive protuberance, with well-defined borders, on the ventral surface of the brainstem (Fig. 2-5). This protuberance is separated from the medulla oblongata by the inferior pontine sulcus and from the cerebral peduncles of the midbrain by the superior pontine sulcus (Fig. 2-5). The ventral prominence consists of transverse strands across the midline. At each side these strands form the middle cerebellar peduncle. There is a shallow midline depression on the ventral surface of the pons, the basilar sulcus. The basilar artery lies in this depression.

In addition to the massive ventral component of the pons, which is also called the *basis pontis,* there is a smaller dorsal component, the tegmentum of the pons. The dorsal surface of the tegmentum forms the upper half of the floor of the fourth ventricle (Fig. 2-4), so the floor of the fourth ventricle is formed in part by the dorsal aspect of the medulla and in part by the dorsal aspect of the pons. These two components form the rhomboid fossa.

The Cerebellum

The cerebellum occupies the greater part of the posterior cranial fossa. It is located on the dorsal aspect of the pons and medulla, separated from these two structures by the cavity of the fourth ventricle (Fig. 2-1B).

The upper surface of the cerebellum lies under the tentorium cerebelli, which separates it from the occipital lobes. As a result of the upward slope of the leaflets of the tentorium toward the midline, the high point of the cerebellum is in the midline anteriorly. The posterior surface of the cerebellum lies against the inner table of the occipital bone. The cerebellum is attached to the brainstem by three cerebellar peduncles. The superior peduncle (brachium conjunctivum) connects it with the midbrain, the middle peduncle (brachium pontis) connects it with the pons, and the inferior peduncle (restiform body) connects it with the medulla. The cerebellum consists of a narrow medial portion, the vermis, and two hemispheres which extend laterally and posteriorly (Fig. 2-7).

The superior part of the vermis begins at the anterior medullary velum, which forms the superior part of the roof of the fourth ventricle. The farthest anterior part of the superior vermis is the lingula, which can be visualized from the ventral aspect of the cerebellum after removal of the brainstem (Fig. 2-7C). The part of the superior vermis behind the lingula is the central lobule, and farther posterior is the culmen. When viewed from the superior aspect (Fig. 2-7A), the cerebellum has a midline shallow concavity anteriorly (the anterior cerebellar fissure)

and a narrow deep groove posteriorly (the posterior cerebellar fissure); the anterior part of the culmen appears at the bottom of the shallow anterior cerebellar fissure (Fig. 2-7A), and the folium lies at the bottom of the narrow and deep posterior cerebellar fissure (Fig. 2-7A). Between the culmen and the folium is the declive. When viewed from the dorsal aspect, the culmen, declive, and folium of the superior vermis appear in continuity with the tuber, pyramid, and uvula of the inferior vermis (Fig. 2-7B). The farthest forward structure of the inferior vermis is the nodulus; this cannot be visualized from the dorsal aspect of the cerebellum but only from the ventral aspect after removal of the brainstem (Fig. 2-7C). In the ventral aspect of the cerebellum (Fig. 2-7C), the lingula and central lobule of the cerebellum lie above the cavity of the fourth ventricle, while the nodulus and uvula lie below the fourth ventricle. On both sides of the fourth ventricle and inferolateral to the cut edges of the middle cerebellar peduncles, the flocculus is seen on each side in relation to the lateral recess of the fourth ventricle (Fig. 2-7C).

The cerebellar tonsils are the most anterior inferior structures of the cerebellar hemispheres (Fig. 2-7B). The rest of the cerebellar hemispheres on the inferior aspect consist of the biventral lobules (Fig. 2-7C), followed posteriorly by the inferior semilunar lobules. The horizontal fissure separating the inferior semilunar lobule from the superior semilunar lobule is best visualized on the dorsal view of the cerebellum (Fig. 2-7B). The superior surface of the cerebellar hemisphere is formed at its posterior end by the superior semilunar lobule (Fig. 2-7A). In front of the superior semilunar lobule and separated from it by the superior posterior fissure is the lobule simplex, which in turn is separated from the quadrangular lobule by the primary fissure (Fig. 2-7A).

Figure 2-7 The cerebellum. **A.** Superior view. (*Modified from Carpenter MB: Human Neuroanatomy, 7th Ed. Baltimore, Williams and Wilkins, 1976.*) **B.** Dorsal view. (*Modified from Nieuwenhuys, Vougd, Van Huijzen: The Human Central Nervous System. Berlin, Heidelberg, New York, Springer-Verlag 1979.*) **C.** Ventral view. (*Modified from Nieuwenhuys, Vougd, Van Huijzen: The Human Central Nervous System. Berlin, Heidelberg, New York, Springer-Verlag 1979.*)

A

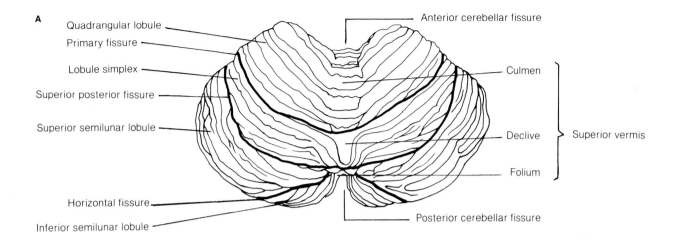

Quadrangular lobule
Primary fissure
Lobule simplex
Superior posterior fissure
Superior semilunar lobule
Horizontal fissure
Inferior semilunar lobule

Anterior cerebellar fissure
Culmen
Declive
Folium
Posterior cerebellar fissure
Superior vermis

B

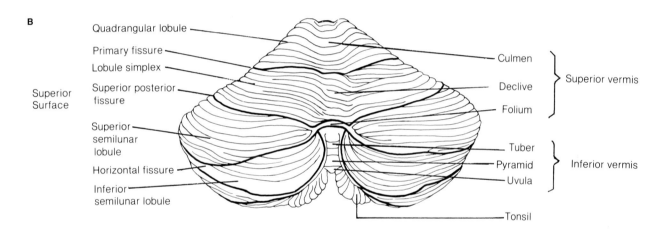

Superior Surface

Quadrangular lobule
Primary fissure
Lobule simplex
Superior posterior fissure
Superior semilunar lobule
Horizontal fissure
Inferior semilunar lobule

Culmen
Declive
Folium
Superior vermis

Tuber
Pyramid
Uvula
Inferior vermis

Tonsil

C

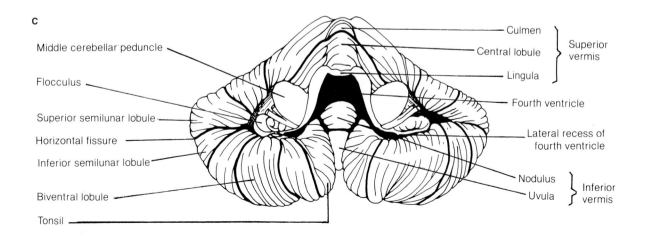

Middle cerebellar peduncle
Flocculus
Superior semilunar lobule
Horizontal fissure
Inferior semilunar lobule
Biventral lobule
Tonsil

Culmen
Central lobule
Lingula
Superior vermis

Fourth ventricle
Lateral recess of fourth ventricle
Nodulus
Uvula
Inferior vermis

THE COMPONENTS OF A COMPLETE SET OF CRANIAL CT IMAGES

The complete set of CT slices of the cranium from foramen magnum to vertex can be conveniently divided into four subsets. For purposes of description, these subsets may be referred to as the infraventricular, low ventricular, high ventricular, and supraventricular. The following discussion is based on slices of 8-mm thickness obtained at a plane of 20° above the orbitomeatal line. Usually, 14 such slices cover the average-size cranium.

In the following text the distinctive features of six slices are described, one each in the infraventricular and supraventricular subsets and two each in the low ventricular and high ventricular subsets. The anatomical features of each of these six slices are so distinct that they can be recognized at a glance.

The *infraventricular series* is the lowest subset (Fig. 2-8). In these slices the petrous bones and the occipital bone delineate the walls of the posterior fossa, while the temporal and frontal bones delineate the remainder of the slice. In the posterior fossa, the fourth ventricle stands out as a landmark that separates the cerebellum posteriorly from the brainstem anteriorly (Fig. 2-8B). In front of the brainstem and situated in the midline is the suprasellar cistern (Fig. 2-8B). On both sides of the brainstem and suprasellar cistern are the inferior parts of the temporal lobes. The tips of the temporal horns may be shown anteromedial to the center points of each temporal lobe (Fig. 2-8B). The uncus of the temporal lobe forms the lateral border of the suprasellar cistern. This cistern has two distinct lateral extensions forming the sylvian cistern on each side. In front of the temporal lobes, and separated from them by the sylvian cisterns, are the frontal lobes (Fig. 2-8A, B). They lie on both sides of the midline separated by the interhemispheric fissure.

The next subset in a cephalad sequence is the *low ventricular series* (Figs. 2-9B and 2-10B). These slices lie above the level of the petrous bones and therefore are bounded peripherally by the occipital, temporal, parietal, and frontal bones; they include

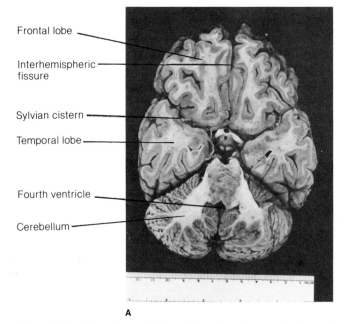

Frontal lobe

Interhemispheric fissure

Sylvian cistern

Temporal lobe

Fourth ventricle

Cerebellum

A

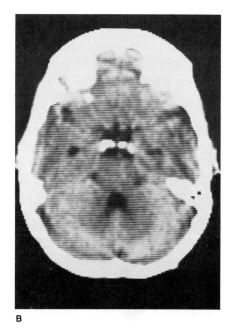

B

Figure 2-8   CT anatomy of the brain at the infraventricular level (see text).   **A.** The cut surface of an antomy specimen.   **B.** CT.

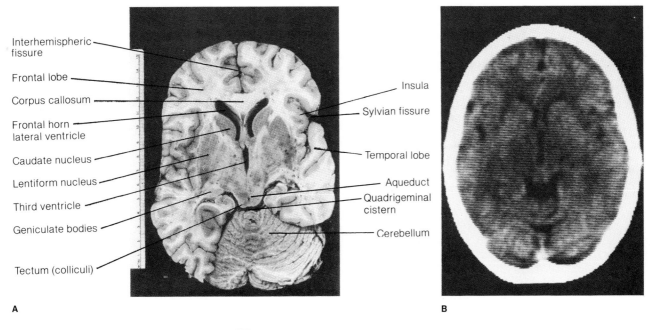

Interhemispheric fissure
Frontal lobe
Corpus callosum
Frontal horn lateral ventricle
Caudate nucleus
Lentiform nucleus
Third ventricle
Geniculate bodies
Tectum (colliculi)

Insula
Sylvian fissure
Temporal lobe
Aqueduct
Quadrigeminal cistern
Cerebellum

A

B

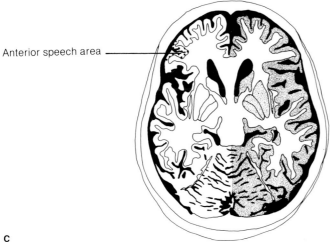

Anterior speech area

C

Figure 2-9　CT anatomy of the brain at the low ventricular level through the midbrain (see text). **A.** The cut surface of an anatomy specimen. **B.** CT. **C.** A diagram showing the location of the anterior speech area of the cerebral cortex of the left cerebral hemisphere. *(Modified from Gado M, Hanaway J, Frank R: Functional anatomy of the cerebral cortex by computed tomography. Journal of Computer Assisted Tomography 3:1–19, 1979.)*

parts of the frontal horns, trigones, and inferior horns as well as posterior horns of the lateral ventricles but not the bodies of the lateral ventricles. In addition, these slices include the superior parts of the cerebellum and brainstem, together with the thalamus and basal ganglia. The lowest (Fig. 2-9B) and uppermost (Fig. 2-10B) of these slices have distinctive features.

The features of the lowest slice in this subset are shown in Figure 2-9B. The CSF spaces lying in the central part of this slice have a consistent pattern (Fig. 2-9B) and include the following structures sequentially from front to back: the interhemispheric fissure, the inferior parts of the frontal horns, the third ventricle, and the quadrigeminal cistern. The inferior parts of the frontal horns appear as oblique

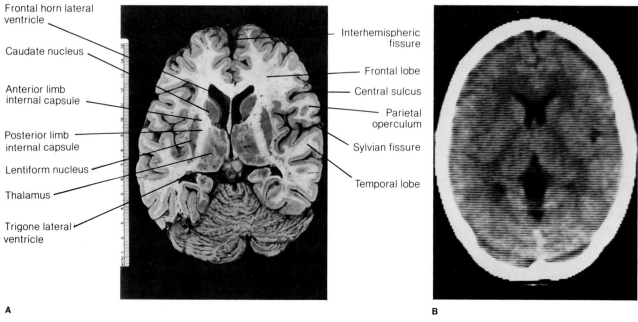

Frontal horn lateral ventricle

Caudate nucleus

Anterior limb internal capsule

Posterior limb internal capsule

Lentiform nucleus

Thalamus

Trigone lateral ventricle

Interhemispheric fissure

Frontal lobe

Central sulcus

Parietal operculum

Sylvian fissure

Temporal lobe

A

B

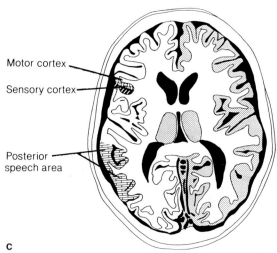

Motor cortex

Sensory cortex

Posterior speech area

C

Figure 2-10   CT anatomy of the brain at the low ventricular level through the thalamus (see text).   **A.** The cut surface of an anatomy specimen. **B.** CT. **C.** A diagram showing the location of the motor and sensory areas as well as the posterior speech area. (*Modified from Gado M, Hanaway J, Frank R: Functional anatomy of the cerebral cortex by computed tomography. Journal of Computer Assisted Tomography 3:1–19, 1979.*)

curved slits that converge on the midline. The interhemispheric fissure and the third ventricle lie in line with each other.

The quadrigeminal cistern lies in a more or less transverse position. It is curved, with the concavity anterior, and it caps the posterior aspect of the tectal plate of the midbrain. For purposes of description,

this slice can be divided into an anterior, a middle, and a posterior third. In the middle third of the slice, the surface of the insula appears buried underneath the surface of the cerebral hemisphere (Fig. 2-9B). The CSF space on the surface of the insula is the circular sulcus. The brain parenchyma separating the circular sulcus and insula from the surface of the hemisphere is formed by the opercula, while deep to the insula the lentiform and caudate nuclei are visualized by their higher density compared with the surrounding white matter (Fig. 2-9B). The thalamus does not appear in this slice. The anterior third of the slice in front of the insula is occupied by the frontal lobes, separated in the midline by the interhemispheric fissure. The posterior third of the slice is occupied by the temporal lobes on both sides and the cerebellum in the midline (Fig. 2-9B). The demarcation between the cerebellum and the temporal lobes is made by the dura and may be visualized on the CT scans after intravenous contrast injection.

The higher slice of the low ventricular subset has distinctive features shown in Figure 2-10B. The CSF structures in the central part of the slice differ in appearance from those of the lower slice just described. The frontal horns each appear as a triangular CSF space with a concave lateral border (Fig. 2-10B). The medial limb of the triangle is straight and lies against the opposite frontal horn, separated by the thin septum pellucidum. The third ventricle lies in the midline, starting at the posterior end of the frontal horns. The foramen of Monro connecting the frontal horns to the third ventricle may be visualized in this slice (Fig. 2-10A). The quadrigeminal cistern in this slice has a rhomboid configuration with four extensions: the anterior extension is in the velum interpositum of the roof of the third ventricle; the posterior extension forms the supracerebellar cistern; and the two lateral extensions form the retrothalamic cisterns. The trigones of the lateral ventricles are situated away from the midline, one each in the depth of a cerebral hemisphere. For purposes of description, the slice may be divided into an anterior, middle, and posterior third. The middle third of the slice contains, in addition to the caudate and lentiform nuclei, the two thalami, one on each side of the third ventricle. On each side, the internal capsule appears as an L-shaped band of lower density separating the caudate nucleus, lentiform nucleus, and thalamus (Fig. 2-10B). The insula is visualized lateral to the lentiform nucleus. The circular sulcus appears on the surface of the insula. The sylvian fissure is shown as a deep fissure that ex-

tends from the surface of the hemisphere to the posterior end of the insula (Fig. 2-10A, B). The posterior third of the slice is occupied by the temporal and occipital lobes, with a component of the cerebellum toward the center. The anterior third of the slice is occupied by the frontal lobes, separated in the midline by the interhemispheric fissure (Fig. 2-10B).

The next (third) subset of slices is the *high ventricular series* (Figs. 2-11 and 2-12). The main distinctive feature of these slices is the presence of the bodies of the lateral ventricles. The lower and the higher slices in this subset are distinguishable by certain anatomic features. In the lower slice of this subset (Fig. 2-11B) the bodies of the lateral ventricles lie close to the midline, separated only by the septum pellucidum. In the posterior part the lateral ventricles diverge away from the midline into the depth of each cerebral hemisphere, where the body of the ventricle joins the trigone (Fig. 2-11B). The cerebellum does not appear in this slice or in any of the slices above this level. The basal ganglia also are not visualized, except perhaps the superior border of the caudate nucleus, which may appear as a narrow band of density at the lateral border of the body of the lateral ventricle (Fig. 2-11B). The rest of the brain parenchyma in this slice consists of the white matter of the centrum semiovale and the overlying cerebral cortex. At the convexity, the sylvian fissure appears in the middle of this slice in the same plane as the trigone of the lateral ventricle (Fig. 2-11B). In the anterior half of the convexity, the central sulcus lies in the same plane as the anterior end of the body of the lateral ventricle. In the midline, the parietooccipital sulcus is seen in the posterior third of the slice separating the parietal lobe from the occipital lobe (Fig. 2-11A, B). The higher slice in this subset is distinct from the lower slice just described by the obvious separation between the bodies of the lateral ventricles (Fig. 2-12B). The gap between the two lateral ventricles is occupied by the corpus callosum and cingulate gyrus. The most remarkable sulcus in the midline is the parietooccipital sulcus in the posterior third of the slice (Fig. 2-12A, B). At the convexity the sylvian fissure and central sulcus may be visualized. The sylvian fissure lies approx-

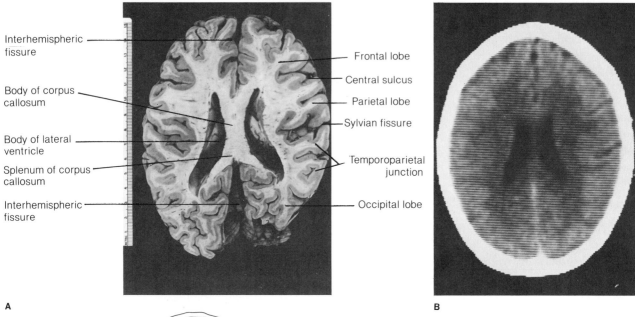

Interhemispheric fissure

Body of corpus callosum

Body of lateral ventricle

Splenum of corpus callosum

Interhemispheric fissure

Frontal lobe

Central sulcus

Parietal lobe

Sylvian fissure

Temporoparietal junction

Occipital lobe

A

B

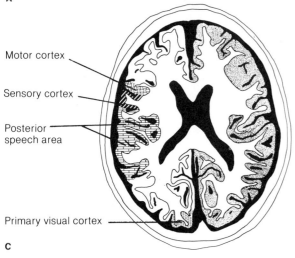

Motor cortex

Sensory cortex

Posterior speech area

Primary visual cortex

C

Figure 2-11   CT anatomy at the high ventricular level through the body of the lateral ventricles (see text).   **A.** The cut surface of an anatomy specimen.   **B.** CT.   **C.** Diagram showing the location of the motor area, sensory area and speech area of the cortex of the left cerebral hemisphere. (*Modified from Gado M, Hanaway J, Frank R: Functional anatomy of the cerebral cortex by computed tomography. Journal of Computer Assisted Tomography 3:1–19, 1979.*)

imately in the same plane as the posterior end of the body of the lateral ventricle (Fig. 2-12A, B), while the central sulcus lies at or in front of the plane of the anterior end of the lateral ventricle (Fig. 2-12A, B).

The last (fourth) subset of slices is the *supraventricular series* (Fig. 2-13B). The slices of this series decrease in size toward the vertex. Also, the higher

the slice the more conspicuous the sulci appear, and they extend farther toward the central part of each hemisphere. The feature common to all slices in this subset is the absence of any central CSF spaces other than the straight midline interhemispheric fissure. On each side, the cerebral hemisphere consists of the centrum semiovale and the overlying cerebral cortex (Fig. 2-13B). The only recognizable feature in

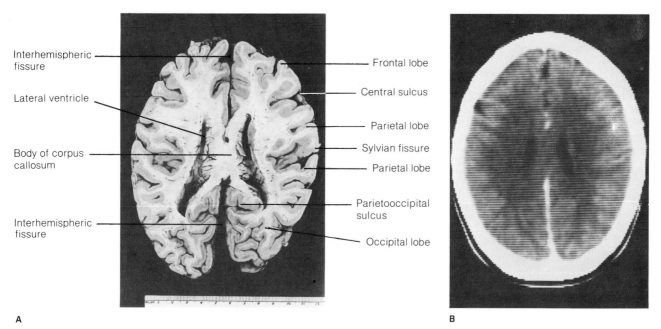

Interhemispheric fissure

Lateral ventricle

Body of corpus callosum

Interhemispheric fissure

Frontal lobe

Central sulcus

Parietal lobe

Sylvian fissure

Parietal lobe

Parietooccipital sulcus

Occipital lobe

A

B

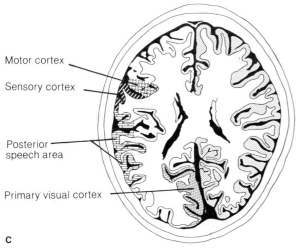

Motor cortex

Sensory cortex

Posterior speech area

Primary visual cortex

C

Figure 2-12 CT anatomy at the high ventricular level through the roof of the lateral ventricle (see text). **A.** The cut surface of an anatomy specimen. **B.** CT. **C.** A diagram showing the location of the motor area, sensory area, posterior speech area and primary visual area of the cerebral cortex in the left cerebral hemisphere. (*Modified from Gado M, Hanaway J, Frank R: Functional anatomy of the cerebral cortex by computed tomography. Journal of Computer Assisted Tomography 3:1–19, 1979.*)

the midline is the interhemispheric fissure. The parietooccipital sulcus is seen near the posterior end of the interhemispheric fissure (Fig. 2-13A, B). Over the convexity, the central sulcus is not distinguishable from the other sulci. Its location is approximately at the junction between the anterior one-fourth and the posterior three-fourths of the convexity.

CT ANATOMY AND FUNCTIONAL ANATOMY

In this section the CT anatomy of the different lobes of the cerebral hemispheres is described, each lobe being dealt with separately. The question of which

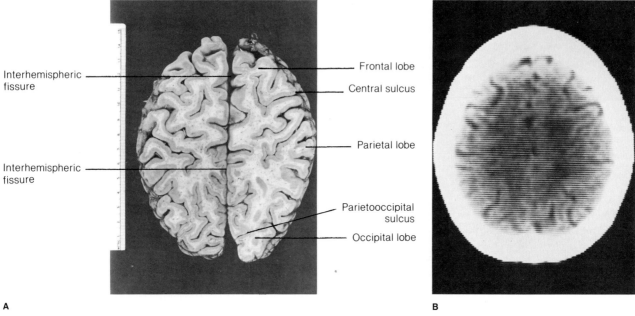

Interhemispheric fissure

Interhemispheric fissure

Frontal lobe

Central sulcus

Parietal lobe

Parietooccipital sulcus

Occipital lobe

A

B

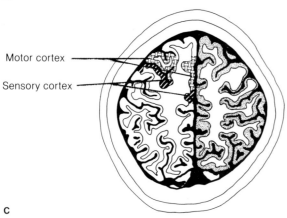

Motor cortex

Sensory cortex

C

Figure 2-13 CT anatomy of the brain at the supraventricular level (see text). **A.** The cut surface of an anatomy specimen. **B.** CT **C.** Diagram showing the location of the motor and sensory areas of the cerebral cortex in the left cerebral hemisphere. (*Modified from Gado M, Hanawy J, Frank R: Functional anatomy of the cerebral cortex by computed tomography. Journal of Computer Assisted Tomography 3:1–19, 1979.*)

slices contain each lobe is addressed, and within each slice the borders of the lobe are defined.

Since the architectonic mapping of the cerebral cortex by Brodmann in 1909, several functional areas of the cerebral cortex have been described (Fig. 2-14A, B). In this section the CT anatomy of the motor, sensory, speech, and visual cortical areas is described.

The Frontal Lobe

Identification of the Borders of the Frontal Lobe

In the *infraventricular subset of slices,* the frontal lobes occupy approximately the anterior third of a slice (Fig. 2-8A, B). Two borders of the frontal lobe can

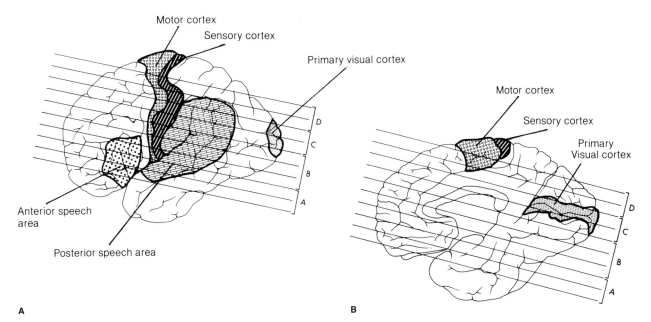

A

B

Figure 2-14 Diagram of the lateral and medial surfaces of the brain showing the motor, sensory, speech and primary visual areas of the cerebral cortex. (*Modified from Gado M, Hanaway J, Frank R: Functional anatomy of the cerebral cortex by computed tomography. Journal of Computer Assisted Tomography 3:1–19, 1979.*) **A.** Lateral surface of the left ce-

rebral hemisphere. **B.** Medial surface of the right cerebral hemisphere. The levels of the CT slices are represented by straight lines across the diagram. The designations A through D refer to the 4 subsets of a complete set of CT slices (see text).

be identified. The lateral border lies against the inner table of the cranium. Anteriorly, it starts at the interhemispheric fissure, where it joins the medial border. Posteriorly, the lateral border of the frontal lobe joins the sylvian cistern, which extends across the slice toward the suprasellar cistern in the midline (Fig. 2-8A). The medial border of the frontal lobe extends in the midline from the inner table of the frontal bone to the suprasellar cistern.

In the *low ventricular subset of slices* (Figs. 2-9A, B and 2-10A, B), the medial borders of the frontal lobes are clearly marked by the interhemispheric fissure which separates them. The interhemispheric fissure occupies only the anterior third of the midline in these slices. The posterior limit of the interhemispheric fissure varies from one slice to the other. In the lower slice of this subset the interhemispheric fissure and the third ventricle appear almost continuous, being separated only by a thin

layer of gray matter, the lamina terminalis. In the higher slice, however, the posterior limit of the interhemispheric fissure is at the corpus callosum, which separates it from the septum pellucidum (Fig. 2-10A, B). The lateral border of the frontal lobe lies against the inner table of the skull. In the lower slice of this subset (Fig. 2-9A, B), the lateral border of the frontal lobe starts anteriorly in the midline at the interhemispheric fissure and extends posteriorly to the sylvian fissure. The sylvian fissure is therefore a definable landmark for the posterior limit of the frontal lobe in this slice (Fig. 2-9A, B). On the other hand, in the higher slice of the subset, the lateral border of the frontal lobe does not extend to the sylvian fissure (Fig. 2-10A, B) but is separated from it by the part of the parietal lobe that contributes to the formation of the operculum, separating the surface of the insula from the inner table of the skull. The central sulcus, which marks the separation of the frontal lobe from the parietal lobe within the operculum, may not be visible. Its location is approximately in the same transverse plane that passes through the anterior end of the septum pellucidum. The sylvian fissure, on the other hand, is clearly recognizable by its extreme depth. At its deepest point, the sylvian fissure marks the posterior limit of the insula (Fig. 2-10A, B).

In the *high ventricular subset of slices* (Figs. 2-11, 2-12), the medial border of the frontal lobe is marked by the interhemispheric fissure extending in the midline between the inner table of the frontal bone and the corpus callosum, which lies between the anterior ends of the two lateral ventricles (Fig. 2-11A, B). The lateral border of the frontal lobe lies against the inner table of the skull, starting anteriorly at the interhemispheric fissure and ending posteriorly at the central sulcus, which separates the frontal lobe from the parietal lobe. The central sulcus is not as easily recognizable as the sylvian fissure. Its location is approximately in the same transverse plane that passes through the anterior ends of the lateral ventricles (Figs. 2-11A, B and 2-12A, B).

In the *supraventricular subset of slices* (Fig. 2-13A, B), the interhemispheric fissure extends through the entire length of the midline, and the lateral ventricles are absent. We therefore have no anatomical landmarks to determine the posterior limits of the frontal lobe at the medial or lateral borders. One may arbitrarily take the frontal lobes to be occupying the anterior one-fourth of the cerebral hemispheres in each slice of this subset (Fig. 2-13A, B).

Functional Localization in the Frontal Lobe

The *anterior cortical speech area* (Broca's speech area) is located in the dominant hemisphere. It occupies the posterior end of the inferior frontal gyrus on the lateral surface of the frontal lobe (Fig. 2-14A). It is thus located in the upper slice of the infraventricular subset and the next slice of the low ventricular subset (Fig. 2-9C). The posterior part of the lateral border of the frontal lobe in both slices forms the anterior cortical speech area.

The *motor cortical area* occupies the precentral

gyrus. It starts inferiorly just behind the speech area (Fig. 2-14A) and extends superiorly to the superior margin of the cerebral hemisphere, with an extension for a short distance downward on the medial surface forming part of the paracentral lobule (Fig. 2-14B). The motor and premotor cortex thus is represented in slices of the low ventricular, high ventricular, and supraventricular subsets.

The Temporal Lobe

Identification of the Borders of the Temporal Lobe

In the *infraventricular slices*, the temporal lobe is limited anteriorly by the sylvian cistern or sphenoid ridge (Fig. 2-8A, B). The lateral border of the temporal lobe lies against the inner table of the cranium. Posteriorly and medially, the temporal lobe lies against the anterior surface of the petrous bone and the lateral border of the clivus, dorsum sella, and/or suprasellar cistern (Fig. 2-8A, B). In the slices of this subset, the temporal lobe occupies a small area in the middle third of the slice on both sides of the clivus.

In the *slices of the low ventricular subset*, the lateral border of the temporal lobe is limited anteriorly by the sylvian fissure (Figs. 2-9A, B and 2-10A, B). Posteriorly, it blends imperceptibly into the occipital lobe. There is no demarcating anatomical structure that separates the lateral border of the temporal lobe from the occipital lobe (Fig. 2-9A). Also, medially, the temporal lobe is continuous with the region of the basal ganglia and thalamus (Figs. 2-9A, B and 2-10A, B).

In the *slices of the high ventricular subset*, the temporoparietal junction is seen at the lateral border of the cerebral hemisphere behind the sylvian fissure, in the lower slice only (Fig. 2-11A, B).

Functional Localization in the Temporal Lobe

The *acoustic cortical area* is located in the superior temporal gyrus. It is located at the lateral border of the temporal lobe, where the border rolls in to form the posterior limit of the sylvian fissure. The slices of the low ventricular subset contain that portion of the superior temporal gyrus.

The *posterior speech area* is located in the dominant hemisphere. It occupies an extensive area of the posterior parts of the superior and middle temporal gyri and extends into the inferior part of the parietal lobe (Fig. 2-14A), being located at the lateral border of the cerebral hemisphere in the slices of the high ventricular subset (Figs. 2-11C and 2-12C). In these slices the posterior speech area extends in front of and behind the sylvian fissure. In addition, part of the posterior speech area is also located in the high slice of the low ventricular subset (Fig. 2-10C), in which, however, it is located only behind the sylvian fissure.

The Parietal Lobe

Because of the orientation of the plane of the CT slices, the anterior inferior part of the parietal lobe appears in the low ventricular slices, anterior to and in line with the superior posterior part of the temporal lobe (Fig. 2-10A, B) and separated from it by the sylvian fissure. We will refer to this part of the parietal lobe as the *parietal operculum,* to distinguish it from the rest of the parietal lobe, which appears in slices of higher levels as one continuous structure extending from the central sulcus anteriorly to the parietooccipital junction posteriorly (Fig. 2-13A).

Identification of the Borders of the Parietal Lobe

In the *slices of the low ventricular subset,* only that anterior inferior part of the parietal lobe referred to above as the parietal operculum is visualized (Fig. 2-10A, B). Its lateral border lies against the inner table of the cranium. Its posterior border is clearly defined by the deep sylvian fissure, which separates the posterior border of that portion of the parietal lobe from the temporal lobe. The slices of the low ventricular subset thus do not include any part of the parietal lobe *behind* the sylvian fissure. This is in contrast to the slices of the high ventricular subset, as discussed below.

In the *slices of the high ventricular subset,* the sylvian fissure is recognized. The central sulcus lies approximately at the same transverse line that passes through the anterior ends of the lateral ventricles (Figs. 2-11A, B and 2-12A, B), so the lateral border of the parietal lobe between these two sulcal landmarks is easily recognized. In the lower slice of this subset (Fig. 2-11A, B), the lateral border of the cerebral hemisphere behind the sylvian fissure belongs to the temporoparietal junction. The lateral border of the temporoparietal junction becomes continuous posteriorly with the lateral border of the occipital lobe. There is no recognizable structure separating the two. In the upper slice of the high ventricular series (Fig. 2-12A, B), however, the parietal lobe forms the lateral border of the cerebral hemisphere from the central sulcus anteriorly to the parietooccipital junction posteriorly. Again, the parietooccipital junction is not defined by an anatomical structure. A clue to the approximate location of the parietooccipital junction may be obtained from the conspicuous parietooccipital sulcus on the *medial* surface of the cerebral hemisphere (Fig. 2-12A, B).

In the *supraventricular slices* (Fig. 2-13), the interhemispheric fissure extends the entire length of the midline. Both the medial and the lateral borders of the parietal lobe are therefore identified in the slices of this subset, the lobe occupying the middle half of the slice, with the frontal lobe occupying the anterior one-fourth and the occipital lobe the posterior one-fourth (Fig. 2-13A, B). The parietooccipital junction is recognized on the medial border of the hemisphere by the parietooccipital sulcus (Fig. 2-13A, B). In the higher supraventricular slices, the extent of the occipital lobe gradually diminishes; the topmost one or two slices of this subset may contain no part of it. In these extremely high levels, the slice consists solely of frontal and parietal lobes. The size of the portions occupied by the frontal and parietal lobes, respectively, would depend upon the orientation of the slice and the slope of the vertex.

Functional Localization in the Parietal Lobe

The *sensory cortex* occupies the postcentral gyrus of the parietal lobe. On the lateral surface of the parietal lobe, this cortical area starts inferiorly in the parietal operculum (Fig. 2-14A) and extends superiorly to the superior border of the cerebral hemisphere, with an extension on the medial surface forming part of the paracentral lobule (Fig. 2-14B). The sensory cortex is thus represented in the slices of the low ventricular (Figs. 2-9C and 2-10C), high ventricular (Figs. 2-11C and 2-12C), and supraventricular (Fig. 2-13C) subsets. Since the localization of the central sulcus may be difficult, the anterior end of the septum pellucidum may be used as a guide to its location in the low ventricular series (Figs. 2-9A, C and 2-10A, C) and the anterior ends of the lateral ventricles in the high ventricular series (Figs. 2-11A, C and 2-12A, C). In the supraventricular series, it lies at the junction of the anterior one-fourth and the rest of the slice. The sensory cortex lies on the posterior side of the central sulcus. In the top slices, the sensory cortex is seen on both the lateral and medial borders of the parietal lobe (Fig. 2-13C).

The posterior speech area is a large area (Fig. 2-14A) curving around the posterior extremity of the sylvian fissure in the dominant hemisphere, occupying the inferior part of the parietal lobe, and extending into a more extensive area of the adjoining parts of the superior and middle temporal gyri (Fig. 2-14A). In the slices of the high ventricular subset (Figs. 2-11C and 2-12C), the posterior speech area is located in the lateral border of the dominant hemisphere extending in front of as well as behind the sylvian fissure. In addition, part of it is also located in the higher slice of the low ventricular subset (Fig. 2-10C), in which it is located only behind the sylvian fissure.

The Occipital Lobe

Identification of the Borders of the Occipital Lobe

Because of the inclination of the plane of the CT slices, the occipital lobe is not visualized in the infraventricular subset of slices nor in some cases in the lowest slice of the low ventricular subset. In these slices, the cerebellum occupies the posterior part of the slice between the temporal lobes (Figs. 2-8A, B and 2-9A, B). In the upper slice of the low ventricular subset (Fig. 2-10B, C), the part of the slice occupied by the cerebellum decreases and the occipital lobe appears in the posterior third of the slice. This upper slice is thus the first slice that shows both the lateral and the medial borders of the occipital lobes (Fig. 2-10B, C). This configuration is also present in the slices of the high ventricular subset (Fig. 2-11A, B) and some of the slices of the supraventricular subset (Fig. 2-13A, B). As previously mentioned, in the topmost one or two slices of the supraventricular subset the occipital lobe may not be represented at all.

In the *low ventricular subset* the occipital lobe can be identified in the uppermost slice of the subset (Fig. 2-10B, C). The anterior limit of the occipital lobe at the medial border is demarcated by the parietooccipital sulcus (Fig. 2-10C). At the occipital pole, the medial border of the occipital lobe is continuous with the lateral border, which lies against the inner table of the skull. The anterior limit of the occipital lobe at the lateral border is not defined by any anatomical structure.

In the slices of the *high ventricular subset* (Figs. 2-11A, B and 2-12A, B), the configuration is the same as just described. The extremely deep convolutions of the visual cortex around the calcarine sulcus may be recognized in slices of this subset. They are situated within the substance of the occipital lobe and encroach upon the white matter in the deep part of the occipital lobe in the slices of this subset.

In the *supraventricular subset*, one has to distinguish between the lower and higher slices. The lower slices show the same configuration just described in the high ventricular slices with one exception: the deep convolutions of the cerebral cortex around the calcarine fissure are not recognizable. It is the cuneus of the occipital lobe that is represented in the slices of this subset. In the higher slices of the supraventricular subset (Fig. 2-13A, B), the distance between the parietooccipital sulcus and the posterior end of the cerebral hemisphere diminishes. This results in a decrease in the length of the portion of the medial border of the hemisphere that belongs to the occipital lobe. In the top one or two slices of the supraventricular subset, the parietooc-cipital sulcus, and hence the occipital lobe, may not be recognizable at all.

Functional Localization in the Occipital Lobe

The *primary visual area,* referred to as the *striate cortex,* occupies the upper and lower lips and the depth of the calcarine sulcus (Fig. 2-14B). It thus lies largely on the medial surface of the occipital lobe, extending posteriorly into the occipital pole and limited laterally by the lunate sulcus (Fig. 2-14A). The primary visual area receives fibers of the optic radiation from the lateral geniculate body. The geniculate radiation spreads out through the white matter of the occipital lobe, terminating in the occipital cortex.

CT Anatomy of the Basal Ganglia

The basal ganglia are parts of the telencephalon. They represent the central gray matter of the telencephalon. They include the caudate nucleus, the lentiform nucleus, the claustrum, and the amygdala. The caudate nucleus consists of an enlarged anterior portion, or head, and a narrow posterior portion, or tail. The head occupies most of the lateral wall of the anterior horn of the lateral ventricle. The tail curves along the lateral aspect of the thalamus. At its terminal portion, the tail forms the amygdala.

The basal ganglia are not visualized in the infraventricular subset of slices. It is the low ventricular subset that includes these deep gray-matter structures (Figs. 2-9A, B and 2-10A, B). In addition, only the superior surface of the body of the caudate nucleus is visualized in the lower slice of the high ventricular subset (Fig. 2-11A, B).

The internal capsule is a thick band of white matter situated between the thalamus, which is part of the diencephalon, and the caudate and lentiform nuclei, which are parts of the telencephalon (Fig. 2-10A, B). As previously stated, both the telencephalon and the diencephalon are parts of the forebrain (prosencephalon). The internal capsule is thus visualized only in the slices of the low ventricular subset (Figs. 2-9A, B and 2-10A, B). The anterior limb of the internal capsule lies between the caudate nucleus and the lentiform nucleus. The posterior limb lies between the thalamus and the lentiform nucleus. The posterior limb contains the motor fibers from the cerebral cortex to the spinal motor nuclei and the sensory fibers from the thalamus to the sensory cortex, as well as fibers of the auditory and optic radiations from the geniculate bodies to the temporal and occipital cortices.

The claustrum appears in the axial section as a thin band of deep gray matter that lies between the lentiform nucleus medially and the cortex of the insula laterally (Fig. 2-10A, B). The white matter between the claustrum and the lentiform nucleus is the external capsule, while that between the claustrum and the insular cortex is the extreme capsule.

Bibliography

CARPENTER MB: *Human Neuroanatomy,* 7th Ed. Baltimore, Williams and Wilkins, 1976.

GADO M, HANAWAY J, FRANK R: Functional anatomy of the cerebral cortex by computed tomography. *J Comput Assist Tomogr* **3**:1-19, 1979.

GOSS CM (ed): *Gray's Anatomy* 29th Am. Ed. Philadelphia, Lea & Febiger, 1973.

HANAWAY J, SCOTT W, STROTHER C: *Atlas of the Human Brain and the Orbit for Computed Tomography.* St. Louis, Warren Green Inc., 1977.

MATSUI T, HIRANO A: *An Atlas of the Human Brain for Computerized Tomography.* Tokyo, New York, Igaki-Shon, 1978.

NIEUWENHUYS, VOUGD, VAN HUIJZEN: *The Human Central Nervous System.* Berlin, Heidelberg, New York, Springer-Verlag, 1979.

WILLIAMS, WARWICK: *Functional Neuroanatomy of Man.* Philadelphia and Toronto, Saunders, 1975.

3

THE ORBIT

Robert A. Zimmerman

Larissa T. Bilaniuk

INTRODUCTION AND TECHNIQUE

The application of computed tomography (CT) to the evaluation of orbital disease constitutes a major advance (Forbes 1980; Glydensted 1977; Trokel 1979; Wende 1977). Computed tomography provides information regarding the presence, location, and extent of intraorbital lesions, as well as the involvement of the orbit by lesions arising in the adjacent bone and paranasal sinuses (Mancuso 1978; Weber 1978). The introduction of scanners with thin sections, short scan times, and high resolution, magnification, and reconstruction capabilities has extended the scope and increased the accuracy of the CT evaluation of orbital lesions.

Technique

The examination of the orbit by CT should be tailored to the clinical problem at hand but should also be anatomically complete. Contiguous thin sections, no larger than 5 mm in thickness, are obtained routinely in at least two planes: (1) transverse, (2) coronal and/or sagittal (Balériaux-Waha 1977; Hoyt 1979; Osborn 1980; Tadmor 1978; Unsöld 1980*a*; Wing 1979). The entire orbit is encompassed, as well as the adjacent portions of brain and of sinus, facial, and pharyngeal soft tissues. The authors' experience indicates that examination is necessary in the transverse plane usually at an angulation of $-10°$ to the orbitomeatal base line (Fig. 3-1) and that the initial examination should be made both before and after the injection of an adequate amount of iodinated contrast material. Coronal sections are made in addition to the transverse section (Fig. 3-2). Where 1.5-mm or 2-mm sections are possible, sagittal reformation, and even satisfactory coronal reformation from the transverse sections, can be made, provided the patient has not moved during the examination. The recent introduction of oblique reformation, so that the plane of the optic nerve (Unsöld 1980*a*) or of the superior ophthalmic vein can be followed, is of value in specific cases.

Because of its sinuous course in two places, the appearance and course of the optic nerve depend on the thickness and plane of the CT section as well as on the direction of gaze (Unsöld 1980*b*). Unsöld recommends a negative angulation of −20° to the orbitomeatal base line with the eye in upgaze position in order to stretch the nerves and have their course parallel to the plane of section.

The adequacy of the CT examination of the orbit can be assured only if the study is carefully monitored and if images that are marred by motion or artifacts are repeated. Following completion of the examination, the study must be carefully reviewed. Such a review is best done on a diagnostic display console, so that the sections may be examined for the osseous and soft-tissue structures at a variety of window widths with different window levels.

NORMAL ANATOMY OF THE ORBIT

Orbital Walls

The orbit is a pyramidal bony compartment that houses the eyeball and its functional components (extraocular muscles, blood vessels, nerves, lacrimal gland, and fat) (Tadmor 1978). The orbital walls separate the intraorbital components from surrounding brain and facial structures (Hesselink 1978).

The *roof* of the orbit (Fig. 3-2) is formed for the most part by the orbital plate of the frontal bone and separates the orbit from the anterior cranial

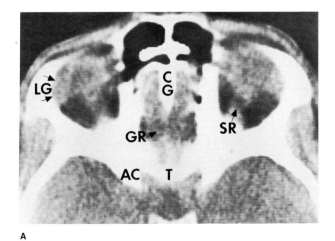

A

Figure 3-1 Transverse CT sections of the orbit parallel to Reid's base line: 5-mm contiguous sections. **A.** Superior section through the orbit shows *SR* (superior rectus). *LG* (lacrimal gland), *GR* (gyrus rectus), *CG* (crista galli), *AC* (anterior clinoid process), and *T* (tuberculum sellae). **B.** Next-lower contiguous section shows *OC* (optic canal), *GWS* (greater wing of sphenoid), *MCF* (middle cranial fossa), and *CP* (cribriform plate). **C.** Next-lower section shows in **C¹** the anatomy unlabeled; in **C²**: *C* (cornea), *AC* (anterior chamber; posterior chamber in continuity but not labeled), *I* (iris), *L* (lens), *V* (vitreous), and *R* (retina). In **C³**: *S* (sphenoid body), *ES* ethmoid sinus air cell), and *LP* (lamina papyracea). In **C⁴**: *OS* (orbital septum), *ON* (optic nerve), *CF* (central fat), *LR* (lateral rectus), *MR* (medial rectus), and *PF* (peripheral fat). In **C⁵**: *CS* (cavernous sinus). **D.** Lowermost section shows *IR* (inferior rectus).

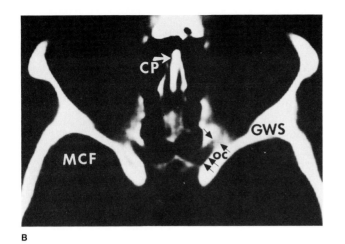

B

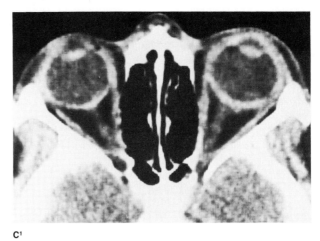

C¹

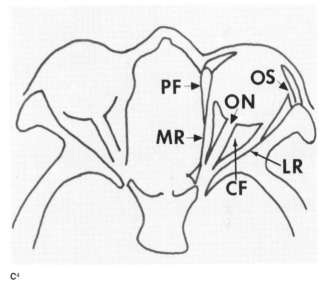

C²   C³   C⁴

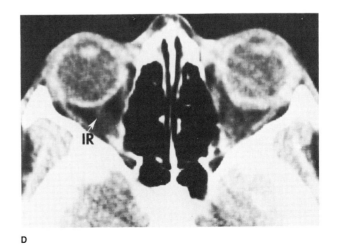

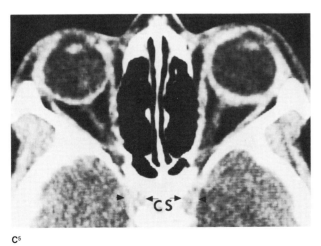

C⁵   D

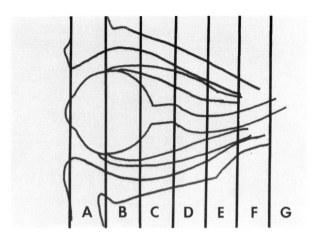

Figure 3-2. Section Diagram.

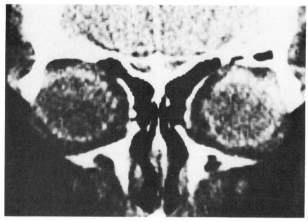

A¹

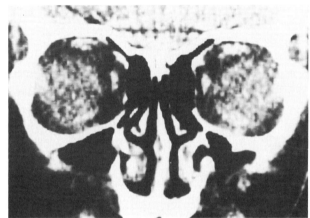

B¹

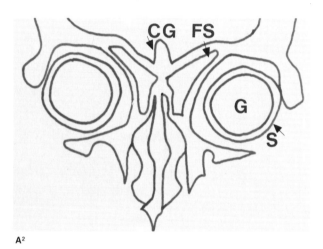

A²

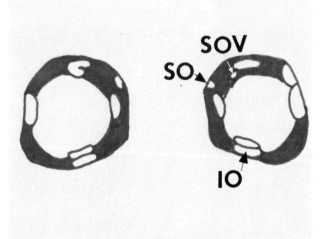

B²

B³

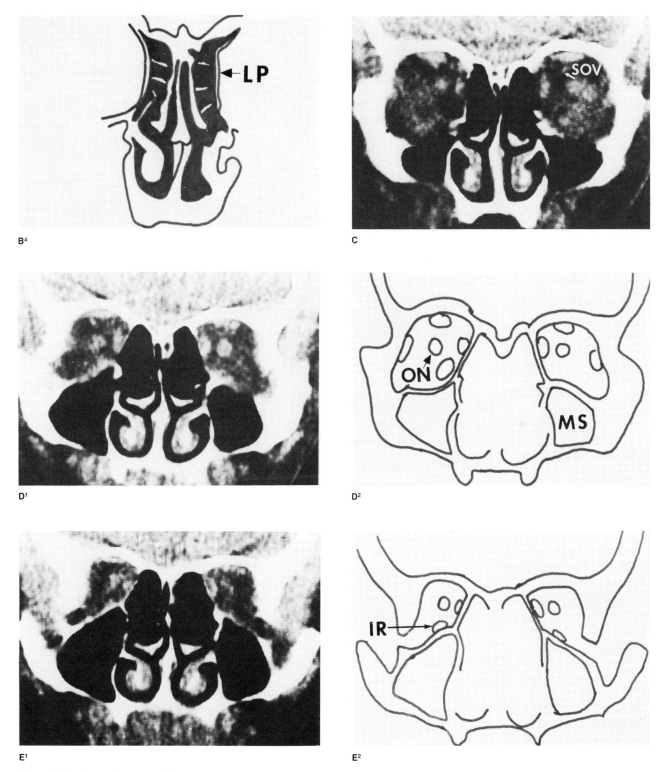

Figure 3-2 Legend on page 76.

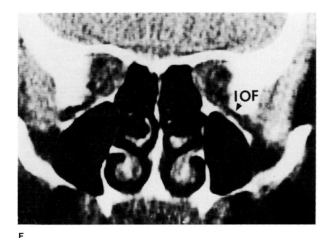

F

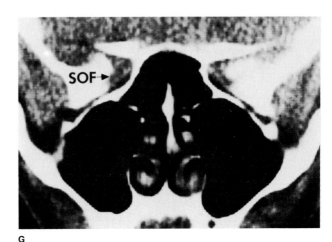

G

Figure 3-2 Coronal CT sections through the orbit. Contiguous 5-mm sections. **A.** Most-anterior section shows, in **A¹**, unlabeled structures of the globe and orbital walls. In **A²**: *G* (globe), *S* (sclera), *FS* (frontal sinus), *CG* (crista galli). **B.** Next-most-posterior section shows, in **B¹**, unlabeled structures of the orbit. In **B²**: *MR* (medial rectus), *SR* (superior rectus), *LG* (lacrimal gland), *LR* (lateral rectus), and *IR* (inferior rectus). In **B³**: *SOV* (superior ophthalmic vein), *SO* (superior oblique muscle), *IO* (inferior oblique muscle). In **B⁴**: *LP* (lamina papy-racea). **C.** Next-most-posterior section shows *SOV* (superior ophthalmic vein). **D.** The most posterior section shows, in **D¹**, the normal structures unlabeled. In **D²**: *ON* (optic nerve), *MS* (maxillary sinus). **E.** Next-most-posterior section shows, in **E¹**, normal structures of the orbit unlabeled. In **E²**: *IR* (inferior rectus muscle). **F.** Next-most-posterior section shows *IOF* (inferior orbital fissure). **G.** Most-posterior section shows the apex of the orbit, containing *SOF* (superior orbital fissure).

fossa. The lacrimal gland (Fig. 3-2B) forms a fossa, the lacrimal fossa, in the superolateral aspect of the orbit. Overall, the bone that forms the roof of the orbit is relatively thin. To a variable extent, the frontal sinus and sometimes the ethmoid sinuses extend into the roof of the orbit. The posterior component of the roof of the orbit that is formed by the lesser wing of the sphenoid may also contain air cells derived from either the posterior ethmoidal air cells or the sphenoid sinus.

The *floor* of the orbit (Fig. 3-2) is composed primarily of the orbital plate of the maxilla. It has a triangular shape, with contributions from portions of the zygoma and the palatine bone. The infraorbital nerve courses along the orbital surface of the floor of the orbit. The orbital floor is thin (Fig. 3-2B–E), except at its most anterior margin, where the orbital rim is formed, which is a thicker osseous structure (Fig. 3-2A) in continuity below with the anterior wall of the maxillary sinus. The floor of the orbit separates the intraorbital structures from the maxillary sinus (Fig. 3-2B–E) which lies beneath.

The *lateral wall* of the orbit is formed by the zygoma (Figs. 3-1A,3-2C) anteriorly and the greater wing of the sphenoid posteriorly (Figs. 3-1C,3-2D). The lateral orbital wall is the thickest and strongest of the orbital walls. Lateral to this structure lies the temporal fossa, which contains the temporal muscle.

The *medial wall* (Figs. 3-1C,3-2B) is the thinnest component of the orbital walls. It serves to separate the orbital contents from the ethmoid and sphenoid air cells. Contributions to the structure of the medial wall are made by the maxilla, lacrimal bone, ethmoid bone, and body of the sphenoid. The largest component is that contributed by the ethmoidal orbital plate (lamina papyracea).

Orbital Fissures and Canals

At the apex of the pyramidal structure of the orbit lie three openings that communicate with adjacent extraorbital areas.

The *optic canal* (Fig. 3-1B) is formed by the sphenoid bone and serves to conduct the optic nerve and ophthalmic artery between the orbit and the middle cranial fossa. The optic nerve is surrounded by a small subarachnoid space which contains cerebrospinal fluid (CSF) and is surrounded by the arachnoid. The ophthalmic artery lies beneath the optic nerve. The roof of the optic canal measures 10 to 12 mm in length and is formed by the lesser wing of the sphenoid. The medial wall of the optic canal is formed by the body of the sphenoid bone, while its inferior and lateral walls are formed by the roots of the lesser wing of the sphenoid (optic strut), which also serves to separate the optic canal from the superior orbital fissure.

The *superior orbital fissure* (Fig. 3-2G) is a space between the greater and lesser wing of the sphenoid. It is separated medially from the optic canal by the optic strut. Transmitted through the superior orbital fissure between the middle cranial fossa and orbit are the superior ophthalmic vein, the third, fourth, and sixth cranial nerves, and the first division of the fifth cranial nerve.

The *inferior orbital fissure* (Fig. 3-2F) permits communication between the orbit and the pterygopalatine and infratemporal fossae. Through it runs the infraorbital nerve and the communication between the inferior ophthalmic vein and the pterygoid venous plexus. The maxilla, palatine bone, and greater wing of the sphenoid bone contribute to its margins.

Periosteum

Periosteum lines the bones of the orbit and is in communication with the periosteum covering the intracranial compartment, through the various fissures.

The septum orbitale (Fig. 3-1C) is a periosteal reflection from the anterior orbital margin which is continuous with the tarsal plates. It serves to separate the orbit into pre- and postseptal components. The intraorbital fat is limited anteriorly by the orbital septum. The eyelids lie anterior to the orbital septum.

Orbital Soft Tissue

The wall of the *globe* consists of three layers (Fig. 3-1C). The innermost, the retina, contains the nerve elements that allow visual perception. The middle layer consists of the choroid, ciliary body, and iris, a set of structures of vascular and nutritive function. The outermost layer is a fibrous protective coating that constitutes the sclera and, anteriorly, the transparent cornea. The lens (Fig. 3-1C) is a transparent crystalline body approximately 1 cm in diameter that serves to transmit light and lies between the iris and the vitreous humor (Fig. 3-1C). Between the cornea and the lens is a space containing aqueous humor that is divided by the iris into an anterior chamber and a posterior chamber.

The *optic nerve* (Figs. 3-1C,3-2D, E), the second cranial nerve, extends from the papilla on the posterior surface of the globe to the optic chiasm. Its length is between 35 and 50 mm, with its intraorbital component 20 to 30 mm, the intracanalicular portion 4 to 9 mm, and the intracranial portion 3 to 6 mm. The diameter of the optic nerve is approximately 3 to 4 mm. Running beneath the optic nerve as it enters the optic canal from the intracranial compartment is the ophthalmic artery, which remains beneath the optic nerve in its intracanalicular segment and in its initial intraorbital segment. Surrounding the optic nerve throughout its intraorbital course is the central orbital fat.

Six *extraocular muscles* (Figs. 3-1,3-2) insert on the sclera. These are the medial and lateral recti, the superior and inferior recti, and the superior and inferior oblique muscles. The superior rectus is the longest, 40 mm, with the medial, lateral, and inferior recti being of progressively shorter length. The medial rectus has the largest diameter of the ocular muscles. The superior oblique muscle is the thinnest muscle and lies in the superomedial aspect of the orbit. The levator palpebrae superioris muscle lies just under the roof of the orbit as a thin flat structure, above the superior rectus. It attaches to the skin of the upper eyelid. Below the superior rectus muscle lies the superior ophthalmic vein, and below it, the optic nerve. The lateral rectus lies adjacent to the periosteum of the lateral orbital wall, and only anteriorly does a slight amount of fat intervene between the periosteum and the muscle. The medial rectus is separated from the lamina papyracea by some peripheral orbital fat. The posterior portion of the inferior rectus muscle lies in contact with the floor of the orbit, but its anterior portion is separated from the roof of the maxillary sinus by peripheral orbital fat.

Orbital fat (Figs. 3-1C,3-2C–E) fills the space that is not occupied by nerve, muscle, or vessels. It extends from the orbital apex to the orbital septum anteriorly and from the optic nerve to the orbital wall. It is divided by the intermuscular membrane into a central portion and a more peripheral (extramuscular) portion. The peripheral fat lies between the periosteum of the orbital walls and the rectus muscles.

The *superior ophthalmic vein* (Fig. 3-2B, C) forms at the root of the nose, at the juncture of the frontal and angular veins, and enters the orbit, passing around the trochlea for the superior oblique muscle. After coursing posterosuperiorly for a very short segment, it passes posterolaterally into the muscle cone and comes to lie adjacent to the inferior surface of the superior rectus muscle. It then turns medially to course between the superior rectus and lateral rectus muscles and at the orbital apex enters the superior orbital fissure. After it passes through the superior orbital fissure it joins the cavernous sinus. The diameter of the superior ophthalmic vein varies in size from 2 to 3.5 mm.

A small space filled with cerebrospinal fluid surrounds the optic nerve. This space lies within the nerve sheath and extends from the optic canal forward to the papilla. The size of the space varies, and its degree of communication with the chiasmatic cistern may also vary (Haughton 1980). Entrance of both Pantopaque (Tabaddor 1973) and air (Tenner 1968) has been reported at the time of myelography and pneumoencephalography. The radiographic visualization of the space has not been a regular phenomenon and has not been without risk of optic nerve injury (Tabaddor 1973). Metrizamide opacifies the *intracranial subarachnoid space,* putting

into relief structures which lie within, such as the optic chiasm. Opacification of the *perioptic subarachnoid space* has been recognized on CT following the intrathecal injection of metrizamide (Fig. 3-3) (Fox 1979, Manelfe 1978).

This has not been a consistent finding at the time of metrizamide CT cisternography. However, its potential usefulness in the evaluation of patients considered for surgical removal of perioptic meningiomas has been pointed out by Fox et al. (1979). Cabanis (1978) noted an increase in the caliber and tortuosity of the optic nerve shadow in patients with papilledema due to increased intracranial pressure. He pointed out that this was usually bilateral and may represent enlargement of the subarachnoid space surrounding the optic nerve. Transmission of the intracranial pressure to the perineural subarachnoid space surrounding the optic nerve may be the mechanism for the production of optic atrophy (through compressive ischemia of the optic nerve) in patients with elevated intracranial pressure.

Thus one of the clinical applications of metrizamide is to evaluate patients with optic nerve atrophy with the CT finding of enlarged optic nerve(s). When on CT the optic nerve appears bilaterally enlarged, in clinically suspected optic atrophy, demonstration of an enlarged subarachnoid space rules out bilateral optic nerve meningiomas and gliomas and implicates transmitted subarachnoid pressure or primary optic atrophy, with distention of the surrounding subarachnoid space. In the case of unilateral optic nerve enlargement as demonstrated by CT, metrizamide offers the potential of distinguishing among nerve enlargement, subarachnoid space enlargement, and enlargement of the perineural arachnoidal structures. In the case of perioptic meningioma, a separation plane between the meningioma and the optic nerve suggests the feasibility of surgical intervention (Fox 1979).

The question of the risk of optic nerve injury with metrizamide has been investigated by Haughton, Davis, Harris, and Ho (1980) in mongrel cats with simulated orbital lesions. The optic nerve and optic nerve sheaths were histologically examined for the presence of developing optic nerve atrophy

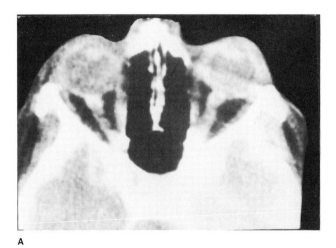

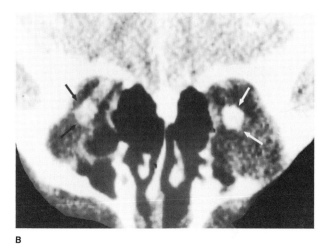

A   B

Figure 3-3 Metrizamide-enhanced perioptic subarachnoid space. CT examination followed intrathecal (lumbar) injection of 4 ml 190 mg/ml metrizamide (Amipaque). **A.** Thin band of increased density outlines both optic nerve shadows in the transverse plane. **B.** Coronal section shows perioptic metrizamide even better (arrows).

and arachnoiditis. Animals receiving 450 mg of iodine or less per milliliter developed no more than slight evidence of arachnoiditis in the optic nerve sheath, but arachnoiditis developed after multiple injections or high concentrations of metrizamide. In clinical practice, successful opacification of the optic nerve sheath requires concentrations of less than 300 mg of iodine per milliliter. Concentrations on the order of 190 to 220 mg of iodine per milliliter with 4 ml total amount used are sufficient. Thus it appears that optic nerve sheath opacification by metrizimide has a low risk of arachnoiditis. However, clinical evaluation in a large series of patients has not been reported, nor has a long-term follow-up on these patients.

ORBITAL INFLAMMATION

Bacterial Infection

Bacterial infection of the orbit is most often due to sinus infection (Gans 1974), foreign body, skin infection, or bacteremia. The orbital septum, the reflected periosteum from the anterior bony margin

of the orbit, functions as a barrier that prevents preseptal cellulitis from extending back into the orbital soft tissues (Fig. 3-4) (Kaplan 1976). The postseptal portion of the orbit may become involved by bacterial infection transmitted through the orbital septum. The infection may extend into the orbit proper along venous pathways or through the orbital wall and then through the periosteum.

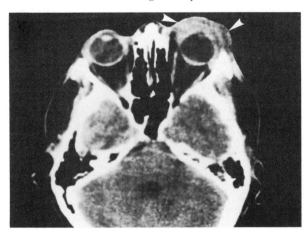

Figure 3-4. Preseptal cellulitis. Thirty-nine-year-old female with 1-day history of swelling of the eye. NCCT study demonstrates marked soft-tissue swelling (arrows) anterior to the septal plate. The retroglobar tissues appear normal.

The chief clinical manifestation of orbital infection is swelling and redness of the eyelids. This may be either edematous swelling or actual cellulitis. In either situation, adequate physical examination of the eye is often difficult or impossible, and the extent of the infection cannot be delineated or its source determined clinically.

The absence of valves in the facial veins (including the orbit and paranasal sinuses) leads to the free transmission of elevated pressure between sinus and orbit. In the child and adolescent, orbital infection is most often a concomitant of sinusitis. Increased pressure in the sinus cavity is transmitted to the orbit and causes preseptal edema. Septic thrombophlebitis leads to cellulitis and possibly to orbital cellulitis. Direct extension of infection through congenital osseous dehiscences or involvement of the thin bony walls of the orbit by osteomyelitis can lead to subperiosteal abscess formation. The orbital periosteum is loosely attached except at the suture lines, so that subperiosteal collections are

easily formed. In the young child with ethmoid sinusitis, the subperiosteal collection is along the medial orbital wall and produces lateral proptosis of the globe. In the adolescent with frontal sinusitis, the subperiosteal collection is in the superior aspect of the orbit (Fig. 3-5) and produces anterior and downward displacement of the globe.

While skull radiographs and pluridirectional tomography of the paranasal sinuses can demonstrate free intraorbital air, osteitis of the sinus wall, and mucosal thickening or sinus opacification, CT is capable of showing not only the bony changes and sinus opacification but the orbital soft tissue changes as well (Figs. 3-1, 3-2). Zimmerman (1980*a*) reported a series of 18 patients with orbital infection with or without cerebral complications studied by CT. In 10 cases of acute periorbital cellulitis, all 10 showed septal swelling (Fig. 3-4), while 7 of the 10 showed proptosis and 6 of the 10 showed scleral thickening. Subperiosteal abscesses were demonstrated in 5, and 1 had an infection of the peripheral surgical space. Frontal lobe cerebritis and epidural inflammation are also well shown by CT. In one patient, who was studied subsequent to the acute process, the CT study showed scarring of the retroorbital soft tissues 2 years after bacterial orbital

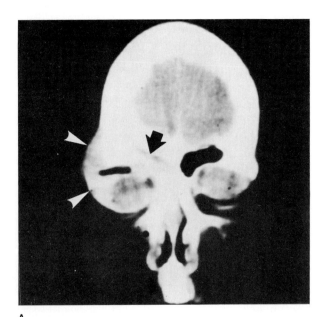

A

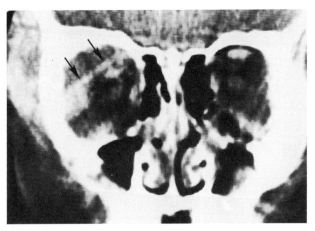

B

Figure 3-5 Orbital subperiosteal abscess secondary to frontal sinusitis. Twelve-year-old female with rapid onset of proptosis and painful ophthalmoplegia. **A.** Coronal CT shows air within the orbit above the left globe. The globe is displaced inferiorly. The left frontal sinus is opacified (arrow), and there is soft-tissue swelling lateral to the orbit (arrowheads). **B.** Coronal section farther back shows the contrast-enhanced periosteum (arrows) displaced away from the orbital wall by a subperiosteal abscess. (*American Journal of Roentgenology 134:45–47, 1980.*)

cellulitis. In seven patients with trauma or foreign body, localization of the radiodense foreign body was achieved and intraorbital, subperiosteal, and intracranial abscesses were demonstrated by CT (Zimmerman 1980*a*).

Infection within the orbit proper can be classified as (1) intraconic, within the muscle cone (central surgical space); (2) extraconic, extrinsic to the intermuscular fibrous septum (within the peripheral surgical space); or (3) subperiosteal, between the orbital wall and its periosteal covering. Infection of the central surgical space obliterates the soft-tissue planes that exist normally between the optic nerve, retroorbital fat, and rectus muscles. Infection in the peripheral surgical space obliterates the plane between the rectus muscles, peripheral fat, and wall of the orbit. Infection in the subperiosteal space is demonstrated by displacement of the contrast-enhanced periosteal membrane away from the orbital wall (Fig. 3-5).

The rapid increase in the use of CT in evaluation of patients with orbital infection at the authors' institution reflects its clinical value in such cases. Treatment of orbital infection, whether medical or surgical, must be timely, specific, and sufficient.It

is imperative that the disease process be recognized quickly and treated aggressively and that operative drainage be carried out whenever indicated. Subperiosteal abscesses need to be drained, and often also the offending infected sinuses. The danger of cavernous sinus thrombosis is real, and it carries with it, even in the antibiotic era, a significant morbidity and mortality. The consequences of inadequate treatment remain potentially catastrophic, because blindness and death may result. The consequences of cerebritis and cerebral abscess formation, even when the condition is adequately treated, may appear as seizures, motor weakness, and psychological aberrations.

Foreign Bodies

Localization of an intraorbital foreign body by routine radiographic means may be difficult. In order to facilitate surgical planning for removal, it is necessary to localize the foreign body accurately. With radiodense foreign bodies this is easier, as they are well shown on routine x-rays, tomography, and CT (Figs. 3-6A, 3-7). CT has the advantage over routine

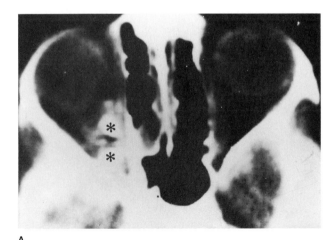

A

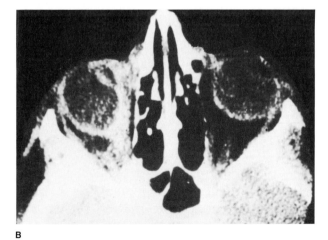

B

Figure 3-6 Scarring of para- and retroglobal soft tissues following removal of a metallic foreign body. Ten-year-old male who fell on an umbrella tip which became embedded in the retroglobal tissues. **A.** Transverse axial CT, 2 years after injury, demonstrates metallic fragments (asterisks) near the apex

of the left orbit.   **B.** CT following surgical removal of the metallic foreign bodies shows the globe to be fixed with the lens facing medially. Scarring obliterates the normal soft-tissue planes between the globe, medial rectus, and medial wall of the orbit.

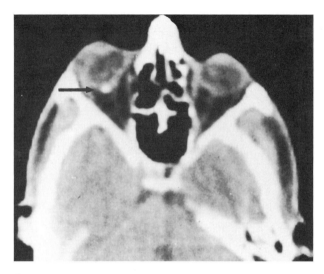

Figure 3-7 Metalllic foreign body. Twenty-five-year-old machinist struck in the eye by metal scrap. NCCT shows position of metallic foreign body (arrow) in posterior sclera of left eye.

radiographic studies of demonstrating the relationship between the radiodense foreign body and the sclera and optic nerve (Fig. 3-7).

With the nonopaque foreign body, such as a wood splinter, CT may show only the granulomatous reaction (Macrae 1979). In the patient who presents with proptosis or with evidence of granulomatous reaction in the vicinity of the orbit, consideration should be given to a forgotten minor trauma produced by an intraorbital foreign body. In such a case, CT is capable of revealing metallic fragments and other radiodense foreign bodies such as pencil lead.

Pseudotumors

Between the ages of 10 and 40, the most common cause of an intraorbital mass is the orbital pseudotumor (Bernardino 1977). The classic clinical triad includes proptosis, soft-tissue swelling, and impaired ocular motility. To a variable degree there may also be diplopia, decreased vision, pain, papillitis, and retinal striae. The symptomatology and clinical signs simulate an intraorbital tumor. Orbital pseudotumor is thought to be one of the most common causes of unilateral exophthalmos (Bernardino 1977). Orbital pseudotumor may be unilateral or bilateral. Bilaterality was reported by Enzmann (1976a) in six of nine patients, and by Bernardino (1977) in from 10 to 15 percent of his patients.

The cause of orbital pseudotumor is not known, but experimental work has implicated an autoimmune response of the retrobulbar tissues to antigens (Wilner 1978). Pathologically two categories of disease exist: (1) an acute form, in which the reaction is that of a vasculitis with vessel wall necrosis and fibrinoid changes and (2) a chronic inflammatory process, with diffuse infiltration of the affected tissues with lymphocytes, plasma cells, macrophages, and occasionally eosinophils (Jones 1979). The changes of orbital pseudotumor may be found in association with certain clinical conditions, including Wegener's midline granuloma (Vermess 1978), fibrosing mediastinitis, thyroiditis, and cholangitis (Bernardino 1978).

The classic CT finding is that of a contrast-enhancing scleral-uveal thickening (Bernardino 1977). The scleral-uveal thickening may obliterate both the

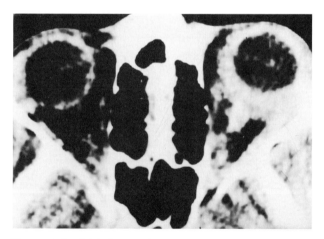

Figure 3-8 Orbital pseudotumor. Fifteen-year-old female with unilateral proptosis, redness of the sclera, and pain in the eye. CECT shows marked thickening and enhancement of the sclera, with obliteration of the normal junction between the lateral and medial rectus and the sclera and between the optic nerve and the sclera.

sharply demarcated insertion of the optic nerve at the papilla and the insertion of the tendons of the rectus muscles onto the sclera (Fig. 3-8). Intraorbitally the involved tissue is usually isodense to slightly hyperdense prior to the injection of contrast. On contrast-enhanced CT (CECT), there is enhancement of the involved tissue. The disease process may present as uveal-scleral thickening

(Fig. 3-8), as an isolated discrete mass without uveal-scleral thickening (Fig. 3-9), as an obliteration of all retrobulbar soft-tissue planes, or as a thickening of the rectus muscles (Fig. 3-10). Single-muscle involvement in the form of a myositis is thought to be a variant in the manifestations of orbital pseudotumor. Uveal-scleral thickening with enhancement may be seen in connection with other causes of intraorbital inflammation (trauma, surgery, and bacterial infection), as well as in connection with infiltrating neoplasm.

Orbital pseudotumor often shows a clinical response to steroids, with evidence of improvement on CT. Pseudotumor may be difficult to differentiate both clinically and on CT from Graves' disease. Orbital pseudotumor may be mimicked clinically by other infiltrative disease processes, including lymphoma and metastatic carcinoma (breast).

Thyroid Exophthalmos

The exophthalmos of Graves' disease is of unknown etiology. Inflammatory infiltration and proliferation of connective tissue occurs in the soft tissues of the orbit, especially the extraocular muscles (Alper 1977).

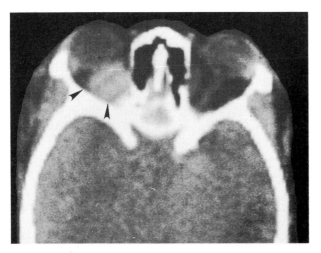

Figure 3-9 Orbital pseudotumor. The intraconic space of the retrobulbar region is filled by a mass lesion (arrowheads).

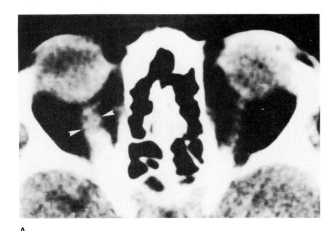

A

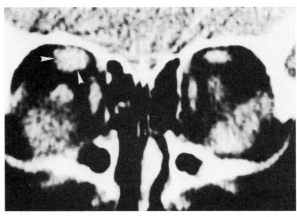

B

Figure 3-10 Superior rectus myositis. Thirty-eight-year-old male with superior rectus dysfunction. **A.** Transverse axial CT shows enlargement of the superior rectus muscle (arrowheads). **B.** Coronal CT demonstrates a large superior rectus muscle (arrows).

The histopathologic picture of the muscles in Graves' disease is similar to that found in orbital pseudotumor (Jones 1979). It is possible that autoimmune responses may be the cause of both the thyroid exophthalmos of Graves' disease and the changes associated with orbital pseudotumor. Most easily recognized is the massive swelling of the extraocular muscles, which may be enlarged volumetrically up to eight times normal size. Interstitial inflammatory edema and lymphocytic infiltration of the muscles account for their enlargement. When the condition occurs in association with thyrotoxicosis, orbital fat content may be increased. The increase in volume of the orbital tissues produces proptosis. Ulceration of the cornea, occlusion of the central retinal vein or artery, and compressive optic neuropathy may be seen as a result. Muscle dysfunction occurs, and ocular motility is impaired.

The exact incidence of thyroid exophthalmos is not known. It occurs in both hyperthyroid and euthyroid patients. Its presentation may be bilateral or unilateral. The classic, mild form is characterized clinically by a prominent stare, mild proptosis, eyelid retraction, and lid lag (Alper 1977). This is most frequently found associated with thyrotoxicosis in young females, and it is bilateral. Most often the patient is asymptomatic (Alper 1977). Typically, the more severe clinical form occurs in the middle-aged patient and is associated with severe proptosis and varying degrees of ophthalmoplegia. Thyrotoxicosis is usually present. Overall, women predominate in the incidence of both thyroid disease (4:1) and Graves' exophthalmos (Alper 1977).

Soon after the introduction of CT, its efficacy in the study of Graves' disease was recognized (Brismar 1976; Enzmann 1976b). In the initial series, Graves' disease accounted for more cases of unilateral and bilateral exophthalmos in the adult than did any other single disease entity (Enzmann 1976b). While CT is not always necessary for the diagnosis of Graves' disease, it has been useful in indicating the degree of muscle involvement and its bilaterality and has proved itself when there is ophthalmopathy without clinical or laboratory evidence or history of thyroid disease (Enzmann 1979).

In the transverse section the inferior and superior recti are cut tangentially (Fig. 3-1). These muscles are better evaluated either in the coronal projection (Fig. 3-2) or on reformed sagittal CT sections. In the direct sagittal CT section the inferior and superior recti are visualized in their entire length, so that minimal changes of Graves' disease can be recognized (Wing 1979).

Enzmann (1979) reported the CT findings in 107 hyperthyroid and 9 euthyroid patients with thyroid exophthalmopathy. The CT revealed bilateral involvement in 85 percent (Figs. 3-11, 3-12), unilateral involvement in 5 percent (Fig. 3-13), and no abnormality in 10 percent. Seventy percent of Enzmann's cases with bilateral involvement had symmetrical muscle disease, whereas 30 percent had asymmetrical muscle involvement. Most commonly, all four of the above-mentioned recti were involved (Fig. 3-12). The inferior and medial recti were involved in approximately three-fourths of the cases and had the most severe degree of enlargement, whereas the

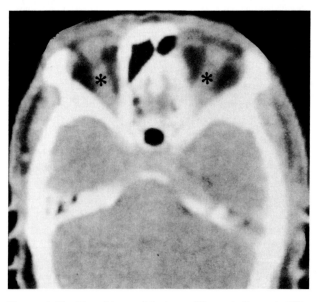

Figure 3-11 Thyroid exophthalmus (Graves' disease). Fifty-one-year-old male with known hyperthyroidism and exophthalmos. Bilateral enlargement of the superior recti (asterisks).

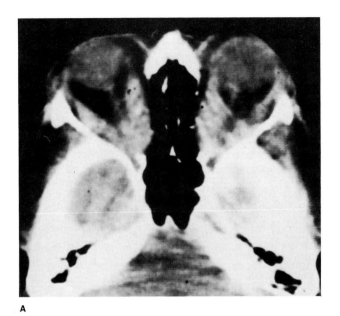

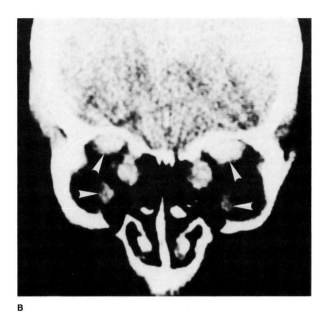

A

B

Figure 3-12 Thyroid exophthalmos. Fifty-three-year-old female with bilateral optic atrophy and proptosis. **A.** Axial CT shows marked enlargement bilaterally of the medial and lateral recti. The globes are proptotic. **B.** Coronal CT also shows enlargement of the superior and inferior recti (arrowheads) bilaterally.

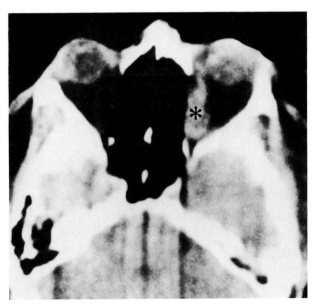

Figure 3-13 Unilateral thyroid exophthalmos. Sixty-year-old male with unilateral medial rectus dysfunction. CT shows enlargement of only the ipsilateral medial rectus (asterisk). Subsequent hormonal studies showed the patient to be hyperthroid.

superior and lateral recti were involved in approximately half the cases and had a lesser degree of enlargement. Enzmann (1979) found a rough linear parallel between the clinical assessment of the degree of ophthalmopathy and the severity of the muscle enlargement. However, no correlation was found between the degree of muscle enlargement and the degree of abnormal thyroid function. Enzmann points out, further, that in 6 of 12 patients who had given a clinical impression of unilateral disease, CT revealed the presence of bilateral disease.

If only transverse sections are available, then the evaluation of the superior rectus muscle may be aided by an additional section through that muscle with the neck slightly more flexed, so that the muscle will be brought parallel to the plane of section. Similarly, the inferior rectus muscle can be better visualized if the head is slightly extended from Reid's base line to bring the inferior rectus into a plane parallel to the plane of section.

ORBITAL TRAUMA

A blow to the face or head may result in injury to the osseous orbit and the orbital soft tissues. Overlying soft-tissue hematoma may preclude adequate physical examination of the orbit. In such circumstances CT is a useful adjunct in demonstrating the presence or absence of underlying osseous and soft-tissue injury (Fig. 3-14). Fractures of the orbit are classifiable as external (e.g., the tripod fracture of the zygoma and anterior orbital rim, Fig. 3-15) or internal (blowout fracture into the maxillary or ethmoid sinuses, Figs. 3-16, 3-17). In fractures of the orbital floor, trapping of the inferior rectus and inferior oblique muscles along with adjacent fat and connective tissue within the comminuted fracture, as the fragment projects into the roof of the maxillary sinus, leads to vertical muscle imbalance. CT is able to demonstrate herniation of the soft-tissue contents into the roof of the maxillary sinus (Fig. 3-16) (Grove 1978). Grove (1978) found that coronal

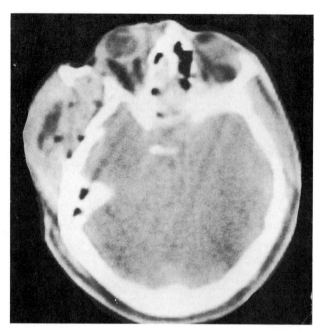

Figure 3-15 Fracture of lateral wall of orbit and depressed fracture of middle cranial fossa. Nineteen-year-old male hit by train. CT shows fracture of the lateral wall of the orbit with the distal fragment rotated laterally and posteriorly. A depressed fracture of the middle cranial fossa is present. The orbit appears intact.

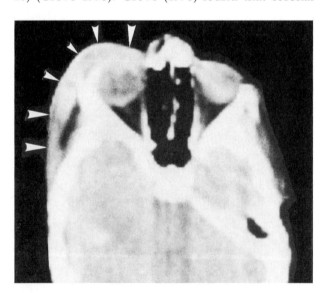

Figure 3-14 Periorbital hematoma. Five-year-old male injured in automobile accident. Examination of the globe was not possible because of overlying periorbital hematoma. CT shows that the globe is intact but surrounded by a hematoma (arrowheads) that involves the periorbital soft tissues as well as the scalp in the temporal fossa.

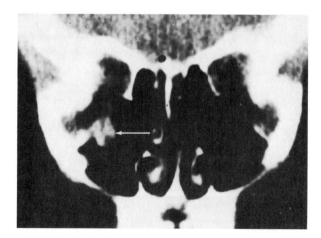

Figure 3-16 Blowout orbital fracture. Thirty-one-year-old male with symptoms of inferior rectus muscle trapping after being punched in the eye. CT shows soft tissue (arrow) extending through the floor of the orbit into the roof of the maxillary sinus.

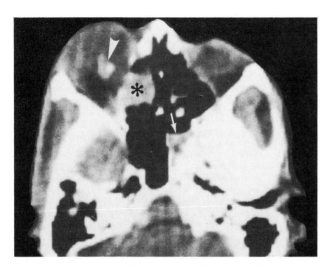

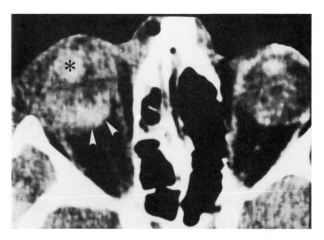

Figure 3-18 Ruptured globe. Thirty-two-year-old male, blind following beating. CT shows the globe to be elongated in shape and surrounded by soft-tissue swelling, with an area of hemorrhage in the anterior and posterior chambers (asterisk) that obscures the lens and an area of hemorrhage in the retina (arrowheads). The eye was enucleated.

Figure 3-17 Blowout fracture of the left ethmoid, with sphenoid sinus blood-air level secondary to basal skull fracture and depressed fracture of roof of orbit. A twenty-nine-year-old male who was hit by an automobile and rendered comatose. Seven days after the automobile accident, marked unilateral proptosis was noted. CT shows an area of hemorrhage in the midethmoid air cells (asterisk) at the site of a blowout fracture. Blood is also present in the opposite sphenoid sinus, with a blood-air level (arrow). The ipsilateral eye is proptotic, and there is an osseous fragment in the retroglobal region (arrowhead). At surgery, the osseous fragment was found to be a depressed fracture from the orbital roof, and the para- and retroglobal soft-tissue mass was an abscess.

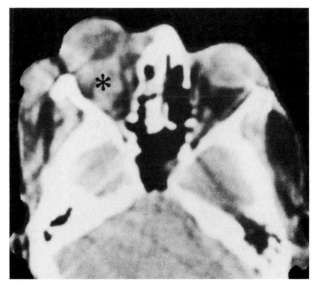

Figure 3-19 Retroorbital hematoma. Sixty-one-year-old male who was mugged and had a rapid onset of proptosis. CT shows a large retrobulbar mass of blood density (asterisk).

CT was better than pluridirectional tomography in depicting the bony fragments in such blowout fractures.

In addition to damage to the bony orbit, trauma of sufficient force and direction can also lead to damage to the globe and optic nerve. Rupture of the optic globe is most often associated with blows to the lateral aspect of the orbit that strike the globe just anterior to the lateral wall. CT demonstrates the deformity of the eyeball shape and the presence of intraocular hemorrhage (Fig. 3-18). Direct damage to the optic nerve and bleeding within the subarachnoid, subdural, or intradural space can lead to loss of vision, due either to the primary optic nerve injury or to secondary optic nerve injury by vascular compression or injury (Fig. 3-19). Fractures in the vicinity of the optic foramen, especially those associated with local subperiosteal hemorrhage, may compress the optic nerve focally. These are an indication for emergency decompression. Intradural hemorrhage in the optic nerve sheath occurs most frequently at the apex of the orbit, where the tendinous attachments insert onto the optic nerve sheath. Intraneural optic nerve hemorrhage occurs also at the apex of the orbit. Subarachnoid and subdural hemorrhage are more frequent just posterior to the papilla, where they are associated with subhyloid retinal hemorrhages (Lindberg 1973).

VASCULAR LESIONS

Hemangioma

Cavernous hemangiomas have an equal sex distribution and occur most frequently from the second to the fifth decade of life. They are characterized by a slowly progressive course. The symptoms consist of proptosis and difficulty with extraocular motility. Hemangioma is one of the most common benign intraorbital lesions and is most often located within the muscle cone.

Cavernous hemangiomas consist of large, dilated, endothelium-lined vascular channels. They are encompassed by a fibrous pseudocapsule. The arterial blood supply is not prominent, and the blood flow is relatively stagnant. Thrombosis, phlebolith formation with calcification, fibrosis, and chronic inflammation are not infrequent.

CT demonstrates the cavernous hemangioma as a homogeneously dense mass (average density 58 HU) within the muscle cone with smooth margins

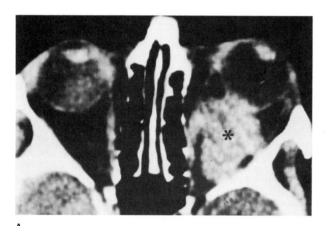

A

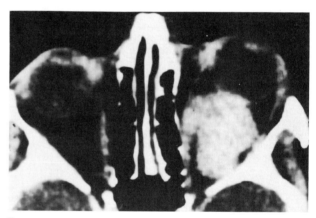

B

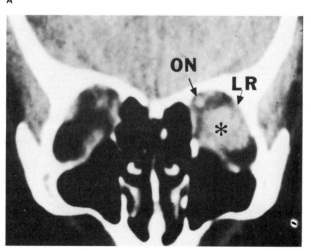

C

Figure 3-20 Hemangioma. Forty-two-year-old male with 18-month history of proptosis without pain. **A.** Transverse CT without contrast enhancement shows a dense mass lesion (asterisk) within the muscle cone of the orbit. **B.** Marked contrast enhancement is present on CECT. **C.** Coronal CT shows intraconic location of the mass (asterisk). *ON* (optic nerve), *LR* (lateral rectus).

and uniform contrast enhancement (Fig. 3-20) (Davis 1980). According to this study, expansion of the adjacent orbital wall is common. In the Davis' series, 83 percent of the cavernous hemangiomas were intraconic, with 67 percent being lateral to the optic nerve; 22 percent of his cases extended to the orbital apex. On CT it is possible to demarcate the cavernous hemangioma from the adjacent optic nerve and muscles. The pronounced contrast enhancement that occurs homogeneously throughout most of the cavernous hemangioma may obliterate this line of demarcation, a disadvantage if only CECT is done (Hilal 1977). The coronal view adds another dimension in visualizing the relationship between the mass and the optic nerve (Fig. 3-20C). This is important in planning for operative removal. Because the cavernous hemangioma is encapsulated, it is easily removed surgically by being peeled off from the extraocular muscles and optic nerves. The tumors show no tendency to recur or to undergo malignant transformation (Jones 1979). It is important to differentiate cavernous hemangioma from lymphangioma of the orbit, a lesion that is not easily removed surgically and is more often extraconic, ill-defined, and less homogeneous in its enhancement (Fig. 3-21).

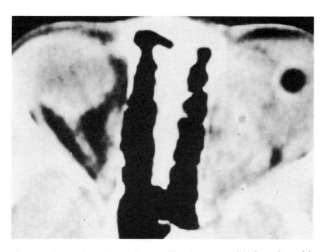

Figure 3-21 Lymphangioma. Twelve-year-old female with proptosis of eye prosthesis. Enucleation for orbital mass at age 1. Large, irregular, poorly defined mass replaces intra- and extraconic structures.

Lymphangioma

Less frequent than cavernous hemangiomas are lymphangiomas. They are most often extraconic in location and present at a younger age (mean age 22) than the cavernous hemangioma (mean age 45). Lymphangiomas have a slow, progressive growth without evidence of regression. They are characterized by thin vascular spaces filled with clear fluid and by lymphoid follicles. Unlike hemangiomas, which have a propensity to thrombosis, lymphangiomas are likely to hemorrhage, producing acute symptoms. They tend to infiltrate along planes without a capsule and for that reason do not lend themselves to surgical extirpation.

On CT, lymphangiomas have the same density before injection of contrast material as do hemangiomas, that is, they appear hyperdense within the orbit. Contrast enhancement is less marked than with hemangiomas. Davis (1980) described lymphangiomas as inhomogeneous masses with irregular margins due to their infiltrative nature (Fig. 3-21). The coronal and transverse CT show them most often to be extraconic (Davis 1980). Bone expansion may be present. Differentiation of lymphangiomas from cavernous hemangiomas is important. The hemangioma may be safely excised because of its encapsulation, whereas the lymphangioma is not removable because it lacks a capsule.

Varix

Vascular malformations of the venous system are infrequent orbital lesions which include orbital varices, varicoceles, and venous angiomas. They are characterized by the production of intermittent exophthalmos, most often associated with activities that produce an increase in venous pressure (coughing, straining, the Valsalva maneuver). The lack of valves within the jugular vein allows back pressure to be transmitted to the orbital veins and the venous malformation. The distention of the vascular spaces within the venous malformation produces the exophthalmus. Recurrent episodes of extreme proptosis have been reported to lead to blindness in as many as 15 percent of patients with orbital varix. Other causes of intermittent exophthalmus are bleeding into lymphangiomas, sinus infection with edema of the orbital soft tissue, and allergic edema. Venous variceal formations associated with arterio-venous fistulas, carotid-cavernous in nature, are usually pulsatile and do not regress.

Routine skull radiographs are usually normal, although phleboliths may be present within the va-

rix. Orbital venography has been the most useful diagnostic modality. Orbital venography performed either through the frontal vein or the angular vein or by reflux through the petrosal vein is now complementary to CT. Rosenblum and Zilkha (1978) reported a case of sudden visual loss secondary to an orbital varix in which the orbital venogram was negative but the lesion was demonstrated by CT. CT demonstrates the location of the soft-tissue mass of the varix (Fig. 3-22) and characterizes it by showing

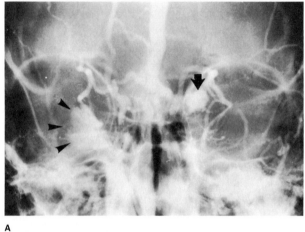

A

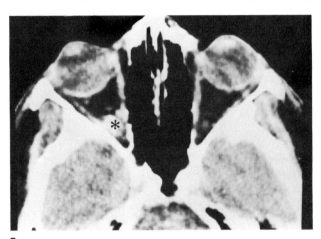

B

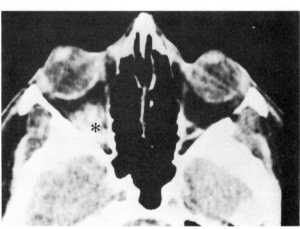

C

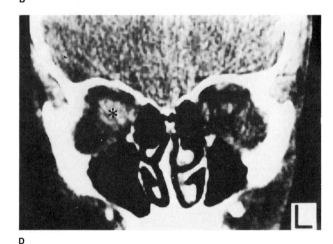

D

Figure 3-22 Bilateral orbital varices. Twenty-nine-year-old female blind in right eye. **A.** Anteroposterior orbital venogram shows the right intraconic orbital varix (arrowheads) and the left medial canthus varix (arrow). **B.** Orbital CT demonstrates a small intraconic mass (asterisk) on Müller maneu-

ver. **C.** Enlargement of the intraconic mass (asterisk) is demonstrated following the Valsalva maneuver. **D.** Coronal CT demonstrates intraconic location of the right orbital varix (asterisk).

enlargement of the varix with the Valsalva maneuver (Fig. 3-22C) and diminution in its size with a Müller (opposite of Valsalva) maneuver (Fig. 3-22B).

Carotid-Cavernous Fistula

A communication between the carotid artery (or branches of the external carotid artery) and the cavernous sinus leads to the development of a fistula in which the veins are under arterial pressure. Valveless venous intercommunication between the cavernous sinus and the superior ophthalmic vein leads to a transmission of arterial pressure into the veins of the orbit. Proptosis, motility disturbances, pulsating exophthalmos (with a bruit), and suffu-

sion of the globe, sclera, and conjunctiva are the hallmarks of the carotid-cavernous fistula. The etiology is most often traumatic, but fistulas may occur spontaneously from communications between dural branches of the external carotid artery and the basilar venous plexus. The exophthalmos and ocular symptoms that accompany the fistula are usually ipsilateral to the site of the fistula but are contralateral in 10 percent.

While carotid arteriography remains the definitive method of demonstrating the site of the fistula and its pattern of venous drainage (Zimmerman 1977), CT is contributory in the initial diagnosis of cases that are not clinically obvious. Enlargement of the superior ophthalmic vein (Fig. 3-23B, C), engorgement of the rectus muscles (Fig. 3-23A), and

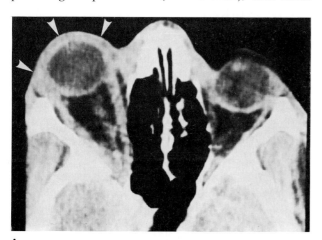

A

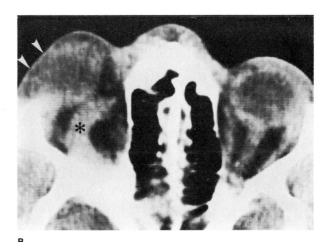

B

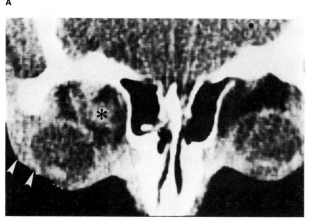

C

Figure 3-23 Carotid-cavernous fistula. Nineteen-year-old male hit in the forehead 5 months before onset of proptosis. Note engorged preseptal soft tissues (arrowheads). **A.** Transverse CT section shows marked proptosis and enlarged ipsilateral medial and lateral rectus muscles. **B.** CECT section immediately above that shown in **A** demonstrates marked enlargement of the right superior ophthalmic vein (asterisk). **C.** Coronal view again shows marked enlargement of the superior ophthalmic vein (asterisk). Arrowheads point to engorged preseptal soft tissues.

distention of the involved cavernous sinus can be demonstrated on CT. Following treatment, CT can be repeated to show resolution of the pretreatment findings.

OCULAR AND ORBITAL TUMORS

Retinoblastoma

Retinoblastoma, an uncommon tumor of childhood, has an incidence of between 1 in 15,000 and 1 in 30,000 (Zimmerman 1978). It accounts for 1 percent of early childhood deaths and 5 percent of childhood blindness (Zimmerman 1979). While the tumor is of congenital origin, it is not necessarily recognized at birth. The average age at time of diagnosis is 18 months (Reese 1976). In 25 to 33 percent of patients with retinoblastoma, the disease is bilateral and represents an autosomal dominant form of genetic transmission that has a variable penetrance (Zimmerman 1979); 50 percent of the offspring of the affected parent are at risk, thus in the bilateral cases there is a frequent familial history.

Retinoblastoma arises in the nuclear layer of the retina as a primary malignant neuroectodermal neoplasm composed of small round or ovoid cells (Russell 1977). It is characterized by multicentric origin, rapid growth, and ability to invade the adjacent tissues. As the tumor outgrows its blood supply, cell necrosis occurs and DNA is released that has a propensity to form a calcified complex. It is this calcified complex that enables the tumor to be identified radiologically (Brant-Zawadski 1979; Klintworth 1978, Zimmerman 1979). X-ray studies of enucleated eyes have shown a characteristic pattern of calcification, consisting of closely packed discrete radiodensities (Klintworth 1978) 1 mm in diameter.

Intraocular spread of retinoblastoma occurs when the malignant cells disseminate throughout the eye and implant at other sites (choroid, retina, posterior surface of the cornea) (Reese 1976). Extension of the tumor along perineural and perivascular spaces results in intraorbital and optic nerve spread of the tumor. Extension of the tumor into the subarachnoid space surrounding the optic nerve allows its dissemination by the cerebrospinal fluid throughout the nervous system. Involvement of the intraorbital vascular system by tumor permits systemic extracranial spread to distant sites such as long bones, lymphatics, and viscera (Jones 1979).

The development of more sensitive diagnostic techniques, including CT, has led in recent years to better detection and prompter treatment. This has led to an increase in survival of patients with retinoblastoma. However, spread beyond the globe carries a poor prognosis.

CT recognition of retinoblastomas is dependent upon the identification of a soft-tissue mass involving the retina without (Fig. 3-24) or with calcification (Fig. 3-25). The presence of calcification helps to differentiate the tumor from other causes of retinal thickening, such as hematoma or retinal detachment. CT is particularly valuable in demonstrating the extension of the tumor to other sites within the globe (or multifocal origins) and bilaterality of the tumor (Fig. 3-25). Thickening of the optic nerve shadow may indicate extension of the tumor into the perineural subarachnoid space. The presence of

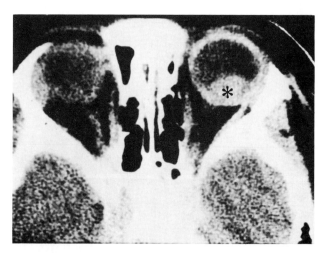

Figure 3-24 Retinoblastoma. Six-month-old infant. NCCT shows a dense but noncalcified mass involving only the retina (asterisk).

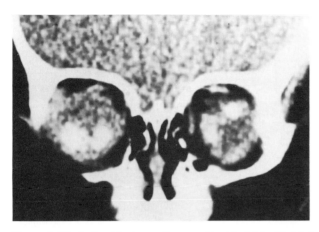

Figure 3-25 Retinoblastoma. Ten-month-old child with bilateral cat's-eye reflexes. Mother became concerned when she thought the child did not see. Coronal CT section shows multiple calcific tumor nodules within both globes.

tumor within the intracranial subarachnoid space can be demonstrated with contrast enhancement (Fig. 3-26).

Concomitant with an improvement in the survival of patients with congenital bilateral retinoblastomas, there has been an appreciation that these patients have a predisposition to the development of radiation-induced neoplasm (Soloway 1966). This occurs in about one-fifth of survivors with bilateral retinoblastomas who have been irradiated. The site of secondary tumor is usually within the field of radiation. These tumors are most commonly manifested within 10 years of radiation therapy. The majority of them are of mesenchymal origin, in the form of sarcomas. However, carcinomas have also been reported (Fig. 3-27) (Zimmerman 1979).

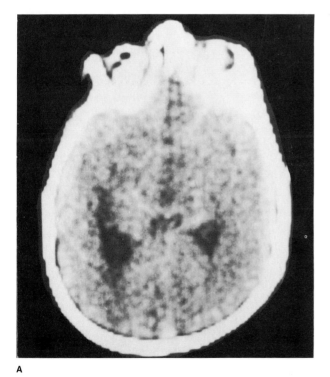

A

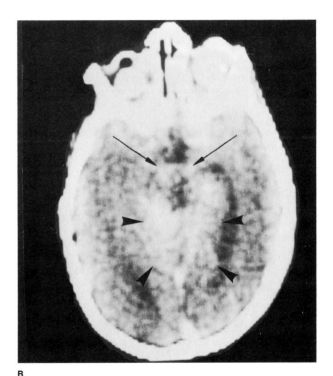

B

Figure 3-26 Subarachnoid spread of retinoblastoma. Four-year-old female with history of bilateral retinoblastomas diagnosed and treated at age 2. Tumor cells were subsequently found in the cerebrospinal fluid and treated with chemotherapy and irradiation. The patient lapsed into coma and a CT examination was performed. **A.** Noncontrast CT. **B.** Contrast-enhanced CT shows enhanced subarachnoid tumor filling the interpeduncular cistern (arrow) and superior cerebellar cistern (arrowheads). (*CT: Journal of Computed Tomography 3:252, 1979.*)

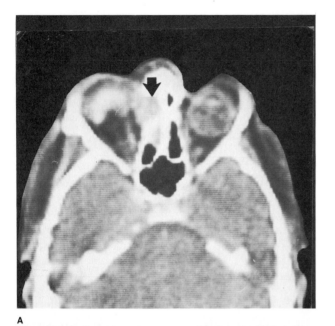

A

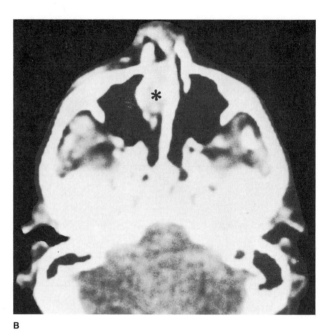

B

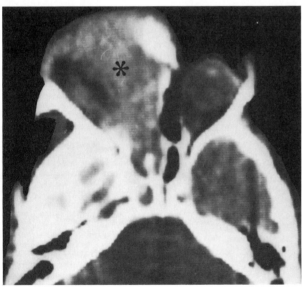

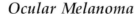

C

Figure 3-27 Papillary adenocarcinoma occurring at the site of irradiation in a patient with previous treatment of bilateral congenital retinoblastomas. Thirty-two-year-old male who had been treated for bilateral retinoblastomas diagnosed at age 2. The patient was examined by CT because of the recent onset of epistaxis and nasal obstruction. **A.** CECT shows contrast-enhanced tumor in the region of the anterior and midethmoid air cells (arrow). The lamina papyracea is destroyed. An eye prosthesis is present on the same side. **B.** A lower CT section shows extension of the tumor inferiorly (asterisk) into the nasal cavity. **C.** Repeat CT 2 months after resection of the ethmoid tumor shown in **A** and **B** shows massive local tumor recurrence (asterisk). The ethmoid sinus, sphenoid sinus, and orbital region are involved. (*CT: Journal of Computed Tomography 3:253, 1979.*)

Ocular Melanoma

Both benign and malignant melanomas arise intraocularly and have been classified according to their site of origin (uveal or retinal). Extraocular extension through the vortex veins occurs in approximately 13 percent of ocular melanomas (Starr 1962). Local recurrence of the melanoma following exenteration is extremely high if extraocular extension has already occurred. The diagnosis of melanoma as a primary tumor in the orbit requires the exclusion of a primary intraocular focus as well as the exclusion of an extracranial primary site (Jones 1979).

The posterior wall of the globe consists of retina, choroid, and sclera. The layers cannot be distinguished by CT, but thickening of the common wall may be shown (Bernardino 1978). Thus retinal melanoma has been recognized on CT examination, and the correlation with pathologic specimens in the three cases reported by Bernardino (1978) was good. On CT, retinal melanoma appears as an irregular thickening of the common wall, with encroachment upon the vitreous. The mass appears slightly hyperdense to brain tissue and shows contrast enhancement (Fig. 3-28). On noncontrast CT (NCCT), differentiation from retinal detachment and intraocular hemorrhage may not be possible (Bernardino 1978). CT may be of value in evaluating extraocular intraorbital extension of the melanoma.

Optic Glioma

Optic gliomas are uncommon tumors of the orbit (1 in 100,000 eye complaints; Jones 1979). The peak age for presentation is between 2 and 6 years, with 75 percent presenting by age 10, 90 percent by age 20. In approximately 12 to 38 percent, there is an association with neurofibromatosis. The symptoms of the intraorbital optic glioma include progressive, nonpulsatile exophthalmos, limitation of eye movement, optic atrophy, and papilledema. The proptosis precedes a decrease in vision and the onset of strabismus.

CT has replaced other radiographic modalities in the diagnostic evaluation of optic gliomas (Byrd 1978), because CT demonstrates the full extent of the optic glioma. A significant number of optic gliomas are part of a more extensive disease process, one that involves the visual pathway, including not only the optic nerve but the optic chiasma, optic tract, lateral geniculate nucleus, and optic radiation. It has been the authors' experience that unsuspected involvement of the chiasmal tract, geniculate nucleus, and optic radiation has been present in one-fourth of patients (Bilaniuk 1982*b*).

Optic gliomas appear most often as irregular nodular enlargements of the optic nerve, or occasionally as fusiform enlargements, most of which show contrast enhancement (Fig. 3-29). In addition to the demonstration of unilateral optic nerve glioma, it is possible to show bilateral involvement, which in some cases is clinically unexpected (Fig. 3-29).

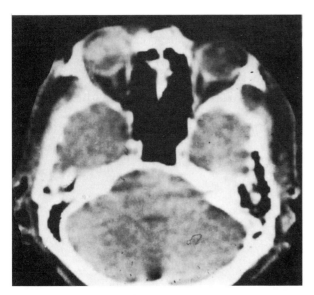

Figure 3-28 Ocular melanoma. Fifty-year-old male with decreased vision. CT shows hyperdense mass in the region of the uvea. On CECT, enhancement is noted.

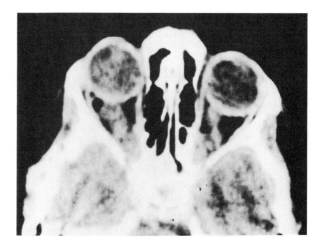

Figure 3-29 Bilateral optic nerve gliomas. Nine-year-old female with known bilateral optic gliomas. CECT shows irregular nodular enlargement of both optic nerves.

Meningioma

Meningiomas may originate within the orbit, most often from the optic nerve sheath (Fig. 3-30) and less frequently from the periosteum of the orbital wall or arachnoidal nests randomly located within the orbit. Meningiomas also secondarily involve the orbit by extension from a primary intracranial meningioma (Fig. 3-31). Primary intraorbital meningiomas (5 percent of primary orbital tumors) are less frequent than those which secondarily involve the orbit. If one considers only primary tumors of the optic nerve, optic nerve meningiomas account for one-third (Reese 1976).

Meningiomas that arise along the course of the optic nerve may do so intraorbitally (sheath meningioma, Fig. 3-30), within the optic canal (intracanalicular meningioma), or at the intracranial opening to the optic canal (foraminal meningioma, Fig. 3-32). Most commonly they occur in females (up to 80 percent) in the third, fourth, and fifth decades of life. The predominant feature of optic nerve sheath meningioma is early visual loss, with proptosis occurring later (Wright 1979). Papilledema or optic atrophy are common accompaniments.

High-resolution CT accurately delineates the size of the optic nerve shadow and its components: subarachnoid space, surrounding arachnoid, and optic nerve. Significant enlargement, whether of the nerve, subarachnoid space, or arachnoidal membrane, is easily visualized. The problem is in differentiating the perioptic meningioma from other lesions that occur at the same anatomical site. To a large extent optic nerve gliomas occur in children, whereas perioptic meningioma occurs in adults. The bilateral enlargement of the optic nerve shadow due to distention of the subarachnoid space by CSF (papilledema) can usually be differentiated from other causes of optic nerve shadow enlargement (optic glioma, perioptic meningioma). Tumor enlargement is more nodular and irregular or fusiform (Bilaniuk 1982*b*) than the smooth, parallel, symmetric enlargement that is seen in distention of the subarachnoid space (Cabanis 1978). The perineural location of the perioptic meningioma may actually be shown on CT as a mass surrounding a relatively less dense center (compressed optic nerve). Contrast enhancement of the optic nerve sheath meningioma is usually present and marked (Fig. 3-30). Changes in the bone of the optic foramen are usually well seen on CT (Fig. 3-32).

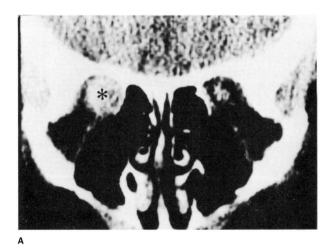

A

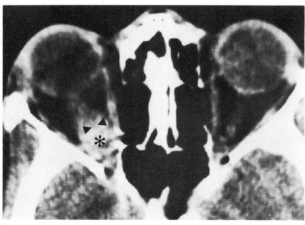

B

Figure 3-30   Perioptic meningioma. Thirty-two-year-old female with proptosis and normal vision.   **A.** Coronal CT shows a contrast-enhanced mass that involves the optic nerve (asterisk).   **B.** Mass (asterisk) surrounds optic nerve (arrowheads), which can be visualized as less dense than the contrast-enhanced mass.

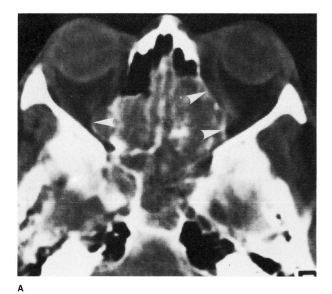

A

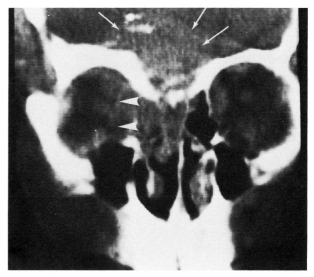

B

Figure 3-31 Extracranial extension of planum sphenoidale meningioma. Fifty-year-old blind female, who had previously had incomplete surgical resection of the planum sphenoidale meningioma.   **A.** Transverse section at the level of the orbits demonstrates an expansile mass filling the sphenoid sinus, posterior ethmoid sinuses, and nasal cavity. The medial walls of the orbits are displaced laterally (arrowheads). The mass contains multiple irregular densities with enhancement on CECT (not shown).   **B.** Coronal CT section shows the anterior extent of the mass projecting into the orbit (arrowheads) through a defect in the lamina papyracea. Tumor is present above the cribriform plate and the roofs of the orbits intracranially (arrows).

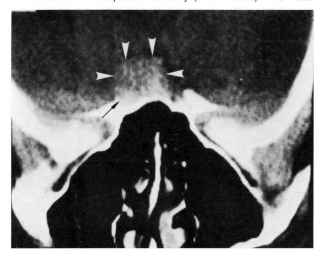

Figure 3-32 Meningioma of the intracranial portion of the optic canal. Forty-seven-year-old male with loss of vision in the right eye for 2 years. Coronal CT shows a contrast-enhanced tumor (arrowheads) involving the intracranial portion of the right optic canal, with extension to the tuberculum. There is erosion of the anterior clinoid process on the right (arrow).

Rhabdomyosarcoma

Orbital rhabdomyosarcoma is one of the more common primary malignant orbital tumors of childhood. It is rarely seen in the adult. The tumor is composed of striated muscle cells and is thought to arise from undifferentiated mesenchymal elements that possess the ability to differentiate into striated muscle. In the orbit, rhabdomyosarcomas appear to arise from the orbital soft tissues and not from the extraocular muscles. The most common clinical presentation is that of rapidly progressive exophthalmos over days to weeks. The superomedial aspect of the orbit is the most common site. In the authors' experience, rhabdomyosarcomas arising in the adjacent paranasal sinuses and extending into the orbit through the thin bony walls, thus presenting with orbital symptoms, have been almost as frequent.

CT is an ideal method of evaluating the location and extent of the sarcoma; differentiation between primary orbital rhabdomyosarcoma and that arising from paranasal sinuses is usually possible (Zimmerman 1978). In one series of craniofacial sarcomas (Zimmerman 1978) there were six orbital rhabdomyosarcomas, and none of these had CT evidence of bone destruction at the time of presentation; the tumors were all confined to the orbital soft tissues (Fig. 3-33). In four paranasal sinus rhabdomyosarcomas which presented with orbital symptoms, the CT scan showed a more extensive process within the paranasal sinus, with destruction of the sinus wall and intraorbital extension (Fig. 3-34) (Bilaniuk 1980). CT is of further use in that it demonstrates intracranial epidural and subarachnoid extension of the tumor, which may be subclinical at the time of presentation (Zimmerman 1978). Intracranial spread into the subarachnoid or epidural space is a poor prognostic sign (Raney 1979), associated with an almost 100 percent recurrence rate. Recurrence of rhabdomyosarcoma is tantamount to subsequent death.

On CT, the rhabdomyosarcoma appears as an isodense to slightly hyperdense mass which infiltrates the retroglobar fat and muscle planes and often involves the posterior aspect of the globe (Fig.

3-33). The contrast enhancement of the tumor is uniform (Fig. 3-33).

The response to chemotherapy is often dramatic, with almost complete disappearance of the tumor following completion of the first cycle (6 weeks) of vincristine, actinomycin, and cyclophosphamide (Raney 1979) (Fig. 3-34C). Six patients who had primary orbital rhabdomyosarcomas have been followed by CT, and there has been no evidence of recurrent tumor for as long as 2 to 5 years after treatment.

Lacrimal Gland Tumors

The lacrimal fossa is located extraconically in the superolateral aspect of the orbit. The lacrimal gland, the size and shape of an almond, lies within the lacrimal fossa, adjacent to the tendons of the lateral and superior rectus muscles. Histologically the lacrimal gland tissue is similar to that of the salivary gland, and pathologically it is affected by similar disease processes. Of the masses that arise within the lacrimal gland, 50 percent are tumors of epithelial origin. Approximately half of these are benign mixed tumors, while the other half comprise a variety of carcinomas. The remaining 50 percent of the

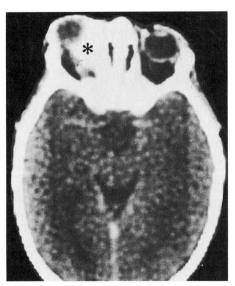

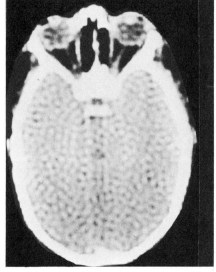

Figure 3-33 Orbital rhabdomyosarcoma. Two-year-old male with a 3-week history of progressive proptosis. **A.** CECT shows a homogeneous enhancing mass (asterisk) occupying the superomedial aspect of the orbit and producing proptosis. **B.** Repeat CT 2 months after institution of chemotherapy shows complete resolution of the intraorbital tumor mass.

A   B

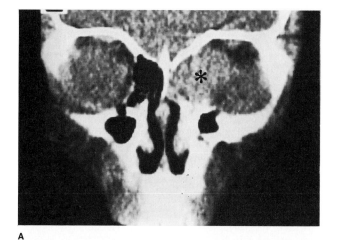

A

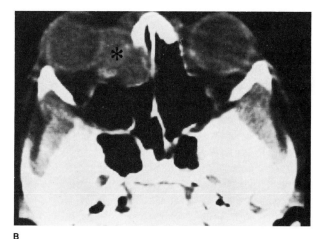

B

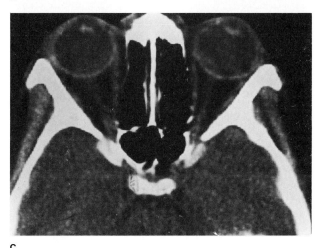

C

Figure 3-34 Rhabdomyosarcoma of the ethmoid sinus. Nine-year-old female with a 7-day history of progressive proptosis. **A.** Coronal scan shows a contrast-enhanced ethmoid sinus soft-tissue mass (asterisk) extending through the lamina papyracea into the orbit. **B.** Transverse section shows the destruction of the anteromedial wall of the orbit, the tumor mass (asterisk), and lateral displacement of the globe. **C.** Transverse section 4 months later, following completion of chemotherapy and radiotherapy, shows complete resolution of the tumor mass and reconstitution of the lamina papyracea. The patient remains well 1 year following completion of therapy. (*A and B from Head and Neck Surgery 2:298, 1980.*)

masses arising in the lacrimal gland are either tumors of lymphomatous origin or are inflammatory masses.

The correct surgical management of the benign mixed lacrimal gland tumor is excision of the whole gland. This avoids the risk of seeding the tumor cells into the adjacent tissues and minimizes the possibility of recurrence (Wright 1979). Other lesions arising in the lacrimal fossa, such as inflammatory pseudotumor, epidermoid, and dermoid cysts, are only biopsied for tissue diagnosis. Thus it is important to know the extent of the disease process and whether the tumor is infiltrative or merely displaces adjacent soft tissues.

Benign mixed lacrimal gland tumors characteristically present in an age range that extends from the late twenties to the early sixties. They present as slowly progressive, painless swellings beneath the upper eyelid, with duration of symptoms usually over 12 months (Wright 1979). Carcinomas of the lacrimal gland characteristically have a rapidly worsening clinical course that usually lasts less than 9 months (Wright 1979).

Both benign and malignant tumors of the lacrimal gland expand and go on to produce unilateral exophthalmos. Because of their location in the superolateral aspect of the orbit, the globe is displaced inferiorly and medially. The mass tends to enlarge

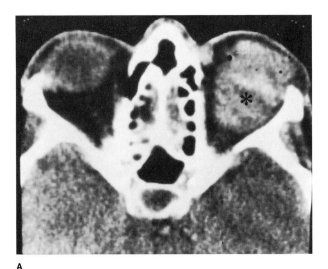

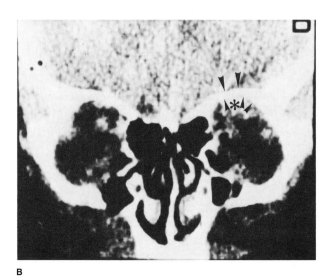

A

B

Figure 3-35 Lacrimal gland tumor. Forty-nine-year-old male with progressive proptosis. **A.** Transverse axial CT shows a soft-tissue mass occupying the superior portion of the orbit (asterisk). **B.** Coronal CT demonstrates the superolateral extraconic location of the lesion (asterisk). Focal thinning of the orbital roof is present (arrowheads).

posteriorly (Fig. 3-35A), so that the muscle cone and optic nerve are displaced along with the globe. The largest lesions extend to the orbital apex. The benign mixed adenomas do not invade the bone nor do they invade the muscle cone. They are usually well-defined masses of the same density as brain tissue, that erode and expand the adjacent lacrimal fossa (Fig. 3-35B). Such erosion is shown both on CT and by skull radiography. Contrast enhancement in the benign mixed adenomas is variable, with only half enhancing (Forbes 1980). Hesselink et al. (1979b) have reported three cases of mucoepidermoid carcinoma of the lacrimal gland that were of high density and contrast-enhanced. Malignant neoplasms of the lacrimal gland have a tendency to invade the muscle cone and to destroy adjacent margins of the orbital wall. They may also produce sclerosis of the adjacent bone and may contain calcifications.

Lymphoma

The incidence of orbital involvement by lymphoma is approximately 1 percent (Jones 1979). The lacrimal gland is the most frequent site of lymphomatous disease within the orbit. Lymphomas presenting in the lacrimal gland may either be due to systemic disease or may indicate the primary site. Bilateral involvement of the lacrimal glands in patients with systemic lymphoma is not unusual. Undifferentiated lymphomas produce symptoms with a duration of weeks to months, while the more differentiated ones often are associated with symptoms of longer duration: months to a year. The patient with involvement of the lacrimal region presents with lid swelling and a palpable mass. Response to radiation therapy and chemotherapy may be in the form of a dramatic reduction in tumor size.

Lymphoma may also present as an infiltrative process in the retroconic space that obliterates the normal soft-tissue planes. Thus it may mimic orbital pseudotumor and may be difficult to differentiate from it histologically, clinically, and by CT.

On CT, the lacrimal gland lymphoma appears as a mass in the lacrimal fossa of increased density that shows contrast enhancement and displaces the globe medially and forward (Fig. 3-36). Not infrequently there is extension of the lacrimal lymphomatous process into the eyelid and into the fossa temporalis.

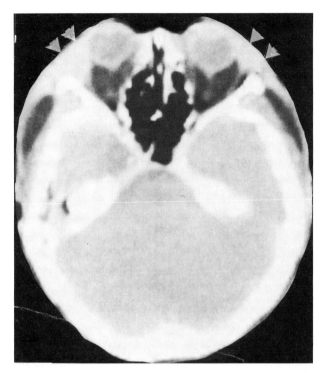

Figure 3-36 Bilateral lacrimal gland lymphoma. Fifty-four-year-old female with known systemic lymphoma, who presented with bilateral proptosis and soft-tissue fullness lateral to proptotic globes. Contrast-enhanced enlarged lacrimal glands (arrowheads) cause medial and forward displacement of both globes. Lymphomatous infiltration was confirmed at biopsy and later at autopsy.

Orbital Metastases from Distant Sites

In a large series of orbital neoplasms, metastases from distant primary sites were relatively rare (5 percent; Albert 1967). This may be a misleadingly low figure, because the orbital structures are rarely examined in patients who die with disseminated metastases. The patterns of orbital metastases differ in children and in adults. The tumors that metastasize most frequently to the orbit in the child are those which arise from embryonal tumors, neuroblastoma, and Ewing's sarcoma (Jones 1979). Leukemia may also involve the orbit. In the child, the orbit is more frequently involved and the globe less often. In the adult, metastases are most often from carcinomas of breast and lung and are most fre-

quently to the globe. In the adult, 70 percent of metastases are ocular, whereas only 30 percent are orbital (Jones 1979). In 50 percent of these orbital metastases, the primary is unknown. In such a situation the site of the unknown primary is more likely to be the lung than the breast.

Symptoms of orbital metastatic disease include an abrupt onset of proptosis, external ophthalmoplegia, and orbital pain early in the course of the disease (Jones 1979).

Metastases to the orbit most often have indistinct boundaries and are diffusely infiltrating. A minority of metastatic lesions are discrete and well circumscribed. Metastatic retroglobar carcinoma from breast carcinoma has been relatively frequent in the authors' experience. This most often appears on CT as a diffusely infiltrative, contrast-enhancing mass lesion without clear-cut margins (Fig. 3-37) (Bilaniuk 1982a). At times it may have a CT appearance similar to that seen with extensive orbital pseudotumors. When the metastasis is from a scirrhous carcinoma, the fibrous response produces enophthalmos.

The intraocular metastases from carcinoma seen in the adult have thus far been better evaluated by

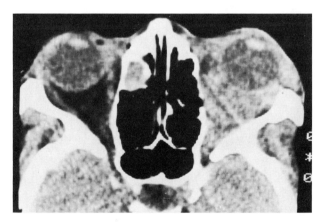

Figure 3-37 Metastasis from carcinoma of the breast. Fifty-seven-year-old female with local recurrence of breast carcinoma and known skin and bone metastases. CECT shows complete replacement of the retroorbital contents by tumor. There is a prominence of the periorbital soft tissues around the globe. Biopsy of the intraorbital contents revealed metastatic adenocarcinoma. The patient was treated with irradiation.

ultrasound and funduscopic examination than by CT. Bernardino et al. (1978) reported one patient with metastatic breast carcinoma to the choroid that was shown by CT. It is possible that with faster, higher-resolution CT scanners and thin sections, ocular metastases will be more easily evaluated by CT.

In children, orbital metastases most often involve the walls of the orbit. The tumors extend subperiosteally into the orbital space. Neuroblastoma frequently presents with simultaneous metastases to both orbits but often also as unilateral metastatic disease. The bone is infiltrated, and the orbital periosteum is displaced (Zimmerman 1980*b*).

Skull radiographs show mixed lytic and hyperostotic bone changes, spiculated periosteal bone reaction, and obliteration of adjacent paranasal sinuses. In addition to revealing similar bone changes, CT demonstrates the subperiosteal portion of the tumor, which shows contrast enhancement (Fig. 3-38) (Zimmerman 1980*b*). The orbital tumor in neuroblastoma may be dense on NCCT, owing to hemorrhage within the tumor.

Distant metastases to the orbital bones and paranasal sinuses also occur in adults and may resemble pediatric neuroblastoma. Metastatic prostate carcinoma is typified by its sclerotic bone reaction and subperiosteal extension.

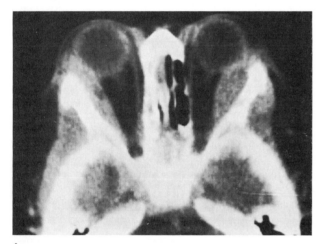

A

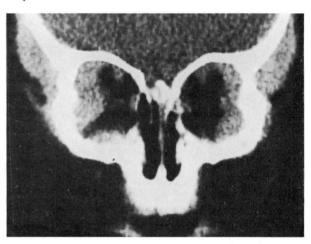

B

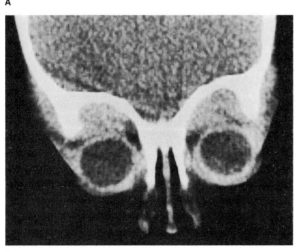

C

Figure 3-38   Bilateral metastatic neuroblastoma to the orbits. Twenty-month-old male who presented with bilateral black eyes and proptosis was found to have a large adrenal neuroblastoma with metastases to the bone marrow and cervical lymph nodes.   **A.** CECT demonstrates bilateral subperiosteal intraorbital metastatic deposits arising from the sphenoidal walls of the orbit. The globes are displaced forward and medially. Tumor also extends subperiosteally into both middle cranial fossae and involves the ethmoid sinuses.   **B.** Coronal section shows the superior-inferior extension of the lateral subperiosteal tumor.   **C.** Coronal section farther forward shows extensive bilateral tumor superior to the globes.   (*A and B from American Journal of Neuroradiology 1:433, 1980.*)

ORBITAL WALL AND PARANASAL SINUS TUMORS

Benign Tumors

Fibrous Dysplasia

Fibrous dysplasia is probably a developmental mesodermal disorder that presents in either a monostotic or a polyostotic form. In its polyostotic form there may be an associated skin pigmentation abnormality and an endocrine disorder (Albright's syndrome). There is no sex predilection. The disease is most often encounted in children and young adolescents. The monostotic facial form presents clinically with headaches, facial asymmetry, and painless swelling of the cheek and periorbital region. When the craniofacial bones are involved it is not unusual to find encroachment upon the paranasal sinuses, orbit, and foramina that transmit nerves. This encroachment can produce visual loss, proptosis, diplopia, and epiphora (tearing) (Liakos 1979). Depending upon the location of the fibrous dysplasia, the symptoms affecting the orbit will differ. Fibrous dysplasia involving the cranial base may produce an extraocular palsy and fifth-nerve neuralgia, whereas fibrous dysplasia involving the optic canal will produce visual loss and optic atrophy. Proptosis and bony prominence are common when there is involvement of the frontal bones.

CT, like skull radiography, reveals obliteration of the medullary canal by expansile homogeneous matrix denser than that of the normal bone but occasionally containing focal sclerotic and lytic areas (Fig. 3-39). CT is excellent in defining the constrictive effect of the osseofibrous lesion upon the orbit, the optic canal, and the adjacent paranasal sinuses (Fig. 3-39). Treatment of fibrous dysplasia is surgical, with unroofing of the optic canal or cosmetic remodeling of the orbit in order to provide adequate room for the intraorbital contents. Radiation therapy is not advised, because osteogenic sarcoma may develop as a result (Jones 1979).

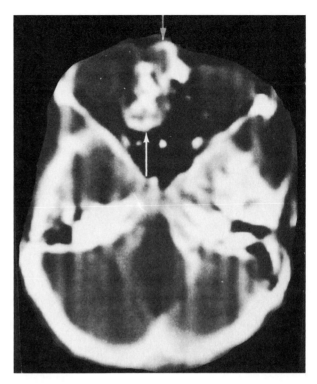

Figure 3-39 Fibrous dysplasia of ethmoid sinus. Seventy-two-year-old female with long-standing proptosis. CT scan shows an osseofibrous expansile lesion involving the ethmoid sinuses (arrows).

Ossifying Fibroma

Ossifying fibromas are controversial lesions, often linked to fibrous dysplasia. They are benign tumors which grow without regard to skeletal maturity and may occur in the mandible, maxilla, and paranasal sinuses. They are found most often after 10 years of age, predominantly in the female. When they arise in the paranasal sinuses adjacent to the orbit, they most often present as painless facial swelling, exophthalmos, and displacement of the eye. Histologically they are highly cellular, with a fibrous stroma, and osteoid, having a calcific matrix. Ossifying fibromas are more apt to show aggressive growth than fibrous dysplasia.

The radiologic picture of an ossifying fibroma reflects the variable composition of the lesion (fibrous tissue, osteoid, and calcific matrix). Conventional roentgenography shows opacification and expansion of the involved paranasal sinus. The lesion is relatively lucent when compared to a typical case of fibrous dysplasia. CT demonstrates the expansion of the paranasal sinus, the homogeneous matrix which shows contrast enhancement, and the admixture of bone spicules within it (Fig. 3-40).

Osteoma

The incidence of osteomas on routine skull radiographs is on the order of 0.3 percent. They are found arising most often within the paranasal si-

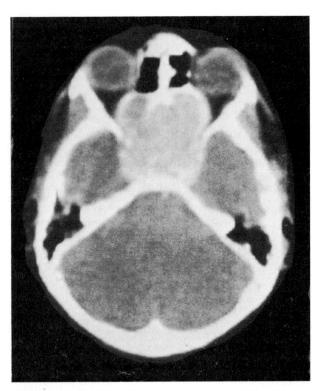

Figure 3-40 Ossifying fibroma of the sphenoid sinus. Eleven-year-old male with abrupt onset of monocular blindness. Transverse computed tomographic section shows an expansile lesion of the sphenoid sinus with bilateral encroachment upon the orbits. A homogeneous matrix is present within the sphenoid sinus. The matrix enhanced on CECT (not shown). (*Computed Axial Tomography 1:27, 1977.*)

nuses (Arger 1977) but on rare occasions may arise from the wall of the orbit. The most frequent location is within the frontal sinuses (40 to 80 percent), with the incidence decreasing in the ethmoid, maxillary, and sphenoid sinuses (2 percent). They are usually found after age 20 and more often in males than females.

The osteoma expands within and conforms to the shape of the sinus. As the osteoma grows, it may produce obstruction of the ostia, which leads to infection or possibly the development of a mucocele. Pneumoencephalus has been reported as a complication of ethmoidal and frontal osteomas that have eroded through the floor of the anterior cranial fossa.

Visual symptoms are due to encroachment on the orbit or compression of the optic nerve. Frontal osteomas may produce both facial asymmetry and downward displacement of the globe. Ethmoidal osteomas can produce lateral displacement of the globe. Sphenoidal osteomas may encroach on the optic canal and orbital apex (Jones 1979).

CT reveals the osteoma to be smoothly demarcated, frequently lobulated, homogeneously hyperdense (Fig. 3-41), and most often lying within the expanded paranasal sinuses. Encroachment on the orbit is graphically demonstrated in the coronal and transverse CT sections (Fig. 3-41).

Inclusion Cyst

Sequestration of ectoderm in the wall of the orbit during embryogenesis leads to the formation of dermoid cysts. These consist of an epidermal lining which contains dermal appendages and ectodermal material (sebaceous glands, hair follicles, and occasional sweat glands) sequestered during embryogenesis. The desquamated contents consist of laminated keratin and cholesterol crystals. Epidermoid cysts are less common than dermoid cysts; they consist of a true epidermis and contain only desquamated keratin. Epithelial cysts also arise in the orbit and in the lacrimal gland as intrinsic lesions due to dilatation of the lacrimal ducts.

Dermoid cysts occur most often in the first dec-

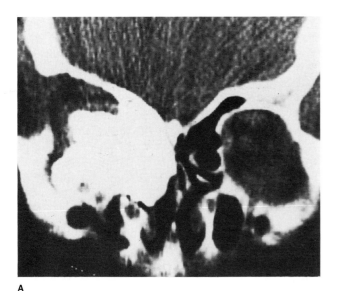

A

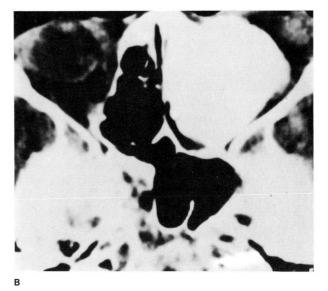

B

Figure 3-41 Osteoma of the ethmoid sinus. Fifty-five-year-old woman with exophthalmos of many years' duration. **A.** Coronal section shows a large ossified mass extending from the ethmoid sinus into the orbit. Defect in the lateral wall of the orbit is due to previous surgical decompression. **B.** Transverse section again shows the osteoma and its lateral extent. (*Head and Neck Surgery 2:299, 1980.*)

ade of life, when they present with physical signs of proptosis or progressive swelling of the upper eyelid. A smooth mass may be palpable in the upper outer quadrant of the orbit.

Dermoid cysts are most often attached to the osseous structures surrounding the orbit. Most frequently they arise in the superolateral portion, in the vicinity of the lacrimal fossa. Extension through the bone, against the dura mater of the anterior cranial fossa, is not uncommon, nor is extension into the orbit with displacement of the orbital periosteum (Fig. 3-42).

On CT the dermoid cysts have well-defined margins and appear cystic, and the density of their center ranges from that of CSF to that of fat (Fig. 3-42) (Hesselink 1979*b*). On CECT the wall is noted to enhance, whereas the central portion remains the same in density. CT is of value in that it identifies a relatively characteristic benign lesion and shows both its intraorbital and its intracranial extent (Fig. 3-42). Surgical treatment is indicated for cosmetic purposes; total removal without dissemination of

the contents is necessary. The contents, if ruptured, may incite a granulomatous inflammatory reaction. Recurrences are unusual.

Mucocele

Mucocele consists of a sac lined by respiratory epithelium, often containing a thin serous fluid but at times showing evidence of hemorrhage or previous infection. There is a history of sinusitis in approximately half the patients with mucocele, a history of trauma in about one-quarter, and a history of allergy in one-eighth. The cause of the mucocele is blockage of the ostium of the involved sinus. The ostium obstruction may be due to inflammation, fibrosis, trauma, prior surgery, anatomic abnormality, or osteoma. The developing mucocele produces an expansion of the sinus, with thinning and remodeling of the sinus wall. The expanded sinus may protrude upon the orbital contents or encroach on the optic canal or cavernous sinus. Mucoceles are uncommon before age 13, as the paranasal sinuses are in the

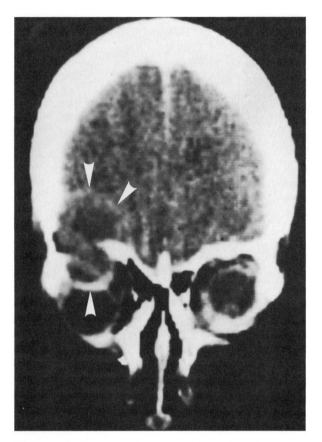

Figure 3-42 Dermoid. Forty-year-old female with proptosis. Coronal CT shows an expansile lesion of the roof of the orbit that has extended both inferiorly to displace the globe and superiorly into the frontal lobe (arrows). Only the margin of the lesion enhances. The central portion is of low density.

(resulting in diplopia). The swelling is usually painless but may be crepitant to palpation.

Skull radiography, pluridirectional tomography, and CT all show the involved sinus to be opacified and expanded and the sinus wall thinned (Fig. 3-43). CT, because of its ability to show both bone and soft tissue, is an ideal method of evaluating the extent of the mucocele. Lateral extension of the frontoethmoidal mucocele produces erosion of the lamina papyracea and lateral displacement of the medial rectus (Fig. 3-44) (Hesselink 1979a). There is preservation of the fat plane between the mucocele and the medial rectus muscle (Som 1980). Proptosis is often evident on the CT. Less commonly there may be medial extension of the ethmoidal mucocele, so that the medial wall of the ethmoid sinus is eroded, with the mucocele projecting into the nasal cavity and against the perpendicular plate of the ethmoid. Superior extension of frontal and ethmoidal mucoceles can occur through the roof of the ethmoid or the cribiform plate. The use of the term *frontoethmoidal* mucocele points to the high incidence of contiguous sinus involvement (Fig. 3-43). The expanded sinus is most often isodense and rarely calcified. Contrast enhancement is infrequent.

Mucoceles that arise in the sphenoid sinus can produce extraocular muscle palsies by involvement of the cavernous sinus and can damage the optic nerve and chiasma by direct compression. They may also interfere with pituitary function and mimic a primary intrasellar tumor (Chap. 13). CT shows expansion and opacification of the sphenoid sinus and may show a soft-tissue mass that extends out of the sphenoid sinus superiorly intracranially, inferiorly into the nasopharynx, or laterally into the cavernous sinus. Destruction of the sellar floor, erosion of the optic canals, widening of the superior orbital fissure, and elevation of the anterior clinoid processes are other manifestations of sphenoidal mucoceles. The clinical picture depends on the direction of expansion: there may be ophthalmoplegia and proptosis (anterolateral expansion into the orbit and cavernous sinus); there may be chiasmal compression and pituitary dysfunction (with superior

process of developing during childhood. Those which occur in the younger child usually do so as a result of problems in sinus drainage (cystic fibrosis). The most frequent location for mucoceles is the frontal sinus; the second-most-frequent site is the ethmoid sinus. The sphenoid and maxillary sinuses are involved considerably less frequently. The type of symptoms depends on the location of the mucocele. Mucoceles that arise in the frontal and ethmoidal sinuses classically present as palpable masses in the superomedial aspect of the orbit. They produce proptosis and limitation of eye movement

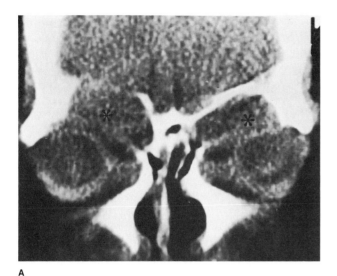

A

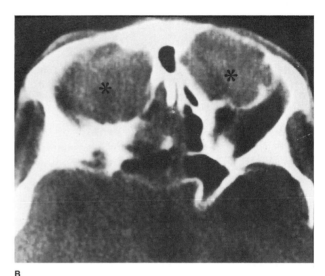

B

Figure 3-43 Bilateral frontal mucoceles. Forty-year-old male with 1-year history of recurrent, bilateral, painful ophthalmoplegia which responded to steroid therapy. **A.** Coronal CT demonstrates bilateral superomedial orbital masses (asterisk) which displaced the globe inferolaterally. **B.** Transverse CT at the level of the frontal sinuses shows expansion of both frontal sinuses by mucoceles (asterisk). (*Head and Neck Surgery 2:296, 1980.*)

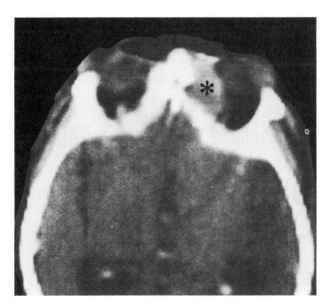

Figure 3-44 Ethmoid mucocele. Fifty-one-year-old male with recent onset of proptosis, 1-year after resection of ethmoid mucocele. CT section shows a soft-tissue mass (asterisk) extending from the region of the ethmoid sinuses into the medial aspect of the orbit.

intracranial extension); there may be airway obstruction (with expansion into the nasopharynx); and there may be multiple cranial nerve (third, fifth, sixth) deficits (with posterolateral extension against the petrous apex) (Osborn 1979).

Malignant Tumors

Sinus Carcinoma

The thin osseous walls separating the orbit from the adjacent four paranasal sinuses offer little resistance to the direct spread of tumor. It has been estimated that in anywhere from 40 to 65 percent of paranasal sinus carcinomas the orbit is at risk. Preoperative management of these tumors necessitates an accurate evaluation of the extent of the malignancy and the presence or absence of orbital involvement. To this extent, CT has added a new dimension to the preoperative evaluation and treatment planning of sinus carcinomas. With CT it is possible to identify osseous involvement of the orbital wall and extension of the tumor extraconically, as well as intraconal extension (Mancuso 1978) (Fig. 3-35B). Any degree of orbital extension is particularly devastating, because it necessitates either orbital exenteration or orbital reconstruction (Jones 1979). This same information is also valuable in postoperative radiotherapy planning. Evaluation of the sinus and orbit should include both transverse sections as well as coronal sections. Sagittal sections, direct or reformation, are also extremely valuable.

Malignant tumors of the paranasal sinuses are relatively rare, constituting between 0.26 and 0.31 percent of cancers. The most frequent site of involvement is the maxillary sinus, with the ethmoid sinus being the next most frequent and the frontal or sphenoid sinus relatively uncommon. The most common forms of paranasal sinus malignancy are squamous cell carcinomas and undifferentiated carcinomas. Less frequent is the lymphoma, and relatively uncommon are melanoma, plasmacytoma, and various sarcomas. Squamous cell carcinoma represents over 50 percent of the lesions in the series reported by Weber et al. (1978), constituting over half of those that arose in the maxillary antrum.

Not infrequently the clinical diagnosis is delayed (over 50 percent of cases) and the tumor is advanced at the time of diagnosis. Frequently more than one of the paranasal sinuses is involved. Early symptoms are often trivial, so the delay between onset of symptoms and histologic diagnosis may be as long as a year. Presenting symptoms depend on the site of origin and the degree of extension of the tumor at the time of diagnosis. The most frequent locations of carcinomas of the maxillary sinus have been described by Baclesse (1952): (1) tumors arising within the inferior portion of the maxillary sinus—these do not involve the orbit; (2) tumors arising in the roof of the antrum—these not infrequently extend posteriorly and laterally to the infratemporal fossa and superiorly into the ethmoid sinuses and orbit; (3) a generalized growth arising from the mucosal surfaces of the antrum and tending not to involve the osseous wall but filling the sinus; (4) medial wall neoplasms which often extend from the maxillary sinuses into the nasal fossa; (5) those which arise in the superior-medial angle at the ethmoidomaxillary septum—these classically have extensive involvement of the medial orbit.

Swelling of the face is the most common symptom with maxillary sinus carcinoma (40 percent). Involvement of the nasal cavity causing pain, unilateral obstruction, and nasal discharge are present in another 35 percent. The orbit is involved at the time of presentation in only 10 percent. Ethmoidal carcinomas have a higher incidence of nasal involvement (55 percent) and a much higher incidence of orbital involvement (35 percent) at the time of initial presentation. Orbital signs are proptosis, diplopia, visual loss, paresthesias, and involvement of such structures as the infraorbital nerve.

The hallmarks of sinus carcinoma, detected by routine radiography, pluridirectional tomography, and CT, are the presence of a sinus soft-tissue mass

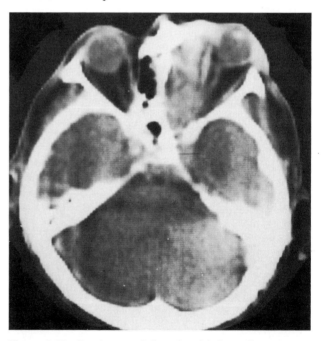

Figure 3-45 Carcinoma of the ethmoid sinus. Seventy-year-old man with progressive exophthalmos, diplopia, and severe orbital pain of several months' duration. CT scan shows a mass lesion destroying the ethmoid air cells and the lamina papyracea, extending into the orbit, and producing proptosis. (*Head and Neck Surgery 2:297, 1980.*)

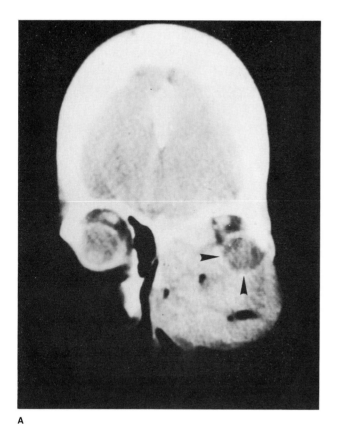

A

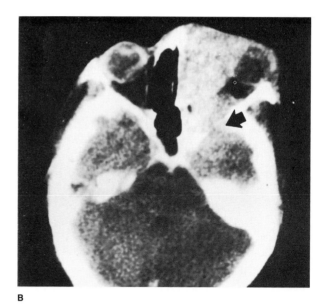

B

Figure 3-46 Carcinoma of the maxillary sinus with orbital involvement. Fifty-year-old female with diplopia and facial disfigurement. **A.** Coronal CT shows a large tumor mass involving the facial soft tissues. The globe (arrowheads) is surrounded by tumor on three sides. The nasal cavity and ethmoid sinuses are replaced by tumor. **B.** Transverse CT shows the tumor involving the ethmoid sinus, with breakthrough into the orbit and retroconic and intracranial extension (destruction of the greater wing of the sphenoid indicated by arrow).

in association with extensive bone destruction (Fig. 3-45). Extension of the mass outside the sinus cavity into the face (Fig. 3-46), other paranasal sinuses (Fig. 3-46A), adjacent orbit (Figs. 3-45, 3-46B), or intracranial contents (Fig. 3-46B) is most typical of a carcinoma, but on rare occasions it can be seen with *Aspergillus* infection or Wegener's granulomatosis (Vermess 1978). It should be noted that opacification of adjacent paranasal sinuses does not necessarily indicate tumor involvement but may merely represent fluid retained within the sinus secondary to ostium obstruction.

Chondrosarcoma

Of the chondrosarcomas occurring in the skeleton, approximately 9.4 percent occur in the bones of the face and cranium. Chondrosarcomas arise from car-

tilaginous rests in the walls of the orbit and paranasal sinuses. The bones of the base of the skull are preformed in cartilage, and rests from this formation give rise to the tumors. Thus the ethmoid region, maxilla, cribiform plate, and sphenoid bone are frequently involved. It is also possible for chondrosarcomas as well as other cartilaginous tumors to arise within the orbit from the cartilage of the trochlea (Jones 1979).

Chondrosarcomas of the craniofacial bones frequently are slowly progressive and form an expansile mass, most often in the maxilloethmoid region. One-third of patients are less than 20 years of age. Unlike osteogenic sarcomas of the facial bones. chondrosarcomas are not known to be painful during their initial growth. In contrast to the chondrosarcoma, osteogenic sarcomas involving the orbit are rare. They occur predominantly in the older

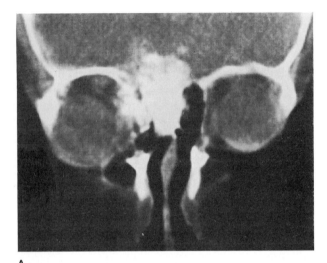

A

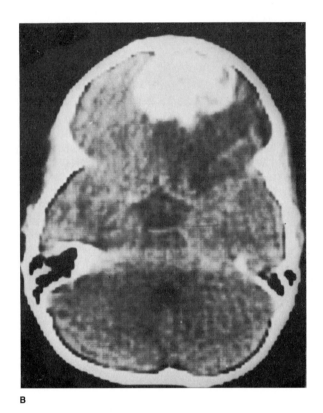

B

Figure 3-47 Chondrosarcoma of the ethmoid sinus. Fourteen-year-old female with a 1-month history of exophthalmos and orbital pain. **A.** Coronal CT demonstrates a heterogeneous lesion of calcific and bony density involving the right ethmoidal sinus, with superior extension into the intracranial space and medial extension into the orbit. The globe is displaced inferiorly and laterally. (*Head and Neck Surgery 2:297, 1980.*) **B.** Transverse CT through the frontal lobe demonstrates a contrast-enhanced and partially calcified intracranial mass lesion, representing the intracranial extension of the chondrosarcoma. Frontal lobe edema is present.

patient (that is, between 20 and 50 years of age), are painful, have a rapid onset of symptoms (less than 3 months), and are much more likely to occur in the mandible or alveolar ridge of the antrum than in the orbital region.

On CT, chondrosarcoma is a densely calcified mass, often showing a whorled pattern (with central hypodensity) and capped by a soft-tissue mass that is not calcified. Both calcified and noncalcified tumor components show contrast enhancement (Fig. 3-47). Adjacent normal bone is destroyed and the local soft-tissue planes are obliterated as a result of invasion (Fig 3-47).

Bibliography

ALBERT DM, RUBENSTEIN RA, SCHEIE HG: Tumor metastases to the eye: I. Incidence in 213 adult patients with generalized malignancy. *Am J Opthalmol* **63**:723–726, 1967.

ALPER MG: Endocrine orbital disease, in Arger PH (ed): *Orbit Roentgenology.* New York, Wiley, 1977.

ARGER PH: Tumor and tumor-like conditions, in Arger PH (ed): *Orbit Roentgenology.* New York, Wiley, 1977.

BACLESSE F: Les Cancers du sinus maxillaire de l'ethmoide et des fosses nasales. *Ann Otolaryngol* **69**:465, 1952.

BACON KT, DUCHESNAU PM, WEINSTEIN MA: Demonstration of the superior ophthalmic vein by high resolution computed tomography. *Radiology* **124**:129–131, 1977.

BALÉRIAUX-WAHA D, MORTELMANS LL, DUPONT MG, TERWINGHE G, JEANMART L: The use of coronal scans for computed tomography of the orbits. *Neuroradiology* **14**:89–96, 1977.

BERNARDINO ME, ZIMMERMAN RD, CITRIN CM, DAVIS DO: Scleral thickening: A sign of orbital pseudo-tumor. *Am J Roentgenol* **129**:703–706, 1977.

BERNARDINO ME, DANZIGER J, YOUNG SE, WALLACE S: Computed tomography in ocular neoplastic disease. *Am J Roentgenol* **131**:111–113, 1978.

BILANIUK LT, ZIMMERMAN RA: Computer-assisted tomography: Sinus lesions with orbital involvement. *Head Neck Surg* **2**:293–301, 1980.

BILANIUK LT, SAVINO P, ZIMMERMAN RA, SCHATZ N: Orbital metastasis from carcinoma of the breast. In press, 1982*a*.

BILANIUK LT, ZIMMERMAN RA, SCHUT L, BRUCE D: Computed tomography of visual pathway gliomas. In press, 1982*b*.

BRANT-ZAWADSKI M, ENZMANN DR: Orbital computed tomography: Calcific densities of the posterior globe. *J Comput Assist Tomogr* **3**:503–505, 1979.

BRISMAR J, DAVIS KR, DALLOW RL, BRISMAR G: Unilateral endocrine exophthalmos. Diagnostic problems in association with computed tomography. *Neuroradiology* **12**:21–24, 1976.

BYRD SE, HARWOOD-NASH DC, FITZ CR, BARRY JF, ROGOVITZ DM: Computed tomography of intraorbital optic nerve gliomas in children. *Radiology* **129**:73–78, 1978.

CABANIS EA, et al: Computed tomography of the optic nerve: II. Size and shape modifications in papilledema. *J Comput Assist Tomogr* **2**:150–155, 1978.

DANZIGER A, PRICE HI: CT findings in retinoblastoma. *Am J Roentgenol Radium Ther Nucl Med* **133**:783–785, 1979.

DAVIS KR, HESSELINK JR, DALLOW RL, GROVE AS JR: CT and ultrasound in the diagnosis of cavernous hemangioma and lymphangioma of the orbit. *CT: J Comput Tomogr* **4**:98–104, 1980.

ENZMANN D et al: Computed tomography in Graves' ophthalmopathy. *Radiology* **118**:615–620. 1976*a*.

ENZMANN D, DONALDSON SS, MARSHALL WH, KRISS JP: Computed tomography in orbital pseudotumor (idiopathic orbital inflammation). *Radiology* **120**:597–601, 1976*b*.

ENZMANN DR, DONALDSON SS, KRISS JP: Appearance of Graves' disease on orbital computed tomography. *J Comput Assist Tomogr* **3**:815–819, 1979.

FORBES GS, SHEEDY PF, WALLER RR: Orbital tumors evaluated by computed tomography. *Radiology* **136**:101–111, 1980.

FOX AJ, DEBRUN G, VINUELA F, ASSIS L, COATES R: Intrathecal metrizamide enhancement of the optic nerve sheath. *J Comput Assist Tomogr* **3**:653–656, 1979.

GANS H, SEKULA J, WLODYKA J: Treatment of acute orbital complications. *Arch Otolaryngol* **100**:329–332, 1974.

GROVE AS JR, TADMOR R, NEW PFJ, MOMOSE KJ: Orbital fracture evaluation by coronal computed tomography. *Am J Ophthalmol* **85**:679–685, 1978.

GYLDENSTED C, LESTER J, FLEDELIUS H: Computed tomography of orbital lesions. *Neuroradiology* **13**:141–150, 1977.

HAUGHTON VM, DAVIS JP, HARRIS GJ, HO KC: Metrizamide optic nerve sheath opacification. *Invest Radiol* **15**:343–345, 1980.

HESSELINK JR, et al: Computed tomography of the paranasal sinus and face: I. Normal anatomy. *J Comput Assist Tomogr* **2**:559–567, 1978.

HESSELINK JR, WEBER AL, NEW PFJ, DAVIS KR, ROBERSON GH, TAVERAS JM: Evaluation of mucoceles of the paranasal sinuses with CT. *Radiology* **133**:397–400, 1979*a*.

HESSELINK JR, DAVIS KR, DALLOW RL, ROBERSON GH, TAVERAS JM: Computed tomography of masses in the lacrimal gland region. *Radiology* **131**:143–147, 1979*b*.

HILAL SK, TROLEL SL: Computerized tomography of the orbit using thin sections. *Semin Roentgenol* **12**:137–147, 1977.

HOYT WF: Coronal sections in the diagnosis of orbital disease, in Thompson HS (ed): *Topics in Neuro-ophthalmology*. Baltimore, London, Williams & Wilkins, 1979, pp 369–371.

JONES IS, JAKOBIEC FA: *Diseases of the Orbit*. Hagerstown, Md., Harper & Row, 1979.

KAPLAN RJ: Neurological complications of infections of the head and neck. *Otolaryngol Clin North Am* **9**:7299–749, 1976.

KLINTWORTH GK: Radiographic abnormalities in eyes with retinoblastoma and other disorders. *Br J Ophthalmol* **62**:365–372, 1978.

LIAKOS GM, WALKER CB, CARRUTH JAS: Ocular complications in craniofacial fibrous dysplasia. *Br J Ophthalmol* **63**:611–616, 1979.

LINDBERG R, WALSH FB, SACHS JG: *Neuropathology of Vision: An Atlas*. Philadelphia, Lea & Febiger, 1973.

MACRAE JA: Diagnosis and management of a wooden orbital foreign body: Case report. *Br J Ophthalmol* **63**:848–851, 1979.

MANCUSO AA, HANAFEE WN, WARD P: Extensions of paranasal sinus tumors and inflammatory disease as evaluated by CT and pluridirectional tomography. *Neuroradiology* **16**:449–453, 1978.

MANELFE C, PASQUINI U, BONK WO: Metrizamide demonstration of the subarachnoid space surrounding the optic nerves. *J Comput Assist Tomogr* **2**:545–548, 1978.

OSBORN AG, JOHNSON L, ROBERTS TS: Sphenoidal mucoceles with intracranial extension. *J Comput Assist Tomogr* **3**:335–338, 1979.

OSBORN AG, ANDERSON RE, WING SD: Sagittal CT scans in the evaluation of deep facial and nasopharyngeal lesions. *CT: J Comput Tomogr* **4**:19–24, 1980.

RANEY RB, et al: Management of craniofacial sarcoma in childhood assisted by computed tomography. *Int J Radiat Biol* **5**:529–534, 1979.

REESE AB: *Tumors of the eye*. New York, Harper & Row, 1976.

ROSENBLUM P, ZILKHA A: Sudden visual loss secondary to an orbital varix. *Surv Ophthalmol* **23**:49–56, 1978.

RUSSELL DS, RUBENSTEIN LJ: *Pathology of Tumors of the Nervous System*. Baltimore, Williams & Wilkins, 1977.

SALVOLINI U, CABANIS EA, RODALLEC A, MENICHELLI F, PASQUINI U, IBA-ZIZEN MT: Computed tomography of the optic nerve: I. Normal results. *J Comput Assist Tomogr* **2**:141–149, 1978.

SOLOWAY HB: Radiation-induced neoplasms following curative therapy for retinoblastoma. *Cancer* **12**:1984–1988, 1966.

SOM PM, SHUGAR JMA: The CT classification of ethmoid mucoceles. *J Comput Assist Tomogr* **4**:199–203, 1980.

STARR H, ZIMMERMAN L: Extrascleral extension and orbital recurrence of malignant melanomas of the choroid and ciliary body. *Int Ophthalmol Clin* **2**:369, 1962.

TABADDOR K: Unusual complications of iophendylate injection myelography. *Arch Neurol* **29**:435–436, 1973.

TADMOR R, NEW PFJ: Computed tomography of the orbit with special emphasis of coronal sections: 1. Normal anatomy. *J Comput Assist Tomogr* **2**:24–34, 1978.

TENNER NS, TROKEL SL: Demonstration of the intraorbital portion of the optic nerves by pneumoencephalography. *Arch Ophthalmol* **79**:572–573, 1968.

TROKEL SL, HILAL SK: CT scanning in orbital diagnosis, in Thompson HS (ed): *Topics in Neuro-ophthalmology.* Baltimore, Williams & Wilkins, 1979, pp 336–346.

UNSÖLD R, NEWTON TH, HOYT WF: Technical note—CT examination of the optic nerve. *J Comput Assist Tomogr* **4**:560–563, 1980*a*.

UNSÖLD R, DEGROOT J, NEWTON TH: Images of the optic nerve: Anatomic CT correlation. *Am J Roentgenol* **135**:767–773, 1980*b*.

VERMESS M, HAYNES BF, FANCI AS, WOLFF SM: Computed assisted tomography of orbital lesions in Wegener's granulomatosis. *J Comput Assist Tomogr* **2**:45–48, 1978.

WEBER AL, TADMOR R, DAVIS R, ROBERSON G: Malignant tumors of the sinuses. *Neuroradiology* **16**:443–448, 1978.

WENDE S, AULICH A, NOVER A, LANKSCH W, KAZNER E, STEINHOFF H, MEESE W, LANGE S, GRUMME T: Computed tomography of orbital lesions. *Neuroradiology* **13**:123–134, 1977.

WILNER HI, COHN EM, KLING G, JAMPEL RS: Computer assisted tomography in experimentally induced orbital pseudotumor. *J Comput Assist Tomogr* **2**:431–435, 1978.

WING SD, HUNSAKER JN, ANDERSON RE, VANDYCK HJL, OSBORN AG: Direct sagittal computed tomography in Graves' ophthalmopathy. *J Comput Assist Tomogr* **3**:820–824, 1979.

WRIGHT JE: Primary optic nerve meningiomas: Clinical presentation and management. *Trans Am Acad Ophthmol Otolaryngol* **83**:617–624, 1977.

WRIGHT JE, STEWART WB, KROHEL GB: Clinical presentation and management of lacrimal gland tumors. *Br J Ophthalmol* **63**:600–606, 1979.

ZIMMERMAN RA, BILANIUK LT, LITTMAN P: Computed tomography of pediatric craniofacial sarcoma. *CT: J Comput Tomogr* **2**:113–121, 1978.

ZIMMERMAN RA, BILANIUK LT: Computed tomography in the evaluation of patients with bilateral retinoblastomas. *CT: J Comput Tomogr* **3**:251–257, 1979.

ZIMMERMAN RA, BILANIUK LT: CT of orbital infection and its cerebral complications. *Am J Roentgenol Radium Ther Nucl Med* **134**:45–50, 1980*a*.

ZIMMERMAN RA, BILANIUK LT: Computed tomography of primary and secondary craniocerebral neuroblastoma. *Am J Neuroradiol* **1**:431–434, 1980*b*.

ZIMMERMAN RA, VIGNAUD J: Ophthalmic arteriography, in Arger PH (ed): *Orbit Roentgenology.* New York, Wiley, 1977.

4

CRANIOCEREBRAL ANOMALIES

Krishna C.V.G. Rao

Derek C. Harwood-Nash

Congenital craniocerebral anomalies of the brain and its coverings are the result of deviation in form and structure during intrauterine development of the nervous system. The combination of genetic and intrauterine environmental factors is the cause of craniocerebral anomalies in nearly 40 percent of intracranial malformations. Of these, chromosomal deviations account for 10 percent, inheritance (either recessive or dominant) for 20 percent, and intrauterine environmental factors such as hypoxia, maternal disease, and infection for 10 percent of the anomalies (Ebaugh 1963). In the remaining 60 percent no single pathogenetic factor has been implicated.

In many of these anomalies a logical cause cannot be deduced, since dysgenesis can occur during the gestational period (initial 3 weeks of intrauterine life), during intrauterine maturation, or during subsequent development. Inflammatory reaction within the fetal brain is uncommon before the sixth month of intrauterine life. Thus most anomalies in which infection is a factor affect the developing fetus during the maturation period, except in unusual situations.

Craniocerebral anomalies have been classified either according to the phases of development (Yakovlev 1959; Adams 1968) or according to anatomical (organogenetic) or cellular (histogenetic) alterations (DeMeyer 1971). Because of the variety of causative factors involved, the etiology in many of the malformations is not clearly established. The classification adopted here (Table 4-1) is the one proposed by DeMeyer.

Prior to the availability of CT, diagnosis of many

Table 4-1   Classification of Cerebral Malformations*

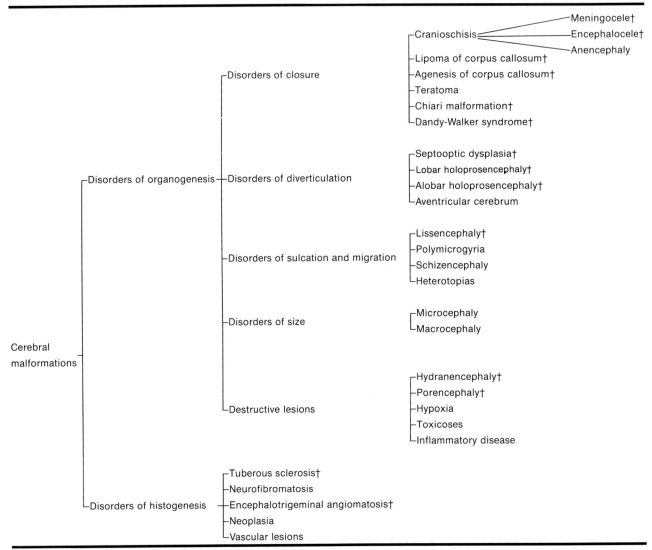

* Modified from DeMeyer 1971.
† Dealt with in this chapter.

of these anomalies was possible only at autopsy or by invasive neurodiagnostic studies such as angiography and air studies. In some cases diagnostic studies were not possible because of a variety of factors, such as unavailability of sophisticated units except in certain institutions, the maturity and size of the infant, or lack of experience in dealing with pediatric-age patients. Computed tomography has provided a noninvasive method of evaluating in vivo the complex structural changes associated with congenital craniocerebral anomalies. A majority of malformations, because of the presence of associated neurological or craniofacial anomaly, are studied in the neonatal period or infancy. A few craniocerebral anomalies, however, may be seen at later ages. Some of the craniocerebral anomalies are detected incidentally by CT. In these patients an understanding of the underlying developmental anomalies may prevent confusion and the need for further diagnostic studies. In pediatric patients, CT studies may be performed for a variety of reasons such as to exclude an associated intracranial malformation when there is a visible structural defect such as midline craniofacial anomaly; the presence of neurological findings although no structural abnormality can be detected clinically, as in septooptic dysplasia; or the presence of an enlarging head or abnormal skull x-rays, with or without evidence of increased intracranial pressure.

In most of the congenital malformations, a precise diagnosis of the anomaly can be made by CT, in both the axial and coronal planes.

Occasionally intraventricular (Fitz 1978*a*) or more commonly intrathecal contrast (Amipaque, brand of metrizamide) followed by CT cisternogram may be necessary to provide detailed morphological visualization of the subarachnoid space and its alterations resulting from or due to the malformation. A combination of the above methods of study will avoid the need for pneumoencephalography or ventriculography in a majority of patients. Angiography is occasionally necessary in spite of the detection of the craniocerebral anomaly by CT; it is useful when enough information is not available on CT to define the craniocerebral anomaly clearly or in situations where a vascular component exists and needs to be defined before surgical treatment. The indications for angiography and air studies will be discussed where appropriate in each of the anomalies, on the basis of our present understanding. These indications may change with further experience and modifications in scanners.

DISORDERS OF ORGANOGENESIS

Chiari Malformations

The hindbrain dysgenesis known as Chiari malformation was first described by Cleland in 1883. Chiari in 1891 described three types of cerebellar malformation and added a fourth type in 1896. The type I malformation consists of tonsillar invagination through the foramen magnum into the spinal canal, with variable degree of displacement of the cerebellum and a normal position of the fourth ventricle. Symptoms are related to the lower cranial and spinal nerves. Symptomatic patients are commonly older children and adults. Although they do not have myelomeningocele, syringohydromyelia is an associated finding.

Chiari II malformation (Arnold-Chiari malformation) is commonly seen in neonates and infants. Along with a more severe hindbrain dygenesis, myelomeningocele and a variety of cerebral malformations are common findings. Chiari's type III and later type IV malformations are variations in the degree of hindbrain dysgenesis. In type III there is a high cervical or occipital encephalocele, and in type IV there is extreme cerebellar hypoplasia without associated downward displacement. In clinical practice the two most common anomalies associated with Chiari's name are the Chiari I malformation in adults and the type II malformation in the pediatric age group.

Chiari I Malformation

In the adult, or Chiari type I, malformation the essential pathology is herniation of the inferior cerebellum and tonsils through the foramen magnum, with peglike projections from tonsils and adhesions, and often associated syringomyelia or hydromyelia. Cranial and skeletal anomalies are uncommon. Very few reports dealing with the CT appearance of Chiari I malformation have appeared in the literature (Forbes 1978; Weisberg 1981), probably because of the difficulty in identifying the cervical spinal cord and cerebellar tonsils, as well as the unreliability in detecting a dilated cord with enlarged central canal or cystic spaces within it by the earlier CT units. With the availability of water-soluble contrast agent (metrizamide) and high-resolution scanners, CT is becoming the primary mode for screening and demonstrating the findings of Chiari I malformation. The two components for a diagnosis of Chiari I malformation are (1) cerebellar tonsillar herniation

Figure 4-1 Chiari type I malformation: CT following intrathecal metrizamide. **A.** Four CT sections demonstrating herniation of the cerebellar tonsil. **B.** Close-up showing the cervicomedullary portion of cord and the tonsil (arrow). **C.** Sagittal reconstructed CT image demonstrates the low position of the cerebellar tonsil (arrow). **D.** Metrizamide myelogram, lateral view, demonstrating the herniated cerebellar tonsil in the same patient.

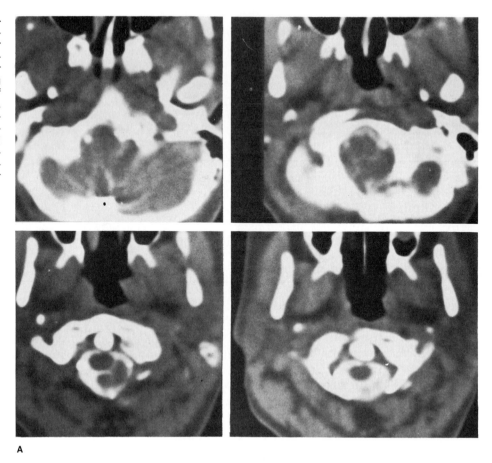

A

and (2) syringomyelia. In the authors' own material, only a few patients have been scanned for whom documentaion was available both by CT and by subsequent surgery. CT of the head and spine was performed before and after intrathecal metrizamide. Delayed CT of the spine was performed 6 to 8 hours later. To prevent high radiation doses, when performing repeat examination at 6 to 8 hours, only the appropriate sections of the spine are scanned.

CT through the posterior fossa and craniocervical junction demonstrates a normal position of the fourth ventricle. The ventricles may not be dilated. None of the changes seen in Chiari II malformation are present intracranially. Metrizamide CT myelography demonstrates the cervicomedullary portion of the cord as a sagittally flat, narrow structure. The tonsils are situated posteriorly and separated from

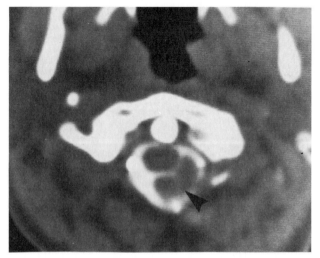

B

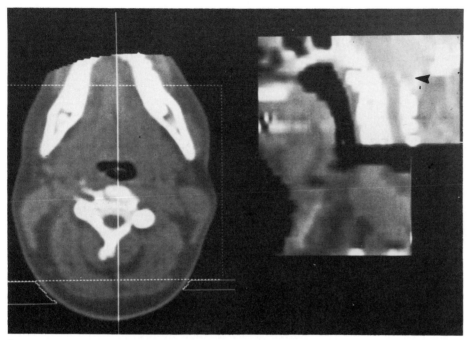

C

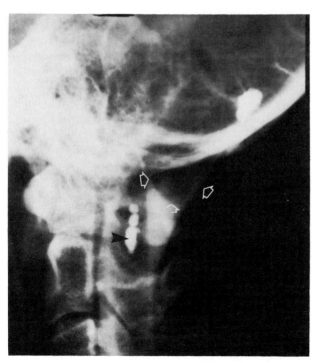

D

the cord by the contrast agent (Fig. 4-1). In the presence of an associated syringomyelia or hydromyelia there is an associated widening of the cord, either localized to the cervical region or extending to the midthoracic region. The CT appearance of syringohydromyelia is well known (Bonafe 1980; DiChiro 1975; Vignaud 1979; Resjo 1979). Delayed CT is helpful in demonstrating the metrizamide, which on initial study is within the subarachnoid space and later concentrates within the central cavity of the cord (Fig. 4-2), further confirming the diagnosis of syringohydromyelia. With the availability of high-resolution CT scanners and safer water-soluble contrast agents, this modality may become the primary form of study and obviate the need for other invasive studies except in unusual situations.

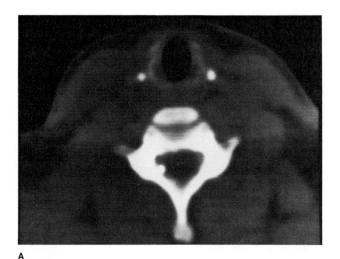

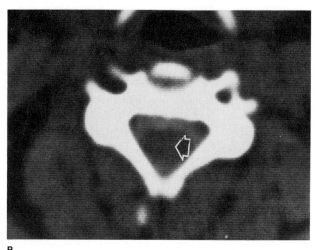

A

B

Figure 4-2 Chiari I malformation. **A.** Dilated cystic cord surrounded by intrathecal metrizamide. **B.** Same patient, 6-hour delayed CT: there is intravasation of metrizamide within the central cavity.

Chiari II Malformation

The hallmark of the Chiari II malformation is dysgenesis of the hindbrain, resulting in a caudally displaced, elongated fourth ventricle and associated caudal herniation of the medulla and vermis. A host of concurrent anomalies involve the neural axis. They include myelomeningocele, mesencephalic beaking, enlarged massa intermedia, accessory anterior commissure, beaking of the frontal horn, absence of the corpus callosum, gyral malformation, and hypoplasia or partial absence of the falx and/or the tentorium. The bony vault is also involved, resulting in the presence of lückenschädel (craniolacunia, lacunar skull), scalloping of the petrous bone as well as the clivus, and enlargement of the foramen magnum.

Not all these findings are necessary for the diagnosis of the Chiari II malformation, and indeed many of them may not be detected on computed tomography except in older children. The computed tomography findings in this anomaly have been reviewed in detail by Naidich (1980*a*, *b*, *c*).

LÜCKENSCHÄDEL Lückenschädel is present in a majority of children with meningocele or encephalocele. The condition is due to dysplasia of the membrane bones. The lacunae disappear after 6 months of age. They do not signify increased intracranial pressure secondary to hydrocephalus. They can be seen in a majority of infants below 6 months by computed tomography. Although obvious in routine CT settings, they are especially easy to identify in wide window settings (Fig. 4-3). They appear as pits which involve predominantly the inner aspects of the calvarium, most prominent in the vertex and upper half of the calvarium involving the parieto-occipital region.

CLIVUS AND PETROUS SCALLOPING Because of the small posterior fossa, as the cerebellum and midbrain develop there is pressure erosion of the clivus and posterior medial aspect of the petrous part of the temporal bone (Kruyffe 1966). Since the changes start in infancy, there is molding of the bones forming the boundaries of the posterior fossa. On computed tomography the characteristic changes involve the petrous pyramids, sparing the jugular tubercles and the petrous ridges. There is resultant shortening of the internal auditory canals, which also appear to be directed posteromedially (Fig. 4-4). These findings are better visualized in older children and may not be significant in infants. The changes in the clivus cannot be appreciated in rou-

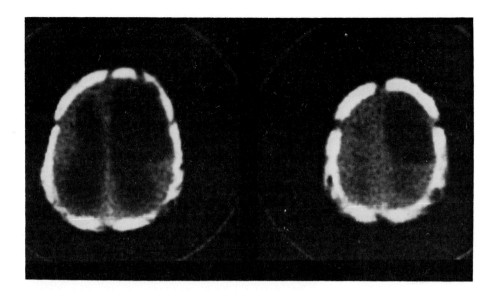

Figure 4-3 Chiari II malformation: craniolacunia appearing on CT as pits involving the inner table of the skull. (See also Fig. 6-8.)

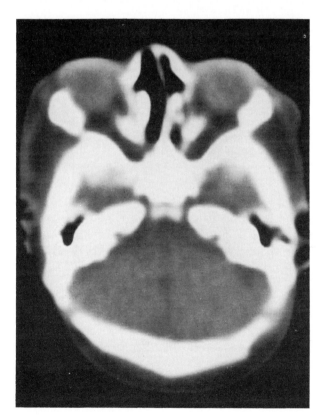

Figure 4-4 Chiari II malformation: mild petrous scalloping with the internal auditory canal directed posteromedially. (See also Fig. 6-9).

tine axial sections unless sagittal reconstruction images can be obtained; they are more commonly seen in infants than in neonates.

ENLARGED FORAMEN MAGNUM The enlarged foramen magnum in the Chiari II malformation is more commonly seen in older children. The enlargement occurs in the sagittal direction (Fig. 4-5). Evaluation of an enlarged foramen magnum by CT may be difficult in the axial plane unless the CT section is done parallel to the foramen magnum. Enlargement can occasionally be appreciated if sagittal and coronal reconstructions are available.

DURAL ANOMALIES

Hypoplasia or Fenestration of Falx Cerebri Pathological specimens demonstrate varying degrees of hypoplasia as well as fenestration of the falx separating the two cerebral hemispheres (Peach 1965) (Fig. 4-6). This finding has been demonstrated on contrast-enhanced CT (CECT) (Naidich 1980*a*). Fenestration can also be demonstrated by CT in the coronal plane. The indirect sign of fenestration of the falx, which can be appreciated on CT in coronal plane, is the close apposition, with interdigitation between the two cerebral hemispheres. In the axial sections the interhemispheric fissure may be narrow

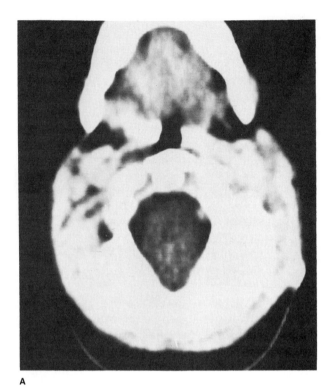

A

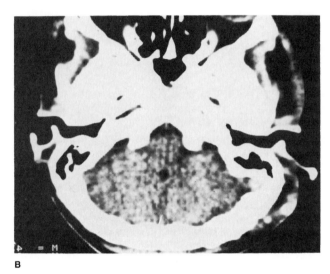

B

Figure 4-5 Chiari II malformation. **A.** Sagittally enlarged foramen magnum. **B.** Slitlike fourth ventricle at a slightly higher level.

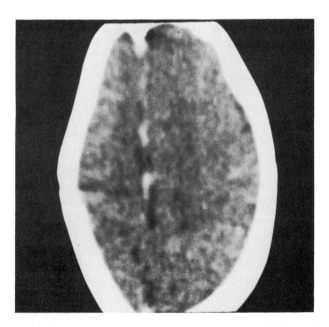

Figure 4-6 Chiari II malformation: interdigitation of the gyri with fenestration in the falx.

in the hydrocephalic infant, although more commonly it is wide following treatment of hydrocephalus. The enhanced falx may not be visualized throughout its length or in segments.

Hypoplasia of the Tentorium On CECT, the normal tentorial hiatus has a V-shaped configuration in nearly 90 percent of normal CT images (Naidich 1977*b*), being wider in the lower sections and becoming narrower until the straight sinus is seen. In Chiari II malformation, hypoplasia of the tentorium and resultant upward direction as well as foreshortening of the straight sinus has a characteristic CT appearance. The free margin of the tentorium, instead of having the normal V configuration, has a U configuration, with the limbs of the U bowed laterally, creating a wide space between the two edges of the tentorium (Fig. 4-7).

HINDBRAIN AND MIDBRAIN ANOMALIES Along with the bony and dural components which form part of the spectrum of Chiari II malformation, the essential

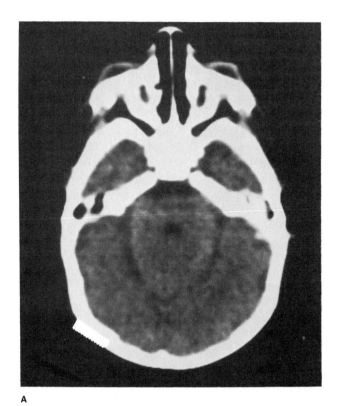
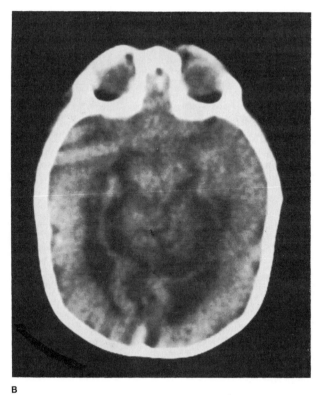

A

B

Figure 4-7 Chiari II malformation. **A.** CECT demonstrates wide tentorial hiatus. **B.** Compressed cerebellar tissue with prominent pericerebellar cistern at a higher level.

feature of this malformation is the pathological downward displacement of the fourth ventricle. This results in an elongated, sagittally flattened fourth ventricle, extending into the cervical canal to a variable extent. Because of these changes, nonvisualization of the fourth ventricle by CT is fairly common. In the series reported by Naidich (1980c), the fourth ventricle was not visualized in 70 percent of cases, was sagittally flattened but identifiable in 15 percent, and in 5 percent was dilated but low in position. The most common feature suggestive of the Chiari II malformation is failure to demonstrate a normal fourth ventricle at or above the level of the petrous pyramids (Zimmerman RD 1979). In infants, even on high-resolution CT the posterior fossa appears full, because of a shallow posterior fossa in which the cerebellum is pushed anteriorly to wrap the surface of the brainstem laterally and anterolaterally fills the cerebellopontine angle cistern. This

finding is more commonly seen in children than in infants (Fig. 4-8). The slitlike fourth ventricle, when visualized, has an appearance of being displaced forward, with a voluminous cerebellar hemisphere. The midline cerebellum in infants with the Chiari II malformation has been found to be denser than the normal cerebellar vermis (Harwood-Nash 1977). The exact cause for the relatively increased density is not known, although this may be a manifestation of a tight posterior fossa.

Because of the low position as well as hypoplasia of the tentorium, the cerebellum projects upward through the wide incisura (Fig. 4-9). Wide or prominent cisternal space called the *pericerebellar cistern* (Naidich 1980b) is commonly seen and is presumed to be due to the large CSF pool created by the shallow posterior fossa. This is more commonly seen following shunting procedures. The portion of the cerebellum visualized through the incisura has

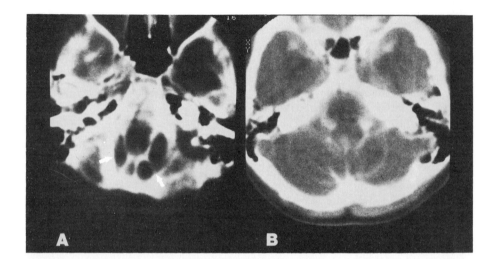

Figure 4-8 Metrizamide CT cisternogram. **A.** CT section shows enlarged foramen magnum. The cervicomedullary portion of the cord is flattened, with the two tonsils (arrows) situated posteriorly. **B.** Section at higher level demonstrating the narrow cisternal space filled with metrizamide. The cerebellar hemisphere wraps the medulla.

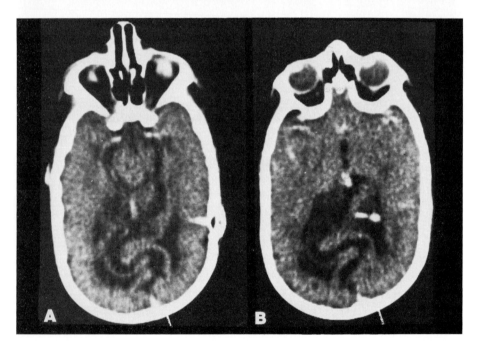

Figure 4-9 A. CECT through midbrain, Chiari II malformation. The cerebellum projects through the wide tentorial incisura. Prominent pericerebellar cistern and deep indentations in the cerebellum are due to infolding of the cerebellum. **B.** At a slightly higher level.

an appearance of prominent sulci, suggestive of an atrophic process but more probably created from invagination of the cerebellum by the midbrain. The third ventricle may show some dilatation. This, however, is less common than dilatation of the lateral ventricles. The massa intermedia is larger and closer to the foramen of Monro (Fig. 4-10). In the majority of cases axial CT demonstrates relatively

small third ventricles with parallel or biconcave side walls, the concavity being maximum at the insertion of the massa intermedia. This has been reported in nearly 80 percent of cases (Naidich 1980c). Similarly, the tectum has a pointed appearance and is best visualized in a section through the superior colliculi (Fig. 4-11). This finding is often seen in the older child and following shunting.

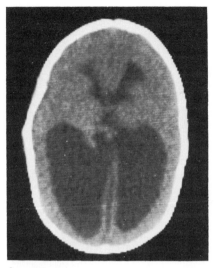

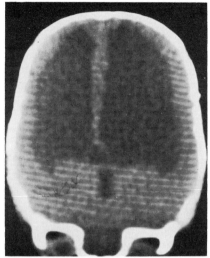

Figure 4-10 Massa intermedia in Chiari II malformation. **A.** Axial. **B.** Coronal noncontrast CT. The massa intermedia bulges into the third ventricle and is situated higher and farther anterior than normal.

A

B

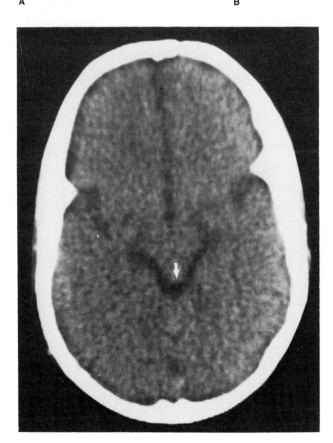

Figure 4-11. Chiari II malformation: pointed tectum (arrow) in a section through level of superior colliculi.

FOREBRAIN ANOMALIES Dilatation of the lateral ventricles is common in the majority of patients. The degree of dilatation is variable and depends to some degree on the time interval between the closure of the myelomeningocele and detection of the cranial enlargement both clinically and by CT. Dilatation is usually bilateral and symmetrical, involving predominantly the atria and occipital horns, the cortical mantle being thinnest in the region of the occipital lobes and vertex. Flattening of the superolateral angle of the frontal horns in spite of significant ventricular dilatation is a common finding (Naidich 1980c). This is better appreciated in direct coronal CT. Although asymmetry of the lateral ventricles has been reported in 42 percent of cases (Naidich 1980c), this has not been the authors' experience in nonshunted infants. Air studies in infants with Chiari II malformation demonstrate a characteristic pointed inferior angle of the frontal horns (Gooding 1967). A similar appearance can be seen on direct coronal CT in sections through the frontal horns (Fig. 4-12). This appearance is due to a prominent caudate nucleus and absence of the forceps major. The septum pellucidum may occasionally be absent. In CT sections above the level of the ventricles the interhemispheric fissure appears narrow, although in some patients before shunting and occasionally afterward this space may be wide (Fig. 4-13). Con-

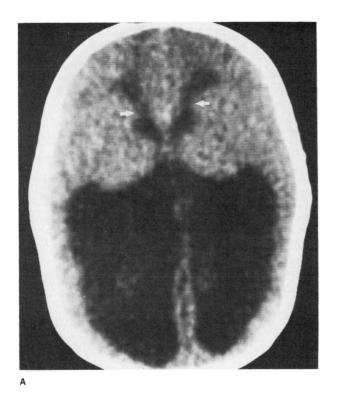

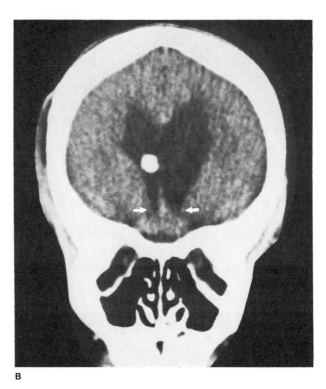

A

B

Figure 4-12 Chairi II malformation: axial image **(A)** shows prominence of the caudate nuclei (arrows). Coronal image **(B)** demonstrates the beaked appearance of the frontal horns along their inferior aspect (arrows). (See also Fig. 6-12.)

trast-enhanced CT in both the axial and the coronal plane demonstrates not only the fenestration and hypoplasia of the falx but also the interdigitation of the gyri between the two cerebral hemispheres (Fig. 4-6). In the majority of cases the various changes described can be diagnosed; however, if surgical intervention other than shunting is being planned, further neurodiagnostic studies for a precise understanding of the anatomical changes in the posterior fossa and the craniovertebral junction are important.

Dandy-Walker Syndrome

Hydocephalus associated with a posterior fossa cyst and atresia of the foramina of Magendie and of Luschka was first described by Dandy and Blackfan in 1914 and subsequently by Taggart and Walker (1942). They also described midline cerebellar hypoplasia, thus the eponym Dandy-Walker cyst. Although the anomaly is well recognized, the pathogenesis is not clearly defined. The posterior fossa cyst which replaces the fourth ventricle may not in all cases be secondary to atresia of the outlet foramina, since patency of the foramina has been shown in some cases (Hart 1972; Gardner 1975). Hydrocephalus, which was part of the original description, may not be present in all cases. Absence of hydrocephalus, however, is more commonly seen in the so-called Dandy-Walker variant. A variety of congenital anomalies may coexist with the posterior fossa cyst. Agenesis of the corpus callosum is the most frequently noted coexisting anomaly. That the anomaly is more complex than the simple atresia of the outlet foramina is well recognized (Benda 1954; Brodal 1959; Gibson 1955; Gardner 1960). Current views indicate the importance of dysgenesis of the

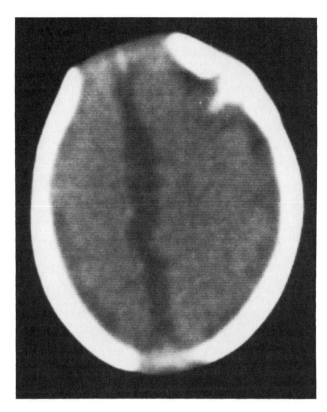

Figure 4-13 Chiari II malformation: wide interhemispheric fissure in a shunted child, also showing the gyral pattern. (Compare with Figs. 4-6 and 6-11.)

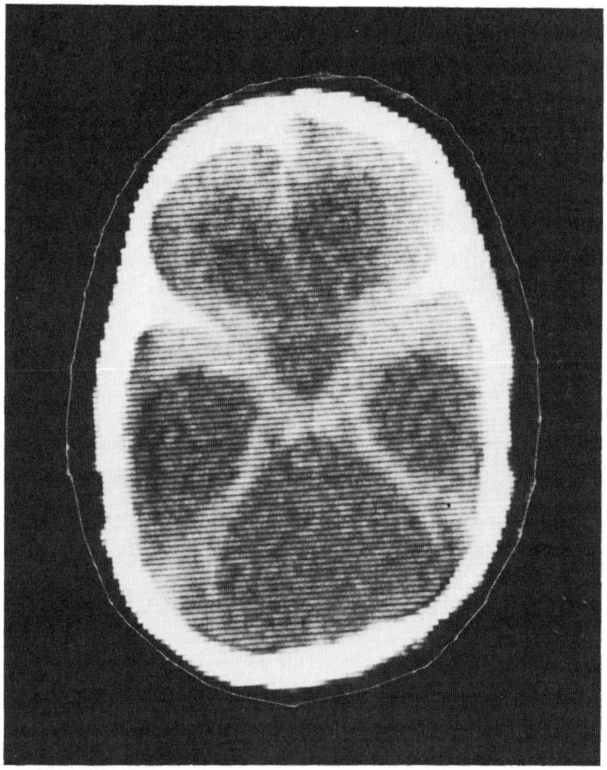

Figure 4-14 Dandy-Walker cyst. Large cystic mass in posterior fossa replaces the fourth ventricle. The lateral and third ventricles are also enlarged.

cerebellar roof rather than the foraminal atresia. Because of the complexity of the anomalies associated with the posterior fossa cyst, the condition is more commonly recognized as Dandy-Walker syndrome.

In its most common form the fourth ventricle is replaced by a symmetrically enlarged midline cyst with hypoplasia of the inferior vermis. The superior vermis is stretched and displaced upward. The aqueduct is foreshortened. The bony calvarium of the posterior fossa is enlarged. The torcular and the transverse sinus are above the lambdoid suture. This results in inversion of the torcular-lambdoid relationship, not seen with posterior fossa intra- or extraaxial cysts (Harwood-Nash 1976) or giant cisterna magna. The tentorium is elevated. The CT appearance of a Dandy-Walker cyst is a large, low-density cystic mass occupying most of the posterior

fossa (Fig. 4-14). The pons and medulla are seen anteriorly, with a thin rim of cerebellar tissue anterolaterally. The cerebellopontine angle cisterns and, in appropriate thin sections, the lateral recess of the fourth ventricle as well as the vallecula cannot be identified. The third and lateral ventricles are usually enlarged, perhaps because of atresia of the outlet foramina of the fourth ventricle, although often there is kinking of the aqueduct which may result in multiple levels of obstruction. This may be of clinical importance, since isolated shutting off of one compartment (lateral ventricle or cystic fourth ventricle) may result in herniation in the opposite direction of the other compartment (Carmel 1977). The relative obstruction of the aqueduct can be easilty resolved by CT study with use of a small amount of dilute metrizamide introduced into the ventricles.

Figure 4-15 Noncommunicating Dandy-Walker cyst. **A.** Axial and reformed sagittal and coronal CT demonstrates the metrizamide within the lateral and third ventricles. **B.** Coronal with reformed axial and sagittal CT following instillation of metrizamide within the dilated cystic fourth ventricle. **C.** Lateral skull x-ray showing the metrizamide within the posterior fossa cyst.

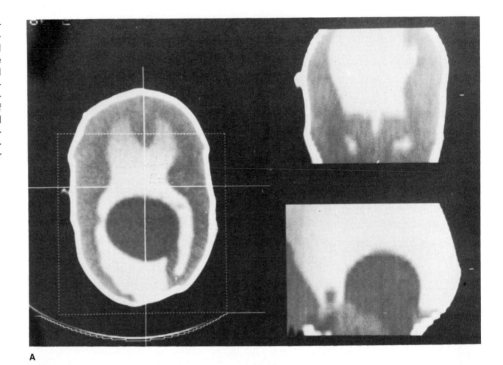

A

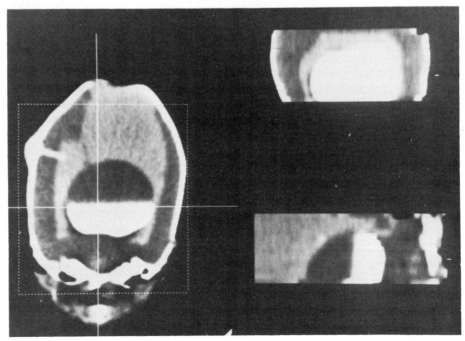

B

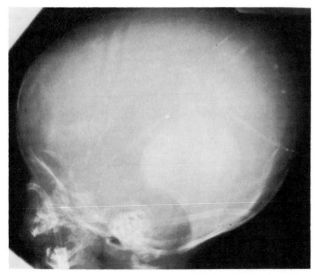

c

The tentorium can be demarcated on noncontrast CT (NCCT) because of the massive cystic dilatation of the posterior fossa midline cyst and resultant thinning of the cerebellar mantle and its compression against the elevated, stretched tentorium. The tentorial margins are elongated and stretched outward (Fig. 4-15). The malpositioned tentorium is seen as diverging bands, usually at a level higher than expected. The tentorial margins have an inverted V configuration. This finding is highly suggestive of Dandy-Walker syndrome and may be seen even in the absence of dilated third and lateral ventricles (Naidich 1977a,b). Similar changes may, however, be seen occasionally with large retrocerebellar arachnoid cysts as well as ependymal cyst.

Dandy-Walker variant is a milder form of the syndrome, in which a diverticular outpouching of varying size and shape extends from the inferior medullary velum, the upper part of the fourth ventricle having a normal shape although being somewhat dilated. The cerebellar hypoplasia is also milder. The incomplete development of the vermis and the nodules results in a wide vallecula. The CT findings in Dandy-Walker variant may often be confusing. The characteristic findings described above

in Dandy-Walker cyst may not be present (Lipton 1978). Unlike Dandy-Walker cyst, which is commonly seen in neonates and infants, the Dandy-Walker variant may not be recognized until later in life. The typical calvarial changes described above may also not be present. CT findings include (Fig. 4-16) a wide vallecula with a cystic space separating the two cerebellar hemispheres. Either because of the extension of the outpouching or the plane of the CT section, the fourth ventricle may be seen separate from the cyst. The fourth ventricle appears in normal position in its upper half but is moderately dilated. The lateral and third ventricles may or may not be dilated.

Dandy-Walker cyst and its variant form may be difficult to differentiate from other midline posterior fossa cystic lesions such as retrocerebellar arachnoid cyst, ependymal cyst, giant or "mega" cisterna magna, trapped fourth ventricle, and, rarely, cystic midline neoplasms.

Giant (mega) cisterna magna is occasionally seen in children and adults, its incidence by CT being 0.4 percent (Adams 1978). Megacisterna magna can extend upward, communicating with the superior cerebellar cistern (Fig. 4-17). It is considered to be a benign developmental anomaly, often identified as an incidental finding (Adams 1968; Harwood-Nash 1977). The adjacent cerebellar hemispheres may show atrophy, although the vallecula is not wide as in Dandy-Walker variant (Fig. 4-18). In megacisterna magna the fourth ventricle is in normal position. The prepontine- and cerebellopontine-angle cisterns are well visualized and occasionally may be prominent. Aqueduct stenosis with resulting hydrocephalus may be associated with megacisterna magna (Fig. 4-19) and mistaken for a Dandy-Walker variant. In occasional cases diagnosis can be established by ventriculography. Enlargement of the third and lateral ventricles secondary to a megacisterna magna, although rare, has been reported (Archer 1978).

Retrocerebellar arachnoid cyst may occasionally be difficult to differentiate from the Dandy-Walker syndrome by CT. The extraaxial cyst may invaginate between the two cerebellar hemispheres, resulting

Figure 4-16 Dandy-Walker variant. **A.** In the axial sections the dilated fourth ventricle with its posterior extension through the widened vallecula is noted. There is associated dilatation of the third and lateral ventricles. **B.** Coronal CT demonstrating the midline dilated fourth ventricle.

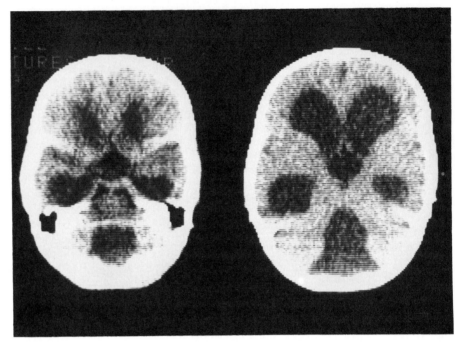

A

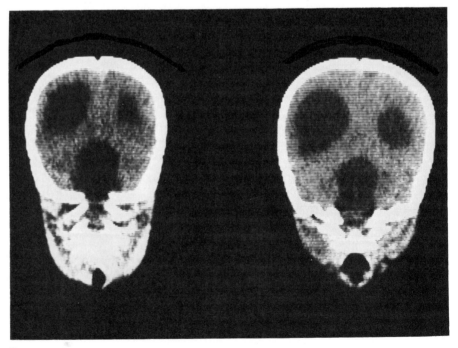

B

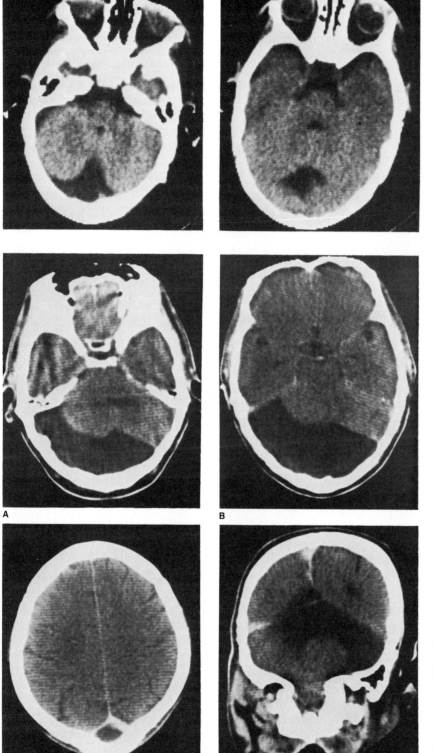

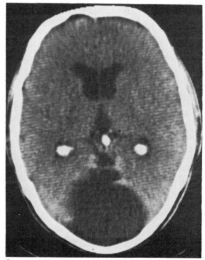

Figure 4-17 Megacisterna magna. The retrocerebellar hypodense area extends upward, but is separate from the normally positioned fourth ventricle. The cerebellopontine and suprasellar cisterns are well visualized.

A

B

C

D

E

Figure 4-18 Megacisterna magna. **A–D.** Axial CT demonstrates the large retrocerebellar cystic area extending up to the tentorium and splitting the posterior margin of the tentorium demarcated by contrast in the venous sinus. The fourth ventricle is in normal position. The ventricles are not significantly dilated. The cisterna magna may communicate with the superior cerebellar cistern, as in this patient. **E.** Coronal CT demonstrating the upward and lateral extension of the giant cisterna magna.

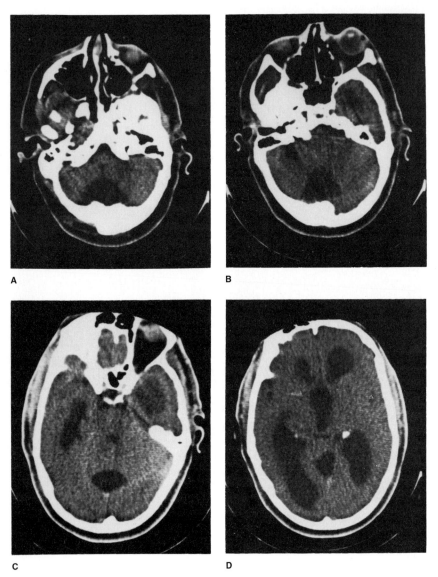

A

B

C

D

Figure 4-19 Giant cisterna magna in association with aqueduct stenosis. Axial CT **(A–D)** demonstrates a large retrocerebellar midline hypodense area. The prepontine cistern is well visualized. The fourth ventricle is not enlarged. Dilatation of the third and lateral ventricles is due to associated aqueduct stenosis.

in nonvisualization of the fourth ventricle. Even when a slitlike fourth ventricle is seen (Fig. 4-20), differentiation from Dandy-Walker variant may be difficult. Metrizamide CT cisternography following intrathecal metrizamide (Drayer 1977) will help in the diagnosis of the noncommunicating arachnoid cyst. Occasionally, a few of the arachnoid cysts communicate with the fourth ventricle or the adjacent subarachnoid space, in which metrizamide CT cisternography may be confusing. Further evaluation

by pneumoencephalography or angiography may become necessary in symptomatic patients. Delayed CT 6 to 8 hours later may demonstrate metrizamide within the cyst. This probably either represents intermittent communication of the cyst or is due to membrane transportation. The belated appearance of metrizamide in the cyst allows differentiation from an epidermoid tumor (Drayer 1977), which can also occur in the midline posterior fossa as a low-density lesion.

Figure 4-20 Retrocerebellar extraaxial cyst.   **A.** The fourth ventricle is sagittally compressed by a large low density retrocerebellar cyst.   **B.** Enlarged third and lateral ventricles. (*Continued on p. 134.*)

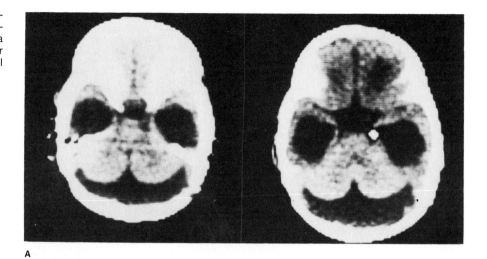

A

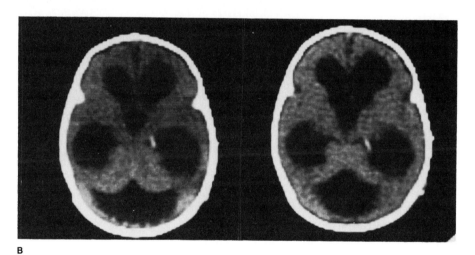

B

Ependymal cysts which are noncommunicating, CSF-containing cavities usually occur in the midline and may be located behind the fourth ventricle.

Blake (1900) indicated that evagination of the roof of the fourth ventricle into an ependyma-lined diverticulum occurs between the eighth and sixteenth week of gestation (Brocklehurst 1969). The so-called Blake's pouch may result in formation of the intraaxial supracollicular cyst. Although in Blake's original description the pouch was lined by cuboidal epithelium, case reports in the literature have used this eponym to designate cysts separate from the fourth ventricle, with different cell types forming the wall (Alvord 1962). It is conceivable that the ependyma-lined cyst located within the cerebellum but close to the normal fourth ventricle may represent a form of Blake's cyst. The extraaxial arachnoid cyst may represent a variation with a similar origin where the orifice of the cyst remains small or separated from the roof of the fourth ventricle. Since some of these cysts are recognized in adult life, their relation to past intracerebellar infarction or hematoma may not be recognized if definite clinical history is not available.

Both axial and coronal CT (Fig. 4-21) will demonstrate the cyst separate from the fourth ventricle.

Figure 4-20 *(Cont)* **C.** Angiogram, lateral view: arterial and venous phases are superimposed to demonstrate the retrocerebellar avascular mass. This angiographic finding is typical of retrocerebellar extraaxial cyst.

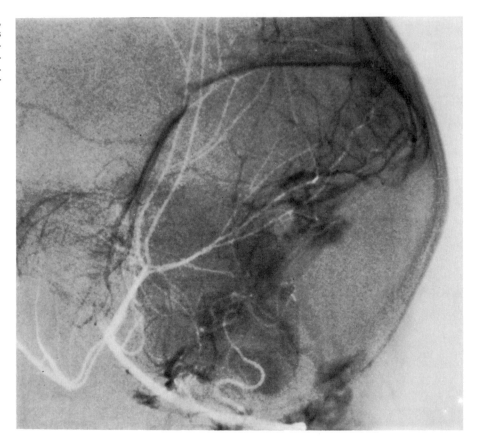

Metrizamide CT cisternography will help differentiate the ependymal cyst from Dandy-Walker variant or retrocerebellar arachnoid cyst. Ependymal cyst may represent a form of Dandy-Walker variant; where it is due to coarctation, the cyst wall, although glia- and ependyma-lined, is separated from the fourth ventricle. Controversy exists as to whether this is a form of arachnoid cyst (Harwood-Nash 1976) or a separate entity (Friede 1973; Bouch 1973). A trapped fourth ventricle (Zimmerman 1978; Scotti 1980) or a dilated fourth ventricle secondary to communicating hydrocephalus (Fig. 4-22) can be easily differentiated from the Dandy-Walker syndrome, since although the fourth ventricle may be markedly dilated, it still retains its shape.

CECT usually does not provide additional information in any of the above entities. The choice of additional studies following conventional NCCT or CECT depends on the clinical history and age of the patient as well as the resultant hydrocephalus.

The most common midline neoplasms which may occasionally be confused with relatively benign cystic conditions are cystic hemangioblastoma (Fig. 4-23) and cystic astrocytoma. They can be differentiated from the above entities following CECT.

Hydranencephaly

Virtual absence of the cerebral hemispheres except for basal parts of the occipital and sometimes the temporal poles is defined as hydranencephaly, the

Figure 4-21 Noncommunicating ependymal cysts. **A.** Axial CE-CT. **B.** Coronal CECT. Neoplasm is excluded by absence of enhancement. The fourth ventricle is compressed in the sagittal plane.

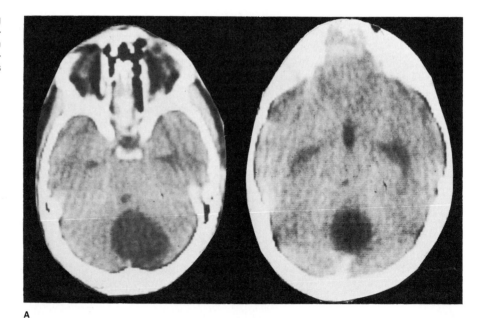

A

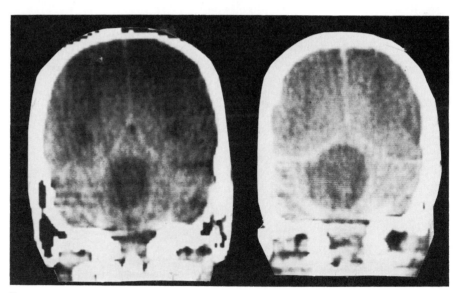

B

most severe form of porencephaly. The walls of the fluid-filled sac consist of pia-arachnoid with an inner lining of glial tissue. These infants have normal falx cerebri, basal ganglia, and infratentorial structures. The exact causative factor or factors are not known. CT demonstrates a fluid-filled cranium with visible falx cerebri and tentorium (Fig. 4-24). CECT accentuates the basal ganglia, the falx, and the tentorium. When these findings are present in a microcephalic infant, hydranencephaly can be easily diagnosed. More commonly, though, infants with hydranencephaly show increase in head circumference. In these children, the condition cannot be differentiated from severe forms of hydrocephalus

Figure 4-22 Dilated fourth ventricle secondary to a communicating hydrocephalus.

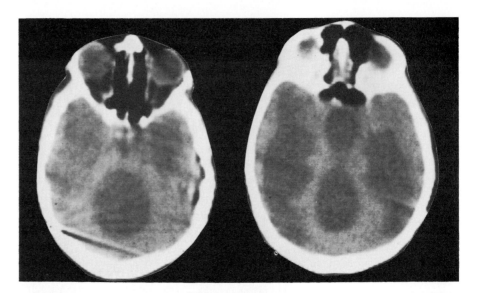

Figure 4-23 Cystic hemangioblastoma. **A.** NCCT. **B.** CECT. Enhancement of the wall of the cystic tumor and the tumor nodule confirmed by angiography and subsequent surgery.

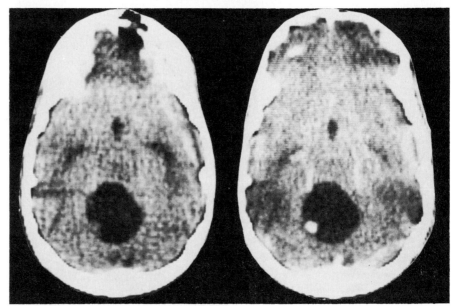

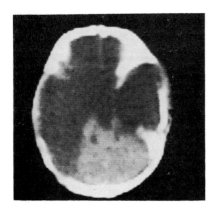

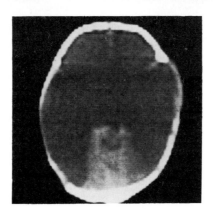

Figure 4-24 CT in hydranencephaly. There is no evidence of cortical mantle. The falx cerebri, the tentorium, and the midbrain structures appear prominent.

(Dublin 1980); it can be definitively differentiated only by angiography. Even in severe hydrocephalus, a normal but stretched complement of middle and anterior cerebral branches can be visualized on angiography; these are usually absent in hydranencephaly (Fig. 4-25). On rare occasions, CECT may show contrast within vascular structures in the sylvian fissures. Presence of contrast in the sylvian fissure is suggestive of massive hydrocephalus, although angiography is still necessary to confirm the diagnosis.

Porencephaly

Porencephaly denotes a cavitation, most often seen on CT as a focal area of low density following infarction and as a result of gliosis. Porencephaly can be due to a variety of etiological factors (Ramsey

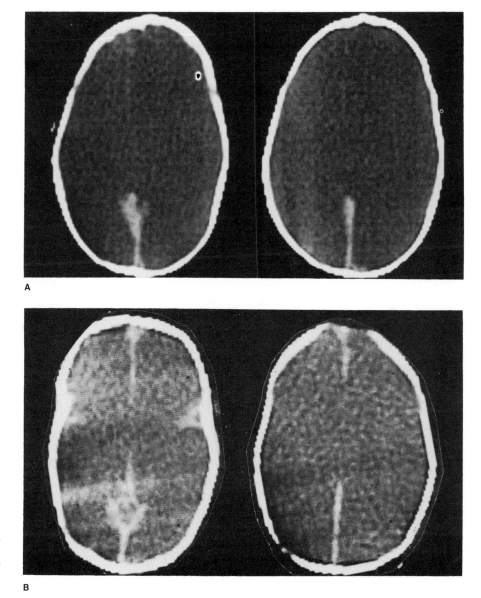

Figure 4-25 A. Hydranencephaly. **B.** Massive hydrocephalus. The CT in these two entities appears similar. (*Continued on p. 138.*)

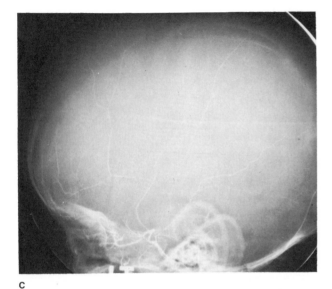

C

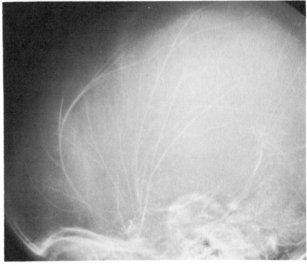

D

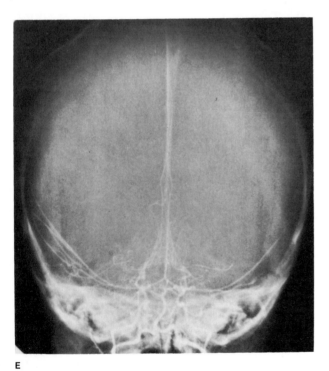

E

Figure 4-25 *(Cont.)* **C.** Angiogram in hydranencephaly: absence of middle and anterior cerebral arteries. **D.** and **E.** Angiogram in hydrocephalus. Both the anterior and middle cerebral arteries are present, although they are stretched from massive ventricular dilatation.

1977), either developmental or acquired. In adults it is almost always acquired (from trauma, hemorrhage, infection, surgery, or a vascular process). The variety seen in neonates and children is probably part of a developmental anomaly, although infection is an added factor, as shown in a few recent reports (DuBois 1979). The porencephalic cavity is often lined with ependymal cells, and the cavitation may be isolated, although more commonly it communicates with either the ventricles or the subarachnoid space. Thus in children and neonates porencephalic cavities may be due to vascular insult (*encephaloclastic*) or may be developmental (*schizencephalic*). The two variants cannot be differentiated on the basis of CT. CT is useful in demonstrating whether the lesion is focal or multiple (*multiple encephalomalacia*), involving one or both cerebral hemispheres (Fig. 4-26). In both these conditions, unlike hydranencephaly, identifiable brain parenchyma and the ventricles can be seen. Communication of the cystic cavities with the ventricular system can also be defined by CT following intraventricular or intrathecal metrizamide, depending on the clinical setting. Most often the developmental variety will show thickening of the calvarium on the side of the cyst. This is secondary to brain atrophy, giving the appearance of Dyke-Davidoff syndrome. The con-

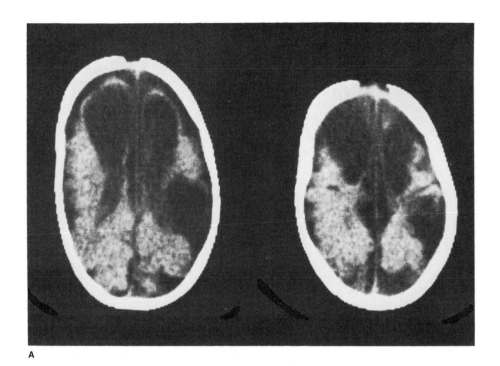

A

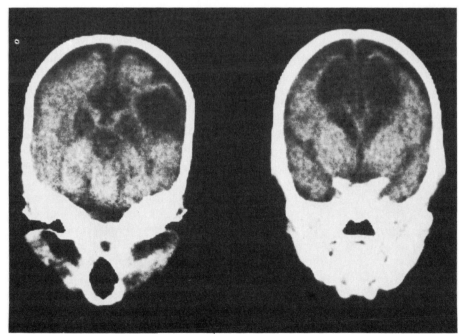

B

Figure 4-26 Encephalomalacia. Contrast-enhanced **(A)** axial and **(B)** coronal CT demonstrate ventricular dilatation with large CSF-containing spaces communicating with the dilated ventricles. The subarachnoid space is prominent, indicating an atrophic process. (*Continued on p. 140.*)

Figure 4-26 (*Cont.*) **C.** Encephalomalacia involving both temporal lobes and left frontal region. The third ventricle is not enlarged.

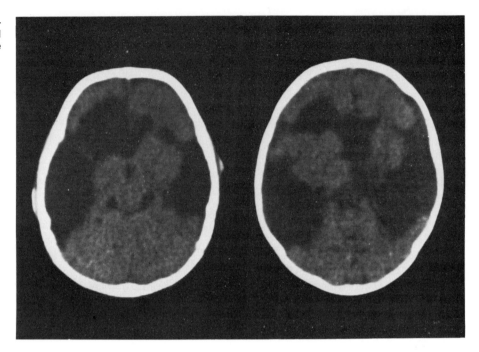

tents of the cystic cavity, whether or not communicating with the ventricles or subarachnoid space, have a density similar to the CSF within the ventricles. Absence of a vascular capsule on CECT excludes the possibility of a necrotic tumor or abscess in isolated porencephalic cavities.

Holoprosencephaly

Holoprosencephaly is the result of failure of normal development of the forebrain (prosencephalon). Failure of the forebrain to divide during the period of differentiation (from three brain vesicles to five) between the fifth and sixth week of embryogenesis results in this complex facial and craniocerebral anomaly (Harwood-Nash 1976). Depending on the severity of the forebrain anomaly, holoprosencephaly has been classified as alobar, semilobar, and lobar. In the alobar and semilobar variety, midline facial anomalies are common. In all three types the septum pellucidum and the olfactory bulb are absent. In all forms of holoprosencephaly the sylvian fissures are poorly developed and the temporal horns may not be clearly defined. Although diag-

nosis can be confirmed by ventriculography (Harwood-Nash 1976), characteristic CT findings have been described (Byrd 1977; Hayashi 1979; Derkhshan 1980).

Alobar Prosencephaly

This is the extreme form of holoprosencephaly, resulting in a single ventricle with thin cortical tissue. Some amount of cerebral tissue can be identified. On CT, alobar holoprosencephaly is seen as a large, low-density area with a thin rim of brain tissue in either the frontal or the occipital region (Fig. 4-27). The thalami are fused. The third ventricle, which cannot be identified, becomes part of the single lateral ventricle. The septum pellucidum and the interhemispheric fissure which separate the two lateral ventricles, as well as the two cerebral hemispheres, are not seen. On coronal CT, there is a single ventricle bounded by a thin rim of cortical mantle, with absence of the midline structures as well as the falx cerebri. Holoprosencephaly can be diagnosed by CT when associated facial anomalies

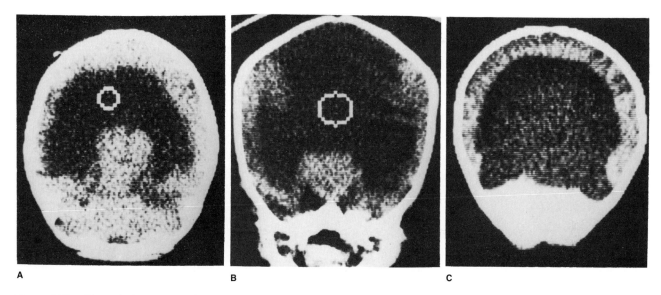

A   B   C

Figure 4-27   Alobar holoprosencephaly: **(A)** axial and **(B** and **C)** coronal CT. A single midline ventricle is noted. Absence of the interhemispheric fissure and falx in the midline is indicative of the alobar form of holoprosencephaly.

such as cleft lip and palate, microophthalmia, anophthalmia, micrognathia, or trigonocephaly are present. Skull x-rays demonstrate absence of the nasal septum, cleft palate, and trigonocephaly. Infants with alobar holoprosencephaly do not usually survive.

Semilobar Holoprosencephaly

CT in infants with semilobar holoprosencephaly differs from the alobar variety in that, although there is a single lateral ventricle, more cerebral tissue is present. An attempt at formation of the frontal and occipital horns is seen (Fig. 4-28). As in the alobar form, midline structures such as the falx cerebri, corpus callosum, and septum pellucidum are not visualized. Although the interhemispheric fissure is not seen on CT, autopsy specimens may show a midline ridging. The facial anomalies are less severe, infants presenting most commonly with cleft palate and cleft lip.

Lobar Holoprosencephaly

In this, the mildest form of holoprosencephaly, CT demonstrates (Fig. 4-29) well-formed lateral ventri-

cles and cerebral hemisphere. The ventricles appear dilated. There is a distinct third ventricle. The roof of the frontal horn appears flat or squared off, in both axial and coronal CT. The septum pellucidum may or may not be present. The falx cerebri, as well as the corpus callosum, may not be present. The sylvian fissures are absent. In the presence of facial anomalies, it is usually possible to differentiate lobar from the semilobar form of holoprosencephaly. When facial anomalies are not seen, differentiation of alobar or semilobar forms of holoprosencephaly from severe forms of hydrocephalus or hydranencephaly may become difficult. However, in both hydranencephaly and severe hydrocephalus the falx cerebri is present (Hayashi 1979); this is not seen in holoprosencephaly.

Lobar holoprosencephaly can be differentiated from simple absence of the septum pellucidum as well as septooptic dysplasia by the absence of the falx cerebri in lobar holoprosencephaly and its presence in the latter two conditions. The CT findings of septooptic dysplasia are detailed separately in the next section.

Occasionally bilateral subdural hygromas may be confused with alobar or semilobar holoprosencephaly (Byrd 1977). Clinical findings usually help

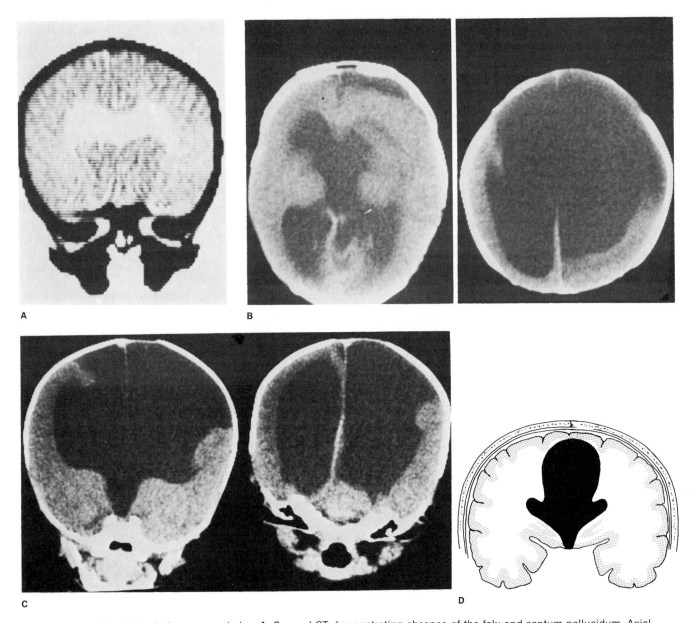

Figure 4-28   Semilobar holoprosencephaly.   **A.** Coronal CT demonstrating absence of the falx and septum pellucidum. Axial **(B)** and coronal **(C)** CT demonstrate semilobar holoprosencephaly in another child. Note absence of cortical tissue and partial absence of falx. There is no evidence of temporal horns or of sylvian fissure.   **D.** Diagrammatic representation of alobar and semilobar holoprosencephaly in which the falx is absent.

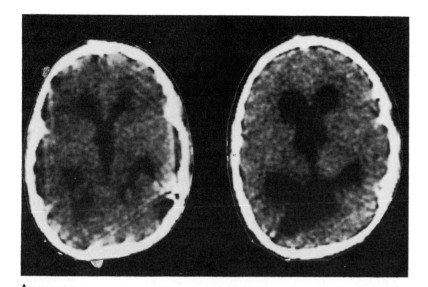

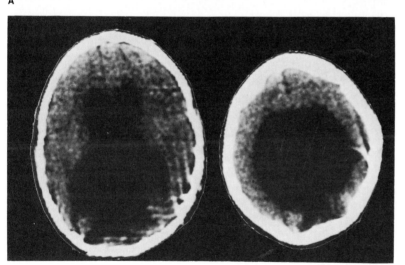

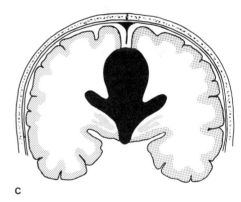

Figure 4-29 Lobar holoprosencephaly. **A.** and **B.** Axial CT demonstrates presence of a third ventricle and well-defined frontal and occipital horns. **C.** Diagrammatic representation in lobar holoprosencephaly.

in the differentiation. In most of the conditions which need to be differentiated from the various forms of holoprosencephaly, the presence of coexisting facial anomalies helps in the CT diagnosis. When no facial anomalies are found, angiography is the next most useful diagnostic modality. In all forms of holoprosencephaly, unlike hydranencephaly, the middle and anterior cerebral arteries are present. In bilateral subdural hygromas, the cerebral vascular architecture is normal but compressed, whereas in holoprosencephaly the vascular architecture has a characteristic appearance (Harwood-Nash 1976).

Septooptic Dysplasia

Septooptic dysplasia is a rare congenital anomaly first described by deMorsier (1956). The anomaly involves anterior midline structures of the brain and consists in absence of the septum pellucidum, primitive optic ventricle, and hypoplasia of the optic nerves, chiasma, and infundibulum, resulting in a prominent chiasmatic recess. On physical examination there is hypoplasia of one or both optic discs and blindness with wandering nystagmus. Hypothalamic-hypopituitary disorders are frequently associated with septooptic dysplasia, the most common being diabetes insipidus. The malformation probably occurs about the fourth to sixth week of gestation. Many of the features seen in septooptic dysplasia appear to be a minor form of lobar holoprosencephaly (Harwood-Nash 1976). Neuroradiological diagnosis has been based on pneumoencephalographic and plain film findings and associated clinical presentation (Harwood-Nash 1976). Very few CT descriptions in septooptic dysplasia have been reported recently (Manelfe 1979a; Byrd 1977; Bush 1978; O'Dwyer 1980). CT demonstrates some or all of the following features (Fig. 4-30). There is absence of the septum pellucidum. The ventricles are enlarged, especially the lateral ventricles. The temporal horns are normal and may not be visualized. The anteromedial aspect of the frontal horns is flat or squared off in both axial and coronal CT. These findings are similar to those seen in lobar holoprosencephaly. With high-resolution CT the

atrophic optic nerve can be demonstrated in both axial and coronal CT. The suprasellar and chiasmatic cisterns are prominent. On coronal CT, beaking of the floor of the lateral ventricles similar to the appearance seen in Chiari II malformation and lobar holoprosencephaly has been noted (Manelfe 1979a). When septooptic dysplasia is associated with diabetes insipidus, enlargement of the pituitary stalk and infundibulum can occur (Manelfe 1979b). This is best seen after contrast enhancement.

Diagnosis of septooptic dysplasia may thus be confirmed by CT examination in the presence of appropriate clinical findings, without the need for invasive studies.

Cavum Septi Pellucidi and Cavum Vergae

The two leaves of the septum pellucidum which separate the lateral ventricle usually fuse in the neonatal period, around the second month. In the majority of neonates and occasionally in older children as well as adults, nonfusion of the two leaves results in a potential space, the cavum septi pellucidi, or cavity of the septum pellucidum. Its posterior extension results in the cavum Vergae. Most often they communicate with the ventricular system

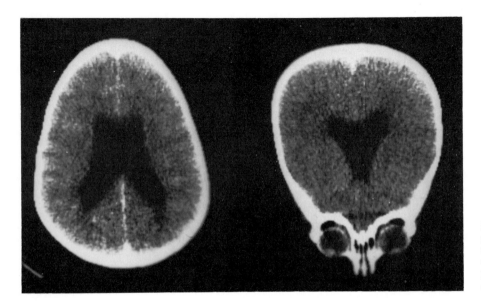

Figure 4-30 Septooptic dysplasia. Axial (*left*) and coronal (*right*) CT demonstrates mildly dilated ventricles with absent septum pellucidum. Normally the suprasellar cistern is prominent.

through the interventricular foramina. Cavum septi pellucidi and cavum Vergae are thus developmental anomalies without any clinical significance, common in children and found in 12 to 15 percent of adults (Shaw 1969; Nakano 1981). Their appearance has been well documented by CT and other diagnostic studies (Berkowitz 1939; Dandy 1931; Dyke 1936; Lowman 1948; Harwood-Nash 1977; Byrd 1978a). Cavum septi pellucidi is seen on CT (Fig. 4-31) as a CSF-containing space separated by thin septi from the frontal horns of the two lateral ventricles. Even though the septi are thin, they are well visualized because of the density of the CSF. The walls are parallel, extending posteriorly up to the foramen of Monro. Unlike the situation in agenesis of the corpus callosum, the lateral walls are not formed by the callosal bundles.

Cavum Veli Interpositi

Cavum veli interpositi, or interventricular cistern, is dilatation of the normal cistern of the velum in-terpositum (cistern of the transverse sinus) (Williams 1975). It is situated over the roof of the third ventricle and communicates with the quadrigeminal cistern. It is frequently seen in infants and children (Byrd 1978a; Harwood-Nash 1977) and has been observed more commonly than cavum septi pellucidi or cavum Vergae (Strother 1978). It has been well documented both by pneumoencephalography (Picard 1976; Harwood-Nash 1976; Amundsen 1978) and by CT (Harwood-Nash 1977; Byrd 1978a). Cavum veli interpositi on CT (Fig. 4-32) usually has a triangular appearance and is situated between the bodies of the lateral ventricles, with its base directed posteriorly. Occasionally it may have a "mitre hat" appearance due to confluence of the adjacent quadrigeminal cistern.

Cyst of the Cavum Septi Pellucidi

Sometimes the cavum septi pellucidi, instead of having a CSF density with parallel walls, may appear distended, with its lateral walls outwardly con-

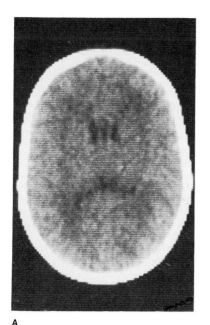
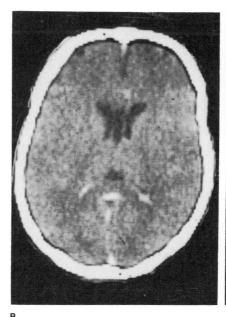
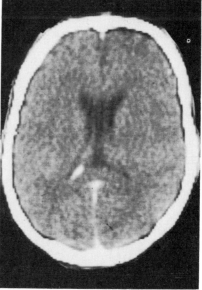

A   B

Figure 4-31   Cava septi pellucidi et Vergae.   **A.** The two frontal horns are separated by a linear CSF-containing cavum septi pellucidi. This is a common finding in infants.   **B.** Axial CT in an adult with cava septi pellucidi et Vergae. The CSF-containing midline space extends posteriorly beyond the foramen of Monro.

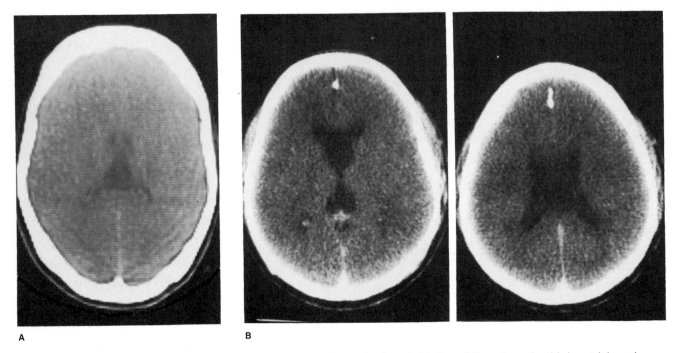

A   B

Figure 4-32   **A.** Cavum veli interpositi. A triangular CSF-containing region is noted in the midline above the third ventricle and between the two lateral ventricles. This is compared with **(B)** cavum septi pellucidi et Vergae.

vex. Cystic dilatation of the septum pellucidum is presumed to be secondary to occlusion at the foramen of Monro. Most often this may be an incidental finding, although occasionally the condition may be symptomatic. The symptoms usually are similar to those of the patient presenting with intermittent obstruction of the foramen of Monro, as can occur with colloid cyst of the third ventricle. There are no criteria which allow a distinction by CT between a dilated cavum septi pellucidi and a cyst of the septum pellucidum (Shaw 1969) or between a symptomatic and a nonsymptomatic cyst. Cystic dilatation of the cavity of the septum pellucidum commonly involves the cavum Vergae. Pathological or symptomatic cyst of the cavity of the septum pellucidum results in dilatation of the lateral ventricles, due to intermittent or complete obstruction of the interventricular foramina, and may require surgical intervention for relief of symptoms (Heiskanen 1973; Berkowitz 1939). On CECT the wall of the bulging cyst is well demarcated by the enhanced choroid plexus (Fig. 4-33) (Cowley 1979). Coronal

CT is useful in demonstrating the cyst associated with enlargement of the lateral ventricles and a normal third ventricle. In symptomatic patients the CT findings can be confirmed either by CT metrizamide ventriculography or by pneumoencephalography, thus differentiating the cyst from atresia or inflammatory obstruction of the interventricular foramina.

Cyst of the cavum septi pellucidi may be mistaken for agenesis of the corpus callosum or arachnoid cyst. In agenesis of the corpus callosum, the interposed third ventricle is separated from the lateral ventricles by the longitudinal columns of the corpus callosum as well as the infolded cerebral tissue. This results in wide separation of the frontal horns and body of the two lateral ventricles, both on axial and on coronal CT. Interhemispheric arachnoid cyst, when small and close to the corpus callosum, may be mistaken for a cyst of the septum pellucidum. The two conditions can be differentiated by coronal CT. Interhemispheric cysts are rare and are commonly associated with partial or complete absence of the corpus callosum (Solt 1980).

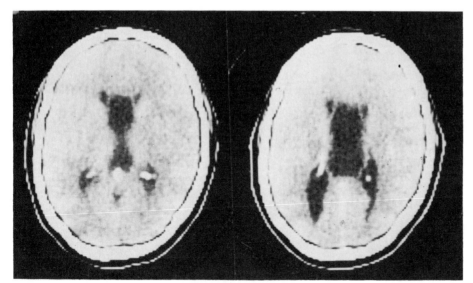

A

Figure 4-33 Cyst of cavum septi pellucidi. Occasionally, due to non-communication, cavum septi pellucidi may become cystic. **A.** Contrast-enhanced CT in axial plane demonstrates the septum pellucidum cyst demarcated by the choroid plexus and the wall of the septum. **B.** Anteroposterior brow-up view during pneumopolytomography: the walls of the cysts (arrow) encroaching on the lateral ventricle demarcates the cyst of the septum pellucidum.

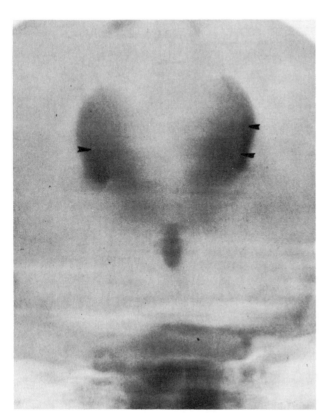

B

Agenesis of Corpus Callosum

The corpus callosum is the transverse commissure connecting the two cerebral hemispheres. The corpus callosum begins to form around the twelfth week of gestation and is fully developed by 18 to 20 weeks. The fibers develop in a medial and longitudinal direction from front to back. The normal anatomy of the corpus callosum is better defined by axial and coronal CT (Fig. 4-34) than by other diagnostic studies (Wing 1977). Absence of the corpus callosum may be complete or partial and may be developmental or acquired. A variety of causes such as genetic, metabolic, and mechanical factors involving the commissural plate early in development have been implicated to explain the defect. Agenesis of the corpus callosum may occur as an isolated lesion or as part of another craniocerebral anomaly, such as the Dandy-Walker cyst. Byrd (1978a) has classified the spectrum of anomalies and variations associated with this dysgenesis (Table 4-2) and the association with other malformations.

CT findings are characteristic and well defined in both axial and coronal CT (Fig. 4-35) (Byrd 1978a; Lynn 1980). CT in the axial plane normally demonstrates wide separation of the frontal horns. The

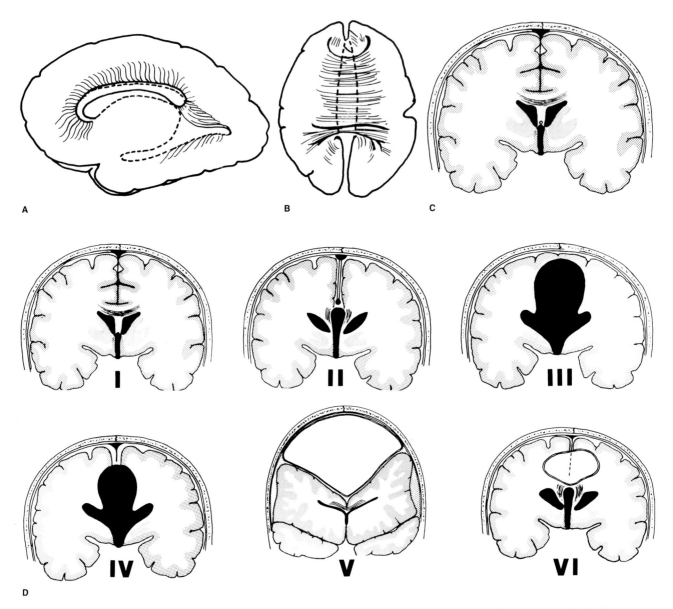

Figure 4-34 **(A)** Sagittal, **(B)** axial, and **(C)** coronal diagrams demonstrating the normal appearance of the corpus callosum. The internal cerebral vein lies over the roof of the third ventricle, separated from the corpus callosum by the medial walls of the lateral ventricles and the septum pellucidum. **D.** Diagrams demonstrating anomalies associated with the corpus callosum: (I) normal appearance, (II) agenesis of corpus callosum, (III) alobar holoprosencephaly, (IV) lobar holoprosencephaly, (V) intradural cyst, and (VI) agenesis of corpus callosum with interhemispheric arachnoid cyst.

Table 4-2   Anomalies Associated with Dysgenesis of Corpus Callosum

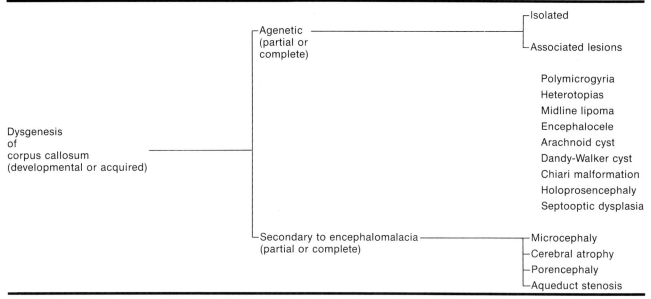

Polymicrogyria
Heterotopias
Midline lipoma
Encephalocele
Arachnoid cyst
Dandy-Walker cyst
Chiari malformation
Holoprosencephaly
Septooptic dysplasia

Modified from Byrd et al: *J Can Assoc Radiol* **20:** 108-112, 1978.

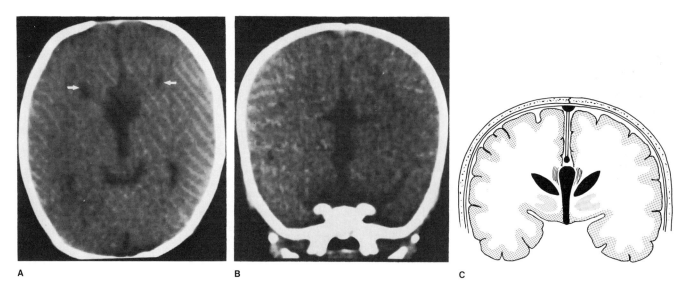

A   B   C

Figure 4-35   Agenesis of the corpus callosum.   **A.** CT in axial section.   **B.** Coronal view. The midline third ventricle extends between the lateral venticles. Characteristically the two frontal horns are widely separated (arrows).   **C.** Diagrammatic representation.

frontal horns also appear narrow, unless there is dilatation secondary to hydrocephalus or associated with other anomalies. The bodies of the lateral ventricles and frontal horns have sharply angled lateral beaks. This is better defined in the coronal CT. Because of the long callosal bundles running longitudinally, the medial walls of the bodies of the lateral ventricles are concave (Fig. 4-36). The occipital horns may show relative dilatation when compared to the width of the bodies of the lateral ventricles. The most important CT finding is interposition of the third ventricle between the bodies of the lateral ventricles. The third ventricle usually appears wider than normal. The height of the interposed third ventricle may vary, sometimes extending upward between the interhemispheric fissure to the vertex.

Differentiation from cavum septi pellucidi and cyst of the cavum septi pellucidi and cavum Vergae

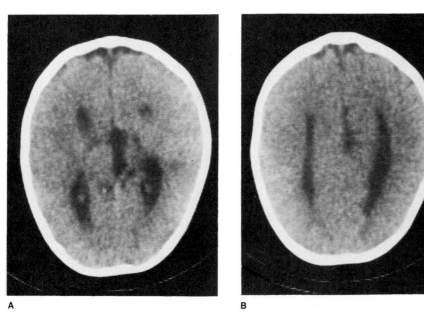

A

B

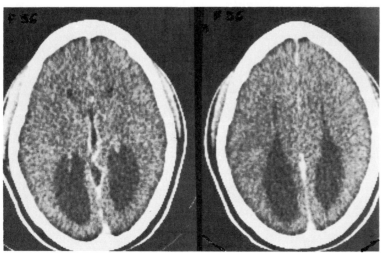

C

Figure 4-36 Agenesis of corpus callosum. **A.** and **B.** CT in axial plane. The bodies of the lateral ventricles are widely separated by the longitudinal rearrangement of the corpus callosum fibers, resulting in the characteristic concave configuration of the bodies of the lateral ventricles. **C.** Contrast-enhanced axial CT in another case of agenesis of corpus callosum demonstrating separation of the internal cerebral veins by the upward displacement of the third ventricle and the characteristic dilated occipital horns.

is possible in most instances when both axial and coronal CT are performed; a distinct separation of the third ventricle from the cavity or cyst of the septum pellucidi and cavum Vergae can be demonstrated. With a cavity or cyst of the septum pelludicum and cavum Vergae the corpus callosum is normally situated both in axial and in coronal CT,

unlike agenesis of the corpus callosum, in which the frontal horn and bodies of the lateral ventricles are separated by the callosal bundles. Rarely, agenesis of the corpus callosum may be associated with an interhemispheric cyst (Solt 1980). On axial CT the appearance may be similar to agenesis of the corpus callosum (Fig. 4-37). Direct coronal CT is

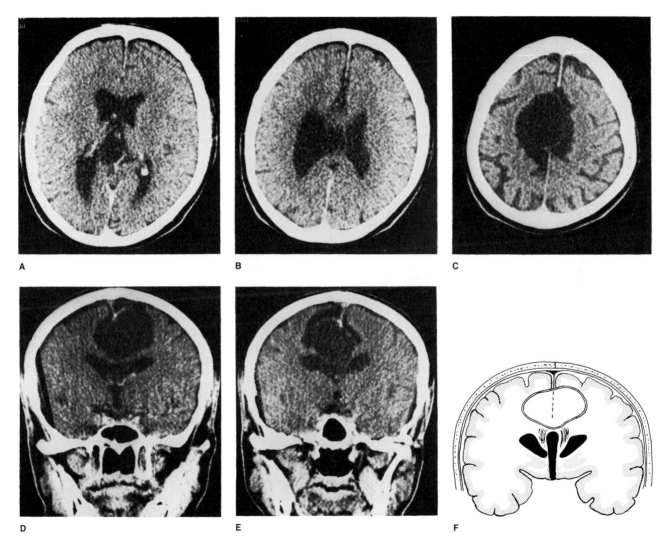

A   B   C

D   E   F

Figure 4-37 Partial agenesis of corpus callosum associated with interhemispheric arachnoid cyst. **A, B,** and **C.** Axial CT demonstrating agenesis of the corpus callosum with a midline hypodense area. **D.** Coronal CT demonstrating the cyst separated from the roof of the lateral ventricles in its anterior position. **E.** Posteriorly the cyst is contiguous with the lateral ventricles. This is due to partial agenesis, which primarily involves the posterior component of the corpus callosum. **F.** Diagrammatic representation. *(Courtesy of Dr. TerBrugge; previously published in Journal of Neurosurgery, vol. 52, 1980.)*

helpful in demonstrating the cyst separate from the roof of the third ventricle. In rare situations there may be difficulty in demonstrating the cyst wall separate from the roof of the third ventricle; metrizamide CT cisternogram then becomes useful. Computed tomography in both axial and direct coronal plane is also helpful in distinguishing porencephalic cavities, when they are close to or communicating with the ventricular system and associated with agenesis of the corpus callosum. Very rarely, a large cyst of the dura (Fig. 4-38) or an intraventricular arachnoid cyst may mimic agenesis of the corpus callosum. Diagnosis can often be made following metrizamide CT cisternography but rarely may require angiography.

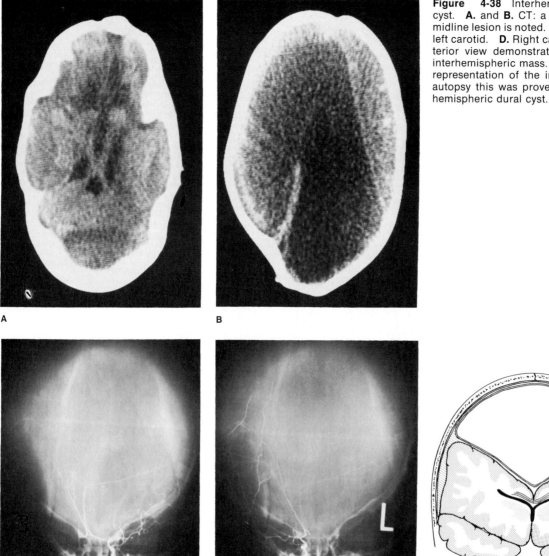

Figure 4-38 Interhemispheric dural cyst. **A.** and **B.** CT: a large low-density midline lesion is noted. **C.** Angiography: left carotid. **D.** Right carotid, anteroposterior view demonstrating an avascular interhemispheric mass. **E.** Diagrammatic representation of the intradural cyst. At autopsy this was proven to be an interhemispheric dural cyst.

A

B

C

D

E

Lipoma of Corpus Callosum

The corpus callosum is the most common site of this fatty tumor of maldevelopmental origin. It is caused by incorporation of the mesodermal adipose tissue into the neural tube during its closure, between the third and fifth weeks of fetal gestation. Intracranial lipomas, although more common in the anterior portion of the corpus callosum, may also be seen in other areas, most commonly close to the midline cisterns. The location of the tumor relative to the midsagittal plane is probably related to the stage of fetal development (Zimmerman RA 1979). Intracranial lipomas have been reported in the suprasellar region, the quadrigeminal cisterns, and the crural cisterns as well as the cerebellopontine-angle cistern (Fukui 1977) (Fig. 4-39).

Lipoma of the corpus callosum is occasionally associated with agenesis of the corpus callosum, another midline dysraphic condition. Calcification

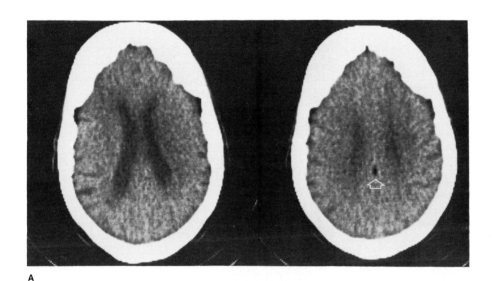

A

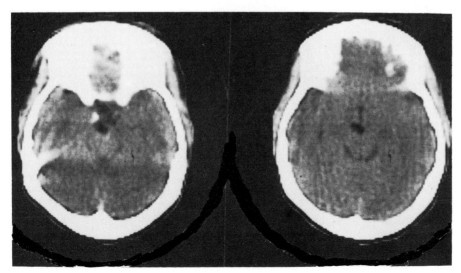

B

Figure 4-39 A. Intracranial lipoma: incidental lipoma (arrow) in posterior aspect of corpus callosum. **B.** Nonsymptomatic lipoma in another patient located in the prepontine cistern.

of the fatty tumor is infrequent and probably depends of the size of the tumor. It is seen most often in large tumors located in the corpus callosum but not at other sites (Zimmerman RA 1979; Faerber 1979; Fukui 1977). When calcification occurs, it is curvilinear and mural in location, although atypical calcification can rarely be encountered (Fig. 4-40). CT diagnosis is characteristic because of the low attenuation values indicative of fat within the tumor. In large lipomas involving the corpus callosum, the anterior cerebral artery is incorporated within the fatty tumor and on angiography is dilated, having the appearance of an elongated fusiform aneurysm. This can be demonstrated within the fatty tumor on CECT (Zimmerman RA 1979). The tumor does not show any change in density on CECT. As with agenesis of the corpus callosum, in which the third ventricle is interposed between the frontal horns and bodies of the lateral ventricles, lipoma of the corpus callosum is seen as a low-density mass between the two lateral ventricles, with the third ventricle situated below the tumor. This can be characteristically seen in coronal CT (Fig. 4-41). Detection of agenesis of the corpus callosum or lipoma of the corpus callosum by CT may be incidental to evaluation of a nonrelated neurological deficit. A history of seizures is the most frequent clinical presentation in patients with agenesis of the corpus callosum or lipoma (Gastaut 1980).

Differentiation of agenesis of the corpus callosum from noncalcified lipoma of the corpus cal-

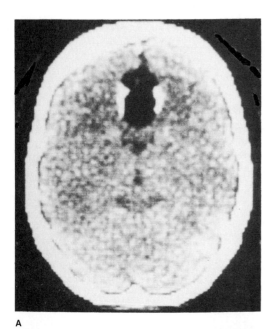

A

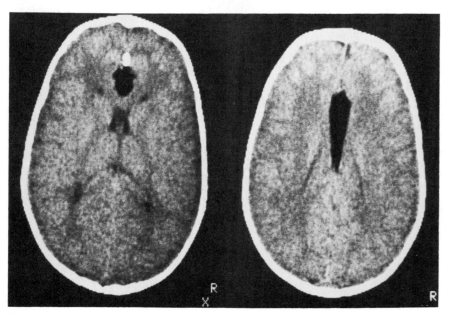

B   C

Figure 4-40 Lipoma of corpus callosum. **A.** The fatty tumor is located anteriorly in the genu of the corpus callosum, with typical calcification in the periphery of the tumor. **B.** Another patient with lipoma of the corpus callosum with minimal calcification. **C.** A third patient with lipoma involving the whole extent of the corpus callosum.

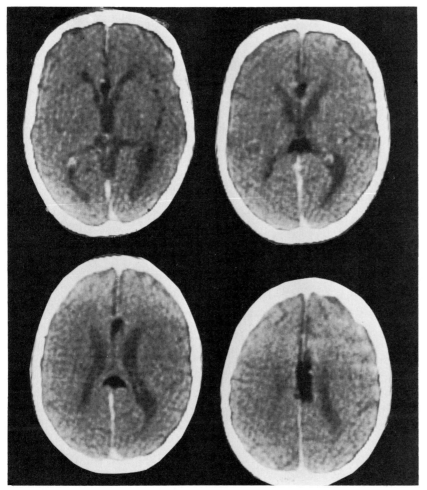

A

Figure 4-41 Noncalcified lipoma of the corpus callosum in **(A)** axial sections and **(B)** coronal sections.

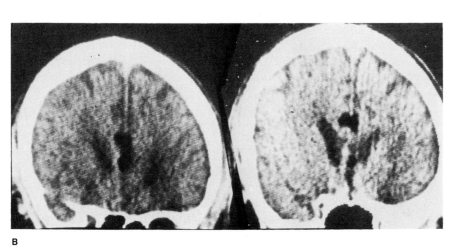

B

losum is usually easy because of the characteristic difference in the CT numbers of fat and CSF, as well as the appearance in axial and coronal CT. Rarely, because of their location, lipomas may result in hydrocephalus, necessitating a shunting procedure (Kazner 1980).

Megalencephaly

Megalencephaly, or enlargement of the head, can be symmetrical, involving both cerebral hemispheres, or, very rarely, unilateral. In symmetrical enlargement of the head, the head circumference is above the ninety-fifth percentile or may show rapid increase in size. A variety of disorders can result in symmetrical enlargement of the head, such as obstructive or communicating hydrocephalus, intracranial neoplasm, tuberous sclerosis, spongy sclerosis (Canavan's disease), Tay-Sach's disease, and Hurler's disease. Excluding the above entities as the causative factor, there remains a rare malformative disorder in which there is symmetrical or unilateral enlargement of the head due to a developmental anomaly. Children with this disorder usually present with seizures, delayed milestones, and mental retardation. The etiology is not known, although the developmental anomaly is presumed to be caused by a defect of cell migration about the third month of gestation (Townsend 1975).

Very few reports have appeared in the CT literature (Fitz 1978b; Michaels 1978). The CT findings in symmetrical enlargement of the head of developmental origin consist in increase in size of the lateral ventricles compared to normal children. The temporal horns are not commonly enlarged. The enlarged lateral ventricles are presumed to be secondary to a cerebral atrophic process. CT diagnosis of megalencephaly is by a process of exclusion of other known pathological processes.

Megalencephaly can, rarely, be unilateral (Fitz 1978b; Townsend 1975); the whole hemisphere or a lobe may be involved. On CT the findings suggest an enlarged hemisphere, occasionally obliterating the ventricles but more commonly associated with dilatation of the ventricles. No change in density is seen following contrast enhancement. Absence of the insula, with a smooth hemispheric surface, is seen at autopsy. This can occasionally be appreciated on high-resolution CT. Even in the presence of these CT findings, the possibility of a neoplasm or nonneoplastic hamartoma such as occurs in tuberous sclerosis cannot be excluded. Angiography or radionuclide brain scan do not provide additional information.

Lissencephaly or Agyria

In lissencephaly there is a lack of gyral formation. The sylvian fissures are wide, with absence of operculation of the insula, resulting in a smooth hemispheric surface lacking primary fissures. The basic mechanism is interruption of neuronal migration from the ventricular matrix to the cortical surface. Since gyral formation occurs between the twenty-sixth and twenty-eighth week of gestation, the anomaly represents cessation of development at that stage.

Children with lissencephaly have microcephaly and micrognathia. They usually present with seizures, psychomotor retardation, decerebrate posture, and failure to thrive. Most children die before 2 years.

Very few cases with well-documented clinical, pathological, and CT findings have been reported (Ohno 1979; Garcia 1978) (Fig. 4-42). CT demonstrates wide sylvian fissures and subarachnoid space. Absence of sulcal pattern over the surface and moderate ventricular enlargement are commonly seen. Differentiation from cerebral atrophy is based on the absence of sulci, with dilated ventricles and sylvian fissures. Angiography has been performed in a few cases but does not provide additional information. A combination of CT and clinical findings should suggest the diagnosis.

Meningoencephalocele

Herniation of glial tissue as well as meninges through a congenital defect in the skull vault results

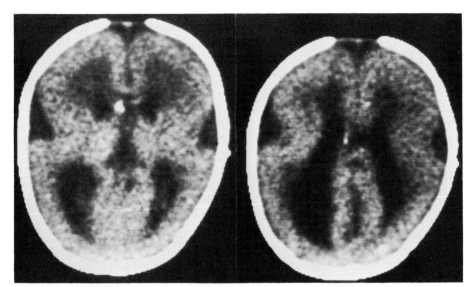

A

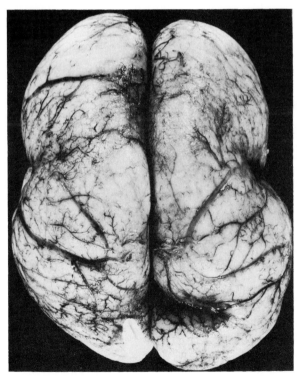

B

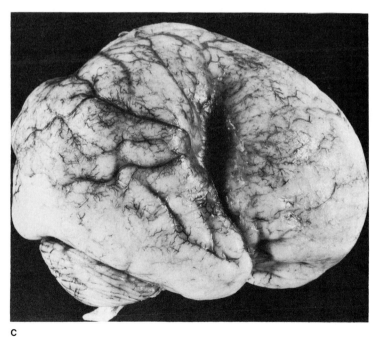

C

Figure 4-42 Lissencephaly. **A.** CT demonstrates absence of gyri, prominent subarachnoid space and sylvian fissures, and moderate ventricular enlargement and punctate calcification of the ependymal lining of ventricle. Autopsy specimen of the same case: **(B)** dorsal and **(C)** lateral views showing the prominent sylvian groove and absence of gyral folds. *(Courtesy of Dr. Powell Williams.)* *(Continued on p. 158.)*

Figure 4-42(D) *(Cont.)* Another case of lissencephaly, with calcification in the region of the caudate nucleus.

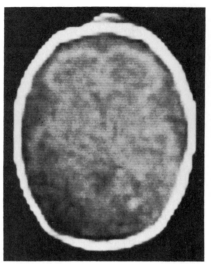
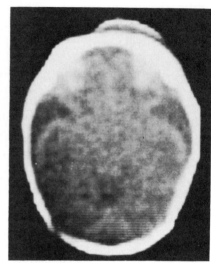

in meningoencephalocele. The contents of the herniated sac may be meninges containing CSF, when the anomaly is defined as *meningocele;* when the contents include brain tissue, it is called an *encephalocele.* This congenital anomaly probably results from a defect in the overlying mesoderm (Emery 1970). Meningoencephalocele may also be acquired, following trauma or surgery. Meningoencephaloceles are midline anomalies, most often involving the occipital region. A variety of classifications have been proposed (Suwanwela 1972; Gisselsson 1947), depending on the site of the cranial defect. Byrd (1978*b*) has modified the classification and described the common associated congenital anomalies of the brain. The encephalocele may be of varying size; sometimes the whole cerebellum may be present within the herniated sac. A large occipital encephalocele may cause hydrocephalus. Frontal encephaloceles produce facial deformities. Evaluation of these anomalies by CT is useful in determining the precise location, extent, and contents of the sac (Fig. 4-43). Encephalocele, although rarely, may also occur at the base of the skull (Manelfe 1978; Byrd 1978*b*; Sakoda 1979). Diagnosis of the basal encephalocele may be more difficult. It may be mistaken for a polyp or soft-tissue mass in the nasal cavity or the nasopharynx. Occult clinical signs which suggest possible basal encephalocele include broad nasal bridge, hypertelorism, wide bitemporal diame-

ter, and, rarely, intermittent CSF rhinorrhea. CT in the routine axial plane may not show the bony defect if the cranial defect is small. Diagnosis requires high-resolution CT in both axial and coronal planes (Fig. 4-44). CT is better than pluridirectional tomography. Metrizamide CT cisternography provides ad-

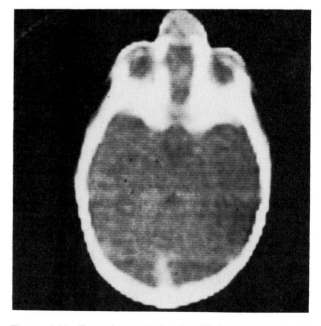

Figure 4-43 Frontal encephalocele: CT demonstrates a soft tissue mass associated with a bony defect at the nasal bridge.

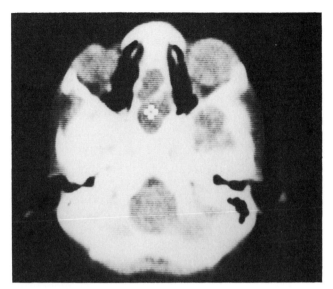

A

Figure 4-44 Ethmoidal encephalocele: CT in the axial **(A)** and coronal **(B)** views demonstrates a bony defect involving the cribriform plate with a soft tissue mass within it. Antero-posterior **(C)** and axial **(D)** polytomography demonstrating the bony defect due to the ethmoidal encephalocele.

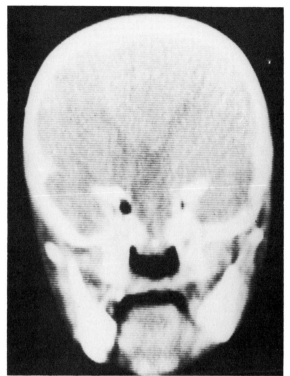

B

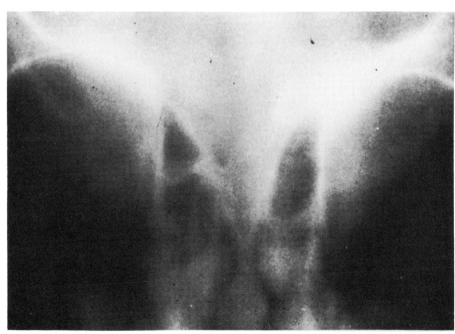

C

(Continued on p. 160.)

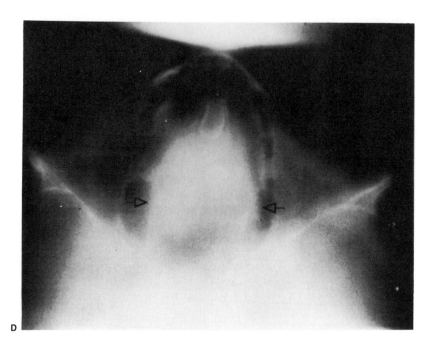

D

ditional information in demonstrating a small encephalocele as well as encroachment of the subarachnoid space into the sac (Manelfe 1978). Once diagnosis of an encephalocele rather than a meningocele has been confirmed by CT, depending on the size of the cranial defect and its contents, angiography may be necessary prior to surgery in evaluating the relationship of the intracranial vasculature to the herniated brain tissue.

DISORDERS OF HISTOGENESIS

Tuberous Sclerosis or Bourneville's Disease

Tuberous sclerosis is a heredofamilial disease with the clinical triad of adenoma sebaceum, seizures, and mental retardation. The condition was first described by von Recklinghausen, and a more detailed description was provided by Bourneville in 1880. The disease is characterized by hamartomas involving virtually all organs, although not commonly in the same patient. Hamartomas in the brain are pres-

ent in every case of tuberous sclerosis. The disease is autosomal-dominant but may skip generations. Sporadic cases thus are common. Occasionally the disease may not be clinically manifested until later in life. Since mental retardation and seizures are the earliest features, definitive diagnosis is useful for genetic counseling of the patient's family. CT, being noninvasive, provides a useful modality for this evaluation.

Intracranially the most common site of the hamartomas is the cerebrum, although the cerebellum, medulla, and spinal cord may be involved (Critcley 1932). The hamartomas may vary in size and number. The vast majority lie adjacent to the CSF pathway, predominantly along the ventricular surface as subependymal nodules close to the foramen of Monro. Obstructive hydrocephalus may result from the location of the hamartomas and change in size. Ten to fifteen percent of the hamartomas have been reported to undergo malignant changes (Fitz 1974; Kapp 1967). These neoplasms are relatively benign, slow-growing, and histologically classified as giant-cell astrocytomas. Malignant change of the hamartomas is common in the subependymal nodules, most commonly in the nodules closest to the foramen of Monro.

CT Findings

CT findings in tuberous sclerosis are characteristic (Gomez 1975; Lee 1978). On NCCT the subependymal nodules appear as rounded projections of varying size. They are denser than the rest of the brain parenchyma. Calcification is fairly common, even faint calcification being well defined by CT (Fig. 4-45). Noncalcified hamartomas within the parenchyma may be difficult to demonstrate. There is normally no change in density following contrast enhancement. When malignant changes have occurred there is significant enhancement (Fig. 4-46). Any change in density following contrast enhancement should arouse suspicion of malignant changes. A few patients will show mild to moderate enlargement of the ventricles with prominence of the cortical sulci, indicative of cerebral atrophy. Thickening of the diploic spaces may also be noted occasionally. This is usually seen in patients who have had severe mental retardation and seizures for a long time. The thickened calvarium may be the result of tuberous sclerosis or, more likely, the effect of prolonged Dilantin medication (McCrea 1980).

The differentiation of the noncalcified subependymal and cortical hamartomas of tuberous sclerosis from cerebral heterotopias may occasionally be difficult. Heterotopias are projections of normal brain tissue in areas where they should not exist. On CT they are seen as projections along the ventricular surface, more commonly along the medial wall. They usually have a density similar to that of the adjacent brain parenchyma and do not enhance on CECT. Presence of associated intracranial congenital anomalies and absence of associated clinical findings of tuberous sclerosis usually help in the diagnosis.

In children below 2 years, calcific nodules in the periventricular area as well as in the parenchyma due to tuberous sclerosis may be difficult to differentiate from an intrauterine infectious process such as toxoplasmosis or cytomegalic inclusion disease. Cerebral atrophy and microcephaly are more commonly associated with these two conditions. Differentiation from a vascular malformation with calcification of the vessels may be difficult when only a few calcific areas of parenchymal density are seen on the same side. CECT usually will show enhancement.

Rarely, when there is only a single nodule in the region of the third ventricle, differentiation from a colloid cyst can be difficult. Most colloid cysts have a higher density than the nodule of tuberous sclerosis. The hamartomas of tuberous sclerosis do not increase in density on CECT unless malignant change has occurred. Similar diagnostic problems

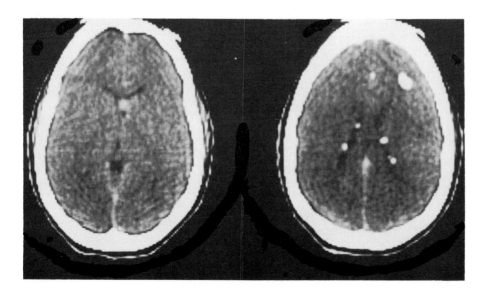

Figure 4-45 Tuberous sclerosis. Calcified hamartomas noted within the parenchyma as well as along the ependymal surface of the ventricles are characteristic.

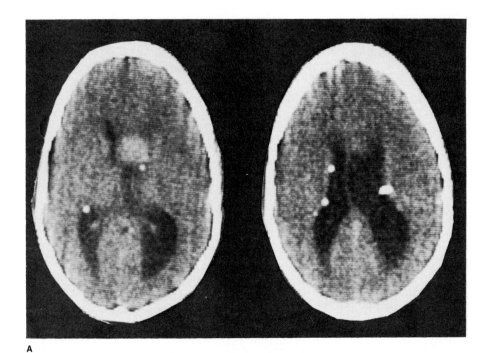

A

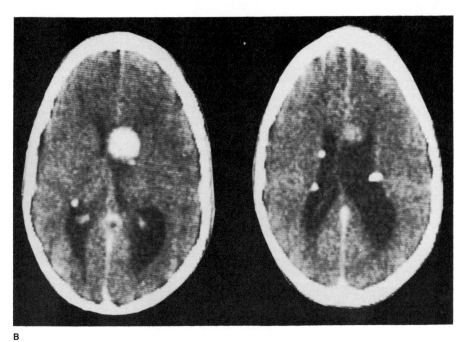

B

Figure 4-46   Malignant transformation in hamartoma of tuberous sclerosis. CT before contrast **(A)** and after contrast **(B)** demonstrates intense enhancement of the large tumor located in the region of the foramen of Monro. This is the typical appearance and location of giant cell astrocytoma.

may also occur when a single nodule enhances on CECT. Differentiation from other varieties of neoplasm such as an ependymoma or other types of glioma is not possible. In these situations other diagnostic studies, short of surgical proof, do not prove helpful.

Sturge-Weber Syndrome

This syndrome, also known as encephalotrigeminal angiomatosis, was first described in 1879. It consists of port-wine nevus of the face, along the first branch of the trigeminal nerve, mental retardation, seizure disorder, leptomeningeal angiomatosis, glaucoma, hemiatrophy, and hemiparesis. The facial nevus and the leptomeningeal angiomatosis are usually on the same side as the cerebral atrophy. Calcification, which starts beneath the leptomeningeal angiomatosis, is rarely seen on routine skull x-rays below 2 years. The angiomatosis and calcification predominantly involve the temporoparietooccipital region. In older children and adults the cranial and facial manifestations are easily identifiable. Skull x-rays demonstrate the dense calcification, with hemiatrophy. The bony changes consist of elevation of the base of the skull and enlargement and increased aeration of the mastoid air cells. These are secondary to the developmental changes in the brain, with resultant remodeling of the calvarium.

CT (Fig. 4-47) usually shows the calcification involving the periphery of the cerebral hemispheres and having a gyral pattern. The sulci on the affected side are prominent, with mild to moderate enlargement of the ventricle, indicating some amount of cerebral atrophy. This finding is more commonly seen in older children and adults. CT is helpful in detecting the intracranial calcification and atrophic process in children less than 2 years of age (Welsh 1980). In older children and adults, CT helps define the extent of the calcification and any associated abnormalities. Calcification has been reported to involve the cerebral hemisphere not only on the same side as the nevus but also on the opposite side, as well as the cerebellum (Kendall 1978). Very rarely, instead of hemiatrophy, enlargement of the hemicranium on the side of the nevus may occur (Enzmann 1977). Contrast-enhanced CT in most cases will show diffuse superficial enhancement on the side of the nevus, extending beyond the calcification. This is similar to the sustained stain seen on

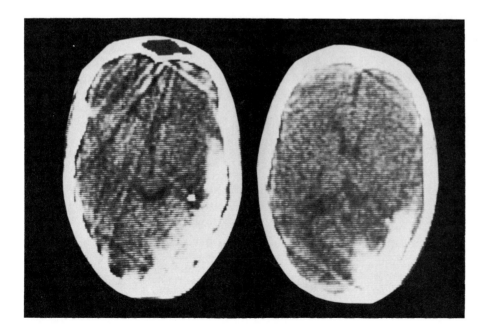

Figure 4-47 Typical calcification in Sturge-Weber syndrome.

angiography (Poser 1957). There is an apparent shift of the falx toward the site of the lesion which reflects calvarium remodeling. The superior sagittal sinus may not be well defined in vertex sections. Non-visualization of the cortical veins on the affected side, associated with resultant tortuous collateral deep venous channels, has been shown by angiography (Bentson 1971). On CECT these tortuous collateral deep veins are seen as linear densities (Kendall 1978; Enzmann 1977).

Most often Sturge-Weber disease can be diag-nosed on the basis of the clinical findings, the skull films, and CT. There are rare instances in which the clinical features of Sturge-Weber syndrome may be present although the CT findings are not character-istic. In the absence of typical gyral calcification on CT, the venous angiomatosis and associated sino-venous thrombosis of Sturge-Weber syndrome (Fig. 4-48) cannot be differentiated from arteriovenous malformation or the CT features of sinovenous thrombosis (Buonanno 1978). Angiography and the clinical features are usually helpful (Wagner 1981).

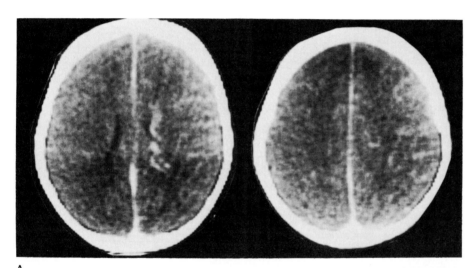

A

Figure 4-48 Sturge-Weber syndrome, atypical presentation. **A.** CECT with enhancing gyral and subependymal vessels. Note slight thinning of the calvarium. **B.** Lateral view of angiograms: note faint vascular stain in arterial phase. **C.** Thrombosed superior sagittal sinus and prominent deep medullary veins.

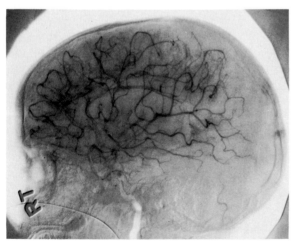

B

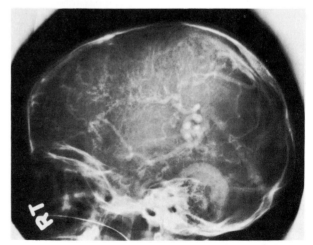

C

Bibliography

ADAMS RD, SIDMAN RL: *Introduction to Neuropathology.* New York, McGraw Hill, 1968.

ADAMS RD, GREENBURG JO: The mega cisterna magna. *J Neurosurg* **48:**190–192, 1978.

ALVORD EC JR., MARCUSE PM: Intracranial cerebellar meningoencephalocele (posterior fossa cyst) causing hydrocephalus by compression at the incisura tentorii. *J Neuropathol Exp Neurol* **2:**50–69 1962.

AMUNDSEN P, NEWTON TH: Subarachnoid cisterns, in Newton TH, Potts DG (eds): *Radiology of the Skull and Brain: Ventricles and Cisterns.* St. Louis, Mosby, vol 4, 1978.

ARCHER CR, DARWISH H, SMITH K: Enlarged cisterna magna and posterior fossa cysts simulating Dandy-Walker syndrome in computed tomography. *Radiology* **127:**681–686, 1978.

BENDA CE: The Dandy-Walker syndrome or so-called atresia of the foramen of Magendie. *J Neuropath Exp Neurol* **13:**12–29, 1954.

BENTSON JR, WILSON GH, NEWTON TH: Cerebral venous drainage patterns of Sturge-Weber syndrome. *Radiology* **101:**111–118, 1971.

BERKOWITZ NJ: Non-communicating cyst of the septum pellucidum with recovery following ventriculography. *Minn Med* **22:**402–405, 1939.

BLAKE JA: The roof and lateral recess of the fourth ventricle, considered morphologically and embryologically. *J Comp Neurol* **10:**79–108, 1900.

BONAFE A, ETHIER R, MELANCON D, BELANGER G, PETERS T: High resolution computed tomography in cervical syringomyelia. *J Comput Assist Tomogr* **4:**(1):42–47, 1980.

BOUCH DC, MITCHELL I, MALONEY AFS: Ependymal lined paraventricular cerebral cyst: A report of 3 cases. *J Neurol Neurosurg Psychiatry* **36:**611–617, 1973.

BROCKLEHURST G: The development of the human cerebrospinal fluid pathway with particular reference to the roof of the fourth ventricle. *J Anat* **105:**467–479, 1969.

BRODAL A, HAUGLIE-HANSEN E: Congenital hydrocephalus with defective development of the cerebellar vermis (Dandy-Walker syndrome): Clinical and anatomical findings in two cases with particular reference to the so-called atresia of the foramina of Magendie and Luschka. *J Neurol Neurosurg Psychiatry* **22:**99–108, 1959.

BUONANNO FS, MOODY DM, BALL MR, LASTER DW: Computed cranial tomographic findings in cerebral sino-venous occlusion. *J Comput Assist Tomogr* **2:**281–290, 1978.

BUSH JA, BAJANDA FJ: Septo-optic dysplasia (deMorsier's). *Am J Opthalmol* **86–**202–205, 1978.

BYRD SE, HARWOOD-NASH DC, FITZ CR, ROGOVITZ DM: Computed tomography evaluation of holoprosencephaly in infants and children. *J Comput Assist Tomogr* **1:**456–463, 1977.

BYRD SE, HARWOOD-NASH DC, FITZ CR: Absence of corpus callosum: Computed tomographic evaluation in infants and children. *J Can Assoc Radiol* **20:**108–112, 1978a.

BYRD SE, HARWOOD-NASH DC, FITZ CR, ROGOVITZ DM: Computed tomography in the evaluation of encephaloceles in infants and children. *J Comput Assist Tomogr* **2:**81–87, 1978b.

CARMEL PW, ANTUNES JL, HILAL SK, GOLD AP: Dandy-Walker syndrome: Clinico-pathological features and re-evaluation of modes of treatment. *Surg Neurol* **8:**132–138, 1977.

COULAM CM, BROWN LR, REESE DF: Sturge-Weber syndrome. *Semin Roentgenol* **11**(1):56–60, January 1976.

COWLEY AR, MOODY DM, ALEXANDER E, BALL MR, LASTER DW: Distinctive C.T. appearance of cyst of the cavum septi pellucidi. *Am J Roentgenol* **133:**548–550, 1979.

CRITCLEY N, EARL CJ: Tuberous sclerosis and allied conditions. *Brain* **55**:311–346, 1932.

DANDY WE, BLACKFAN KD: Interval hydrocephalus: An experimental, clinical and pathological study. *Am J Dis Child* **8**:406–482, 1914.

DANDY WE: Congenital cerebral cysts of the cavum septi pellucidi (fifth ventricle) and the cavum Vergae (sixth ventricle). *Arch Neurol Psychiatry* **25**:44–66, 1931.

DEMEYER W: Classification of cerebral malformations. *Birth Defects* **7**:78–93, 1971.

DEMORSIER G: Etudes sur les dysraphies cranioencéphaliques: III. Agénésie du spetum lucidum avec malformations du tractus optique: La Dysplasie septo-optique. *Schweiz Arch Neurol Neurochir Psychiatr* **77**:267–292, 1956.

DERKHSHAN I, SABOUR-DEYLAMI M, LOTTI J: Holoprosencephaly: Computed tomographic and pneumographic findings with anatomical correlation. *Arch Neurol* **37**:55–57, 1980.

DICHIRO G, AXELBAUM SP, SCHELLINGER D, TWIGGS HL, LEDLEY RS: Computerized axial tomography in syringomyelia. *N Engl J M* **292**:13–16, 1975.

DRAYER BP, ROSEBAUM AE, MAROON JC, BANK WO, WOODFORD JE: Posterior fossa extra-axial cyst: Diagnosis by metrizamide C.T. cisternography. *Am J Roentgenol* **128**:431–436, 1977.

DUBLIN AB, FRENCH BN: Diagnostic image evluation of hydranencephaly and pictorially similar entities with emphasis on computed tomography. *Radiology* **137**:81, 1980.

DUBOIS P, HEINZ ER, WESSEL HB, ZAIAS BW: Multiple cystic encephalomalacia of infancy: Computed tomographic findings in two cases with associated intracerebral calcification. *J Comput Assist Tomogr* **3**:97–102, 1979.

DYKE CG, DAVIDOFF LM: The pneumoencephalographic diagnosis of tumors of the corpus callosum. *Bull Neurol Inst NY* **4**:602–623, 1936.

EBAUGH FG, HOLT AW: Congenital malformations of the nervous system. *Am J Med Sci* **246**:106–113, 1963.

EMERY JL, KALHAN SC: The pathology of exencephalus. *Develop Med Child Neurol* **12**(suppl. 22):51–64, 1970.

ENZMANN DR, HAYWARD RW, NORMAN D, DUNN RP: Cranial C.T. scan appearances of Sturge-Weber disease: Unusual presentation. *Radiology* **122**:721–724, 1977.

FAERBER EN, WOLPERT SM: The value of computed tomography in the diagnosis of intracranial lipoma. *J Comput Tomogr* **2**:297–299, 1979.

FITZ CR, HARWOOD-NASH DC, THOMPSON JR: Neuroradiology of tuberous sclerosis in children. *Radiology* **110**:635–642, 1974.

FITZ CR: Metrizamide ventriculography and computed tomography in infants and children. *Neuroradiology* **16**:6–9, 1978a.

FITZ CR, HARWOOD-NASH DC, BOLDT DW: The radiographic features of unilateral megalencephaly. *Neuroradiology* **15**:145–148, 1978b.

FITZ CR, HARWOOD-NASH DC: Computed tomography in hydrocephalus. *Comput Tomogr* **2**:91–108, June 1978c.

FORBES W, ISHERWOOD I: Computed tomography in syringomyelia and the associated Arnold-Chiari Type I malformation. *Neuroradiology* **15**:73–78, 1978.

FRIEDE RL, YASARGIL MG: Supratentorial intracerebral (ependymal) cysts: Review, case reports, and the fine structure. *J Neurol Neurosurg Psychiatry* **36**:611–617, 1973.

FUKUI M, TANAKA A, KITMURAK K, OKUDERA T: Lipoma of the cerebellopontine angle: Case report. *J Neurosurg* **46**:544–547, 1977.

GARCIA CA, DUNN D, TREVOR R: The lissencephaly (agyria) syndrome in siblings: Computerized tomographic and neuropathological findings. *Arch Neurol* **35**:608–611, 1978.

GARDNER WJ, MCCORMACK LJ, DOHN DF: Embryonal atresia of the fourth ventricle, the cause of arachnoid cyst of the cerebellopontine angle. *J Neurosurg* **17**:226–237, 1960.

GARDNER E, O'RAHILLY R, PROLO D: The Dandy-Walker and Arnold-Chiari malformation. *Arch Neurol* **32**:393–407, 1975.

GASTAUT H, REGIS JL, GASTAUT E, YERMENOS E, LOW MD: Lipomas of the corpus callosum and epilepsy. *Neurology* **30**:132–138, 1980.

GIBSON JB: Congenital hydrocephalus due to atresia of the foramen of Magendie. *J Neuropathol Exp Neurol* **14**:244–262, 1955.

GISSELSSON L: Intranasal forms of encephalomeningocele. *Acta Otolaryngol (Stockh)* **35**:519–531, 1947.

GOMEZ MR, MELLINGEN JF, REESE DF: The use of computerized transaxial tomography in the diagnosis of tuberous sclerosis. *Mayo Clin Proc* **50**:553–556, 1975.

GOODING CA, CARTER A, HOARE RD: New ventriculographic aspects of the Arnold-Chiari malformation. *Radiology* **89**:626–632, October 1967.

HART MN, MALAMUD N, ELLIS WG: The Dandy-Walker syndrome: A clinicopathological study based on 28 cases. *Neurology* **22**:771–780, 1972.

HARWOOD-NASH DC, FITZ CR: *Neuroradiology in Infants and Children.* St. Louis, Mosby, 1976.

HARWOOD-NASH DC: Congenital cranio-cerebral abnormalities and computed tomography. *Semin Roentgenol* **12**(1):39–51, 1977.

HAYASHI T, YOSHIDA M, KURAMOTO S, TAKYA S, HASHIMOTO T: Radiological features of holoprosencephaly. *Surg Neurol* **12**:261–265, 1979.

HEISKANEN O: Cyst of the septum pellucidum causing increased intracranial pressure and hydrocephalus. *J Neurosurg* **28**:771–773, 1973.

KAPP JP, PAULSON GW, ODOM GL: Brain tumors with tuberous sclerosis. *J Neurosurg* **26**:191–202, 1967.

KAZNER E, STOCHDORP O, WENDE S, GRUMME T: Intracranial lipoma: Diagnostic and therapeutic considerations. *J Neurosurg* **52**:243–245, 1980.

KENDALL BE, KINGSLEY D: The value of computed axial tomography (CAT) in cranio-cerebral malformations. *Br J Radiol* **51**:171–190, March 1978.

KRUYFFE E, JEFF SR: Skull abnormalities associated with the Arnold-Chiari malformation. *Acta Radiol [Diagn] (Stockh)* **5**:9–24, 1966.

LEE BCP, GAWLER J: Tuberous sclerosis: Comparison of computed tomography and conventional neuroradiology. *Radiology* **127**:403–407, 1978.

LIPTON HL, PREZIOSI TJ, MOSES H: Adult onset of the Dandy-Walker syndrome. *Arch Neurol* **35**:672–674, 1978.

LOWMAN RM, SHAPIRO R, COLLINS LC: The significance of the widened septum pellucidum. *Am J Roentgenol* **59**:177–196, 1948.

LYNN RB, BUCHANAN DC, FENICHEL GM, FREEMON FR: Agenesis of the corpus callosum. *Arch Neurol* **37**:444–478, 1980.

MANELFE C, ROCHICCIOLE P: C.T. of septo-optic dysplasia. *Am J Roentgenol* **133**:1157–1160, 1979*a*.

MANELFE C, LOUVET JP: Computed tomography in diabetes insipidus. *J Comput Assist Tomogr* **3**:309–316, 1979*b*.

MANELFE C, STARLING-JARDIM D, TOUIBI S, BONAFE A, DAVID J: Transsphenoidal encephalocele associated with agenesis of the corpus callosum: Value of metrizamide computed cisternography. *J Comput Assist Tomogr* **2**:356–361, 1978.

MCCREA ES, RAO KCVG, DIACONIS JN: Roentgenographic changes during long-term diphenylhydantoin therapy. *South Med J* **73**(3):310–311, 1980.

MEDELEY BE, MCLEOD RA, WAYNE HO: Tuberous sclerosis. *Semin Roentgenol* **11**(1):33–54, January 1976.

MILLER EM, NEWTON TH: Extraaxial posterior fossa lesions simulating intraaxial lesions on computed tomography. *Radiology* **127**:675, 1978.

MICHAELS LG, BENTSON JR: Computed assisted tomography and pneumoencephalography in nonhydrocephalic, nontumorous head enlargement. *J Comput Assist Tomogr* **2**:439–447, 1978.

NAIDICH TP: Primary tumors and other masses of the cerebellum and fourth ventricle: Differential diagnosis by computed tomography. *Neuroradiology* **14**:153–174, 1977*a*.

NAIDICH TP, LEEDS NE, KRICHETT II, PUDLOWSKI RM, NAIDICH JB, ZIMMERMAN RD: The tentorium in axial section: I. Normal C.T. appearance and non-neoplastic pathology. *Radiology* **123**:631–638, 1977*b*.

NAIDICH TP, PUDLOWSKI MR, NAIDICH JB, GORNISH M, RODRIGUEZ FJ: Computed tomographic signs of the Chiari II malformation: I. Skull and dural portions. *Radiology* **134**:65–71, 1980*a*.

NAIDICH TP, PUDLOWSKI MR, NAIDICH JB: Computed tomographic signs of the Chiari II malformation: II. Midbrain and cerebellum. *Radiology* **134**:391–398, 1980*b*.

NAIDICH TP, PUDLOWSKI MR, NAIDICH JB: Computed tomographic signs of the Chiari II malformation: III. Ventricles and cisterns. *Radiology* **134**:657–663, 1980*c*.

NAKANO S, HOJO H, KATAOKA K, YAMASAKI S: Age-related incidence of cavum septi pellucidi and cavum Vergae on CT scans of pediatric patients. *J Comput Assist Tomogr* **5**:348–349, 1981.

O'DWYER JA, NEWTON TH, HOYT WF: Radiologic features of septooptic dysplasia. *Am J Neuroradiol* **1**:443–448, 1980.

OHNO K, ENOMOTO T, IMAMOTO J, TAKESHILA K, ARIMA M: Lissencephaly (agyria) on computed tomography. *J Comput Asst Tomogr* **3**(1):92–95, 1979.

OSBORN AG, WILLIAMS RG, WING SD: Low-attenuation lesions in the midline posterior fossa: Differential diagnosis. *Comput Tomogr* **2**(4):319–329, 1978.

PEACH B: Arnold-Chiari malformation: Anatomic features of 20 cases. *Arch Neurol* **12**:613–621, 1965.

PICARD L, LEYMARIE F, ROLAND J, SIGIEL M, MASSON JP, ANDRE JM, REARD M: Cavum veli interpositi: Roentogen anatomy-pathology and physiology. *Neuroradiology* **10**:215–220, 1976.

POSER CM, TAVERAS JM: Cerebral angiography in encephalotrigeminal angiomatosis. *Radiology* **68**:327–336, 1957.

RAMSEY RG, HUCKMAN MS: Computed tomography of porencephaly and other cerebrospinal fluid–containing lesions. *Radiology* **123**:73–77, 1977.

RAO KCVG, GUNADI IK, DIACONIS JN: Congenital interhemispheric dural cyst: A case report. In press.

RAO KCVG, KNIPP H, WAGNER E: Computed tomographic findings in cerebral sinus and venous thrombosis. *Radiology* **140**:391–398, 1981.

RESJO IM, HARWOOD-NASH DC, FITZ CR, CHUANG S: Computed tomographic metrizamide myelography in syringohydromyelia. *Radiology* **131**:405–407, 1979.

SAKODA K, ISHIKAWA S, VOZUMI T, HIRAKAWA K, OKAZAKI H, HARADA Y: Sphenoethmoidal meningoencephalocele associated with agenesis of the corpus callosum and median cleft lip and palate: Case report. *J Neurosurg* **51**:397–401, 1979.

SCOTTI G, MUSGRAVE MA, FITZ CR, HARWOOD-NASH DC: The isolated fourth ventricle in children: CT and clinical review of 16 cases. *Am J Neuroradiol* **1**:419–424, 1980.

SHAW CM, ALVORD EC: Cava septi pellucidum et verge: Their normal and pathological studies. *Brain* **92**:213–224, 1969.

SOLT LC, DECIC JHN, BAIM RG, TERBRUGGE K: Interhemispheric cyst of neuroepithelial origin in association with partial agenesis of the corpus callosum: Case report. *J Neurol* **52**:399–403, 1980.

STROTHER CM, HARWOOD-NASH DC: Congenital malformations in radiology of the skull and brain, in Newton TH, Potts DG (eds): *Radiology of the Skull and Brain: Ventricles and cisterns.* St. Louis, Mosby, 1978, vol 4, pp 3712–3748.

SUWANWELA C, SUWANWELA N: A morphological classification of sincipital encephalomeningocele. *J Neurosurg* **36**:201–211, 1972.

TAGGART JK, WALKER AE: Congenital atresia of the foramens of Luschka and Magendie. *Arch Neurol Psychiatr* **48**:583–594, 1942.

TOWNSEND JJ, NIELSON SL, MALAMUD N: Unilateral megalencephaly: Hamartoma or neoplasm. *Neurology* **25**:448–453, 1975.

VIGNAUD J, AUBRIN ML, JARDIN C: Computed tomography in 25 cases of syringomyelia. Presented at the American Society of Neuroradiology meeting, Toronto, 1979.

WAGNER E, RAO KCVG, KNIPP H: Sturge-Weber syndromes. CT angiographic correlation. CT: *J Comput Tomogr* **5**:324–327, 1981.

WEISBERG L, STRABERG D, MERIWETHER RD, ROBERTSON H, GOODMAN G: Computed tomography findings in the Arnold Chiari type I malformation. *Comput Tomogr* **5**:1–11, 1981.

WELSH K, NAHEEDY MH, ABROMS IF, STRAND RD: Computed tomography of Sturge-Weber syndrome in infants. *J Comput Assist Tomogr* **4**:33–36, 1980.

WILLIAMS PL, WARWICK R: *Functional Neuroanatomy of Man*. Philadelphia, Saunders, 1975.

WING SD, OSBORN AG: Normal and pathological anatomy of the corpus callosum by computed tomography. *Comput Tomogr* **1**:183–192, 1977.

YAKOVLEV PI: Pathoarchitectonic studies of cerebral malformation. *J Neuropathol Exp Neurol* **18**:22–55, 1959.

ZETTNER A, NETSKY MG: Lipoma of the corpus callosum. *J Neuropathol Exp Neurol* **19**:305–319, 1960.

ZIMMERMAN RA, BILANIUK LA, GALLO E: Computed tomography of the trapped fourth ventricle. *Am J Roentgenol* **130**:503–506, 1978.

ZIMMERMAN RA, BILANIUK LT, DOLINSKAS C: Cranial computed tomography of epidermoid and congenital fatty tumors of maldevelopmental origin. *Comput Tomogr* **3**(1):40–47, 1979.

ZIMMERMAN RD, et al: Cranial C.T. findings in patients with meningomyelocele. *Am J Roentgenol* **132**:623–629, April 1979.

5

HYDROCEPHALUS AND ATROPHY

Karel G. TerBrugge

Krishna C.V.G. Rao

Hydrocephalus (nonatrophic ventricular enlargement) is defined as ventricular enlargement secondary to an increase in the intracranial content of cerebrospinal fluid, associated with an elevation in intracranial CSF pressure which may be intermittent or present at some times. Hydrocephalus is a dynamic process in which there is an active and progressive increase in the volume of the ventricles because of relative obstruction of the passage of CSF between its place of origin and the site of absorption.

The term *hydrocephalus ex vacuo* has been used in the past where increased intracranial CSF spaces are associated with enlarged ventricles secondary to a destructive process involving brain parenchyma. In this chapter the term *atrophy*, which is synonymous with hydrocephalus ex vacuo, is used.

Nonatrophic ventricular enlargement (hydrocephalus) in the adult population may be caused by increased CSF production or decreased CSF absorption. Increased production of CSF, such as occurs in patients with choroid plexus papillomas, is an extremely rare cause for ventricular enlargement in the adult population. Nonatrophic distention of the cerebral ventricles in adults is most commonly the result of obstruction somewhere along the pathway of the CSF circulation. If the obstruction is within the ventricular system, which may be as far distal as the outlet foramina of the fourth ventricle, then it is defined as obstructive (noncommunicating) hydrocephalus. In communicating hydrocephalus, the obstruction in the CSF pathway can be due to causes between the outlet foramina of the fourth ventricle, or involving the various compartments of the subarachnoid spaces, or secondary to pathological processes involving the arachnoid villi and the venous sinuses.

If the condition develops acutely, it is usually accompanied by headaches, vomiting, papilledema, and obtundation; but if the mode of onset is slower, these symptoms may be absent. Depending on the location and etiology of the obstructing lesion, localizing neurological symptoms and signs may be present.

COMPUTED TOMOGRAPHY IN HYDROCEPHALUS AND ATROPHY

Computed tomography has proved a reliable method in evaluating the ventricular system and intracranial cerebrospinal fluid (CSF) spaces. A variety of characteristic CT findings have been described which help in distinguishing nonatrophic ventricular enlargement (hydrocephalus either communicating or noncommunicating) from ventricular enlargement due to atrophy. Presence of sulcal prominence, as well as the cisternal spaces, provides features which are useful in distinguishing the CT findings as being due to an atrophic process rather than secondary to hydrocephalus. A variety of measurements have been described utilizing pneumoencephalography in determining the normal range of measurements of the ventricular and CSF spaces. Unlike pneumoencephalography, CT provides a reliable noninvasive method to evaluate the size of the ventricles and the sulcal prominence (Epstein 1977).

Linear measurements of the ventricular system utilizing either the axial sections or direct coronal sections in the different age groups have been established (Barron 1976; Gyldensted 1975; Gyldensted 1977; Hahn 1976; Haug 1977; Huckman 1975; Meese 1980; Pedersen 1979; Wolpert 1977). Another method has been to calculate the area using planimetry, comparing ventricles to brain volume from single sections (Synek 1976). Synek et al. (1976) felt the reliability of measurements of the ventricular system by CT to be similar to that obtained by pneumoencephalography. However, the measurements can be in error because of a variety of factors such as the partial-volume averaging and the spatial resolution of the scanner. The measurements are less precise when the ventricles are not enlarged (Wolpert 1977) or when they are rapidly enlarging (Penn 1978). Penn et al. (1978) suggested that even though there was a discrepancy of 16 percent, a more reliable analysis could be done on the basis of estimating the volume of the ventricles. The ventricular system increases only slightly in size from the second to the sixth decade. A significant increase in the size of the ventricular system is apparent after the sixth decade, together with a progressive increase in width of the cerebral sulci, as part of the normal aging process (Zatz 1982). In most cases, experience will suffice to judge the size of the ventricular system and sulci, but in borderline cases one still has to rely on certain measurements which have been established. Utilizing the EMI scanner, the combined width of the anterior horns of the lateral ventricles normally does not exceed 45 mm on the transaxial CT scan. The normal intercaudate distance measures about 15 mm, with an upper limit of 25 mm. The normal width of the third ventricle is 4 mm, with an upper limit of 6 mm. The normal width of the fourth ventricle is about 9 mm. Since actual measurements utilizing different scanners may differ, it is better to use an index system. This also may be more reliable, since slight change in angulation of the patient's head may result in different values in each study. The frontal-horn ratio which divides the maximum width of the anterior horns by the transverse inner diameter of the skull at that level is normally not more than 35 percent. In cases of atrophic ventricular enlargement, the ratio is above 40 percent, with an upper limit of 50 percent. In obstructive hydrocephalus the frontal-horn ratio is more than 45 percent in the majority of cases and frequently exceeds 55 percent.

Several morphological features may help to distinguish ventricular enlargement in noncommunicating hydrocephalus from that in atrophy (Fig. 5-1). Distention of the ventricular system in obstructive hydrocephalus is symmetrical and characterized by concentric expansion. The ventricular

Ventricular
size
index

$$V.S.I. = \dfrac{\text{Bifrontal diameter}}{\text{Frontal horn diameter}}$$

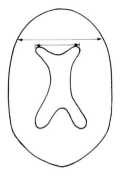

Normal	30%
Mild enlargement	30-39%
Moderate enlargement	40-46%
Severe enlargement	47%

	Atrophy		Obstructive hydrocephalus		Remarks
Angle of frontal horn		Obtuse		Acute	
Frontal horn ratio		Small		Wide	FHR: Measured at the widest part of the frontal horn perpendicular to the long axis of the frontal horn.
Temporal horn ratio		Not visible or small		Wide	Width of temporal horn measured at the genu.
Sulci and cistern		Wide		Obliterated	

Figure 5-1 Differentiating features between atrophic and obstructive ventricular enlargement. *(Adapted from Heinz et al., J Comput Assist Tomogr 4:320–325, 1980.)*

walls bulge as if they were expanded by multiple vectors of force radiating from a central axis (Heinz 1970). This causes a change in the appearance of, in particular, the anterior horns of the lateral ventricles, which become balloon-shaped (Fig. 5-2), as opposed to cerebral atrophy, which enlarges the ventricles without significantly changing their shape (Fig. 5-3). In cerebral atrophy, all parts of the ventricle may be affected equally, while in obstructive hydrocephalus, the larger parts of the ventricular system become distended first (anterior horns), to be followed by distention of the smaller parts (temporal horn, fourth and third ventricles). Enlargement of the temporal horns as a sign of obstructive hydrocephalus was noted by Sjaastad in 1969. LeMay et al. (1970) further defined this sign for CT and suggested that obstructive hydrocephalus is probable when the temporal horns are enlarged and the sylvian and interhemispheric fissures are normal in appearance or not visible (Fig. 5-4). A discrepancy between the ventricular enlargement and the degree of cortical cerebral atrophy is strongly suggestive of obstructive hydrocephalus.

Periventricular decreased density has been noted as an important but sometimes transient feature of obstructive hydrocephalus (Di Chiro 1979; Hopkins 1977; Hiratsuka 1979; Mori 1980). It is most often present in acute noncommunicating hydrocephalus but has been recognized in as high as 40 percent of cases with communicating hydrocephalus (Mori 1980). The periventricular hypodensity starts and is best recognized along the dorsolateral and dorsomedial angles of the anterior horns of the lateral ventricles (Fig. 5-5). Di Chiro et al. in 1979 attempted to characterize the periventricular hypodensity phenomenon in a variety of pathological

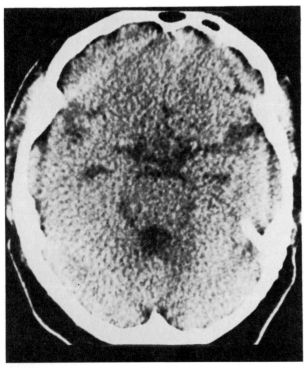

A

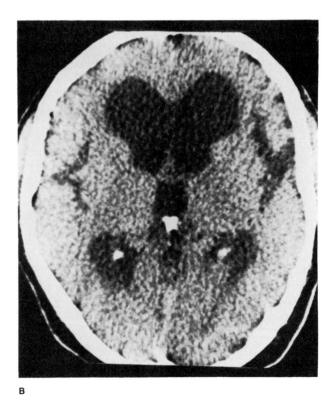

B

Figure 5-2 A and **B.** Primary communicating hydrocephalus in a 71-year-old male who presented with a 6-month history of dementia, ataxia, and urinary incontinence. Note generalized ventricular enlargement with ballooning of the anterior horns, as well as slightly prominent sylvian fissures. Dramatic relief of symptoms occurred after ventricular shunting.

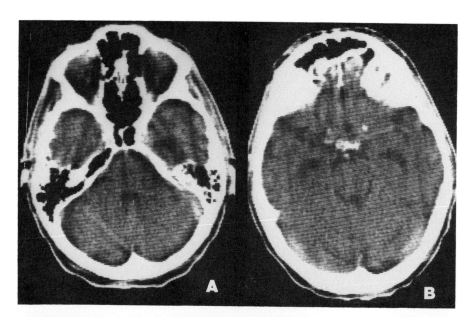

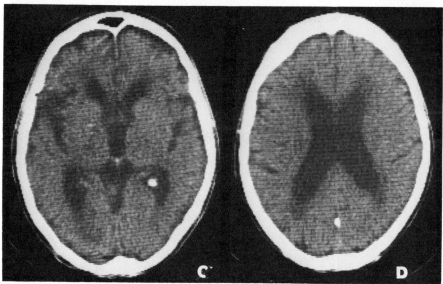

Figure 5-3 Cerebral atrophy, with dilatation of the lateral ventricle and the cisterns. The cortical sulci over the convexity are also dilated. The fourth ventricle is normal size. Even though the ventricles are enlarged, they retain their shape.

conditions. When density measurements were done from the anterior horn toward the cortex in acute hydrocephalus, most often a linear pattern was noted; that is, the ventricular wall was not evident and the density increased linearly toward the cortex. When the hydrocephalus had been present for some time, a double-slope pattern was evident, that is, a moderately steep increase in density at the

ventricular wall was present, followed by a slower increase in density in the parenchyma. The steeper initial slope presumably reflected partial restoration of the damaged wall. The periventricular hypodensity patterns in the leukoencephalopathies were different because of nonuniform involvement of the white matter, although sometimes overlap occurred when secondary hydrocephalus was present

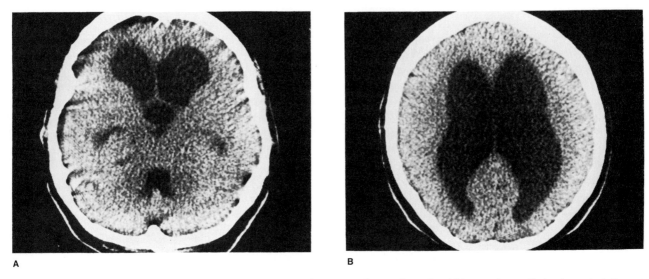

A   B

Figure 5-4 **A** and **B.** Communicating hydrocephalus secondary to previous subarachnoid hemorrhage. Note characteristic generalized ventricular enlargement with absent sulci in this 53-year-old female who underwent aneurysm surgery 8 months prior to the CT scan. Gait disturbance and dementia disappeared after ventricular shunting.

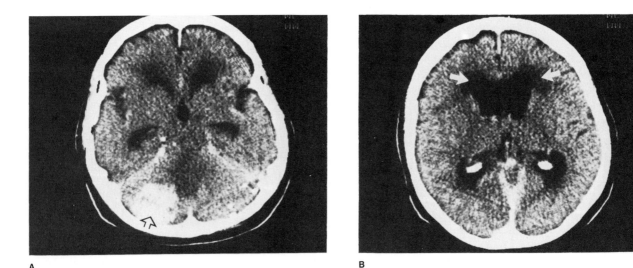

A   B

Figure 5-5 Noncommunicating (obstructive) hydrocephalus caused by metastasis of lung carcinoma to the right cerebellar hemisphere (open arrow), with obliteration of the fourth ventricle. Note the symmetrical enlargement of the third ventricle and both lateral ventricles, as well as the periventricular hypodensity adjacent to the anterior horn (white arrow) in this 68-year-old male.

(Di Chiro 1979). Periventricular hypodensity is sometimes present in elderly patients with cerebral atrophy (Mori 1980), but it differs from the appearance in noncommunicating hydrocephalus in that the ventricular wall is usually preserved on the CT scan (Fig. 5-6).

The etiology of the periventricular hypodensity in obstructive hydrocephalus is still under investigation. It can be inferred, however, that if the drainage of the CSF from the ventricular system is inhibited, as in noncommunicating hydrocephalus, there will be progressive ventricular enlargement with ependymal changes due to the pressure and rupture of cell junctions, in particular at the dorsolateral angles of the anterior horn (James 1980). Water and salts pass freely across the ependyma into the periventricular tissue, causing decreased density on the CT scan. In communicating hydrocephalus, a steady state may be obtained when proteins pass through the damaged ependyma into the subependymal tissue, leading to a fall in effective intraventricular colloid osmotic pressure, and the ventricular protein concentration will reach a normal level characterized by an increased amount of CSF (Jensen 1979). In time, repair mechanisms take effect, with a glial and ependymal scar covering the previously

exposed brain parenchyma in an incomplete manner (James 1980). This possibility explains why in most cases of long-standing communicating hydrocephalus the periventricular hypodensity is no longer present.

Noncommunicating Hydrocephalus

In noncommunicating hydrocephalus there is symmetrical distention of the ventricular system proximal to the obstruction and a ventricular system of normal or less than normal size distal to the obstruction. The possible site of the obstruction should be examined in detail with thin slices and if necessary overlapping cuts, using the transaxial and possibly the coronal mode as necessary to establish the pathogenesis of the obstruction. In noncommunicating hydrocephalus, depending on the nature and location of the obstructing process, the ventricular dilatation may be focal or generalized (Table 5-1). The lesion may be located within the lumen of the ventricle (colloid cyst, meningioma) (Fig. 5-7), the wall of the ventricular system (ependymal cyst, ependymoma) (Fig 5-8), or the adjacent brain tissue (primary and secondary brain tumors) (Fig. 5-9).

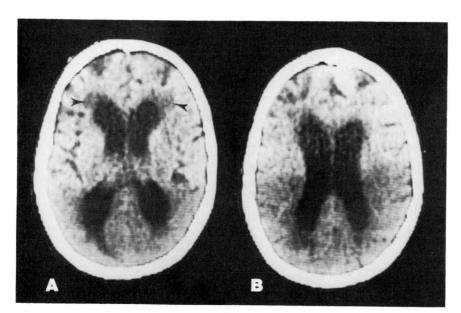

Figure 5-6 Periventricular hypodensity in atrophic ventricles. The ventricles are dilated, with rounded frontal horns. Periventricular hypodensity is present around both frontal horns (arrows), although the margins of the ventricles are well defined. The sulci are prominent.

Table 5-1   Hydrocephalus: Classification and Causative Factors

Overproduction	*Noncommunicating*	*Communicating*
Choroid plexus papilloma	1. Postinflammatory 2. Congenital anomalies 3. Posthemorrhagic 4. Tumors	Infection Neoplastic Subarachnoid hemorrhage Congenital anomalies Dural venous thrombosis Normal-pressure hydrocephalus

Anterior third ventricle		*Posterior third ventricle*
Intraaxial	*Extraaxial*	Pinealoma
Trauma	Pituitary adenoma	Teratoma
Colloid cyst	Craniopharyngioma	Collicular/paracollicular cysts
Arachnoid cyst	Giant aneurysm	Galenic venous aneurysm
Hypothalamic glioma	Arachnoid cyst	
Ependymoma	Ectopic teratoma	
	Dermoid	

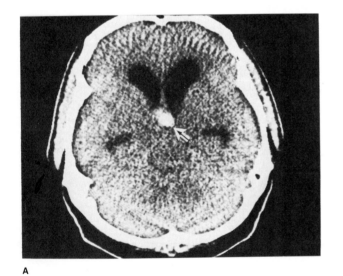

A

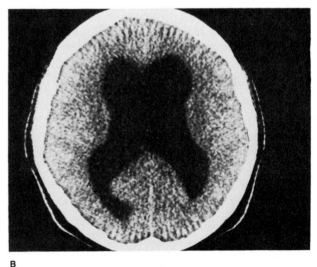

B

Figure 5-7 Noncommunicating hydrocephalus caused by a colloid cyst (arrow) within the third ventricle. Note the symmetrical distention of both lateral ventricles in this 29-year-old female, who presented with a 5-month history of increasing headaches. The third and fourth ventricles were less than normal in size.

The effectiveness of CT for reliably demonstrating such lesions has been established, and CT is without doubt the method of choice in the investigation of patients and noncommunicating (obstructive) hydrocephalus. The role of ventriculography and pneumoencephalography after an intraventricular drain has been installed is limited to the demonstration of intraventricular webs, aqueduct stenosis, and fourth-ventricle outlet obstruction, if one wants to pursue the probable cause of the hydrocephalus demonstrated on CT (Fig. 5-10). Similar information can also be obtained by CT examination

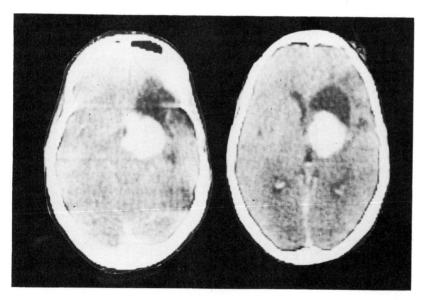

Figure 5-8 Hydrocephalus due to intraventricular obstruction. An enhancing mass obstructs the foramen of Monro, with resulting obstructive dilatation of both lateral ventricles. At subsequent survey, the mass was proved to be an ependymoma.

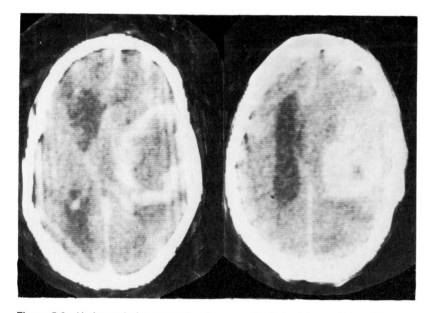

Figure 5-9 Hydrocephalus secondary to mass at a distant focus. Enhancing mass, which turned out to be glioblastoma, is present in the left temporoparietal region. Because of the bulk of tumor and the associated edema, the left lateral ventricle is not only compressed but pushed across the midline. Hydrocephalus in this patient is due not only to the mass but also to the associated obstruction at the foramen of Monro as well as the uncal herniation.

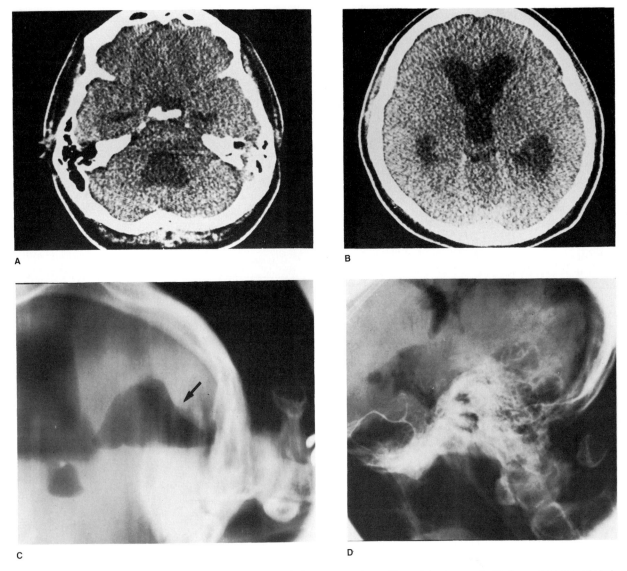

A

B

C

D

Figure 5-10 **A** and **B.** Noncommunicating hydrocephalus caused by outlet obstruction of the fourth ventricle in a 38-year-old male who presented with positional vertigo. Note the generalized symmetrical enlargement of the entire ventricular system. Air ventriculogram in **C** showed no exit of air from the enlarged fourth ventricle (arrow). **D.** subsequent pneumoencephalogram revealed air within the basal cisterns, but no entry into the ventricular system.

following intrathecal instillation of a small amount of metrizamide. The treatment of these conditions, however, would still be ventricular shunting, and most institutions would probably omit ventriculography and pneumoencephalography and perform a shunting procedure, to be followed by a repeat CT scan to examine the ventricular size and the possible development of complications such as extracerebral fluid collections. Cerebral angiography is indicated to evaluate the vascularity of the lesion if surgery is contemplated.

Communicating Hydrocephalus

In communicating hydrocephalus, the ventricular enlargement is due to obstruction in the normal CSF pathway distal to the fourth ventricle. The obstruction usually involves the subarachnoid space between the basal cisterns and cisterns over the convexity of the brain, and may involve the Pacchionian granulations of the venous sinuses as well. The entity of symptomatic hydrocephalus in adults with normal CSF pressure was first described by Hakim in 1964 and subsequently by Adams et al. in 1965. The patients presented with symptoms of ataxia, dementia, and urinary incontinence. At pneumoencephalography a communicating type of hydrocephalus was demonstrated, and dramatic relief of

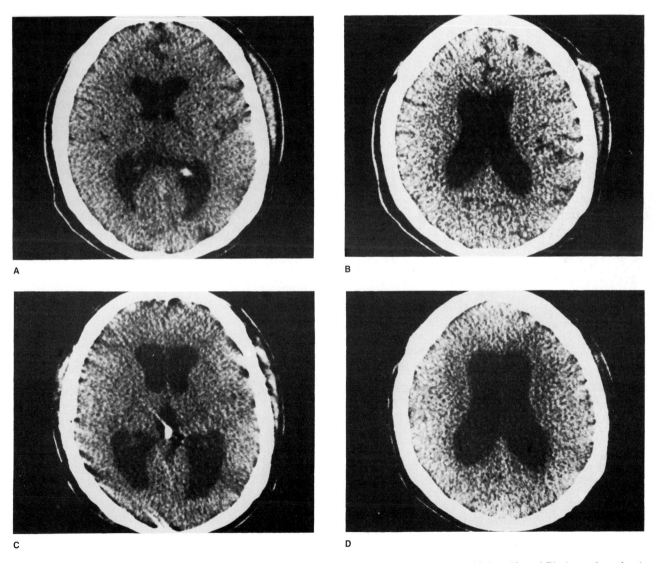

Figure 5-11 Communicating hydrocephalus secondary to trauma. CT at the time of the head injury (**A** and **B**) showed moderate diffuse cortical atrophy in this 40-year-old male. CT scan done 4 days later (**C** and **D**) shows progressive generalized ventricular enlargement and absent sulci. The clinical condition improved after ventricular shunting.

symptoms occurred after ventricular shunting had been carried out. Subsequently, two types of communicating hydrocephalus were identified. In the primary, or idiopathic, form, no cause for the hydrocephalus is apparent (Fig 5-2). In the secondary form, a previous history of trauma (Fig. 5-11), subarachnoid hemorrhage (Fig. 5-4), meningitis (Fig. 5-12), or meningeal carcinomatosis is supposedly responsible for the defect in absorption of CSF and subsequent development of communicating hydrocephalus.

Unfortunately, not all patients with the clinical triad suggestive of so-called *normal pressure hydrocephalus* have responded favorably to shunting. Pneumoencephalography (LeMay 1970; Benson 1970), Risa cisternography (Tator 1968; Benson 1970; Heinz 1970; McCullough 1970), metrizamide cisternography (Hindmarsh 1975; Enzmann 1979), and cerebral blood flow studies (Greitz 1969a; Greitz 1969b) have all been used to identify those patients who would benefit from ventricular shunting. The predictive value of these tests has been disappointing (Black 1980; Coblentz 1973; Jacobs 1976b; Salmon 1972; Shenkin 1973; Stein 1974; Wolinsky 1973). Encouraging treatment results have been reported in patients with a positive lumbar CSF infusion test (Katzman 1970; Coblentz 1973; Nelson 1971; Ter-Brugge 1980, Wolinsky 1973). This test examines the compliance (CSF volume change per unit change of CSF pressure) of the cerebral and spinal compartments, which is in part governed by the collapsibility of the cerebral venous vascular system (Marmarou 1975). It has also become apparent that the intracranial pressure in patients with occult hydrocephalus is not necessarily low or normal at all times; high-pressure waves have been demonstrated during prolonged intracranial-pressure monitoring (Gunasekera 1977; Symon 1977; Ter-Brugge 1980).

Generalized ventricular enlargement on CT with normal or absent sulci has proved to be a useful sign indicative of communicating hydrocephalus (Gunasekera 1977; Black 1980). Gado et al. (1976) proposed a scoring system in which lateral ventricular enlargement was scored as mild ($+1$), moderate ($+2$), or severe ($+3$); the third ventricle as normal (0) or enlarged ($+2$); and the sulci as normal (0) or enlarged (-2). Communicating hydrocephalus was suggested if the algebraic sum of the score was 3 or more. TerBrugge et al. (1980) showed that in a group of patients with clinical evidence of normal pressure hydrocephalus (NPH) who responded

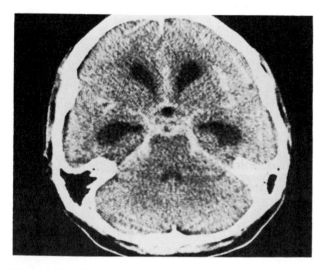 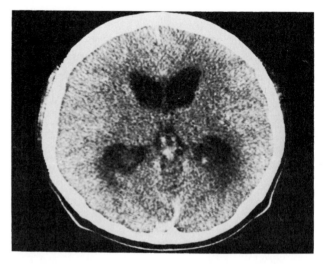

Figure 5-12 Obstructive hydrocephalus in a 49-year-old female with previous history of tuberculous meningitis. Note symmetrical enlargement of the lateral ventricles and, in particular, the temporal horns. The fourth ventricle is relatively normal in size. Obliteration of the basal cisterns is due to previous inflammatory disease. The obstruction of CSF is probably at the level of the midbrain.

favorably to shunting , only 56 percent had CT evidence of communicating hydrocephalus, while 24 percent showed evidence of atrophy and 20 percent had a normal CT scan. The findings were identical for the primary and secondary types of communicating hydrocephalus.

Computed tomography, because of its proven ability in evaluating the size of the ventricular system and the cortical sulci, should be the first investigative procedure when clinically the diagnosis of NPH is suspected. While generalized ventricular enlargement and normal or absent sulci represent excellent CT evidence of communicating hydrocephalus, the diagnosis should not be rejected when the CT is normal or reveals evidence of cerebral atrophy. In such cases further investigations, such as the lumbar CSF infusion test, intraventricular pressure monitoring, and possibly radionuclide (Risa) or metrizamide cisternography, should be carried out to assess whether the patient may benefit from CSF shunting. In the investigation of patients with possible communicating hydrocephalus, pneumoencephalography has been replaced by CT.

ATROPHY OF THE BRAIN

Brain atrophy is defined as loss of substance within the brain, which may involve the white matter, the gray matter, or both. Depending on the etiology (Table 5-2), brain atrophy can be focal or diffuse (generalized).

Focal Brain Atrophy

Focal brain atrophy presents on CT as a region of low density within the brain parenchyma or as focal dilatation of a part of the ventricle or subarachnoid space. Most often there is a combination of components. Occasionally the pathogenesis of the atrophy is suggested by the location of the focal atrophic process, but more often a clinical history is necessary for correlation with the CT findings.

Table 5-2   Brain Atrophy

Focal	Diffuse
Posttrauma	Alzheimer's disease
Postinfarction	Pick's disease
Postinflammatory	Multifocal infarct
Postvascular anomalies	Huntington's disease
Cerebellar	Parkinson's disease
	Wilson's disease
	Cerebral anoxia
	Binswanger's disease
	Jakob-Creutzfeldt disease
	Neoplasia and metabolic disorder
	Drug related atrophy
	Demyelinating disease
	Chronic schizophrenia

Posttraumatic Atrophy

The atrophic process is usually seen 3 to 6 months following the trauma (Kishore 1980; see also Chapter 12 in this book). Focal atrophy is common when a hemorrhagic contusion is present in the acute phase. Surgical evacuation of a large hematoma or spontaneous resolution of an intracerebral hematoma may result in focal atrophy. Although hemorrhagic contusions or hematoma may involve any portion of the brain, they are often located peripherally, predominantly involving the frontal lobe and the anterior temporal lobes (Fig. 5-13). When hemorrhagic contusion or hematoma involves the parenchyma close to the ventricular margins or subarachnoid space, they appear as porencephaly. Posttraumatic atrophy may occasionally be diffuse.

Postinflammatory Atrophy

Postinflammatory atrophy secondary to brain abscess is most often due to necrosis of the brain, although surgical drainage may also, indirectly, be a factor, resulting in focal atrophy even when resolution of the abscess has been achieved with medical treatment. Diffuse cerebral atrophy may occasionally be seen in patients surviving low-grade infection, as in Reye's syndrome.

Figure 5-13 Focal atrophy following trauma: CT in a young man who had a head trauma 4 months earlier and who presented with seizures. There is focal atrophy involving the left temporal lobe. The left lateral ventricle is larger than the right.

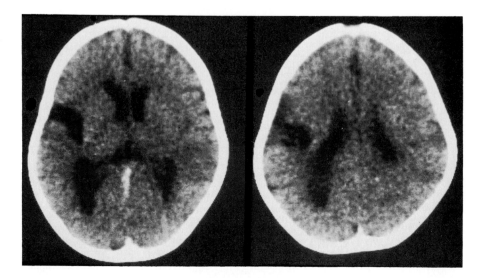

Figure 5-14 Focal atrophy following cerebral infarction: CT 3 months after stroke in a 58-year-old female. There is mild prominence of the cortical sulci. The ventricles are slightly enlarged. Focal low density in the left occipital pole is noted, indicating parenchymal loss rather than mass. The clinical history was consistent with cerebral infarction.

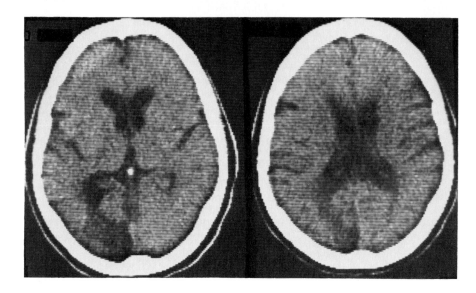

Postinfarction Atrophy

Cerebral infarction can be ischemic or hemorrhagic. Usually there is an antecedent history of frequent transient ischemic attacks and of hypertension. Since infarcts, both ischemic and hemorrhagic, involve major arterial branches, the atrophic process tends to be confined to their distribution. Post-ischemic infarcts tend to be evident on CT as early as 3 to 6 months after the episode (Fig. 5-14). It is not surprising to find a discrepancy between the neurologic deficit and the volume of focal atrophic process demonstrated by CT. CT may show mild ventricular dilatation with prominence of the cortical sulci without a focal low density in the parenchyma, although the patient may have a profound neurological deficit.

Cerebral Hemiatrophy

Cerebral hemiatrophy (Davidoff-Dyke syndrome) usually manifests itself during adolesence. The hemiatrophy is secondary to neonatal or intrauterine vascular occlusion, resulting in massive infarction. Rarely, the vascular occlusion may occur in childhood. CT demonstrates atrophy involving almost the entire hemisphere, with the ventricles shifted toward the side of the atrophy (Fig. 5-15). The sulci on the involved side are widened and occasionally may not be visible. Thickening of the calvarium on the involved side is common. CT will also occasionally show elevation of the roof of the orbit on the involved side, associated with prominent mastoid and adjacent paranasal sinuses. Focal cerebral atrophy associated with calcification of the cortical surface is seen in Sturge-Weber syndrome, in which a capillary angioma of the cortical surface is associated with a cutaneous facial nevus on the ipsilateral side (see Chapter 14). The cause of the atrophy is the angioma combined with the associated cortical venous thrombosis.

Atrophy Associated with Vascular Anomalies

Arteriovenous malformation may occasionally be associated with focal atrophic changes, usually located distal to the vascular malformation (see Chapter 14). On CT this is most often seen as prominence of the cortical sulci in a focal area adjacent to the vascular malformation, predominantly over the cortical surface (Fig. 5-16). Ventricular dilatation on the same side as the vascular malformation may be seen when the vascular anomaly is located deep within the parenchyma. The atrophy is most often due to ischemia of the adjacent parenchyma, probably resulting from a "steal" or from repeated small hemorrhages within the vascular malformation, or a combination of these factors.

Diffuse Atrophy

Diffuse cerebral atrophy may involve primarily the gray matter or the white matter, but most often it is mixed. Diffuse atrophy has also been classified as

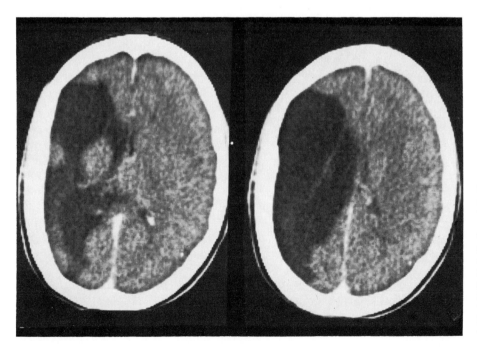

Figure 5-15 Cerebral hemiatrophy: enhanced CT in a young male with uncontrolled seizures. There is extensive loss of parenchyma involving the right cerebral hemisphere. The volume loss is partly compensated by an apparent shift of the opposing cerebral hemisphere. There is also compensating thickening of the calvarium on the affected side. These changes indicate a process that occurred during the neonatal period.

Figure 5-16 Focal atrophy in vascular malformation. Enhanced CT demonstrates focal loss of brain, with an irregular enhancing component on a higher section. Angiography confirmed the posterior parietal arteriovenous malformation.

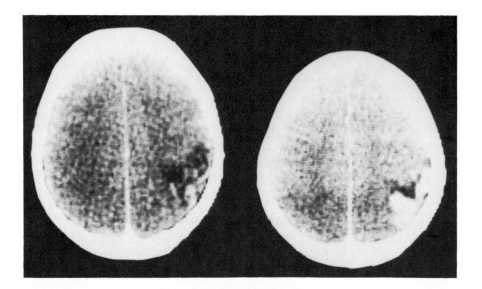

Figure 5-17 Cortical atrophy: CT in a 68-year-old male. The cortical sulci over the periphery are prominent. The ventricles are relatively well preserved.

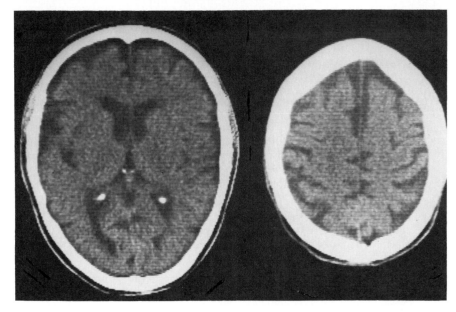

either central atrophy, in which the ventricular enlargement is more prominent than widening of the sulci (Fig. 5-3), or cortical atrophy, in which the sulci are wide relative to the enlarged ventricles (Fig. 5-17).

Diffuse cerebral atrophy can be due to a variety of entities (Table 6-2). The atrophic process, although diffuse, may involve the ventricle, sulci, or both (Fig. 5-18).

Numerous studies have been conducted evaluating the role of CT in predicting the degree of intellectual impairment in persons demonstrating evidence of cerebral atrophy (Huckman 1975; Fox 1975; Gado 1976; Roberts 1976; deLeon 1979; Jacoby 1980*b*, *c*), as well as CT correlation with aging (Barron 1976; Brinkman 1981; Hughes 1981; Jacoby 1980*a*; Yamaru 1980). All previous studies have shown that an increase in the size of ventricles and

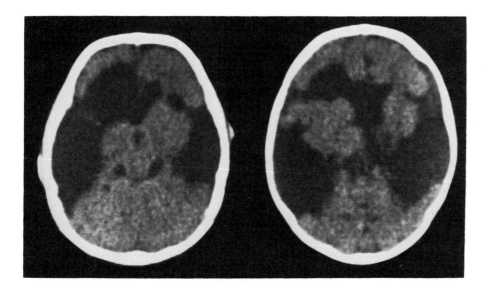

Figure 5-18 Diffuse cerebral atrophy. A 2-year-old child with large CSF spaces involving the temporal poles as well as the frontal pole on the right side. The CSF space between the ventricles and subarachnoid space are communicating. The lateral ventricle is dilated. The third ventricle is normal. This is another form of diffuse cerebral atrophy and does not require ventricular subarachnoid shunting.

cerebral sulci occurs with aging and results from loss of brain substance. The decrease in brain substance involves both gray and white matter. Neuropathological studies indicate that the decrease in brain volume is due to progressive neuronal loss (Brody 1955) as well as decrease in Betz cells (Scheibel 1975). Decrease in brain volume and weight, however, may be more significant in patients with dementia (Tomlinson 1970). In the earliest CT study dealing with the subject Huckman et al. (1975) felt that there was a correlation between the severity of atrophy detected by CT and the dementia, though they were cautious in their analysis of the inconsistency between the CT pattern and the clinical rating of dementia. Hughes et al. (1981) have utilized linear measurements on CT in patients over 60 years old in defining the demented group as distinguished from the normal control group. They found that linear indices (measurements of ventricular space and sulcal width at appropriate levels) which have been utilized by other authors were not, in their own evaluation, useful in separating the two groups. More recently, Gado (1981) has shown that although linear indices may not be useful, volumetric indices derived from CT can be utilized in identifying dementia. In evaluating patients over 60, while the CT may show ventricular and sulcal prominence indicative of cerebral atrophic process,

volumetric analysis from CT will show greater loss of brain substance in demented patients than in a control group of the same age, sex, and socioeconomic status.

Other methods of quantifying dementia by means of CT include measuring the mean Hounsfield number in the centrum semiovale. In patients over 60 years old Naeser et al. (1980) found a mean CT number below 40 HU for patients with dementia while normal individuals had a mean CT number above 41. George et al. (1980) noted a loss in discriminability of gray and white matter by CT in patients demonstrating cognitive impairment, and did not find this to be age-related.

CT is useful in demonstrating treatable causes of dementia, and thus is a useful screening test (Huckman 1975; Jacobson 1979; Hughes 1981). With the limitations discussed above borne in mind, CT features found in some of the causes of diffuse cerebral atrophy are described below.

Alzheimer's Disease

Alzheimer's disease, or presenile dementia, is a diffuse form of cerebral atrophy, although there is predominant involvement of the gray matter. Senile dementia is considered to be a progression of the presenile stage. The latter is one of the most common forms of dementia encountered in clinical practice. Neuropathological studies demonstrate atrophy of the brain secondary to neuronal loss, vascular degeneration, neurofibrillary tangles, and plaques within the perikaryon of the cerebral cortex. The CT findings are nonspecific. The most common CT findings are symmetrically enlarged ventricles with prominence of the cortical sulci (Fig. 5-19), which, as shown earlier, are not characteristic of Alzheimer's disease and may not be confirmed on pathological studies. Occasionally the cortical sulci may appear more prominent, and in other instances the ventricles are significantly increased in size. It is not usual to have a normal CT in a demented patient with abnormal psychometric test and cognitive functions. In a few cases, further studies such as radioisotope cisternography may be indicated to evaluate for normal-pressure hydrocephalus—a treatable cause of dementia.

Pick's Disease

Clinically, differentiation of Pick's lobar atrophy from the diffuse atrophy of Alzheimer's disease may be difficult. In both, the clinical progression is gradual and downhill. Pick's disease is more commonly seen in females. The disease is occasionally familial and may be inherited. The atrophic process, although diffuse, predominantly involves the temporal and frontal lobes. CT findings include dilatation of frontal and temporal horns (McGeachi 1979). The cisterns and sylvian fissure also appear prominent. Significant cortical atrophy over the convexity may be absent.

Huntington's Disease

Huntington's disease is characterized by choreiform movement and dementia. It is autosomal dominant, predominantly involving males and manifesting itself in the fourth and fifth decade. The disease starts with choreiform movement of the extremities, followed by dementia and personality changes. The hallmark in neuropathologic studies is atrophy of the caudate nucleus and putamen. In later stages diffuse atrophy of frontal and temporal regions occur. CT in this disease is characterized by atrophy of the caudate nucleus, resulting in increased bicaudate diameter of the ventricles (Fig. 5-20). This may or may not be associated with enlargement of the

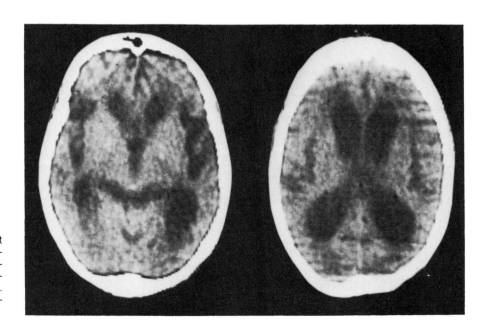

Figure 5-19 CT in a patient proven to have Alzheimer's disease. The ventricles are dilated, especially the body of the lateral ventricle. The sulci are also prominent. Note the periventricular hypodensity.

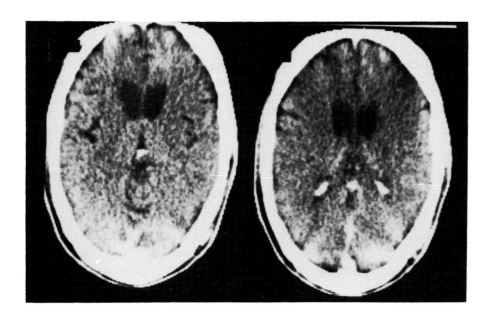

Figure 5-20 Huntington's disease: enhanced CT demonstrating focal dilatation of the frontal horn secondary to atrophy of the caudate nucleus. This is characteristic of Huntington's disease.

ventricles and cortical sulci. Presence of this CT picture confirms the clinical diagnosis, although in the authors' series, four of nine patients did not show CT evidence of caudate nucleus atrophy.

Parkinson's Disease

Brain atrophy in Parkinson's disease predominantly involves the subcortical regions, primarily resulting in degeneration of the cells and fibers of the corpus striatum, the globus pallidus, and the substantia nigra. Postencephalitic Parkinson's disease is presently uncommon. Most cases present in the sixth and seventh decades. CT in Parkinson's disease is associated with enlarged ventricles and calcification of the basal ganglia. Isolated calcification of the basal ganglia per se is not an indication of Parkinson's disease, since it can be seen in the normal population; and CT findings of enlarged ventricles and prominent cortical sulci associated with aging are difficult to differentiate from those caused by the disease process. No significant correlation between the severity of the tremor and akinesia and the severity of the cerebral atrophy as shown by CT has been documented. Numerous studies, however, have shown that the atrophic process on CT is more marked in patients with Parkinson's disease

than in persons in the same age group without the disease (Schneider 1979; Becker 1979; Johnstone 1976; Weinberger 1979). A higher degree of cognitive impairment, not age-related, has been associated with severity of the atrophic process as detected by CT (Johnstone 1976). Other studies have shown that patients with Parkinson's disease demonstrating basal ganglia calcification respond poorly to L-dopa therapy.

Wilson's Disease

Wilson's disease is due to impairment in copper metabolism. Pathologic changes in the brain consist of loss of neurons and fibrillary gliosis involving the basal ganglia and cerebral cortex. Because of deficiency of ceruloplasmin there are deposits of copper both in the liver and within the basal ganglia in the brain. The authors have not seen any CT findings in two cases of proven Wilson's disease. Harik (1981) and Ropper et al. (1979) have described hypodense regions within the basal ganglia, occasionally involving the cerebellar nuclei and adjacent white matter. There was, however, no correlation between the severity of dementia and the degree of atrophic process on CT in a majority of their cases.

Cerebral Anoxia

Anoxia results in neuronal loss associated with gliosis and edema. The end result in persons surviving anoxia is diffuse cortical atrophy disproportionate to the dilatation of the lateral ventricles. A few reports of cerebral anoxia in neonates have shown predominant involvement of the basal ganglia and cerebellum. A focal low-density region within the basal ganglia probably represents necrosis. In children and adults who survive the acute episode, the CT shows diffuse cortical and ventricular enlargement. Changes similar to those seen in neonates are also seen in adults exposed to carbon monoxide poisoning. In the acute stage the CT may appear normal, or there may be an increase in hypodensity of the white matter. Some have described symmetrical necrosis involving the globus pallidus, usually in those surviving beyond 48 hours. Late changes include enlargement of the ventricles and cortical sulci (see Chap. 15).

Binswanger's Disease

Binswanger's disease (Binswanger 1894) is progressive dementia associated with periods of remission and exacerbation. The disease is usually manifested in the fifth or sixth decade of life, usually in the form of intellectual impairment and alteration of personality progressing to dementia. The gradual but progressive course of the disease is presumed to be due to arteriosclerotic involvement of the small vessels in the subcortical region, with sharply demarcated areas of necrosis and demyelination involving the white matter. The CT findings described in Binswanger's disease (Rueck 1980; Zeumer 1980; Rosenberg 1979) consist of hypodense lesions in the periventricular white matter, lacunar infarcts in the basal ganglia, and dilatation of the ventricles. Similar CT findings are also seen in dementia secondary to multifocal infarcts. The diagnosis of Binswanger's disease is based on the clinical progression of the dementia and findings on CT (see Chap. 15).

Jakob-Creutzfeldt Syndrome

Jakob-Creutzfeldt disease is characterized by rapidly progressive dementia. Other neurological findings include altered perception, myoclonus, increased response to startle stimulus, and cerebellar dysfunction. It is now known to be caused by a transmissible agent, a slow virus (Gajdusek et al. 1977). Neuropathological studies demonstrate enlarged ventricles, with atrophy predominantly involving the gray matter. Spongiform changes of the cerebral cortex predominantly involve the temporal and occipital lobes. In the few cases in which CT findings have been reported (Rao 1977), the pattern is that of diffuse cerebral atrophy (Fig. 5-21). Although this finding is not characteristic, diagnosis is based on rapid clinical deterioration and progression of the atrophic process on sequential CT (Chap. 16).

Neoplasia and Metabolic Disorder

Huckman (1975) reported on patients with neoplasia without metastatic brain disease, enlarged ventricles, and cortical sulci, indicative of atrophy, matched with a control group of similar age and sex. The atrophic appearance is believed to be related to nutrition; similar findings have been reported in patients with anorexia nervosa (Enzmann 1977). The atrophy is reversible following restoration of proper nutrition. Prominence of the cortical sulci with apparent ventricular enlargement is also seen in patients with chronic renal failure who are on hemodialysis.

Drug-Related Atrophy

Atrophic changes have been reported on CT studies with a variety of drugs such as steroids, Dilantin, methotrexate, amphetamines, and cannabis (including marijuana) and in alcoholics.

Persons on steriods for a prolonged period demonstrate enlarged ventricles with prominence of the cortical sulci. In addition, an increase in hypodensity

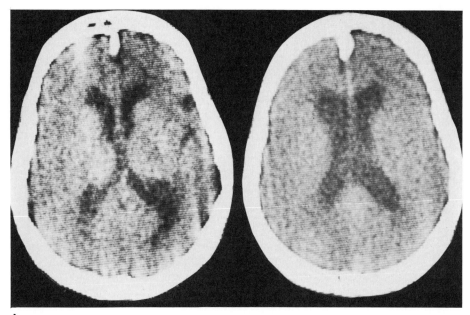

A

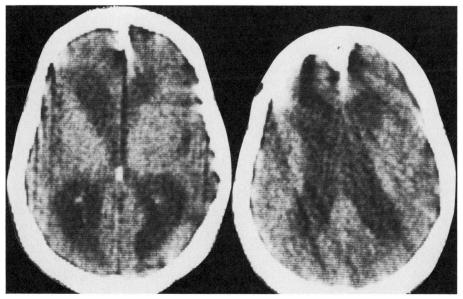

B

Figure 5-21   Jakob-Creutzfeldt disease. The rapid change in ventricular size is a characteristic feature in this disease.   **A.** Initial CT.   **B.** CT a few weeks later, demonstrating rapid progression of atrophic process.

(Continued on p. 192.)

Figure 5-21 (Cont.) **C.** Significant loss of grey matter (arrows) characteristic of this disease at autopsy in the same patient.

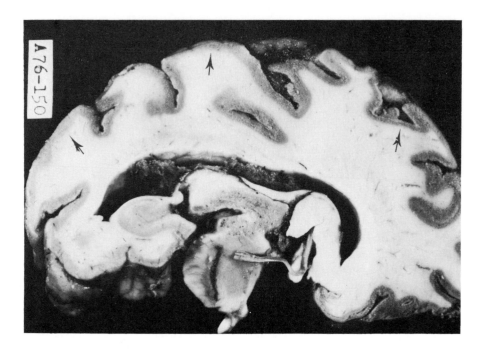

of the white matter has been reported (Bentson 1978). Return to normal ventricles and sulci has been documented when the steriod medication is stopped (Heinz 1977; Bentson 1978; Okuno 1980).

Increase in periventricular hypodensity and focal ventricular enlargement may also be seen in patients on methotrexate. But with methotrexate, focal enhancement of the white matter occurs in periventricular regions. The enhancement is presumed to be due to focal areas of drug-induced vasculitis.

A few reports have dealt with the CT findings in patients who are on amphetamines, cannabis, and marijuana (Rambaugh 1980; Co 1977; Kuehnle 1977). Patients on amphetamines were reported to have changes indicative of cerebral atrophy. However, in these cases, since there was an associated history of head trauma and use of alcohol, amphetamine may not have been the cause of atrophy. Animal studies do, however, suggest that chronic use of intravenous amphetamines can produce cerebral atrophy (Rambaugh 1980).

Prolonged use of Dilantin has been shown to result in atrophy predominantly involving the cerebellar hemisphere. This finding has been shown both by pneumoencephalography and by CT stud-

ies (Ghatak 1976; McCrea 1980) (Fig. 5-22). Dilantin in toxic doses, however, does not result in cerebral atrophy.

Numerous studies document the effect of chronic alcoholism by CT studies. Chronic alcoholism results in enlargement of the ventricles and sulci when compared to controls of similar sex and age. It is possible that in a few patients the cerebral atrophic process may be due also to hepatic encephalopathy, since studies have shown liver damage in a majority of patients who are chronic alcohol abusers. Chronic alcohol abusers show not only cerebral but also cerebellar atrophy (Fox 1976). It has also been shown that the degree of cerebral atrophy correlates with impairment of the nondominant hemisphere functions but not of the intelligence quotient (Cala 1978). There have been a few studies in which, following abstinence from alcohol, there was a reversal of the atrophic process as documented by CT (Carlen 1978; Artmann 1981). The reversal involved the cortical sulci more than the ventricles. In one series, the reversal in CT appearance occurred and corresponded to the clinical improvement between 9 and 20 months following abstinence (Artmann 1981).

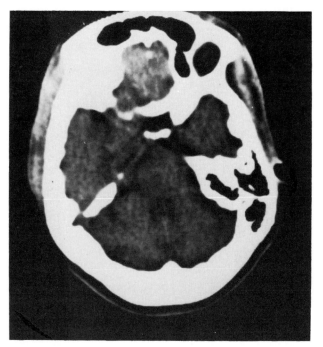

A

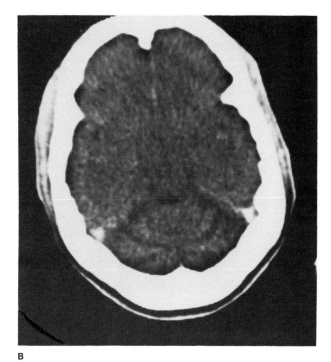

B

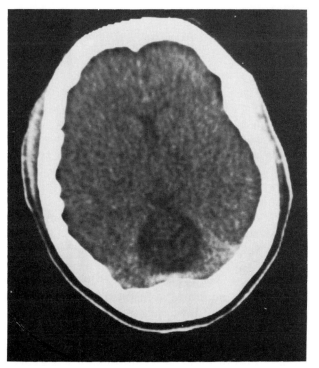

C

Figure 5-22 Drug-related cerebellar atrophy: CT in a patient on prolonged diphenylhydantoin medication. The folia of the vermis and to a lesser extent the cerebellar folia are prominent. The fourth ventricle and the cerebellopontine cisterns are mildly dilated. Prolonged use of diphenylhydantoin results in cerebellar atrophy predominantly involving the vermis. Similar changes can also be seen with chronic ethanol use.

Cerebellar Atrophy

Isolated atrophy of the cerebellum is seen in a variety of degenerative disorders, as well as being secondary to the toxic effect or prolonged use of drugs such as alcohol and diphenylhydantoin. In chronic alcoholism, cerebellar degeneration primarily involves the vermis and, to a lesser extent, the cerebellum (Allen 1979). Prolonged use of diphenylhydantoin in toxic doses has been shown to produce degeneration of the Purkinje cells of the cerebellum in animals. Similar findings can also be seen with CT (Fig. 5-22). In olivopontocerebellar degeneration, one form of spinocerebellar degeneration,

Figure 5-23 Cerebellar atrophy in olivopontocerebellar degeneration. There is prominence of the folia of both the cerebellum and the vermis. The cerebellopontine cisterns are prominent. The fourth ventricle is dilated, although retaining its shape.

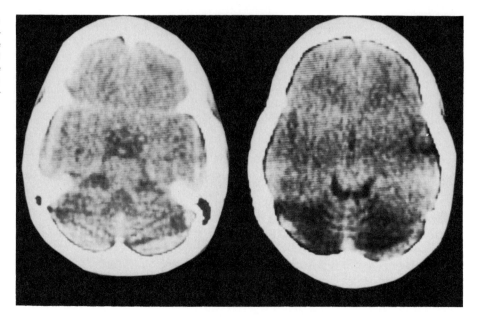

atrophic changes involve the inferior olive, pons, and cerebellum (Fig. 5-23).

The CT changes are similar in all the above-described clinical processes. Atrophy of one component may be more significant than the other. CT diagnosis of cerebellar atrophy is based on demonstrating two or more of the following features (Allen 1979):

1. Enlargement of the cerebellar sulci by more than 1 mm
2. Enlargement of the cerebellopontine cisterns by more than 1.5 mm, the measurement being taken at the superior lateral margin of the cerebellar hemisphere and adjacent petrous bone
3. Enlargement of the fourth ventricle by more than 4 mm
4. Enlargement of the superior cerebellar cistern

Isolated enlargement of the fourth ventricle and presence of a giant cisterna magna, as proposed by Baker et al. (1976), do not signify cerebellar atrophy.

Focal cerebellar atrophy is most often secondary to a vascular process or trauma (Fig. 5-24).

ANCILLARY NEUROIMAGING STUDIES

Skull Radiographs

Skull radiographs in obstructive hydrocephalus are often normal, since not enough time has elapsed to allow for pressure changes to occur on the inner table of the cranial vault. Normal physiological calcifications may be displaced, indicating mass effect, and in particular one should search for possible downward displacement of the pineal gland on lateral skull radiographs. Slightly raised or intermittently increased intracranial pressure which has been present for more than 2 months may cause demineralization of the inner table of the cranial vault and, in particular, the sella turcica. If the obstructive hydrocephalus is due to a lesion distal to the third ventricle—that is, a lesion blocking the aqueduct or the fourth ventricle—the resultant dilatation of the third ventricle may cause amputation of the dorsum sella. Skull radiographs therefore may reveal important information but are frequently normal and therefore do not suffice as a screening

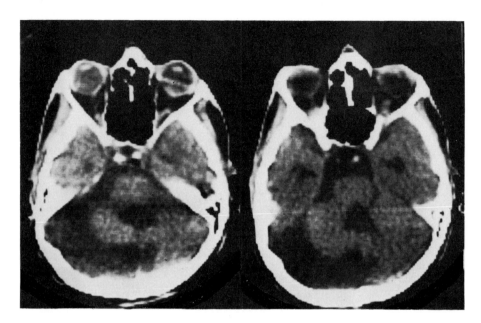

Figure 5-24 Cerebellar atrophy secondary to vascular occlusion. There is focal loss of cerebellar parenchyma on the right side with resulting widening of the cerebellopontine cistern. The fourth ventricle is dilated. Absence of deformity and contralateral displacement of the dilated fourth ventricle excludes the possibility of a cerebellopontine angle mass.

technique in the evaluation of nonatrophic ventricular enlargement. In atrophic ventricular dilatation, skull roentgenograms are not useful in the majority of cases. Occasionally, skull roentgenograms may demonstrate and provide an etiological basis for focal cerebral atrophy, such as thickening of one side of the calvarium as seen in cerebral hemiatrophy (Dyke-Davidoff syndrome) or the diffuse calvarial thickening that may rarely occur in patients on diphenylhydantoin who also have cerebellar degeneration.

Radionuclide Studies

Radionuclide scans are rarely performed these days, with the availability of CT. Rarely, they may be indicated when a focal process is present or when hydrocephalus due to carcinomatous meningitis is clinically suspected and contrast infusion is contraindicated because of a history of definite allergic reaction in the past.

Radioisotope cisternography is occasionally used in the evaluation of normal-pressure hydrocephalus. The results of this study, at least in the authors'

experience, are equivocal, but in conjunction with other studies it may help in the selection of patients for shunting.

Cerebral Angiography

Cerebral angiography is rarely indicated in the evaluation of atrophy. In patients with obstructive hydrocephalus in which a mass is the cause, angiography is occasionally necessary to determine whether the mass is a vascular structure or, if it is a tumor, to evaluate its vascularity.

Positron-Emission Tomography

In the future, with the availability of positron-emission tomography, a better appreciation of the biochemical changes associated with various forms of dementia and organic brain syndromes will result in improving our understanding of the underlying pathological process in many of the degenerative disorders of the brain.

Bibliography

ADAMS RD, FISHER CM, HAKIM S, OJEMANN RG, SWEET WH: Symptomatic occult hydrocephalus with "normal" cerebrospinal fluid pressure. *N Engl J Med* **273**:117–126, 1965.

ALLEN JH, MARTIN JT, MCLAIN LW: Computed tomography in cerebellar atrophic processes. *Radiology* **130**:379–382, 1979.

ARTMANN H, GAIL MV, HACKER H, HERRHICH J: Reversible enlargement of cerebral spinal fluid spaces in chronic alcoholics. *Am J Neuroradiol* **2**:23–27, 1981.

BAKER HL, HOUSER OW: Computed tomography in the diagnosis of posterior fossa lesions. *Radiol Clin N Am* **14**:129–147, 1976.

BANNA M: The ventriculo-cephalic ratio on CT. *J Can Assoc Radiol* 1977.

BARRON SA, JACOBS L, KINKEL WR: Changes in size of normal lateral ventricles during aging determined by computerized tomography. *Neurology* **26**:1011–1013, 1976.

BECKER H, SCHNEIDER E, HACKER H, FISCHER PA: Cerebral atrophy in Parkinson's disease—represented by CT. *Arch Psychiat Nervenkr* **227**:81–88, 1979.

BENSON DF, LEMAY M, PATTEN DH, RUBENS AB: Diagnosis of normal pressure hydrocephalus. *N Engl J Med* **283**:610–615, 1970.

BENTSON J, REZA M, WINTER J, WILSON G: Steroids and apparent cerebral atrophy on computed tomography scans. *J Comput Assist Tomogr* **2**:16–23, 1978.

BINSWANGER O.: Die Abgrenzung der allgemeinen progressive Paralyse. *Berl Klin Wochenscher* **31**:1103–1105, 1137–1139, 1180–1186, 1894.

BLACK PM: Idiopathic normal-pressure hydrocephalus. *J Neurosurg* **52**:371–377, 1980.

BRINKMAN SD, SARWAR M, LEVINE HS, MORRIS HS: Quantitative index of computed tomography in dementia and normal aging. *Radiology* **138**:89, 1981.

BRODY H: Organization of the human cerebral cortex: III. A study of aging in the human cerebral cortex. *J Comp Neurol* **102**:511–556, 1955.

CALA LA, JONES B, MASTAGLIA FL, WILEY B: Brain atrophy and intellectual impairment in heavy drinkers—a clinical, psychometric and computerized tomography study. *Aust NZ J Med* **8**:147–153, 1978.

CALA LA, MASTAGLIA FL: Computerized axial tomography in the detection of brain damage. *Med J Aust* **2**:616–620, 1980.

CARLEN PL, WORTZMAN G, HOLGATE RC, WILKINSON DA, RANKIN JG: Reversible cerebral atrophy in recently abstinent chronic alcoholics measured by computed tomography scans. *Science* **200**:1076–1078, 1978.

CO BT, GOODWIN DW, GADO M, MIKHAEL M, HILL SY: Absence of cerebral atrophy in chronic cannabis users–evaluation by computerized transaxial tomography. *JAMA* **237**:1229–1230, 1977.

COBLENTZ JM, MATTIS S, ZINGESSER LH, KASOFF SS, WISNIEWSKI HM, KATZMAN R: Presenile dementia. *Arch Neurol* **29**:299–308, 1973.

DELEON MJ ET AL: Correlations between computerized tomographic changes and behavioural deficits in senile dementia. *Lancet* **2**:859–860, 1979.

DI CHIRO G, REAMES PM, MATHEWS WB: RISA ventriculography and RISA cisternography. *Neurology* **14**:185–191, 1964.

DI CHIRO G, ARIMITSU T, BROOKS RA, MORGENTHALER DG, JOHNSTON GS, JONES AE, KELLER MR: Computed tomography profiles of periventricular hypodensity in hydrocephalus and leukoencephalopathy. *Radiology* **130**:661–666, 1979.

ENZMANN DR, LANE B: Cranial computed tomography findings in anorexia nervosa. *J Comput Assist Tomogr* **1**:410–414, 1977.

ENZMANN DR, NORMAN D, PRICE DC, NEWTON TH: Metrizamide and radionuclide cisternography in communicating hydrocephalus. *Radiology* **130**:681–686, 1979.

EPSTEIN F, NAIDICH T, KRICHEFF I, CHASE N, LIN J, RANSOHOFF J: Role of computerized axial tomography in diagnosis, treatment and follow-up of hydrocephalus. *Child Brain* **3**:91–100, 1977.

FOX JK, KASZNIAK AW, HUCKMAN M: Computerized tomographic scanning not very helpful in dementia—nor in craniopharyngioma. *N Engl J Med* **300**:437, 1979.

FOX JK, RAMSEY RG, HUCKMAN MS, PROSKE AE: Cerebral ventricular enlargement: Chronic alcoholics examined by computed tomography. *JAMA* **236**:365–368, 1976.

FOX JH, TOPEL JL, HUCKMAN MS: Use of computerized tomography in senile dementia. *J Neurol Neurosurg Psychiatry* **8**:948–953, 1975.

GADO MH, COLEMAN RE, LEE KS, MIKHAEL MA, ALDERSON PO, ARCHER CR: Correlation between computerized transaxial tomography and radionuclide cisternography in dementia. *Neurology* **26**:555–560, 1976.

GADO MH, HUGHES CP, DANZIGER W, CHI D, JOST G, BERG L: Volumetric measurements of the cerebrospinal fluid spaces in subjects with dementia and controls. Presented in the Neuroradiology Section of the 67th Annual Meeting of the Radiological Society of North America, December 1981.

GAJDUSEK DC, GIBBS CJ, ASHER DM, BROWN P, DIWAN A, HOFFMAN P, NEMO G, ROBWER R, WHITE L: Precautions in medical care of, and in handling materials from, patients with transmissible virus dementia (Jakob-Creutzfeldt disease). *N Engl J Med* **297**:1253–1258, 1977.

GEORGE AE, DELEON MJ, FERNS SH, KRICHEFF II: Parenchymal CT correlates of senile dementia (Alzheimer's disease)—loss of grey-white matter discriminability. *Am J Neuroradiol* **2**:205–213, 1981.

GHATAK NR, SANTOSO RA, MCKINNEY WM: Cerebellar degeneration following long-term phenytoin therapy. *Neurology* **26**:818–820, 1976.

GLUCK E, RADU EW, MUNDT C, GERHARDT P: A computed tomographic protective study of chronic schizophrenics. *Neuroradiology* **20**:167–169, 1980.

GREITZ TVB: Cerebral blood flow in occult hydrocephalus studied with angiography and the xenon 133 clearance method. *Acta Radiol* **8**:376–384, 1969a.

GREITZ TVB, GREPE AOL, KALMER SF, LOPEZ J: Pre- and postoperative evaluation of cerebral blood flow in low-pressure hydrocephalus. *J Neurosurg* **31**:644–651, 1969b.

GUNASEKERA L, RICHARDSON AE: Computerized axial tomography in idiopathic hydrocephalus. *Brain* **100**:749–754, 1977.

GYLDENSTED C, KOSTELJANETZ M: Measurements of the normal hemispheric sulci and computer tomography. *Neuroradiology* **10**:147–149, 1975.

GLYDENSTED C, KOSTELJANETZ M: Measurements of the normal ventricular system with computer tomography of the brain. *Neuroradiology* **10**:205–213, 1976.

GYLDENSTED C: Measurements of the normal ventricular system and hemispheric sulci of 100 adults with computed tomography. *Neuroradiology* **14**:183–192, 1977.

HACKER H, ARTMANN H: The calcification of CSF spaces in CT. *Neuroradiology* **16**:190–192, 1978.

HAHN FJY, KEAN RIM: Frontal ventricular dimensions on normal computed tomography. *Am J Roentgenol Radium Ther Nucl Med* **126**:593–596, 1976.

HAKIM S: Some observations on C.S.F. pressure: Hydrocephalic syndrome in adults with "normal" CSF pressure. Thesis No. 957, Javeriana University, School of Medicine, Bogota, Colombia, 1964.

HARIK SI, POST MJD: Computed tomography in Wilson's disease. *Neurology* **31**:107–110, 1981.

HAUG G: Age and sex dependence of the size of normal ventricles on computed tomography. *Neuroradiology* **14:**201–204, 1977.

HEINZ E, DAVIS DO, KARP HR: Abnormal isotope cisternography in symptomatic occult hydrocephalus. *Radiology* **95:**109–120, 1970.

HEINZ E, MARTINEX J, HAWNGGELI A: Reversibility of cerebral atrophy in anorexia nervosa and Cushing's syndrome. *J Comput Assist Tomogr* **1:**415–418, 1977.

HINDMARSH T, GREITZ T: Computer cisternography in the diagnosis of communicating hydrocephalus. *Acta Radiol* **346:**91–97, 1975.

HIRATSUKA H, FUJIWARA K, OKASA K, TAKASATA Y, TSUYUMU M, INABA Y: Modification of periventricular hypodensity in hydrocephalus and ventricular reflux in metrizamide CT cisternography. *J Comput Assist Tomogr* **3:**204–208, 1979.

HOPKINS LN, BAKAY L, KINKEL WR, GRAND W: Demonstration of transventricular CSF absorption by computerized tomography. *Acta Neurochir (Wien)* **39:**151–157, 1977.

HUCKMAN MS, FOX J TOPEL J: The validity of criteria for evaluation of cerebral atrophy by computed tomography. *Radiology* **116:**85–92, 1975.

HUGHES CP, GADO M: Computed tomography and aging of the brain. *Radiology* **139:**391–396, 1981.

JACOBS L, KINKEL WR: Computerized axial transverse tomography in normal pressure hydrocephalus. *Neurology* **26:**501–507, 1976*a*.

JACOBS L, CONTI D, KINKEL WR, MANNING EL: Normal pressure hydrocephalus. *JAMA* **235:**510–512, 1976*b*.

JACOBSON PL, FARMER TW: The "hypernormal" CT scan in dementia: Bilateral isodense subdural hematoma. *Neurology* **29:**1522–1524, 1979.

JACOBY RJ, LEVY R, DAWSON JM: Computed tomography in the elderly: 1. The normal population. *Br J Psychiatry* **136:**249–255, 1980*a*.

JACOBY RJ, LEVY R: Computed tomography in the elderly: 2. Senile dementia: Diagnosis and functional impairment. *Br J Psychiatry* **136:**256–269, 1980*b*.

JACOBY RJ, LEVY R: CT scanning and the investigation of dementia: A review. *J Roy Soc Med* **73:**366–369, 1980*c*.

JAMES AE, FLOR WJ, NOVAK GR, RIBAS JL, PARKER JL, SICKEL WL: The ultrastructural basis of periventricular edema: Preliminary studies. *Radiology* **135:**757–760, 1980.

JENSEN F: Acquired hydrocephalus: III. A pathophysiological study correlated with neuropathological findings and clinical manifestations. *Acta Neurochir (Wien)* **47:**91–104, 1979.

JOHNSTONE EC, CROW TJ, FRITH CD, HUSBAND J: Cerebral ventricular size and cognitive impairment in chronic schizophrenia. *Lancet* **30:**924–926, 1976.

KATZMAN R, HUSSEY F: A simple constant-infusion manometric test for measurement of CSF absorption. *Neurology* **20:**534–544, 1970.

KISHORE PRS, LIPPER MH, DASILVA AAD, GUDEMAN SK, ABBAS SA: Delayed sequelae of head injury. *Comput Tomogr* **4:**287–295, 1980.

KUEHNLE J, MENDELSON J, DAVIS K, NEW P: Computed tomographic examination of heavy marijuana smokers. *JAMA* **237:**1231–1232, 1977.

LEMAY M, NEW PFJ: Radiological diagnosis of occult normal pressure hydrocephalus. *Radiology* **96:**347–358, 1970.

LEMAY M, HOCHBERG FH: Ventricular differences between hydrostatic hydrocephalus and hydrocephalus ex vacuo by computed tomography. *Neuroradiology* **17:**191–195, 1979.

MARMAROU A, SHULMAN K, LAMORGESE J: Compartmental analysis of compliance and outflow resistance of the cerebrospinal fluid system. *J Neurosurg* **43:**523–534, 1975.

MCCREA ES, RAO KCUG, DIACONIS JN: Roentgenographic changes during long-term diphenylhydantoin therapy. *South Med J* **73**(3):310–311, 1980.

MCCULLOUGH DC, HARBERT JC, DICHIRO G, OMMAYA SK: Prognostic criteria for cerebrospinal fluid shunting from isotope cisternography in communicating hydrocephalus. *Neurology* **20**:594–598, 1970.

MCGEACHI RE, FLEMING JO, SHARER LR, HYMAN RA: Diagnosis of Pick's disease by computed tomography. *J Comput Assist Tomogr* **3**:113–115, 1979.

MEESE W, KLUGE W, GRUMME T, HOPFENMULLER W: CT evaluation of the CSF space of healthy persons. *Neuroradiology* **19**:131–136, 1980.

MORI K, HANDA T, MURATA T, NAKANO Y: Periventricular lucency in computed tomography of hydrocephalus and cerebral atrophy. *J Comput Assist Tomogr* **4**:204–209, 1980.

NAESER MA, GEBHARDT C, LEVINE HC: Decreased computerized tomography numbers in patients with presenile demintia. *Arch Neurol* **37**:401–418, 1980.

NARDIZZI LR: Computerized tomographic correlate of carbon monoxide poisoning. *Arch Neurol* **36**:38–39, 1979.

NELSON JR, GOODMAN SJ: An evaluation of the cerebrospinal fluid test for hydrocephalus. *Neurology* **21**:1037–1053, 1971.

OKUNO T, MASATOSHI I, KONISHI Y, MIEKO Y, NAKANO Y: Cerebral atrophy following ACTH therapy. *J Comput Assist Tomogr* **4**:20–23, 1980.

PEDERSEN HM, GYLDENSTED M, GYLDENSTED C: Measurement of the normal ventricular system and supratentorial subarachnoid space in children with computed tomography. *Neuroradiology* **17**:231–237, 1979.

PENN WD, BELANGER MG, YASNOFF WA: Ventricular volume in mass computed from CT scans. *Ann Neurol* **3**:216–223, 1978.

RAMBAUGH CL et al: Cerebral CT findings in drug abuse: Clinical and experimental observations. *J Comput Assist Tomogr* **4**:330–334, 1980.

RAMSEY RG, HUCKMAN MS: Computed tomography of porencephaly and other cerebrospinal fluid–containing lesions. *Radiology* **123**:73–77, 1977.

RAO KCVG, BRENNAN TG, GARCIA JH: Computed tomography in the diagnosis of Creutzfeldt-Jakob disease. *J Comput Assist Tomogr* **1**:211–215, 1977.

ROBERTS MA, CAIRD FL: Computerized tomography and intellectual impairment in the elderly. *J Neurol Neurosurg Psychiatry* **39**:986–989, 1976.

ROPPER AH, HATTEN HP, DAVIS KR: Computed tomography of Wilson's disease: Report of two cases. *Ann Neurol* **5**:102–103, 1979.

ROSENBERG GA, KORNFELD M, STOVRING J, BICKNELL JM: Subcortical arteriosclerotic encephalopathy (Binswanger) and computerized tomography. *Neurology* **29**:1102–1106, 1979.

RUDICK RA, JOYUT RT: Normal pressure hydrocephalus: A treatable dementia. *Tex Med* **76**:46–49, 1980.

RUECK JD, CREVITS L, COSTER WD, SIEBEN G, ECKEN H: Pathogenesis of Binswanger chronic progressive subcortical encephalopathy. *Neurology* **30**:920–928, 1980.

SALMON JH: Adult hydrocephalus: Evaluation of shunt therapy in 80 patients. *J Neurosurg* **37**:423–428, 1972.

SCHEIBEL ME et al: Progressive dendritic changes in aging human cortex. *Exp Neurol* **47**:392–403, 1975.

SCHNEIDER E, BECKER H, FISHER PA, GRAU H, JACOBY P, BRINKMAN R: The course of brain atrophy in Parkinson's disease. *Arch Psychiatr Nervenkr* **227**:89–95, 1979.

SHENKIN HA, GREENBERG J, BOUZARTH WF, GUTTERMAN P, MORALES JO: Ventricular shunting for relief of senile symptoms. *JAMA* **225**:1486–1489, 1973.

SJAASTAD O, SKALPE IO, ENGESET A: The width of the temporal horn in the differential diagnosis between pressure hydrocephalus and hydrocephalus ex vacuo. *Neurology* **19**:1087–1093, 1969.

STEIN SC, LANGFITT TW: Normal pressure hydrocephalus: Predicting the results of cerebrospinal fluid shunting. *J Neurosurg* **41**:463–470, 1974.

SYMON L, HINZPETER T: Enigma of normal pressure hydrocephalus. *Clin Neurosurg* **24**:285–315, 1977.

SYNEK V, REUBEN JR, GAWLER J, DUBOULAY GH: Comparison of the measurements of the cerebral ventricles obtained by CT scanning and pneumoencephalography. *Neuroradiology* **17**:149–151, 1976.

TATOR CH, FLEMING JFR, SHEPPARD RH, TURNER VM: A radioisotope test for communicating hydrocephalus. *J Neurosurg* **28**:327–340, 1968.

TERBRUGGE KG, SCHUTZ H, CHIU MC, TAYLOR F: CSF dynamics in adults with hydrocephalus. Presented at the 18th annual meeting, American Society of Neuroradiology, March 16-21, 1980, Los Angeles.

TERRENCE CF, DELANEY JF, ALBERTS MC: Computed tomography for Huntington's disease. *Neuroradiology* **13**:173–175, 1977.

TOMLINSON BE, BLESSED G, ROTH M: Observations on the brains of demented old people. *J Neurol Sci* **11**:205–242, 1970.

WEINBERGER DR, TORREY EF, NEOPHYTIDES AN, WYATT RJ: Lateral cerebral ventricular enlargement in chronic schizophenia. *Arch Gen Psychiatry* **36**:735–739, 1979.

WOLINSKY JS, BARNES BD, MARGOLIS MT: Diagnostic tests in normal pressure hydrocephalus. *Neurology* **23**:706–713, 1973.

WOLPERT S: The ventricular size on computed tomography. *J Comput Assist Tomogr* **1**:222–226, 1977.

YAMARU H, ITO M, KUBOTA K, MAFSUZAWA T: Brain atrophy during aging: A quantitative study with computer tomography. *J Gerontol* **35**:492–497, 1980.

ZATZ LM, JERNIGAN TL, AHUMADA AJ Jr: Changes on computed cranial tomography with aging: intracranial fluid volume. *Am J Neuroradiol* **3**(1):1–12, 1982.

ZEUMER H, SCHONSKY B, STRUM KW: Predominant white matter involvement in subcortical arteriosclerotic encephalopathy (Binswanger disease). *J Comput Assist Tomogr* **4**:14–19, 1980.

ZILKHA A: CT of cerebral hemiatrophy. *Am J Roentgenol Radium Ther Nucl Med* **135**:263–267, 1980.

THE VENTRICLES AND SUBARACHNOID SPACES IN CHILDREN

Charles R. Fitz

HYDROCEPHALUS

Ventricular dilatation does not necessarily mean hydrocephalus. Several other causes of ventricular dilatation can be identified by CT. Physiologic dilatation occurs in premature infants (Fig. 6-1), being greatest in those born early in the mother's pregnancy and approaching normal size in those born after approximately 36 weeks of gestation. Mild ventricular enlargement occurs in some megalencephalies such as Soto's syndrome (Fig. 6-2). Congenital malformations may have a developmental or dysplastic ventricular enlargement. Atrophic ventricular enlargement, to be discussed later in this chapter, may be present with or secondary to hydrocephalus.

The definition of hydrocephalus as a dynamic process (Harwood-Nash and Fitz, 1976, Chap. 10) due to a blockage of CSF flow somewhere along its pathway or an overproduction of CSF remains valid. Because it is a dynamic process, the static image of a single CT examination may not be sufficient to indicate clearly whether the ventricular enlargement is secondary to hydrocephalus. Experience, however, often offers the physician clues to help decide whether true hydrocephalus is present.

CT Evaluation of Suspected Hydrocephalus

Most hydrocephalus in childhood begins and is diagnosed in early infancy. Most cases are congenital, though they result from a variety of causes. Given

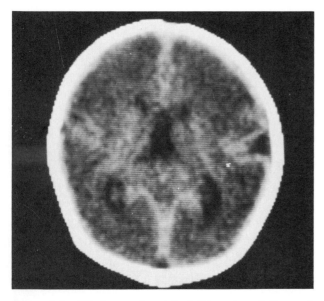

Figure 6-1   CT of premature infant (30-week gestation age) showing physiologic mild dilatation of the lateral ventricles. The sylvian fissures are also wide. CT done without contrast.

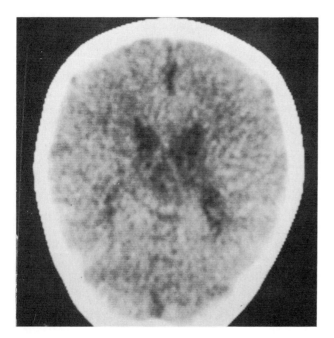

Figure 6-2   Soto's syndrome. A 5-year-old child with large head and mild retardation shows mild ventricular and sulcal enlargement suggestive of Soto's syndrome. There was no evidence of increased intracranial pressure.

a short history of enlarging head in an infant under 3 months of age, with no obvious preceding event such as infection or hemorrhage, it is the author's routine practice to perform the CT examination without contrast, using 10-mm slices. If the results of the initial examination are unusual or suggestive of a disease process that would become clearer with intravenous contrast injection, this is given and the examination is repeated. Other views, especially coronal or clival perpendicular, may be obtained, as well as thinner, 5-mm slices in areas where greater detail is needed, though this is uncommon.

The radiation dose should be kept as low as possible in the newborn. Most examinations of infants are done at the author's institution at a dose of approximately 1 rad (GE 8800 third-generation scanner) if extra views or contrast enhancement are not required. The dose is even lower for premature infants.

In a child of 6 months or more, intravenous contrast is always part of the examination, since congenital causes for hydrocephalus are less common at that age and tumor in particular must be excluded as a cause of hydrocephalus. Signs of inflammation or trauma, such as subdural membranes, may also be seen.

Intraventricular contrast thus continues to have a limited, though important, role in the diagnosis of hydrocephalus. It is no longer necessary to outline the ventricles with air, but air or metrizamide can give important information as to the sites of obstruction and the location of cysts that are the occasional cause of hydrocephalus (Marc 1980) and can be introduced via the shunt reservoir after treatment of hydrocephalus. An average of 1 to 3 ml of 210 to 220 mg I per ml metrizamide is injected very slowly through the shunt tubing so as to layer on the floor of the frontal horns or directly into the third ventricle, with the patient in a sitting position. The head is flexed slightly forward to hold the metrizamide in the frontal horns if it has not already entered the third ventricle. The head is slowly extended or rotated toward the supine position to allow the contrast to drain into the third ventricle and outline its floor, the aqueduct, and the fourth ventricle if the aqueduct is patent. The initial part

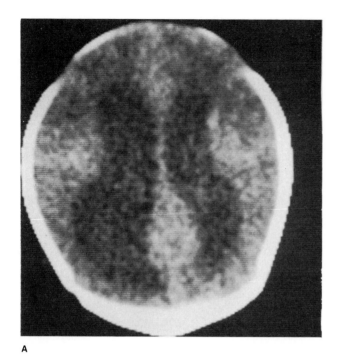

A

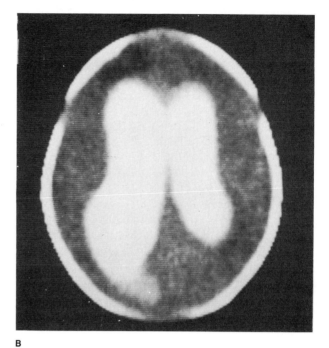

B

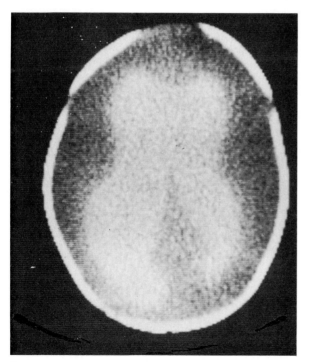

C

Figure 6-3 Transependymal absorption of metrizamide. **A.** CT without contrast in an infant with aqueduct stenosis shows large lateral ventricles. **B.** CT immediately following metrizamide ventriculogram shows the contrast agent within the ventricular system. **C.** Examination 24 hours later using the same window setting shows transmission of ventricular contrast through the entire brain. Further examination showed continued decrease in ventricular density and increase in brain density.

of this examination is best done on a conventional pneumoencephalographic unit. If an obstruction is encountered, CT can be done to see if any metrizamide passes the obstruction. If the ventricular system is patent, CT can be used to follow the metrizamide flow into the subarachnoid space and to watch for any block. The examination can in this way substitute for a radionuclide study of the cerebral spinal fluid flow. In an infant with bulging fontanelle, injection of similar amounts of metrizamide following a ventricular tap may provide the diagnosis in occasional cases.

A serendipitous observation in examinations done in this manner has been the transependymal absorption of the metrizamide through the brain parenchyma (Fig. 6-3) (Fitz 1978*b*), confirming the conclusion of others that periventricular hypodensities are due to transependymal passage of CSF (Milhorat 1970, Hiratsuka 1979).

Metrizamide has little or no place in the primary CT investigation of hydrocephalus.

Intraventricular Obstructive Hydrocephalus

This term refers to the obstruction of CSF flow anywhere along the ventricular pathways from the lateral ventricles to the fourth ventricular outlets, commonly called *noncommunicating hydrocephalus*. The cause of congenital intraventricular obstructive hydrocephalus (IVOH), excluding toxic, infectious, and posthemorrhagic causes, is usually aqueduct stenosis, often associated with the Chiari II malformation.

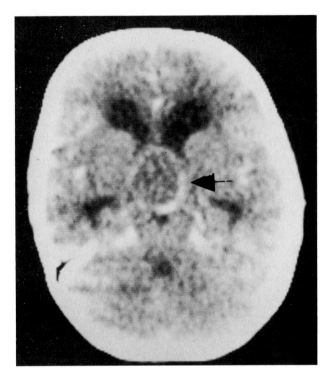

Figure 6-4   Occlusion of the foramen of Monro. CT with intravenous contrast shows ring enhancement of suprasellar craniopharyngioma (arrow) partially blocking the foramen of Monro and causing hydrocephalus.

OCCLUSION OF THE FORAMEN OF MONRO   IVOH due to occlusion of one or both of the foramina of Monro is uncommon. Intraventricular hemorrhage from trauma or other causes of bleeding, such as arteriovenous malformation or hemophilia, can cause a temporary clot in the foramen with resulting hydrocephalus, but this is usually temporary in children. Infection is also an uncommon cause of obstruction at this site. Congenital atresia is extremely rare (Taboada 1979).

The most common obstructing lesion is tumor of various types. Suprasellar masses, especially craniopharyngiomas, extend upward and sometimes compress the third ventricle and cause a partial obstruction of the foramen of Monro (Fig. 6-4). Intraventricular tumors or cysts and arachnoid cysts of the suprasellar cistern (Fig. 6-5) may also obstruct the foramen of Monro.

In the case of tumors in the midline, the obstruction is usually bilateral but not always equal on both sides. Unilateral tumors, such as those arising in the hypothalamus, basal ganglia, or cerebral parenchyma may obstruct only one side (Fig. 6-6), but a large tumor can compress both foramina. In the latter case it is common for the ipsilateral ventricle to be compressed by the tumor mass and the opposite ventricle dilated.

AQUEDUCT STENOSIS   Congenital aqueduct stenosis, or occlusion without the Chiari malformation, does occur but is uncommon (Table 6-1). A hereditary type has also been reported (Edwards 1961) but is, in the author's experience, extremely rare.

Hydrocephalus, especially that following repair of the meningocele, is invariably associated with the Chiari II malformation. It is by far the most common cause of hydrocephalus and aqueduct stenosis seen in early childhood. Most aqueduct occlusions in association with the Chiari malformation were previously thought, on the basis of air or Pantopaque ventriculography, to be total. Metrizamide examination has shown, however, that a majority have some contrast flow through the aqueduct and fourth ventricle, with a significant blockage of CSF flow within the subarachnoid cisterns at the tentorial

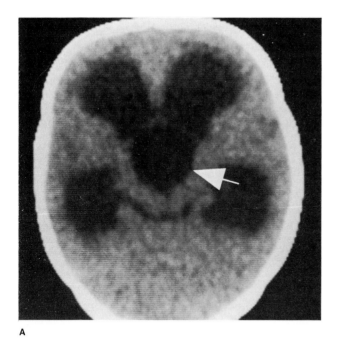

A

Figure 6-5 Occlusion of the foramen of Monro. **A.** Five-month-old with suprasellar cyst obstructing the third ventricle and causing severe hydrocephalus. Even in severe hydrocephalus the third ventricle is usually not this wide. **B.** Metrizamide ventriculogram, lateral view. Metrizamide is visible in the

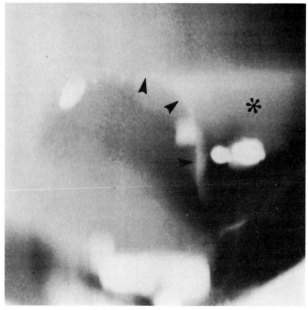

B

frontal horns (asterisk) and in the anterior third ventricle, which is compressed upward by the large suprasellar cyst (arrows). Denser contrast material is a small amount of Pantopaque also injected.

Table I   Lesions Causing Aqueduct Obstruction

Intrinsic
Infection
Congenital factors
Hemorrhage
Chiari II malformation

Extrinsic
Neoplasm
Dilated vein of Galen
Quadrigeminal cyst
Brainstem edema

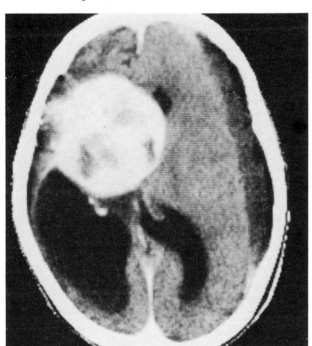

Figure 6-6 Occlusion of the foramen of Monro. The right lateral ventricle is totally obstructed by a huge thalamic tumor. There is partial obstruction of the left lateral ventricle. A large subacute subdural hematoma is also present on the left side secondary to previous shunting and operative procedures.

level (Fig. 6-7) (Fitz 1978*a*). Other specific abnor-malities of the Chiari malformation that can be iden-tified on CT are dealt with in greater detail in Chap-ter 4. The bony abnormalities of the lacunar skull (Fig. 6-8) are seen in the neonatal period, usually up to 3 to 6 weeks. Scalloping of the posterior wall of the petrous bones (Fig. 6-9) can be seen from birth onward. The steep tentorium and low trans-verse sinuses are visible with intravenous contrast enhancement in clival perpendicular views (Fig. 6-10).

Features of the brain and ventricular system are also identifiable (Naidich 1980*b*). As the falx is de-ficient, the medial cortices of the cerebral hemi-sphere are not separated and may show interdigi-tation (Fig. 6-11). This is better defined in the older child. The lateral ventricles have a peculiar config-uration, best seen when they are not grossly en-larged. The occipital horns are relatively larger than the ventricular bodies in many cases, and the bodies of the lateral ventricles are parallel, as seen in agen-esis of the corpus callosum. The frontal horns also have a peculiar configuration (Fig. 6-12), visible in

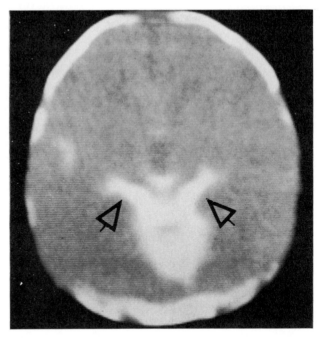

Figure 6-7 Chiari II malformation. CT 2 hours after metriza-mide ventriculography shows most of the contrast trapped in the quadrigeminal cistern and against the hiatus (arrows). A small amount of contrast is visible in one sylvian fissure.

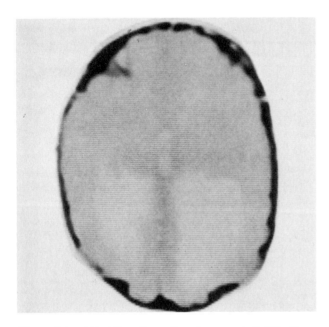

Figure 6-8   Chiari II malformation: lacunar skull. CT with re-versed gray scale shows scalloping of the inner table of the skull in 5-day-old infant.

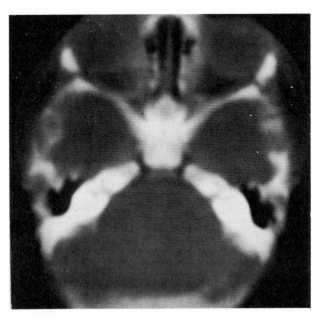

Figure 6-9   Chiari II malformation. Scalloping of the petrous bones due to compression of the hindbrain is visible in a two-week-old infant.

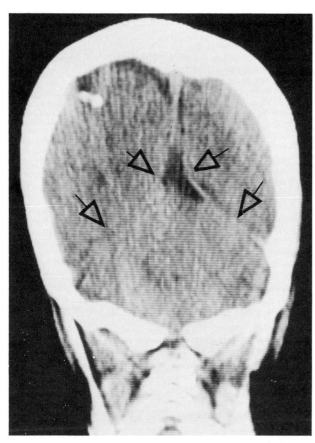

Figure 6-10 Chiari II malformation. Clival perpendicular view with contrast in 2-year-old shows the steepness of the tentorium (arrows).

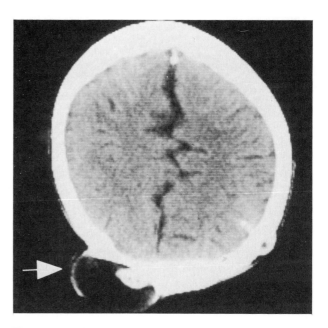

Figure 6-11 Chiari II malformation. Interdigitation of the sutures across the interhemispheric fissure is easily visible in this shunted child. An unusual shunt complication—leakage of CSF along the shunt into the scalp around the reservoir—is also visible (arrow).

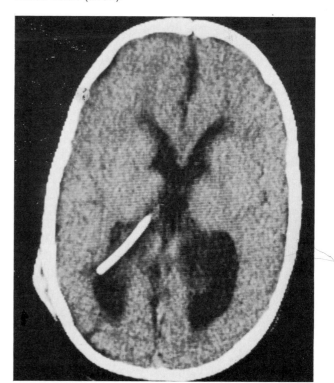

Figure 6-12 Arnold-Chiari malformation: frontal horns. Prominent caudate nuclei give the frontal horns their characteristic appearance, as though they are being compressed from their lateral surfaces.

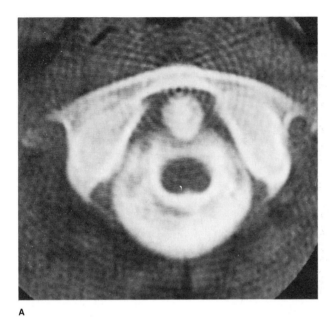

A

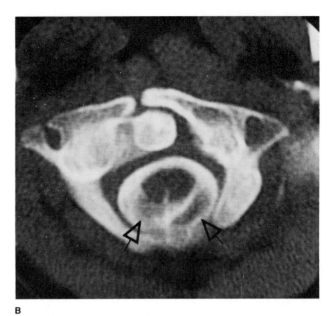

B

Figure 6-13   Chiari II malformation: tonsillar herniation.   **A.** CT metrizamide myelogram through C1 shows the cerebellar tonsils as slight posterior bulges not separable from the cervical cord.   **B.** A CT metrizamide myelogram of an 11-year-old child. At the C1–C2 level CT image shows larger tonsils that can be seen separate from the cord (arrows). The right tonsil is more poorly seen because of averaging of the CT numbers between the inferior tip of the tonsil and metrizamide below it. Also note bony anomaly.

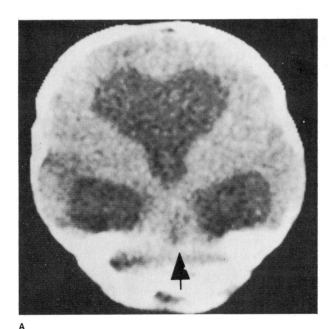

A

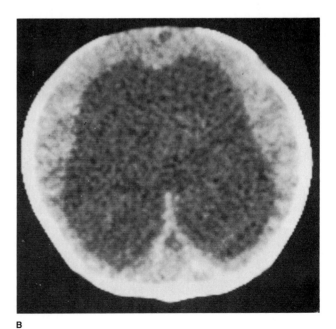

B

Figure 6-14   Congenital aqueduct stenosis.   **A.** Inferior CT slice shows marked enlargement of the lateral and third ventricles, with a normal-size fourth ventricle (arrow).   **B.** Marked enlargement of the lateral ventricles on a higher cut.

both standard and coronal views, due to the prominence of the caudate nuclei. Such findings were previously described from air studies (Gooding 1968; Harwood-Nash and Fitz 1976, Chap. 16.). The fourth ventricle is usually small and can be missed if the CT sections are 10 mm or thicker. The cerebellar tonsils may be seen below the foramen magnum, especially if they are outlined with metrizamide (Fig. 6-13). The larger-than-normal foramen magnum may also be recognizable. The beaking of the tectum, the inverted V shape of the tentorial hiatus, and other features (Naidich 1980a) are best seen after shunting in older children.

Congenital aqueduct stenosis without the Chiari malformation is most often a structural lesion of unknown cause. It is not known to be commonly related to any specific insult. In aqueduct stenosis, or in any IVOH for that matter, the ventricles are usually larger than in extraventricular obstructive hydrocephalus (communicating hydrocephalus), in-

dicating that the obstruction is more severe. The lateral and third ventricles are moderately to severely enlarged (Fig. 6-14). The shapes of the ventricles are not specific. However, in neonates and infants with hydrocephalus, the occipital horns appear more dilated than the frontal horns. Subsequently, in the untreated infant, progressive enlargement of all segments of the lateral ventricles takes place. If a Chiari malformation is not present the fourth ventricle is usually normal in size, but on occasion it, too, is mildly enlarged for unknown reasons.

Delayed aqueduct stenosis of childhood is a relatively specific entity. It is usually diagnosed around ages 8 to 11 years. The head is mildly enlarged. The patient may present with signs or symptoms of hydrocephalus of relatively recent onset. On CT, the ventricles resemble those seen in infantile aqueduct stenosis. Usually only moderately large, they can sometimes be quite sizable (Fig. 6-15). The skull

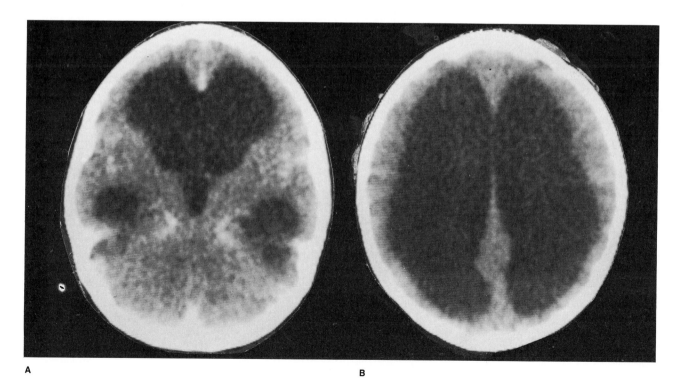

A   **B**

Figure 6-15   Delayed-onset aqueduct stenosis. **A** and **B** resemble the findings in Figure 6-14 in this 10-year-old. The **A** view is slightly above the fourth ventricle.

usually shows signs of chronic increased intracranial pressure, with sutural splitting and prominent digital markings of the inner table.

CT after intravenous contrast should always be performed to rule out enhancing masses or acute inflammation, though these are uncommonly found in hydrocephalus without specific neurological signs in children. Because CT spatial resolution does not show the aqueduct well enough, contrast ventriculography with air or metrizamide should also be done. The simplest method is the injection of metrizamide via a shunt reservoir into the ventricular system to outline the posterior third ventricle and aqueduct. In the author's experience, the posterior third ventricle and proximal aqueduct commonly have some irregularity suggesting previous inflammation (Fig. 6-16), and care is required to avoid overdiagnosis of tumor in such cases. For this portion of the examination, CT has not been an adequate substitute. In many cases the cause of the stenosis may not be known (Chuang 1981); most probably it is inflammatory and of post-neonatal onset.

Tumors causing aqueduct stenosis are not uncommon, though rare in the first 3 months, when most aqueduct stenosis is found. Any posterior fossa mass may obstruct the aqueduct, usually by a forward displacement and kinking of the passage. Brainstem gliomas do not usually cause aqueduct stenosis or significant hydrocephalus except when they are exophytic and growing superiorly into the cerebellum. Direct compression by pineal tumors has the same result as posterior fossa masses.

Cysts of the quadrigeminal cistern likewise cause aqueduct obstruction (Fig. 6-17). In the author's experience, nearly all quadrigeminal cysts have occurred in children with the Chiari malformation who have had previous shunts. The tumor or cyst is nearly always clearly visible on CT as the cause of aqueduct stenosis in such cases. If the tumor can be successfully removed, the hydrocephalus will not require shunting in most cases.

Aqueduct stenosis may also be secondary to edema, with uncal herniation or generalized swelling and downward compression of the midbrain into the posterior fossa. The stenosis is self-limited

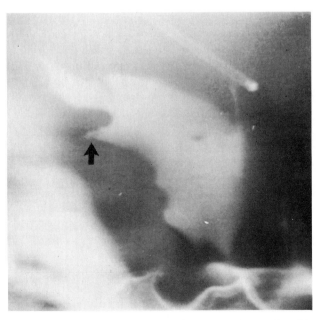

Figure 6-16   Delayed-onset aqueduct stenosis: metrizamide ventriculogram. Lateral view shows some irregularity of the third ventricle–aqueduct junction area (arrow).

and temporary if the edema is treatable. In association with vascular malformation, aneurysmal dilatation of the vein of Galen is one of the less common causes of aqueductal obstruction and resulting hydrocephalus.

Acute infection is usually not a cause of aqueduct stenosis, but it may be suspected, inasmuch as the aqueduct is the narrowest and longest intraventricular passage. Neonatal hemorrhage as a cause of aqueduct stenosis is dealt with separately in a later section of this chapter.

OBSTRUCTION OF THE FOURTH VENTRICULAR OUTLETS
Although it is relatively uncommon in childhood, obstruction of the fourth ventricular outlets is second to aqueduct stenosis as a cause of hydrocephalus in infancy. Most often, regardless of age, the fourth ventricle is quite dilated and proportionately slightly larger than the third ventricle (Fig. 6-18) in this condition. Occasionally the fourth ventricle can be of normal size in spite of the outlet obstruction (Fig. 6-19). Such discrepancy is not easily explainable by CSF dynamics, as it is most com-

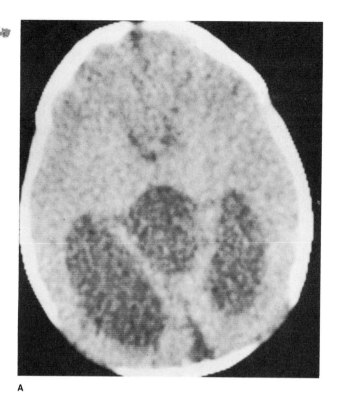

A

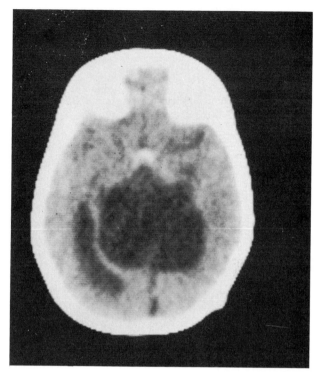

B

Figure 6-17 Aqueduct stenosis: quadrigeminal cyst. **A.** CT slice through level of the quadrigeminal cistern shows CSF space betwen occipital horns interpreted as a large quadri-geminal cistern in this infant with Chiari malformation. **B.** CT at 1 year shows marked enlargement of the quadrigeminal cyst.

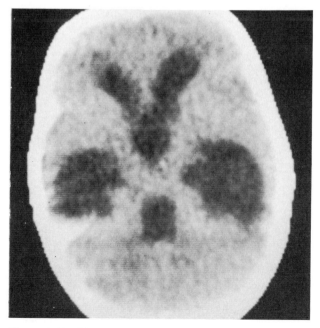

Figure 6-18 Obstruction of the fourth ventricular outlet. CT show typical enlargement of the entire ventricular system.

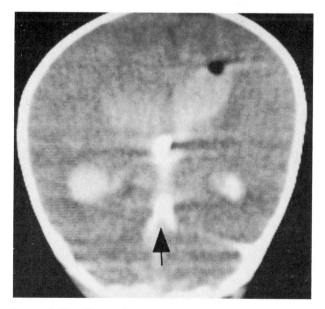

Figure 6-19 Obstruction of the fourth ventricular outlet. CT in clival parallel position following metrizamide ventriculo-graphy shows dense collection of metrizamide in obstructed fourth ventricle (arrow). Artifacts due to motion are present.

monly the ventricle closest to the obstruction that is the most dilated.

The specific causes of fourth ventricular outlet obstruction are similar to those of other ventricular narrowings. Ventricular hemorrhage or infection can obstruct the foramina, though proven cases are uncommon. Tumors are usually not located in such a position as to cause this obstruction, though inferior vermis medulloblastomas, brainstem tumors of the inferior medulla, and congenital or malignant extraaxial tumors may rarely do this.

Extraaxial cysts such as arachnoid cysts of the cisterna magna may cause hydrocephalus by occluding the fourth ventricular outlets (Fig. 6-20). The specific diagnosis is of some importance, since permanent collapse of the cyst may obviate the need for ventricular shunting. Enlargement of the cisterna magna or a CSF space is obvious in such cases, but the cause may not be. A congenitally large cisterna magna and some Dandy-Walker malformations may also resemble an arachnoid cyst (Fig. 6-21). Unless one sees an obvious mass effect and compression of the cerebellar hemispheres, radionuclide or contrast material such as metrizamide should be injected. If the contrast is injected into the ventricles, CT will usually show contrast within the ventricles with demonstration of the extraaxial arachnoid cyst (Fig. 6-20*B*). If injected by the lumbar subarachnoid space, it will either not enter the posterior fossa or entry will be delayed.

In the Dandy-Walker cyst, a developmental obstruction of the fourth ventricular outlets with ab-

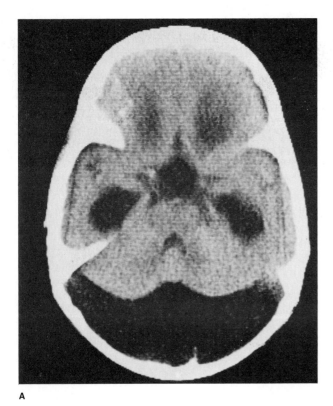

A

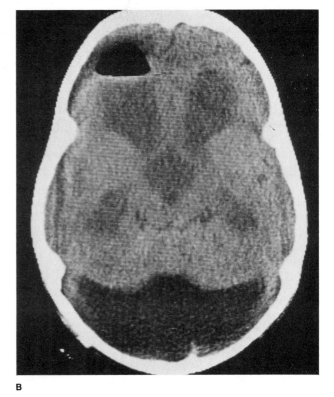

B

Figure 6-20   Posterior fossa arachnoid cyst.   **A.** CT in a 9-year-old shows a large posterior fossa cyst with enlargement of the lateral and third ventricles but a normal-size, possibly compressed, fourth ventricle.   **B.** After metrizamide ventriculography, CT shows metrizamide in the ventricular system but none in the arachnoid cyst. A small amount of air is present in the right frontal horn.

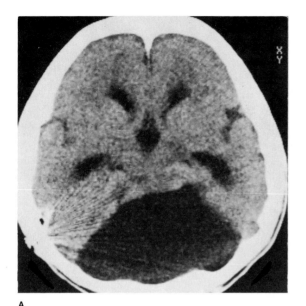

A

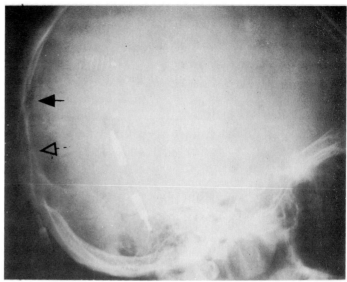

B

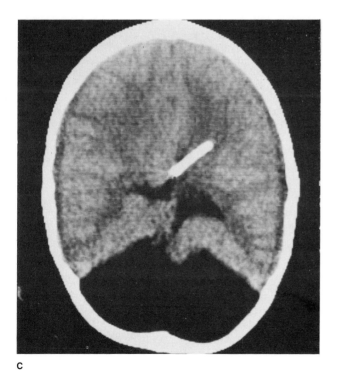

C

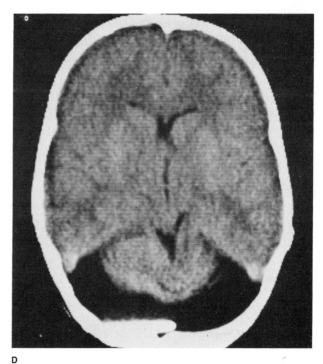

D

Figure 6-21 Posterior fossa cyst. **A.** Twelve-year-old with Dandy-Walker cyst and shunted hydrocephalus. **B.** In spite of extreme cerebellar hypoplasia, the torcular (open arrow) is not higher than lambda (closed arrow). **C.** Posterior fossa arachnoid cysts resemble **A** at higher level. **D,** at lower levels, shows compressed fourth ventricle and more development of the cerebellum. Both the hydrocephalus and the cyst are shunted (**C** and **D**).

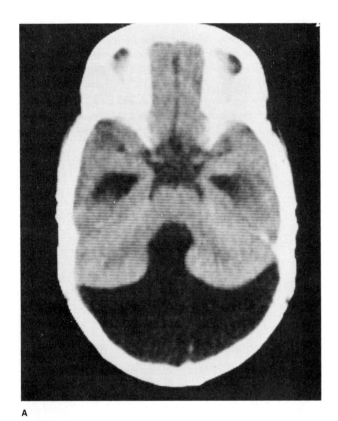

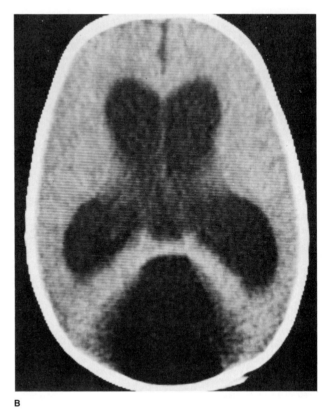

A   B

Figure 6-22   Dandy-Walker cyst.   **A.** Enlarged fourth ventricle opening directly into the posterior fossa cyst owing to absence of the vermis.   **B.** Higher cut shows hydrocephalus and lack of cerebellar tissue.

sence or hypoplasia of the vermis (Hart 1972), a large fourth ventricle that empties directly into a cystic cavity resembling the cisterna magna is common (Fig. 6-22). The vermis is not visible, and the cerebellar hemispheres are hypoplastic. The cyst is nearly always in direct communication with the fourth ventricle.

The Dandy-Walker variant is a less well-defined lesion in which the fourth ventricle has a wide but formed foramen of Magendi. Some inferior vermis may also be visible. The torcular-lambdoid inversion of the classical Dandy-Walker cyst is usually not present. Differentiation from an arachnoid cyst may be quite difficult (Archer 1978) without ventricular instillation of contrast that fills the cyst in the Dandy-Walker variant and the normal fourth ventricle in the extraaxial arachnoid cyst. Even this is not a completely reliable sign, with variations re-

ported. Dandy-Walker cysts are said to have open foramina at times (Raimondi 1969), and arachnoid cysts may communicate with the ventricular system or subarachnoid space (di Rocco 1981).

Extraventricular Obstructive Hydrocephalus

In extraventricular obstructive hydrocephalus (EVOH), or *communicating hydrocephalus*, the obstruction is distal to the ventricles and may be anywhere along the subarachnoid space. The basal cisterns, the tentorial hiatus, the spaces over the cerebrum and arachnoid granulations, or any combination of these may be sites of obstruction. Identification of the sites is usually not of clinical importance except in certain situations. If a shunt from the lumbar arachnoid space to the peritoneum is planned, one must be sure that the obstruction is at least above the basal cisterns. If IVOH is to be treated by ventriculotomy—most commonly puncture of the third ventricle (Hoffman 1980)—one would like to know that the subarachnoid space is not obstructed.

Children with hydrocephalus, unlike adults, may show dilatation of the subarachnoid space over the hemisphere. Most commonly this occurs in EVOH (Fig. 6-23), and it is, in the author's experience, a reasonably reliable sign that the obstruction is outside the ventricular system.

The lateral ventricles are usually only moderately dilated in EVOH, and the third and fourth ventricles also show mild dilatation. There are, of course, exceptions to this rule, and considerable dilatation of all ventricles or of only the lateral and third ventricles occasionally occurs (Fig. 6-24). The reasons for these variations are not certain, though one may speculate that the cause of the hydrocephalus may currently or previously have been affecting the outlets of the more dilated ventricles. Generally, this information is not of much clinical significance.

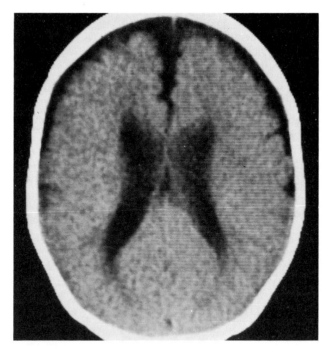

Figure 6-23   EVOH: dilated sulci. Five-month-old with mild to moderate hydrocephalus showing enlargement of the sulci. Compare with normal sulcal prominence in Figure 6-55.

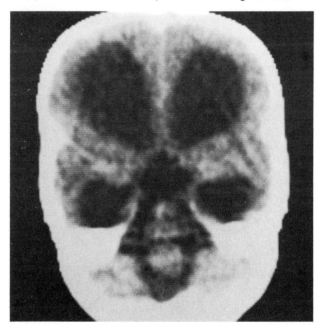

A

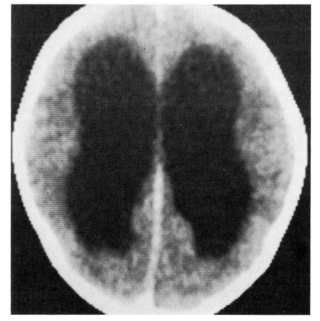

B

Figure 6-24   EVOH. Clival parallel projection in **A** shows large suprasellar cistern and cisterns around the brainstem. This may occur in spite of marked ventricular dilatation, as noted in **B**.

Because the appearance of EVOH is similar no matter what the level of obstruction, this entity is discussed here by cause rather than by site. For the most part the causes are the same as in IVOH, but they are more likely to be documented. This is because EVOH more frequently is diagnosed after the neonatal period and after a clinically evident causal event. Because the ventricles are less enlarged, the head is relatively less enlarged. In an older child the head also will not expand as rapidly as in an infant. Symptoms may be mild, and the obstruction to CSF flow is usually incomplete.

TUMORS   Primary brain tumors do not obstruct the subarachnoid space. The possible exception to this might be a large posterior fossa mass that compresses the cerebellum against the tentorium and causes obstruction at the hiatus at the same time as it occludes the aqueduct.

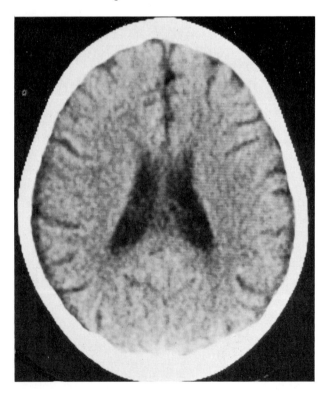

Figure 6-25   Leukemia. CT in 8-year-old child being treated for acute lymphocytic leukemia shows mild enlargement of the sulci and lateral ventricles.

In children, secondary seeding of the subarachnoid space from almost any malignant disease except leukemia is rare. In leukemia, a blockage of the basal cisterns or subarachnoid space (or both) over the hemispheres may occur. Contrast examination should be carried out to confirm this leukemic spread, though in the author's experience, enhancement of the subarachnoid space is uncommon in spite of the presence of hydrocephalus and of visible leukemic cells in the CSF on microscopy.

Ventricular and sulcal dilatation in leukemia presents a problem to the radiologist. It is a common event, even in leukemic children who do not have symptoms of hydrocephalus (Fig. 6-25). A possible cause other than hydrocephalus in such cases is treatment with methotrexate and/or radiation, producing atrophic enlargement. Treatment with steroids is also known to give the brain an atrophy-like appearance (Okuno 1980).

Primary tumor of the subarachnoid space is a very rare cause of hydrocephalus. The author has seen only one such case, a primary melanosarcoma of the meninges. Here the contrast enhancement of the meninges could not be distinguished from that caused by metastases or inflammation (Flodmark 1979).

INFECTION   Acute meningitis can cause permanent or temporary obstruction of the flow of CSF by inflammatory reaction and later adhesions. In the acute stage one will usually see contrast enhancement in the cisterns or other subarachnoid spaces along with the ventricular enlargement (Chap. 13). After treatment only the history may suggest the cause of hydrocephalus.

Subdural or extradural empyema is also a cause of EVOH. In the acute phase, contrast enhancement is visible (Fig. 6-26). The hydrocephalus is secondary to both the inflammatory reaction and the pressure, which may compress a portion of the subarachnoid space.

NEONATAL HEMORRHAGE   Before the availability of CT and ultrasound, it was thought that intraventricular hemorrhage was a common cause of hydrocephalus in infants. Experience has shown that this

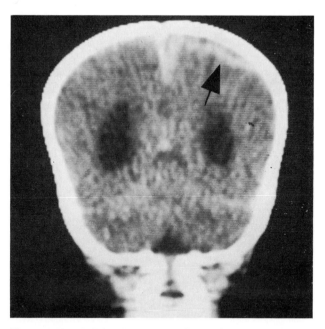

Figure 6-26 Subdural empyema. Coronal projection following intravenous contrast shows enhancing membrane (arrow) of thin subdural empyema which displaces cortex inward from the calvarium and extends into the interhemispheric fissure. Note dilatation of the occipital horns.

is not a common sequela, especially in our own series of patients (Flodmark 1980). While intraventricular hemorrhage usually causes temporary dilatation of the ventricles and hydrocephalus, the condition most often resolves. It has also been found that intraventricular hemorrhage is usually accompanied by subarachnoid hemorrhage (Flodmark 1980), and hydrocephalus that occurs after ventricular bleeding can be a combination of partial obstruction in both areas. Subarachnoid hemorrhage as a primary event in neonates usually occurs only in the term infant who has had a traumatic delivery. Here too, hydrocephalus is not necessarily a subsequent condition.

SUBDURAL HEMATOMA Subdural hematoma, especially in the chronic stage, is commonly a cause of EVOH. From about 1 week after the hematoma occurs, an inflammatory membrane is often visible on the inner surface of the hematoma after contrast enhancement. This can persist for an indefinite pe-

riod. Subdural hematoma also causes dilatation of the subarachnoid space over the cortex, presumably because the CSF accumulates in the subarachnoid space near the site of obstruction.

In the author's experience, subdural hematoma fairly quickly reaches the density of the brain in about 4 to 7 days, then appears decreasingly less dense and reaches a chronic appearance that is of approximately CSF density in about 4 weeks. It may be possible to see evidence of recurrent subdural hematoma bleeding by visualization of layers of different density (Fig. 6-27).

The hydrocephalus caused by subdural hematoma is usually mild to moderate, though nonetheless clinically significant.

CONGENITAL FACTORS Communicating hydrocephalus is often seen in children with achondroplasia. The ventricles are dilated moderately in association with prominent subarachnoid spaces, especially over the convexity. Although the exact mechanism is not known, the condition is presumed to be secondary to a relative outlet obstruction from the narrow foramen magnum. More recently it has been postulated that the communicating hydrocephalus is secondary to decreased venous outflow at outlet foramina such as the sigmoid sinus (Yamada 1981). Similar patterns of communicating hydrocephalus have also been reported in craniometaphyseal dysplasia (Fig. 6-28) (Allen 1982). Communicating hydrocephalus possibly due to hypoplasia of the arachnoid granulations has also been reported (Gilles 1971).

Increased Production of CSF

Overproduction of CSF in children is a rare event caused by choroid plexus papilloma or carcinoma. In the adult these are usually in the fourth ventricle; in children, in the lateral ventricle. When these tumors are large, they are fairly easy to diagnose on CT (Fig. 6-29), and can be differentiated from other intraventricular masses by their choroid location and typical choroidal contrast enhancement. With a small tumor, diagnosis by CT may be difficult, because the tumor may not be obviously larger than

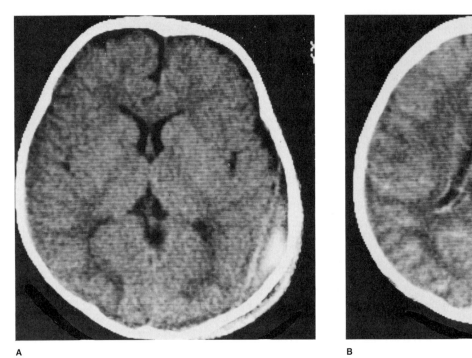

A   **B**

Figure 6-27   Subdural hematoma. CT before intravenous contrast **(A)** and after contrast **(B).** Marked enhancement of inner membrane of subacute or chronic subdural hematoma is seen in **B** (arrow). Recurrent nonenhancing bleeding is seen as increased density in both **A** and **B** within the isodense hematoma. No hydrocephalus is present in this 7-year-old.

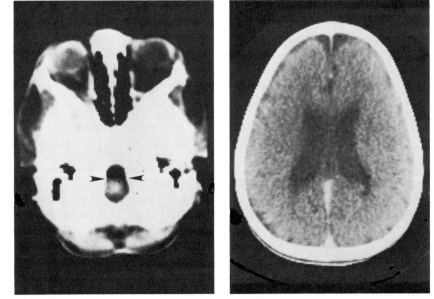

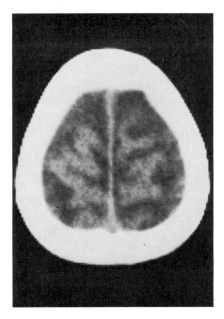

A

Figure 6-28   **A.** Cranial CT. Thickening of skull base; normal ventricular size with prominent frontal subarachnoid space; frontal bossing; dilated cortical sulci.   **B.** Right side: narrowing at the origin of the jugular vein (arrowhead).

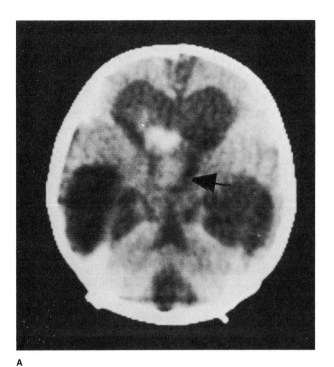

A

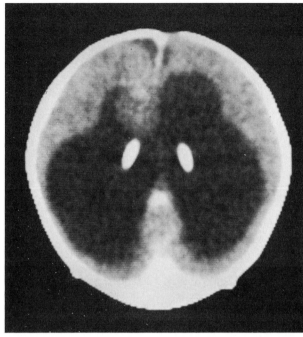

B

Figure 6-29 A large choroid plexus papilloma visible in contrast-enhanced CT in a 3-month-old. Papilloma is unusual in that it extends in **A** from the third ventricle (arrow) into the frontal horn in both **A** and **B.** Only a portion of the papilloma adjacent to the third ventricle shows enhancement. Note the marked hydrocephalus in spite of the biventricular shunts.

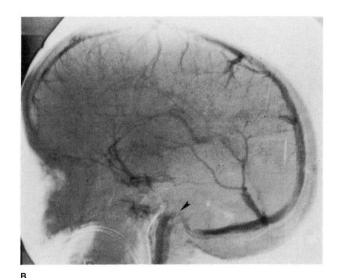

B

Figure 6-28B (Legend on facing page)

the prominent choroid plexus on the normal side. This usually occurs in children under the age of 2 years, a group that has prominent choroid plexuses even in the normal situation (Fig. 6-30). When the tumors are small, angiography may be needed to visualize an abnormal choroid vasculature. In some cases measurement of CSF output by ventricular catheterization may be necessary to be certain of the diagnosis.

Normal-Pressure Hydrocephalus

Normal-pressure hydrocephalus, a condition that occurs in older adults, is not a diagnosis made in children. It may be that children investigated for hydrocephalus who have mild ventricular and sulcal dilatation on CT but no definite clinical symptoms of raised intracranial pressure have a condition that is equivalent to the adult normal-pressure hy-

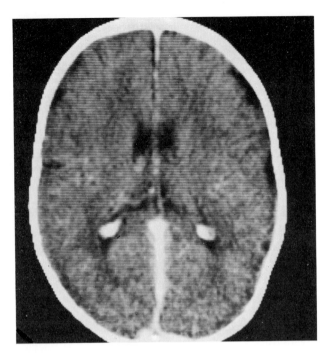

Figure 6-30   CT with intravenous contrast shows prominence of the normal choroid plexus in an 8-month-old child.

drocephalus. They do not, however, have the clinical triad of gait ataxia, urinary and fecal incontinence, and dementia.

Arrested Hydrocephalus

It may be said in some seriousness that the only arrested hydrocephalic is one who is under police custody. A better term is *compensated hydrocephalus,* since a person with hydrocephalus, treated or untreated, may have an activation of the disease even though it has been asymptomatic for several years. It must again be emphasized that a single CT examination may be noninformative as to the dynamic state of the patient's hydrocephalus. This is especially true when the first CT examination available to the radiologist is made after treatment or there has been an interval of 2 or more years between examinations. Ventricular size may change considerably over a short period of time—a week to a month (Fig. 6-31).

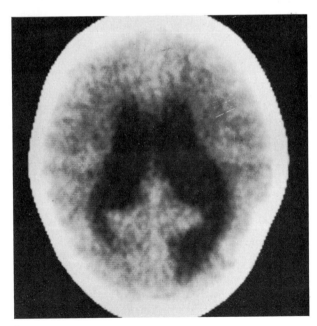

A

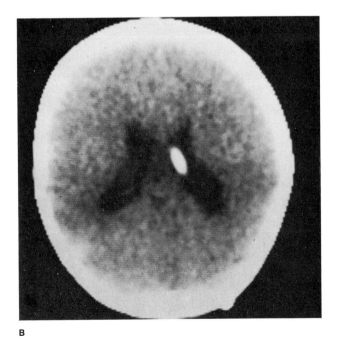

B

Figure 6-31   **A.** Moderate hydrocephalus before shunting in a 7-year-old.   **B.** One week after shunting, the lateral ventricles have shrunk to nearly normal size.

Treated Hydrocephalus

Normal Posttreatment Status

The ideal situation following shunting is a decrease in intracranial pressure and ventricular size. The amount of change in ventricular size and apparent gain in brain tissue can be significant (Fig. 6-32). On CT it may be unclear whether the ventricular size after treatment is ideal, as patients with small normal or mildly enlarged ventricles may be asymptomatic. Most treated children in either of these states show enlargement of the sulci following shunting (Fig. 6-33). This is probably mostly brain remolding to the smaller ventricular size but may reflect some degree of atrophy. It is especially common when shunting has been done after age 2, when the skull is less compliant.

In a recent study of uncomplicated hydrocephalus, there was surprisingly little difference in IQ levels between most treated hydrocephalic patients and normal children (Dennis 1981) and no relationship between the IQ and the number of shunt revisions, indicating that the complications of shunt blockage may not be as severe as usually thought.

Complications

Blocked shunts are the most common problem in treated hydrocephalus. An abnormal shunt position is easily diagnosed on CT, though the significance is not always known when several shunts are present. Indeed, it is not too uncommon to see an extraventricular shunt tip in a patient who no longer needs a shunt or where there is CSF going along

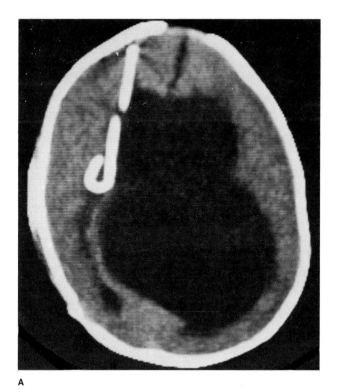

A

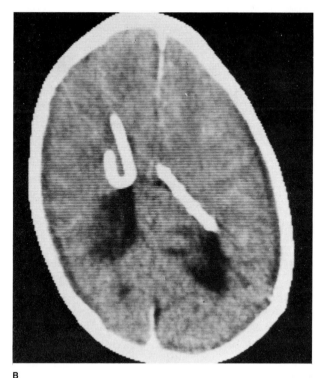

B

Figure 6-32 Ventricular shunting. **A.** Huge encysted lateral ventricle in a 6-month-old with thinning of the cortex on both ipsilateral and contralateral side. The contralateral ventricle is small, with a fuctioning shunt. **B.** Five months later, after shunting of the encysted ventricle, both ventricles are small and there is an apparent thickening of the cortex. Note that some of this increased brain volume is actually due to a narrowing of the calvarium.

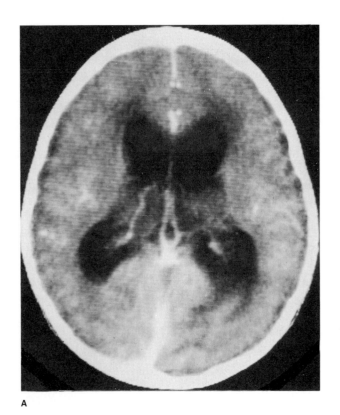
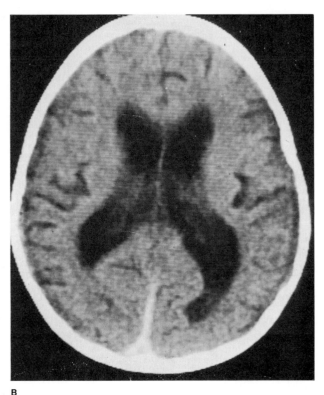

A   **B**

Figure 6-33 Ventricular shunting. **A.** Four-year-old child with hydrocephalus secondary to posterior fossa tumor. **B.** Two weeks after shunting and tumor removal, there is some decrease in ventricular size and visibly dilated sulci. The patient had not received chemotherapy or radiation.

the shunt tract to its tip. With a suspected shunt block, a previous CT is most helpful to confirm the change in ventricular size and thus the obstruction in CSF flow.

Shunt types change from year to year as neurosurgeons continue to look for the ideal shunt that will find its way into the proper position and never block. All intracranial shunts are visible on CT, even if not seen on plain skull x-ray. A short shunt in the subdural space against the inner table can be missed unless the window settings are adjusted to see it.

Shunt disconnection between the reservoir and intracerebral tubing is quite uncommon, because there is no motion between these two parts. It may be missed because of its proximity to the inner table, or it may be overlooked when multiple tubes are present (Fig. 6-34). Plain radiographs are of great help in such cases.

When no previous knowledge of ventricular size is available and the shunt system is connected and in good position, two other clues are sometimes available for the radiologist. One is the periventricular hypodensity of transependymal absorption of CSF. This is usually most visible at the tips of the frontal horns and the lateral atrial regions. It is uncommon following shunt blockage unless there is a rapid and large change in intracranial pressure. The other clue is the plain film finding of split sutures or resplit sutures in the older child. Because a child's skull, even up to age 14 or 15, responds quickly to changes in increased intracranial pressure, x-ray should be done along with CT. Usually a posteroanterior and a lateral film are sufficient to evaluate sutural changes.

Excessive shunt function is a complication at the opposite end of the spectrum. This is nearly always

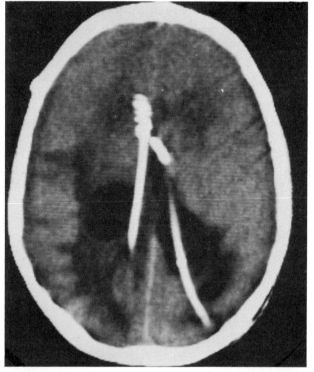

A

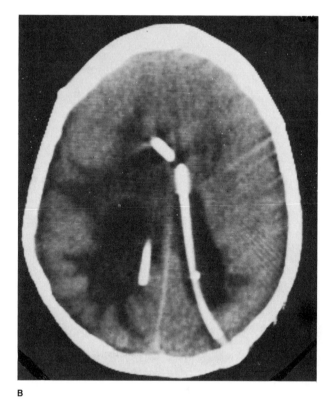

B

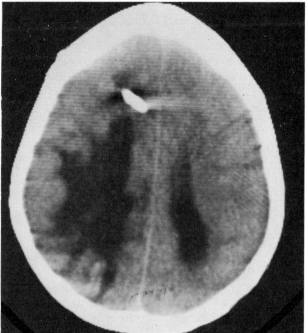

C

Figure 6-34 Ventricular shunting: seven-year-old hydrocephalic child with multiple shunts and clinical signs of a blocked shunt. **A.** Ventricular catheters are noted in both lateral ventricles. **B.** Left-sided catheter can be followed to the calvarium, while right-sided catheter is disconnected and does not reach the inner table. A third Hakim catheter is seen anteriorly in **B** and **C**. This catheter was seen to be connected in higher cuts. Note periventricular edema due to right-sided block and encystment of a portion of the right lateral ventricle.

an acute phenomenon following shunting in children or infants for the very large ventricles. It is especially a danger in the child beyond infancy, where the decreased compliance of the calvarium (and perhaps the brain) no longer allows as much physiological "collapse" in response to the decreased ventricular size. In such a case the ventricles quickly get smaller, allowing the brain to "shrink" and enlarging the subdural-subarachnoid space. Stretching of the bridging veins occurs, and subdural hematomas, often of large size and extent, may result (Fig. 6-35). If this occurs, the surgeon is

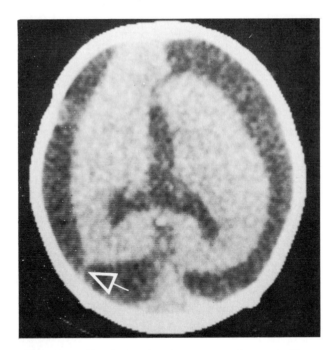

Figure 6-35 Ventricular shunting: same patient as in Figure 6-29. After removal of the choroid plexus papilloma and shunting of the ventricles, the patient developed huge bilateral subdural hematomas. A bridging vein (arrow) is visible posteriorly.

often in the position of trying to balance the two spaces—ventricular and subdural-subarachnoid—and may be forced to allow the ventricles to reexpand in order to prevent recurrence of the subdural hematoma. Shunting of the subdural space itself is sometimes necessary in such cases.

Intracerebral hematomas and subdural hematomas from shunt insertion are quite uncommon, and have no features that distinguish them from other hemorrhages in the same regions of other etiology.

ISOLATED FOURTH VENTRICLE This complication occurs only in shunted hydrocephalus, usually as a result of repeated infection. The fourth ventricle becomes blocked at both the aqueduct and its outlets, causing the ventricle to expand in spite of good shunt function in the lateral ventricles (Fig. 6-36). Often the patients are those with Chiari malformation and previous aqueduct stenosis, but the condition can also occur in EVOH (Scotti 1980).

Treatment is by shunting of the fourth ventricle. It is often difficult to pass a shunt into this dilated ventricle in spite of its size and closeness to the skull vault. This complication has been diagnosed only since CT became available (see Chap. 13).

SLIT-VENTRICLE SYNDROME Also known as *shunt dependency,* this is said to occur when shunting allows the ventricles to become very small. Either by adhesions or other mechanisms, the ventricles lose their compliance and ability to reexpand. Neither the clinical symptoms nor the CT appearance are necessarily clearcut, and small ventricles may reexpand (Fig. 6-37). When the problem is clinically diagnosed and the ventricles are slitlike on CT, one possible treatment is decompression of the temporal lobe by so-called subtemporal craniectomy. This may allow both expansion of the temporal horn and bulging of the brain when shunt blockage occurs (Fig. 6-37) (Holness 1979).

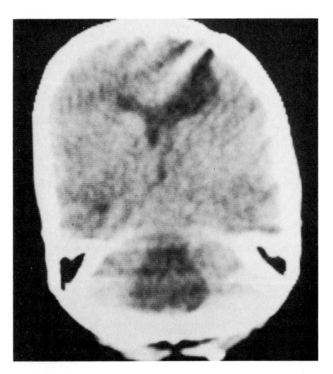

Figure 6-36 Isolated fourth ventricle. CT in a shunted 5-year-old hydrocephalic child shows normal-size frontal horns and marked enlargement of a somewhat pear-shaped fourth ventricle.

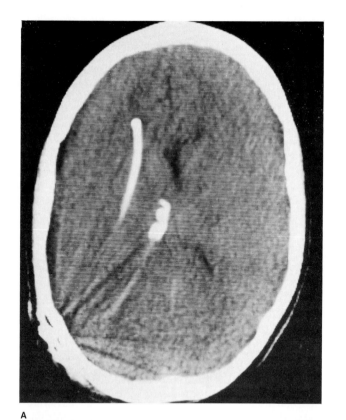

A

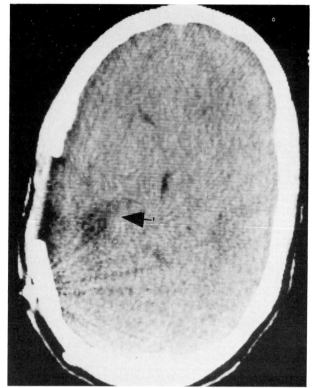

B

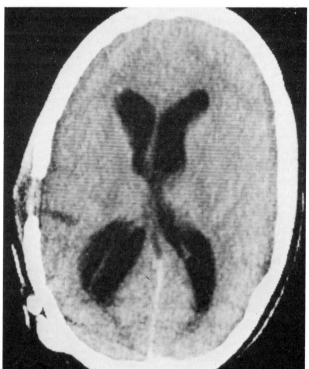

C

Figure 6-37 Slit-ventricle syndrome. **A.** This 9-year-old shunted hydrocephalic child had symptoms of increased intracranial pressure and small ventricles on CT. **B.** Five-and-a-half months later, after temporal decompression, there is some enlargement of the right temporal horn (arrow). **C.** Approximately 1 year later, child again returned with signs of increased intracranial pressure. CT at this time showed that the entire vascular system had reexpanded.

INFECTION On occasion, especially following shunt revision, the shunt system becomes infected and causes a ventriculitis. This can be diagnosed by contrast enhancement of the ventricular walls (Fig. 6-38). Although usually suspected clinically, it is sometimes masked by the symptoms of shunt obstruction.

MISCELLANEOUS Migration of shunt tubing outside the cranial vault is not a common occurrence, but radiologists and neurosurgeons are familiar with it. Intracranial migration of shunt tubing is extremely rare but may also occur. The author has experience in one such case, in which the tubing migrated intracranially. In this case there was no reservoir, and neck motion was assumed to have caused the shunt tubing to move continually upward.

In shunting in the older child with very large ventricles, considerable thickening of the skull may be seen, caused by the decrease in brain size and growth of the bone on the inner table to fill the space. Because skull thickness is not accurately demonstrated on CT without using a very wide window (Fig. 6-39), mild thickening is often overlooked unless accompanying skull x-rays are done.

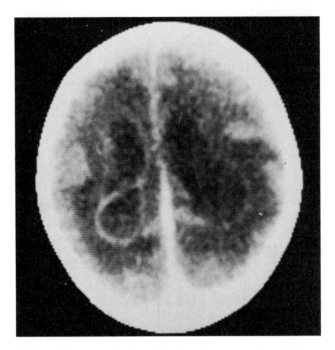

Figure 6-38 Ventriculitis. CT following intravenous contrast shows enhancement of the ventricular walls secondary to an infected shunt which had been removed. Hydrocephalus and white-matter edema are present. The picture is the same as that seen in ventriculitis from other causes.

ATROPHY

As stated at the beginning of this chapter, ventricular enlargement is not necessarily hydrocephalus. The same condition causing hydrocephalus may cause atrophy. The two abnormalities may also be seen combined in the same patient. This is especially true for ventricular dilatation secondary to hemorrhage or infection. On a single CT examination it may be impossible to state whether the abnormal findings are due to hydrocephalus alone, atrophy alone, or a combination of the two problems.

There are signs to help distinguish atrophy from hydrocephalus. If the subarachnoid space and sulci are relatively larger than the ventricles, it is fairly certain that hydrocephalus is not the primary diagnosis (Fig. 6-40). Local areas of enlargement of the ventricles are a sign of focal atrophy and suggest that atrophy is the predominant condition, especially if combined with the above-mentioned relatively large sulcal dilatation.

Calcifications of the brain secondary to infection, radiation, or other insult are signs of damage. There is usually an accompanying sulcal or ventricular enlargement or both.

Heinz et al. (1980) noted that in atrophy the frontal horns keep their normal shape but expand, whereas in hydrocephalus the angle formed by the corners of the tips of the frontal horns become much more obtuse. The author believes that while this is usually the case, it is not a completely reliable criterion, as atrophic ventricular dilatation may mimic hydrocephalus on occasion (Fig. 6-40). One must make use of the clinical information available: if a child has clinical evidence of brain damage and no evidence of hydrocephalus, the radiological diag-

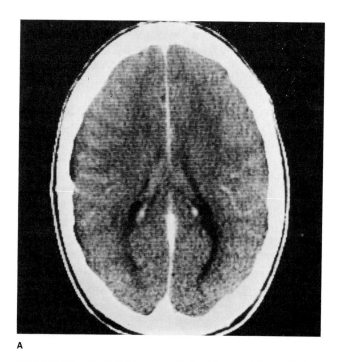

A

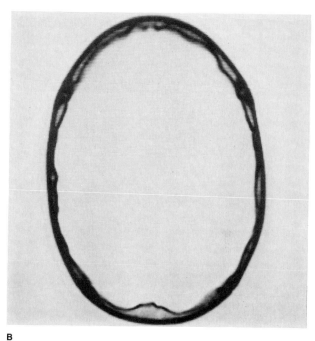

B

Figure 6-39   Skull thickness.   **A.** An 11-year-old retarded child with a thickened skull vault that is not especially prominent with the standard window.   **B.** Wide windows and reverse gray scale show true skull thickness, which is greater than normal but again not appreciated unless one is used to this window setting.

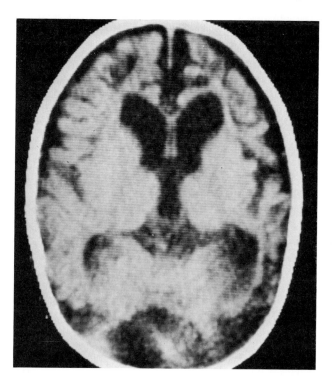

nosis should take such information into account even if the ventricular enlargement appears to be hydrocephalic on CT.

Hemiatrophy

This can occasionally be difficult to tell from a mass effect on CT, though differentiation is much less of a problem with better scanners. In hemiatrophy, the atrophic side usually has the larger ventricle, the midline shift, if present, is to the atrophic side, and the sulci on that side are equal to or larger than those on the contralateral side (Fig. 6-41), although infrequently the larger ventricle is seen on the more normal side (Fig. 6-42). With hemiatrophy, it is dif-

Figure 6-40   Severe atrophy. CT in a 10-month-old with marked atrophy shows both enlargement of the lateral ventricles with rounding of the frontal horns and marked dilatation of the sulci disproportionate to what would be seen in EVOH.

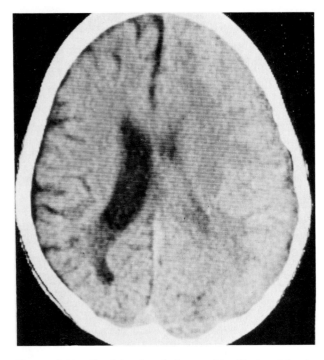

Figure 6-41 Hemiatrophy. A 6-year-old with hemiatrophy shows mild dilatation of the lateral ventricle and sulci on the affected side. The affected hemisphere is smaller.

ficult to tell how much damage is also present on the opposite side or how much any ventricular and sulcal dilatation is simply a reaction to occupy the atrophic space.

Focal Atrophy

This is usually easy to diagnose on CT. It can be seen as local ventricular enlargement or local sulcal enlargement or a combination of the two (Fig. 6-43). The term *infarction* usually refers to atrophy resulting from a vascular accident, but probably most atrophy is the result of a partial or complete loss of blood supply to the area involved. Exceptions are direct toxic insults, infection, and perhaps edema.

Figure 6-42 Hemiatrophy. A 5-year-old with hemiatrophy shows slight enlargement of the sulci on the right side in both **A** and **B.** The left frontal horn is slightly larger in **A.** The left lateral ventricle is slightly larger in **B,** in spite of the fact that the right hemisphere is visibly smaller, with a shift of the straight sinus **(A)** and falx **(B)** from the atrophy.

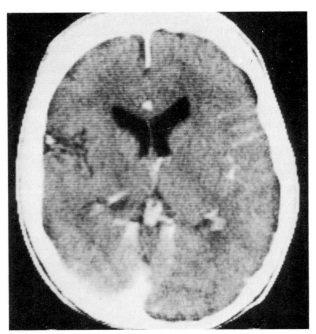

A

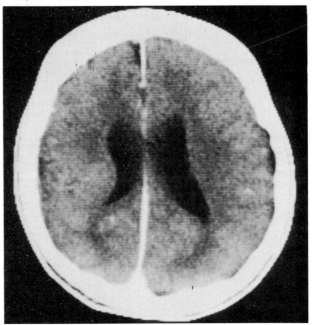

B

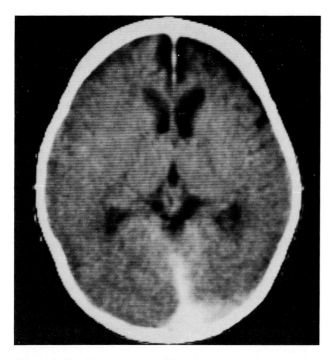

Figure 6-43 Focal atrophy. CT following intravenous contrast shows focal enlargement of the left frontal horn, with enlargement of the sulci over much of the left frontal area and the right frontal region at the midline. The atrophy was secondary to birth anoxia.

Central Atrophy

This term usually refers to a condition in which a child shows mild ventricular enlargement with no sulcal enlargement and has clinical signs of delayed development or brain injury or similar evidence not compatible with hydrocephalus.

Cortical Atrophy

This term refers to enlargement of the sulci without enlargement of the ventricles, with a clinical condition similar to that described in the above paragraph. In the author's experience, these two radiological diagnoses, though affecting very different areas of the brain, do not have significant differences in clinical symptoms or history.

Microcephaly

Microcephaly is often due to brain damage, yet it is surprising that there is often no enlargement of the ventricles or sulci on CT. The reason for this is not known, though one may speculate that the damage occurred very early in utero and retarded the overall growth rate of the brain. An interesting finding in microcephaly is the frequent visualization of normal brain markings of the inner skull table despite obvious lack of brain growth (Fig. 6-44). Some microcephalic children, however, show obvious ventricular and sulcal enlargement, and at least some of these enlargements are secondary to severe postnatal damage such as neonatal meningitis.

Total Brain Infarction

A very small number of infants undergo what can probably be best described as total brain infarction. This is an unusual postnatal or perinatal event, usually secondary to a severe insult, most often infection but occasionally birth anoxia or intracranial hemorrhage. In such cases one initially sees ventricular and sulcal enlargement due to hydrocephalus from the active process such as encephalitis or infarctions. Following this there is a decrease in the density of the brain to that of the enlarged ventricles, or nearly so. If this is due to anoxia, there is initial severe edema and small ventricles (Fig. 6-45A), followed by marked ventriculomegaly and continued low brain density with sparing of the basal ganglia and cerebellum (Fig. 6-45B). It may become nearly impossible to distinguish brain from ventricle on CT. In most cases the subarachnoid space is not visibly large, but occasionally the brain may shrink considerably, leaving only a thin rim around the enlarged ventricles and a huge subarachnoid space.

Porencephaly

Porencephaly is a condition defined in different ways in different specialties and by medical dictionaries (Anderson 1977, Dorland's 1974, Blakiston's Gould 1979, Stedman's 1976). To the neuroradiolo-

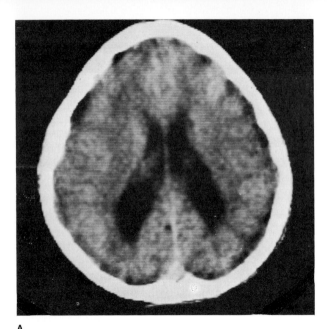

A

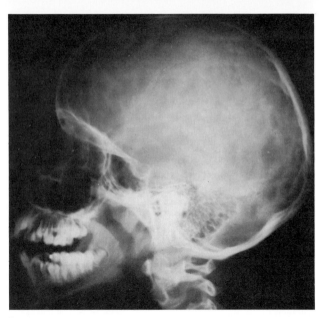

B

Figure 6-44 Microcephaly. **A.** CT in an 11-year-old child with severe microcephaly shows mild dilatation of the lateral ventricles and sulci. **B.** Lateral skull x-ray in the same patient.

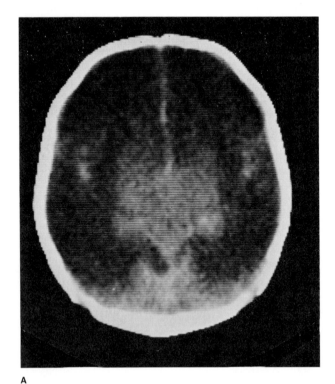

A

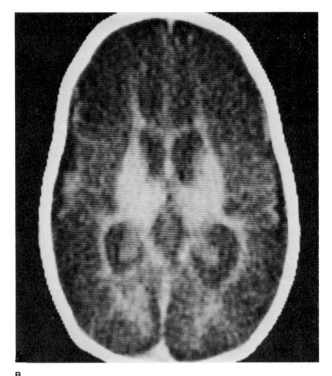

B

Figure 6-45 Brain infarction. **A.** CT in a 2-day-old full-term infant who suffered marked birth asphyxia. The brain is of low density except for the central basal ganglia and thalami, the posteriorly located cerebellum, and a small portion of cortex in the area of each sylvian fissure. **B.** Repeat CT at 17 days of age shows mild ventricular enlargement. The apparent increased density of the basal ganglia and thalami is due to the marked decrease in density in the remainder of the brain, which can be seen to be of nearly the same density as the ventricular CSF.

gist it is a fluid-filled cavity (presumably CSF-filled) in the brain secondary to local infarction. It may be noncommunicating—that is, separate from the ventricles—or communicating—that is, connecting to the ventricles and most often a portion of one of the lateral ventricles. It may be associated with hydrocephalus as discussed earlier. It is thought to be usually due to vascular occlusion and can arise from a variety of insults, varying from neonatal anoxia (Fig. 6-46) to infection to simple vascular occlusion. When the porencephalic defect connecting the ventricles is associated with hydrocephalus and expands from the transmitted increased ventricular pressure, it becomes a porencephalic cyst.

Developmental defects may leave underdeveloped areas of brain. These may form cavities that are usually considered to be porencephaly and are indistinguishable from the type caused by damage of an already developed area.

Puncture porencephaly is an uncommon condition that occurs when hydrocephalus dilates the tract of the ventricular needle (Fig. 6-47); it will usually not occur if shunting is done or other means are taken to control the increased pressure within 1 or 2 days of puncture. Such cysts more commonly occur when repeated ventricular punctures are performed for instillation of antibiotics in ventriculitis when shunting is not feasible because of existing infection.

Hydranencephaly

This may be thought of as a gross polyporencephaly. It is usually believed to be due to a vascular accident early in utero with complete or nearly complete infarction of the territories of the brain supplied by the middle cerebral and anterior cerebral arteries (Crome 1972). Evidence of other malformations of the brain, however, suggests anomalous development (Halsey 1971). Typically, the basal ganglia are spared and a collapsed strip of occipital lobe is visible against the tentorium (Fig. 6-48). The cranial cavity is mostly filled with CSF, but no ventricles except the fourth ventricle can be identified

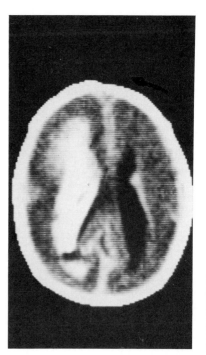 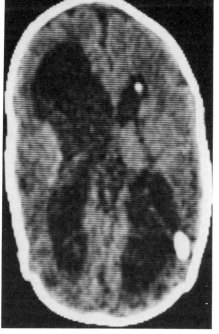

Figure 6-46 Porencephaly. **A.** A 6-day-old infant born after 27 weeks of gestation with large ventricular hemorrhage and hemorrhagic infarct in the right frontal region. **B.** At age 2 months, the patient has a large right frontal porencephaly communicating with the frontal horn. Shunted hydrocephalus is also present. Note the marked change in head size from the hydrocephalus.

A   B

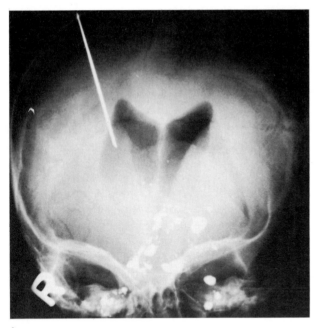

A

on CT. Occasionally a partial hydranencephaly can occur, with sparing of portions of the inferior, frontal, and temporal lobes (Fig. 6-49). Patients usually present in infancy, sometimes with a large head but often with a normal head and normal brainstem function but with transillumination over the entire skull.

In extreme hydrocephalus, on rare occasions, the cortex is so thin as not to be clearly visible on CT. In such cases the resemblance to hydranencephaly may be so great that angiography is needed to distinguish the two entities. At angiography, hydrocephalus, no matter how severe, will show cortical arteries and veins over the brain surface beneath the inner table.

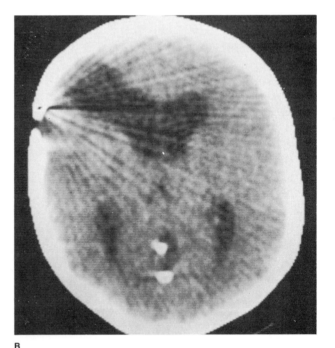

B

Figure 6-47 Puncture porencephaly. **A.** Anteroposterior film during a ventriculogram shows the needle in the right frontal horn in a 1½-year-old child. **B.** CT after shunting and 5-year interval shows a large porencephalic cyst in the frontal horn. *(Fitz CR and Harwood-Nash DC 1978a. Reprinted with permission from the publisher.)*

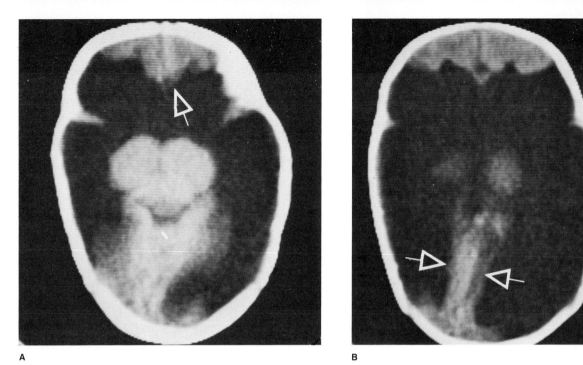

Figure 6-48 Hydranencephaly. **A.** CT at level of the tentorium shows small amount of residual frontal lobe anteriorly (arrow), central thalami, and cerebellum and inferior occipital lobes posteriorly. **B.** Slightly higher cut shows residual frontal cortex, tops of the thalami, and thin strips of occipital lobe (arrow) on either side of the falx.

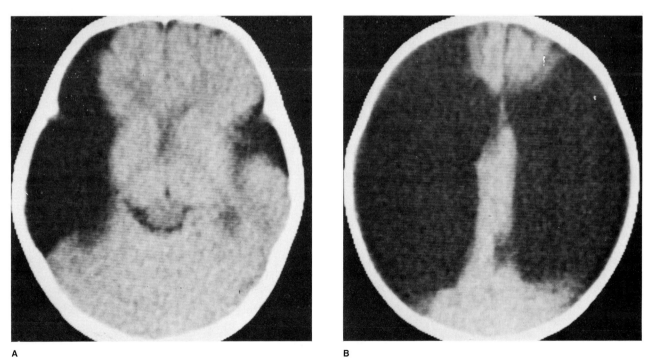

Figure 6-49 Partial hydranencephaly. The child presented with an enlarging head at 6 months. **A.** CT shows far better preservation of the brain than in Figure 6-48, although there is considerable damage on the right. **B.** CT through the level of the ventricular bodies shows severe damage but some preservation of brain in the midline to a greater degree than in Figure 6-48.

MISCELLANEOUS CONDITIONS

Encephalocele

This anomaly, a disorder of the midline closure, is rare, being said to occur in 4 of 10,000 births (Leck 1966). It is most commonly seen in the occipital region. When large, it is easily diagnosed clinically and by CT. The exact contents of the encephalocele may be difficult to determine if brain has herniated into it (Fig. 6-50). Enlargement of the ventricles invariably accompanies large encephaloceles, though this is probably in part developmental rather than hydrocephalic.

Small encephaloceles that present only with a small lump on the scalp can be difficult to diagnose on CT. Since they are only 1 to 3 cm in size outside the cranial vault, the Hounsfield numbers are usually not accurate enough to determine whether they contain CSF. Those in the occipital region will usually show an enlarged interhemispheric space from vault to quadrigeminal cistern (Fig. 6-51), and this is a reliable indication that the mass is an encephalocele.

Arachnoid Cyst

Arachnoid cysts causing hydrocephalus have been discussed in the hydrocephalus section. It is the location of the cyst in or beneath the third ventricle,

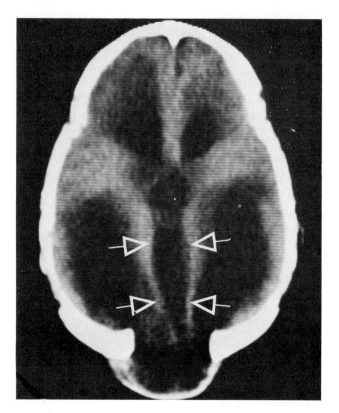

Figure 6-51 Encephalocele. Six-month-old infant with occipital bony defect and moderate encephalocele protruding posteriorly. Tract of encephalocele (arrows) extends to the quadrigeminal cistern.

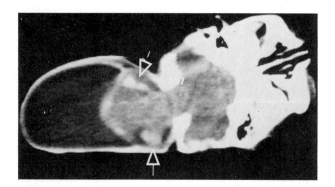

Figure 6-50 Encephalocele. CT shows a large occipital encephalocele containing considerable brain and CSF. In spite of inferior location, there are two enhancing regions suggestive of lateral ventricle choroid plexus (arrows). The infant had to be examined on its side because of the large encephalocele.

in the quadrigeminal cistern, and in the cisterna magna region that is the cause of the hydrocephalus rather than any other quality of the cyst itself. Arachnoid cysts are probably congenital lesions that arise in utero. Their exact cause is not known.

The most common location for arachnoid cyst is in the region of the sylvian fissure. A gradual dilatation of the cyst is thought to occur over a period of months or years until it becomes clinically evident by local enlargement of the skull vault, seizures, or bleeding into the subdural space outside the cyst following an injury. CT shows the enlarged sylvian fissure and cystic space (Fig. 6-52). It often goes beneath the temporal lobe to the midline and is occasionally bilateral (Fig. 6-53). The brain adjacent to the cyst, especially the temporal tip, is usually atrophic in appearance on CT (Fig. 6-54) and hy-

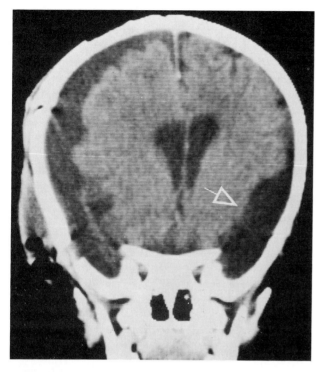

Figure 6-52 Arachnoid cyst. Coronal view in a 14-month-old shows a left-sided unoperated temporal arachnoid cyst (arrow) and a right-sided arachnoid cyst with superimposed large subacute subdural hematoma that has reaccumulated after evacuation. The hematoma causes a shift of the ventricles to the left.

Figure 6-54 Arachnoid cyst. Coronal view of a 3-year-old with a large left temporal arachnoid cyst shows deepening of the temporal fossa in comparison with the normal side. Temporal lobe is replaced by cyst back to the level of this slice at the sella.

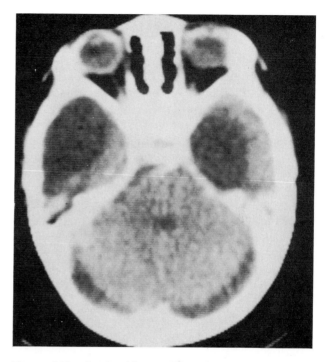

Figure 6-53 Arachnoid cyst. Bilateral temporal arachnoid cysts are seen in this inferior CT slice in a 6-year-old child examined for behavior problems. The cisterna magna is prominent but normal.

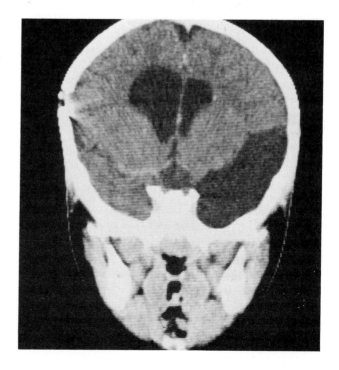

povascular on angiography. Although surgical treatment is usually given to create communication between the cyst and the normal subarachnoid space and to remove any abnormal vasculature of its covering that might reintroduce bleeding, the brain often will not reexpand to fill the space even though it is no longer under pressure, or this may occur only over a period of several years.

Subdural Hygroma

The sulci are normally visible up to 6 months of age and probably up to 1 year (Fig. 6-55). A subarachnoid space showing more sulcal separation or displacement of the cortex farther away from the inner table than seen in Figure 6-55 is abnormal. It is not uncommon to see on CT large subarachnoid spaces, especially frontally in children examined for possible hydrocephalus, who usually present with increased head size and no other symptoms (Fig. 6-56). If there is no contrast enhancement of membranes to indicate a traumatic or infectious cause, the diagnosis is often perplexing. The ventricles frequently are minimally enlarged (Robertson 1979, Mori 1980). It is the author's belief that these lesions are subdural hygromas which are benign accumulations of CSF of unknown cause.

At the author's hospital, these patients usually have a radionuclide CSF flow study to evaluate the dynamics of CSF absorption. There is frequently a mild abnormality involving fourth ventricle reflux and slight delay of passage of radionuclide over the cerebral hemisphere but no clear-cut evidence of EVOH. These children are usually followed without treatment. Followup studies including CT demonstrated either no change or decrease in the size of the wide subarachnoid spaces. A few have undergone tapping of the fluid collection, which reaccumulated fairly quickly. The psychomotor development and neurologic examinations have been normal in the majority of these children.

The collections tend to be located over the frontal lobes. It was our original thought that examination of such children in the prone position might differentiate a loculated collection from a simple atrophy, because an atrophic brain might change position

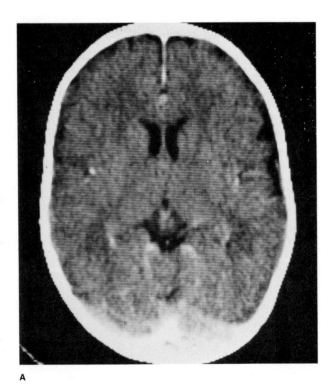

A

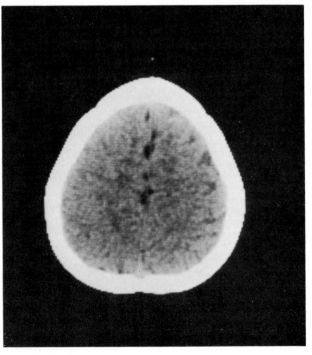

B

Figure 6-55   Normal subarachnoid space.   **A.** The frontal sulci and interhemispheric fissure are slightly visible in this 8-month-old.   **B.** At the level of the vertex, the sulci are also slightly visible in another child of 8 months.

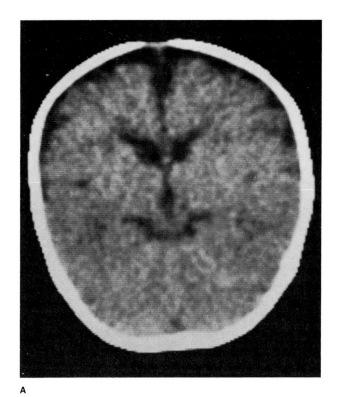
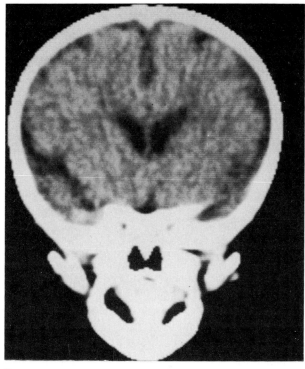

A

B

Figure 6-56 Subdural hygroma. Enlargement of the extracerebral space is seen, especially in the frontal region, in **(A)** the standard semiaxial view and **(B)** the coronal view. No enhancing membrane was visible following intravenous contrast.

and sink forward in the prone position. This, however, did not prove to be the case, and such examination could not reliably differentiate the two conditions. Though the radiologist can easily diagnose the enlarged extracerebral space, it can sometimes be hard to tell whether it is in the subdural or the subarachnoid compartment and whether it is clinically significant.

Bibliography

ALLEN HA, HANEY P, RAO KCVG: Vascular involvement in cranial hyperostosis. *Am J Neuroradiol* **3:** 193–195, 1982.

ANDERSON WAD, KISSANE JM: *Pathology,* 7th ed. St. Louis, The C.V. Mosby Company, 1977, chap. 48.

ARCHER C, DARWISH H, SMITH K JR: Enlarged cisternae magnae and posterior cysts simulating Dandy-Walker syndrome on computed tomography. *Radiology* **127:** 681–686, 1978.

Blakiston's Gould Medical Dictionary, 4th ed. New York, McGraw-Hill Book Company, 1979.

CHUANG SH, FITZ CR, HARWOOD-NASH DC: The use of metrizamide ventriculography in pediatric hydrocephalus. Presented at the Society of Pediatric Radiology, March, 1981.

CROME L: Hydraencephaly. *Dev Med Child Neurol* **14:** 224–234, 1972.

DENNIS M ET AL: The intelligence of hydrocephalic children. *Arch Neurol* **38:** 607–615, 1981.

DI ROCCO C, CALDARELLI M, DI TRAPANI G: Infratentorial arachnoid cysts in children. *Child's Brain* **8:** 119–133, 1981.

Dorland's Illustrated Medical Dictionary, 25th ed. Philadelphia, W.B. Saunders Company, 1974.

EDWARDS JH: The syndrome of sex-linked hydrocephalus. *Arch Dis Child* **36:** 486–493, 1961.

FITZ CR, HARWOOD-NASH DC: Computed tomography in hydrocephalus. *CT: Comput Tomogr* **2:** 91–108, 1978*a*.

FITZ CR, HARWOOD-NASH, DC, CHUANG S, RESJO M: Metrizamide ventriculography and computed tomography in infants and children. *Neuroradiology* **16:** 6–9, 1978*b*.

FLODMARK O ET AL: Correlation between computed tomography and autopsy in premature and full-term neonates that have suffered perinatal asphyxia. *Radiology* **137:** 93–103, 1980.

FLODMARK O, FITZ CR, HARWOOD-NASH DC, CHUANG S: Neuroradiological findings in a child with primary leptomeningeal melanoma. *Neuroradiology* **18:** 153–156, 1979.

GILLES FH, DAVIDSON RI: Communicating hydrocephalus associated with deficient dysplastic parasagittal arachnoidal granulations. *J Neurosurg* **35:** 421–426, 1971.

GOODING, CA, CARTER A, HOARE RD: New ventriculographic aspects of the Arnold-Chiari malformation. *Radiology* **89:** 626–632, 1968.

HALSEY JA, ALLEN N, CHAMBERLIN HR: The morphogenesis of hydraencephaly. *J Neurol Sci* **12:** 187–217, 1971.

HART MN, MALAMUD N, ELLIS WG: The Dandy-Walker syndrome: A clinicopathological study based on 28 cases. *Neurology* **22:** 771–780, 1972.

HARWOOD-NASH DC, FITZ CR: *Neuroradiology in Infants and Children.* St. Louis, C.V. Mosby Company, 1976.

HEINZ ER, WARD A, DRAYER BP, DUBOIS PJ: Distinction between obstructive and atrophic dilatation of ventricles in children. *J Comput Assist Tomog* **4:** 320–325, 1980.

HIRATSUKA H ET AL: Modification of periventricular hypodensity in hydrocephalus with ventricular reflux in metrizamide CT cisternography. *J Comput Assist Tomog* **2:** 204–208, 1979.

HOFFMAN HJ, HARWOOD-NASH DC, GILDAY DL: Percutaneous third ventriculostomy in the management of non-communicating hydrocephalus. *Neurosurgery* **7:** 313–321, 1980.

HOLNESS RO, HOFFMAN HJ, HENDRICK EB: Subtemporal decompression for the slit-ventricle syndrome after shunting in hydrocephalic children. *Child's Brain* **5:** 137–144, 1979.

LECK I: Changes in the incidence of neural tube defects. *Lancet* **2:** 791–793, 1966.

MARC JA ET AL: Positive contrast ventriculography combined with computed tomography: Technique and applications. *J Comput Assist Tomog* **4:** 608–613, 1980.

MILHORAT TH, CLARK RG, HAMMOCK MK, MCGRATH PP: Structural, ultrastructural, and permeability changes in ependyma and surrounding brain favoring equilibration in progressive hydrocephalus. *Arch Neurol* **22:** 397–407, 1970.

MORI K, HANDA H, ITOH M, OKUNO T: Benign subdural effusions in infants. *J Comput Assist Tomgr* **4** (4)466–471, 1980.

NAIDICH TP, PUDLOWSKI RM, NAIDICH JB: Computed tomography signs of Chiari II malformation: II. Midbrain and cerebellum. *Radiology* **134:** 391–398, 1980*a*.

NAIDICH TP, PUDLOWSKI RM, NAIDICH JB: Computed tomography signs of Chiari II malformation: III. Ventricles and cisterns. *Radiology* **134:** 657–663, 1980*b*.

OKUNO T, ITO M, YOSHIOKA M, NAKANO Y: Cerebral atrophy following ACTH therapy. *J Comput Assist Tomogr* **4:** 20–23, 1980.

RAIMONDI AJ, SAMUELSON G, YARZAGARAY L, NORTON T: Atresia of the foramina of Luschka and Magendie: The Dandy-Walker cyst. *Neurosurgery* **31:** 202–216, 1969.

ROBERTSON WC JR., CHUN RWM, ORRISON WW, SACKETT JF: Benign subdural collections of infancy. *J Pediatr* **94:** 382–385, 1979.

SCOTTI G, MUSGRAVE MA, FITZ CR, HARWOOD-NASH DC: The isolated fourth ventricle in children. *Am J Neuroradiol* **1:** 419–424, 1980.

Stedman's Medical Dictionary, 23d ed. Baltimore, Williams & Wilkins Company, 1976.

TABOADA D, ALONSO A, ALVAREZ JA, PARAMO C, VILA J: Congenital atresia of the foramen of Monro. *Neuroradiology* **17:** 161–164, 1979.

YAMADA H, NAKAMURA S, TATIMA M, KAGEYAMA N: Neurological manifestations of pediatric achondroplasia. *J Neurosurg* **54:** 49–57, 1981.

PRIMARY TUMORS IN ADULTS[*]

Seungho Howard Lee

Krishna C.V.G. Rao

GENERAL CONSIDERATIONS

After Roentgen's discovery of x-rays, the first radiographic means of evaluating intracranial pathology, apart from plain skull roentgenograms, was pneumoencephalography. This consisted in injection of small amounts of air or inert gas into the ventricular and subarachnoid spaces so as to study the effects of intracranial masses on these structures and to localize the masses. The limited information obtained was enough for carrying out appropriate treatment. With the availability of angiography and development of more sophisticated pneumoencephalographic equipment, there was significant improvement in the diagnosis of intracranial disease. By judicious use of these two study tools, a mass could be diagnosed and its vascular anatomy defined in a majority of cases; one provided information dealing with the encroachment of intracranial masses on the CSF compartments, either directly or indirectly, and the other provided the vascular topography. In fact, specificity as defined then related to the ability to specify the nature of an intracranial lesion by utilizing these two techniques.

Craniocerebral radionuclide studies provided an added dimension, since the radionuclide accumulated in tissues, cerebrospinal fluid spaces, or vascular structures altered by various pathological processes. Thus radionuclide studies, although not specific, were more sensitive than pneumoencephalography or angiography. Specificity in the past could not be attributed to any single study but was a function and outcome of the judicious utilization of a combination of studies.

Sensitivity and Specificity

Sensitivity and specificity have a slightly different connotation when applied to CT images. As used in the CT literature, *sensitivity* is defined as the ability to distinguish between two similar objects of a certain size or to differentiate a single object from an adjacent or surrounding region. In CT parlance, it is the ability to detect a single lesion (or more than one lesion) within the brain parenchyma which is slightly more dense or less dense than the surrounding parenchyma. Extending this concept further, it is the ability, as applied to tumors, to discern a small lesion (less than 1 cm) within the brain parenchyma. Several factors contribute to the detectability of such a lesion (Table 7-1), most of them by an instrument-related characteristic designated *resolution capacity.* The resolution capacity of the most recent scanners is excellent when viewing a dense object such as a 1-mm pinhead, but it may not be adequate to detect an object with a density slightly greater or less than water.

Since the detection of a given lesion also depends on the linear attenuation of the x-ray beam, certain lesions may be better visualized if the study is performed with different energies (kilovoltages).

Table 7-1 Factors Influencing Sensitivity

Instrument-related	
Spatial resolution:	Detector aperture
	Tube focal spot size
	Magnification geometry
	Radiation dose
Contrast resolution:	Spatial sampling frequency
	Slice thickness
	Reconstruction algorithm
	Target reconstruction
Patient-related	Size of body organ
	Size of lesion
	Nature of pathological process
	Patient motion
Observer-related	Visual perception
	Level of expertise

Section thickness also plays an important part in the detectability of a lesion, inasmuch as a larger section thickness (10 mm) may obscure a lesion because of partial volume averaging, while the lesion may be visible when a smaller (2 to 5 mm) section thickness is used. In evaluating sellar and petrous bone, the process of target reconstruction, which involves reconstruction of the detector readings, results in an image with better spatial resolution (Shaffer 1980). These factors are explained in greater detail in Chapter 1. Patient-related factors such as the size of the organ in relation to the size of the lesion can also result in decreased sensitivity, as can the type of lesion. A small or pinhead-size hematoma can be detected by CT, whereas a hematoma having a density similar to the brain parenchyma can easily be missed. Patient motion resulting in artifacts may also be responsible for nonvisualization of a lesion.

Sensitivity has also been used in CT literature to compare CT with other diagnostic modalities, that is, to evaluate the ability of procedures to distinguish between normal and abnormal processes. After the introduction of CT, several investigators compared the sensitivity of CT with cranial radionuclide studies and indicated that the two modalities were equally sensitive in the detection of acute lesions, with almost the same rate of accuracy (Pendergrass 1975; Clifford 1976; Alderson 1976). The sensitivity of CT for the detection of certain lesions can also be increased significantly by utilizing intravenous iodinated contrast. Lesions which are small or isodense may be detected by their vascularity and their disruption of the blood-brain barrier. The amount of iodinated contrast also appears to play a role in increasing the sensitivity of CT. Initially, small volumes of contrast (50 ml of 60% iodinated contrast) were felt to be adequate. Davis (1979) and Hayman (1980) have shown that certain lesions, because of either their small size or their ultrastructure, may be seen only if very large amounts of contrast (300 ml of 60% iodinated contrast; close to 80 g of iodine) are utilized.

Even without the use of high doses of contrast, the sensitivity of CT in the detection of intracranial neoplasms is uniformly high, varying between 85 and 98 percent in the different series (Ambrose 1975*a;* Wende 1977; Claveria 1977*b;* Evens 1977; Baker 1980). With presently available scanners and judicious utilization of iodinated contrast, the detection rate in neoplastic processes may approach 100 percent.

Numerous similar studies have evaluated the specificity of CT. *Specificity* can be defined as the ability to determine the exact nature of the lesion and, if possible, its histological nature. The approaches adopted by various authors have been to correlate the pathology data with the histological variance. A variety of factors influence the attempt to be specific about a given lesion (Table 7-2). Some are related to the CT equipment and the utilization of different software, others depend on the pathological process itself.

The specificity of CT in establishing histologic types and grades of intracranial tumors has not proved nearly as high as its sensitivity in the careful qualitative analysis of CT patterns (Steinhoff 1976; Thomson 1976; Tchang 1977; Butler 1978; Tans 1978; Hilal 1978*b;* Oi 1979). Qualitative analyses have utilized the structural composition of tumors as seen on CT both before and after contrast enhancement. Circular or irregular homogeneous contrast enhancement was noted in 89 percent of meningiomas, mixed or ring enhancement in 77 percent of glioblastomas, and no enhancement in 100 percent

of grade I atrocytomas (Steinhoff 1977). Although these contrast-enhancement CT characteristics are of assistance in histologic diagnosis, others have not been able to duplicate these results (Tans 1978). The specificity is somewhat limited because of significant overlap among different tumors.

Different methods of quantitative analysis have also been attempted. Huckman (1977) utilized quantitative measurement of the mean values of CT numbers to delineate the different varieties of intracranial lesions. Hilal et al. (1978) attempted histological diagnosis by correlation between the initial density on NCCT and the extent of uptake on CECT. Their study revealed an often inverse relationship between the degree of enhancement and the grade of malignancy: the higher the initial density the less the contrast uptake and usually the lower the grade of malignancy, whereas the lower the density on NCCT the higher the contrast uptake and the grade of malignancy. However, it is doubtful that a consistent linear relationship exists between the initial density of a tumor and the degree of enhancement which is specific for each group of tumors. The use of histograms in the region of interest have been reported to be an additional help in the pathologic definition of tumors when careful analysis of pre- and postcontrast curves is carried out (Dorsch 1978; Vonofakos 1978; Mances 1978; Gardeur 1977).

Contrast-enhancement response as a function of time has been investigated in various types and grades of intracranial tumors as an aid to diagnostic specificity (Steinhoff 1976; Lewander 1978). The time-response curve of enhancement has been divided into an initial and a delayed phase. Rapid early rise of the curve is noted in the initial phase and slow minimal variation in the late phase extending from ½ hour to 3 hours. Although delayed scanning is at least minimally useful in the grading of certain tumors, its practicality in many institutions is limited. CT numbers on the CECT may not be dependable, since multiple variables such as the amount of contrast injected, the mode of injection, and variation in scanner calibration may compound the difficulty in evaluation of the contrast-enhancement pattern. Several authors have shown that when the same lesion is scanned at different volt-

Table 7-2 Factors Influencing Specificity

Instrument-related	Differences in linear attenuation coefficient
	Effective atomic number
	Dual energy
Patient-related	Clinical history (mode of onset, etc.)
	Age and sex
Pathological process	Size and shape of lesion
	Location of lesion
	Extent of mass effect
	Presence or absence of Ca^{++} or hemoglobin
	Nature of enhancement (ring, homogeneous, etc.)
	Time/density curve of CECT

ages before and after contrast enhancement, the effective atomic numbers change. Latchaw (1978b, 1980) has shown that the percentage change in the effective atomic number following contrast enhancement can be helpful in differentiating major categories of intracranial neoplasms such as gliomas, meningiomas, and metastases. A potential role of the new-generation scanners with extremely fast scanning time (dynamic CT study) is to help divorce the intravascular and extravascular elements in the early phase of contrast enhancement, although the usefulness of the response curve in various tumors remains to be proved. The rapid-high-dose (80 g of iodine) infusion technique (Hayman 1979, 1980) may be of further help in defining tumor pathology when combined with delayed scans; it needs to be further evaluated.

Histologic diagnosis and grading of a tumor as a means of estimating its biologic behavior have intrinsic problems. The fraction of tissue histologically examined may not be representative of the total tumor; also, mixed grades and types may occur in a tumor. The gross pathology of a tumor observed at operation or autopsy frequently suggests its histology. Correct diagnosis based on gross pathology is possible, especially after consideration of the location of the tumor, which may indicate cells of origin in some cases. A similar dilemma in making a histologic diagnosis on the basis of CT characteristics is to be expected, since CT depicts very closely the gross pathology of a tumor as seen at autopsy or surgery.

Nevertheless, one of the advantages, and a significant contribution, of CT is its ability to distinguish a tumor mass from surrounding edema, which can be accomplished only with some difficulty and limited accuracy by cerebral angiography. Cerebral edema is associated with most, if not all, primary and metastatic tumors and is present in the distribution of the white matter. Malignant intracerebral tumors, specifically glioblastoma and metastatic tumor, usually incite the greatest degree of edema. Slow-growing intracerebral tumors have been considered to incite less edema and extradural tumors the least edema. But edema is notably absent in intraventricular and some midline tumors,

probably because of lack of contact with the white matter. However, the frequency, extent, and degree of edema are not pathognomic and, taken alone, lack specificity.

Technical Considerations

The earlier CT scanners with fixed section thickness and other limitations in flexibility resulted in nonvisualization of neoplasms less than 8 to 10 mm in size, particularly when the tissue density of the lesion did not change significantly on CECT. Some of the larger lesions were also not detected, either because of their location or because of motion artifacts resulting from the long scanning time. With the present generation of scanners, which are not only faster but have more flexible options (slice thickness, scanning time, and high resolution), very small lesions can be easily detected. Most centers have evolved protocols for CT studies, with guidelines for contrast enhancement (Latchaw 1978a; Kramer 1975). Most centers perform CT studies in the noncontrast mode (NCCT) followed by the contrast-enhanced mode (CECT), although others (Latchaw 1978a; Butler 1978) believe that NCCT does not add further information, and its omission will decrease the radiation dose to the patient. Cost-saving factors such as more patient throughput in a given unit are also a consideration in deciding not to perform the NCCT. Eliminating the NCCT, however, may cause the examiners to miss fresh hemorrhage or calcification in a tumor—findings that may be of immediate clinical importance or may help to characterize the tumor histologically. Occasionally, thinner sections (2 to 5 mm) following a high dose of contrast are necessary to demonstrate smaller lesions, especially when the decision as to treatment modality depends on the CT findings.

Contrast Enhancement

When CT first became available, Ambrose (1975b) observed that intravenous iodinated contrast enhanced the visualization of brain tumors. Contrast enhancement can be attributed to two mechanisms, (1) extravascular and (2) intravascular accumulation of contrast material (Gado 1975). Contrast enhancement in tumors depends to a significant extent on the contrast agent accumulation in an extravascular compartment due to the leakage of contrast medium across the blood-brain barrier, analogous to that of radionuclide (Gado 1975). The portion contributed by increased intravascular accumulation of contrast agent in tumors may not be as significant as in cerebrovascular anomalies. In the early period of CT utilization, there were significant differences of opinion regarding the necessity of and indications for contrast enhancement (New 1975; Paxton 1974). The total dosage of iodine, its concentration, and the mode of administration (bolus, infusion, or both) were set arbitrarily by different groups. At present the consensus (Norman 1978; Davis 1976) is to use a dose which provides about 40 g of intravenous iodine (150 ml of 60% iodinated contrast), given intravenously as a bolus (Deck 1976) in 4 to 5 minutes, or else 300 ml of 30% solution as a drip infusion (Kramer 1975; Butler 1978; Huckman 1975) for an adult patient of average weight. Even larger amounts of up to 80 g of iodine have been utilized (Kramer 1975; Davis 1979; Hayman 1979) and have been useful in detecting very small neoplasms. The only contraindication to the use of a large volume of contrast appears to be poor renal function. Various studies have shown that the incidence of untoward reactions is not dose-related (Hayman 1979). As a guideline, Table 7-3 gives the total amount of iodine at different volumes and concentrations.

Table 7-3   Iodine Content Based on Volume and Concentrations

Volume, ml	Concentration, %	Total amount of iodine, grams
50	60	14.1
100	60	28.2
100	76	35.7
150	60	42.3
300	30	42.3
300	60	84.6

The time interval between administration of intravenous iodinated contrast and CT has also been debated. In general, CECT, when performed immediately following injection of contrast, demonstrates enhancement of the lesion unless the patient is on large doses of steroids. Delayed CT studies may occasionally be helpful in demonstrating smaller lesions or for those patients who are on high doses of steroids. Although the exact mechanism is not clearly understood, it is presumed that steroids restore the normal blood-brain barrier and reverse the abnormal capillary permeability associated with metastatic and primary brain tumors. Hayman (1980) has shown that in patients on heavy doses of steroids, the smaller metastases can be demonstrated by CT immediately following large doses of intravenous contrast (80 g of iodine), suggesting that visualization of certain neoplasms, regardless of their size or histology, may be related to the volume of contrast material. The authors believe that both the disruption of the blood-brain barrier and the volume of contrast influence detection of the lesion. CECT may also show varying degrees of enhancement of the cisternal spaces in leptomeningeal carcinomatosis (Enzmann 1979). Enhancement of epidural and subdural metastases is common on CECT. Delayed examination is useful in determining whether a lesion is truly cystic or is solid and necrotic (Afra 1980).

Approach to Diagnosis

When an intracranial neoplasm is suspected, certain features are helpful in identifying the mass, its location, and the effect of the mass on the normal intracranial contents.

A neoplasm, whether it is enhancing or nonenhancing, most often will produce a mass effect, which may be focal or hemispheric. There is often distortion or obliteration of the adjacent CSF-containing spaces such as the sulci, subarachnoid cisterns, or ventricles. Enhancement of the neoplasm often helps in defining its precise location and its remote effects on the adjacent structures. Focal areas of hemorrhage or calcification on NCCT often provide information on the nature of the tumor.

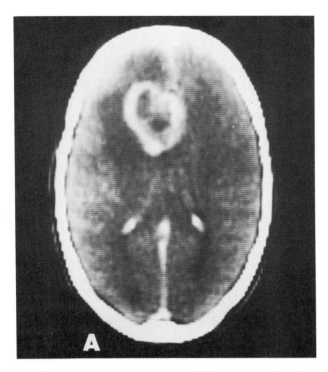 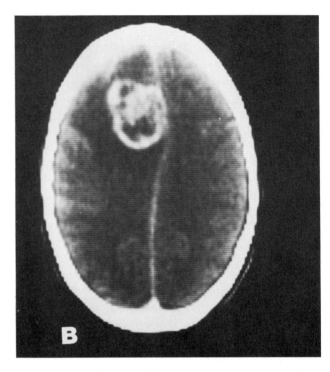

Figure 7-1   Subfalcine herniation. CECT demonstrating the bowing of the free margin of the falx secondary to the large glioblastoma involving the corpus callosum and extending to the frontal lobe.

CT also provides evidence of brain herniation within the rigid compartments resulting from the attachment of the dural folds. In herniation across the falx, the characteristic CT findings consist of slight bowing of the falx (since only the inferior margin is free), associated with distortion of the various components of the lateral ventricles (Fig. 7-1). This effect is most often seen when the mass is located below the level of the corpus callosum. In lesions located at a higher level, the only evidence is obliteration of the sulcal pattern.

In masses located in the temporal lobe, there is first medial and then downward herniation of the temporal lobe through the tentorial hiatus (Fig. 7-2). The earliest sign of transtentorial herniation consists of encroachment on the lateral recess of the suprasellar cistern, resulting in flattening of the normal pentagonal cistern (Osborn 1977; Stovring 1977). With further herniation of the hippocampus and uncus, there is widening of the crural, ambient,

and lateral pontine cisterns on the ipsilateral side of the lesion. Because of associated rotation of the brainstem, the opposite cistern is obliterated (Fig. 7-2). Widening of the contralateral temporal horn is a common feature, caused by downward herniation and compression of the mesencephalon with resulting hydrocephalus (Stovring 1977).

If the condition is unrelieved, the uncus and hippocampus are forced through the tentorial hiatus by the combination of the mass and the associated hydrocephalus. This results in nonvisualization of the interpeduncular and parasellar cistern, with anteroposterior elongation of the brainstem (Fig. 7-3). The posterior cerebral artery, which travels in the mesencephalic cistern, if caught between the tentorial margin and the herniating brain tissue, can become occluded, with resultant infarction.

In massive transtentorial downward herniation which is rapid, as in diffuse cerebral edema, the CT findings may indicate slitlike ventricles and absence

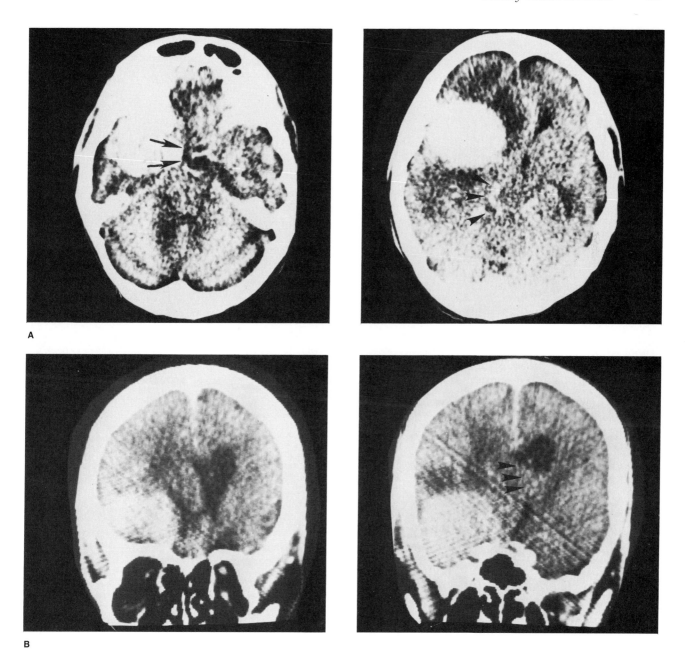

A

B

Figure 7-2 Uncal herniation. CECT. **A.** Axial section. A large glioblastoma involving the temporal pole has resulted in deformity of the suprasellar cistern (arrows), as well as mild rotation of the brainstem (arrowheads). **B.** Coronal section not only demonstrates the encroachment of the cistern but also the associated subfalcine herniation (arrowheads).

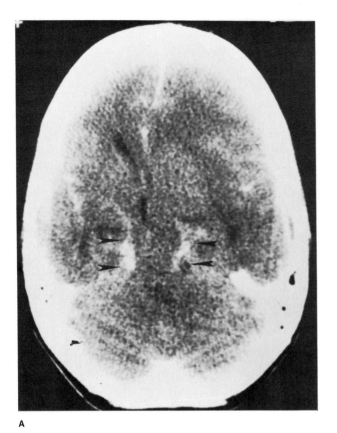

A

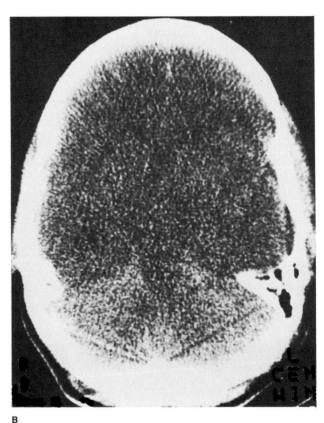

B

Figure 7-3 Transtentorial downward herniation. **A.** Left temporoparietal glioma with transtentorial downward herniation. Compression, displacement, and elongation of the brainstem (arrowheads) are shown on CECT. **B.** Complete obliteration of the quadrigeminal cistern due to diffuse severe cerebral edema in the supratentorial compartment.

of the gyral pattern, associated with obliteration of the suprasellar cistern anteriorly. The crural and ambient cisterns are obliterated laterally and the superior cerebellar cisterns posteriorly (Fig. 7-3).

Similarly, masses located in the infratentorial compartment may result in upward herniation of the midline posterior fossa structures through the tentorial incisure. The highly variable size and configuration of the tentorial incisure, as well as the size of the superior cerebellar cisterns, determine the CT appearance.

The earliest sign of upward herniation of the vermis may be compression or asymmetry of the quadrigeminal cistern (Fig. 7-4). In later stages, obliteration of the superior cerebellar cistern and flattening of the quadrigeminal cistern occur. With

massive upward herniation, the "toothy smile" configuration of the quadrigeminal cistern changes to a "toothless frown" (Osborn 1978a). The resulting flattening of the posterior aspect of the third ventricle, with associated obstructive hydrocephalus, is the end stage of the upward herniation (Fig. 7-4). Associated with the above findings there is usually

Figure 7-4 Transtentorial upward herniation. The CT findings ▶ of upward herniation are demonstrated in a malignant ependymoma growing through the tentorial hiatus. **A.** A large hemangioblastoma in the right cerebellar hemisphere compresses and obliterates the quadrigeminal cistern (arrows). **B.** CECT in another patient with ependymoma growing through the tentorial hiatus. The prepontine and superior vermian cisterns are obliterated.

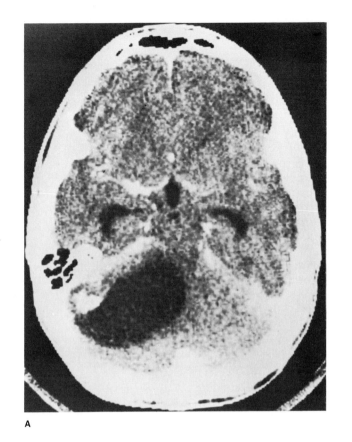
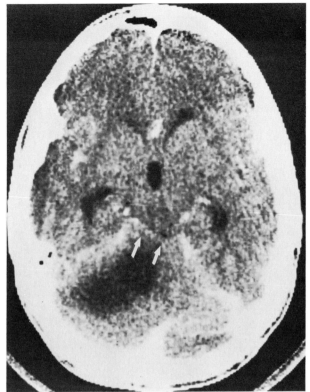

A

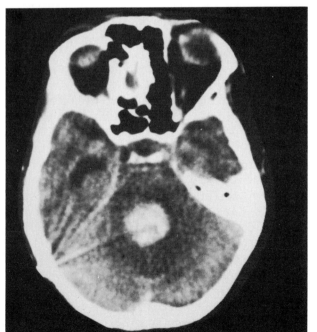
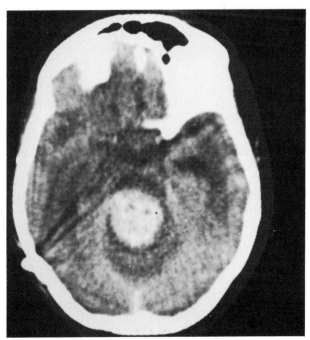

B

(Continued on p. 250.)

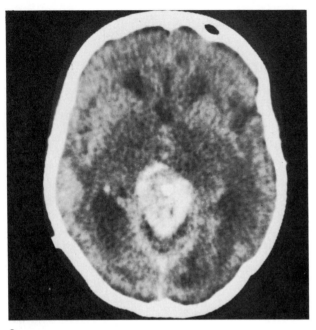

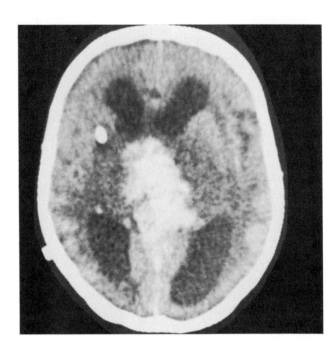

c

Figure 7-4   C. The tumor is growing through the incisura, with resulting hydrocephalus.

obliteration of the cerebellopontine angle cistern and the prepontine cistern and anterior displacement of the brainstem. Depending on the pathological process and the location of the mass, there may also be distortion or nonvisualization of the fourth ventricle.

CT, however, is not useful in demonstrating tonsillar herniation, unless intrathecal metrizamide has been injected. In most situations where tonsillar herniation is suspected as a secondary effect rather than as the primary pathological process (e.g., Chiari I malformation), lumbar puncture and thus use of intrathecal metrizamide are contraindicated. In such a situation, angiography is usually helpful in documenting tonsillar herniation.

Other Diagnostic Modalities

The diagnostic accuracy of angiography has proved to be slightly inferior to that of CT, and the latter provides considerably more information. However, cerebral angiography of high quality has a role to play even in this sophisticated era of CT. Preoper-

ative cerebral angiography has certain advantages. These include its ability to delineate (1) exact and accurate arterial anatomy—multiple feeding vessels, tumor infiltration and arterial encasement, aneurysm formation, and stenosis or occlusion; (2) tumor angioarchitecture—vascularity and blush and arteriovenous shunting; and (3) venous anatomy—thrombosis, collateralization, and variations in the vascular filling and draining pattern. Frequently angiography is necessary in order to obtain detailed anatomic information relating the lesion to familiar angiographic landmarks for satisfactory therapeutic planning and also to assess the histologic diagnosis preoperatively. More important, whenever vascular anomalies are a consideration in the differential diagnosis of a tumor, angiography should be performed prior to surgery in order to prevent potential catastrophe. Angiography should be utilized when CT alone may not be sufficient to determine the pathophysiologic changes of a suspected tumor.

The detectability of cerebral tumors by radionuclide scan ranges from 84 to 93 percent (Alderson 1977; Buell 1977). Perhaps the major problems with radionuclide scan are its nonspecificity and, to a lesser degree, its lack of sensitivity. Pneumoencephalography and ventriculography utilizing air or metrizamide are rarely needed in elucidating detailed relationships with other structures, as in the midline situations of posterior fossa lesions, because, with recent technologic improvements, such as CT reformation in multiple planes, CT images can yield exquisite details with demonstration of precise anatomic relationships.

TYPES OF ADULT PRIMARY INTRACRANIAL TUMORS

The major categories of primary intracranial tumor in the adult population are astrocytoma and meningioma. Other histologic varieties of tumor are less common. Diagnosis of the specific histology of a tumor purely on the basis of CT is often difficult. In the authors' experience, certain CT features are helpful in identifying the type of neoplasm (Table 7-4), but variations from the usual pattern are not uncommon.

Congenital Intracranial Tumors

This group of tumors makes up less than 5 percent of all intracranial tumors. Epidermoids are the most common within the group, followed closely by lipomas, dermoids, and teratomas (Russell 1977). Embryologically, these tumors arise from incorporation of one or more of the three germ layers (ectoderm, mesoderm, and endoderm) into the neural tube during its closure. This closure occurs at 3 to 5 weeks' gestation. The stage of fetal development during which the incorporation takes place determines the location of the tumor. If inclusion is early (3 weeks), the lesion is usually midline. Later inclusions place the tumor further from the midline, and if extremely late, the lesion becomes intradiploic (Toglia 1965).

Epidermoid

The incidence of this tumor ranges from 0.2 to 1.8 percent of all intracranial neoplasms (Banerjee 1977). The age of occurrence encompasses the years from 25 to 60. Males are affected at a rate of 2 to 1. Ectodermal inclusion of the neural tube gives rise to this lesion, which occurs in the midline or laterally.

Epidermoids may have a multilobulated and grayish white appearance suggesting a pearl. They may be intradural, extradural, or intraventricular but are predominantly intradural and occur most commonly at the cerebellopontine angle. Other sites, in order of frequency, include the parapituitary and midposterior cranial fossa. Intradural lesions rarely calcify and are difficult to diagnose because of minimal neurological findings and normal skull radiographs. Extradural masses make up 25 percent of all epidermoids and are easier to recognize because of well-marginated radiolucent defects and bone erosion of the base of the skull or diploe. Their edges are sclerotic and may be scalloped (Chambers 1977). This radiographic appearance is not specific and may require differentiation from neuroma, meningioma, aneurysm, chordoma, and metastatic lesion (Tadmor 1977). Some epidermoids are found in the ventricles: the fourth ventricle is the most common location, followed by the temporal horn of the lateral ventricles (Chambers 1977). Epidermoids may also rupture into the ventricular system, exhibiting a fat–CSF fluid level (Laster 1977; Zimmerman 1979a).

On CT, epidermoids most frequently show low density similar to that of the CSF (Fig. 7-5). The tumor density reflects the composition of the two major contents, keratinized cellular debris and cholesterin (Davis 1976b; Zimmerman 1979a). Frequently, the density on CT is greater than the negative value of lipids, which is accounted for by the presence of a large amount of nonlipid material (keratin) compared to the chief lipid content, cholesterin. Less often, the cholesterin is present in greater proportion than the keratin, so that the tumor density falls into the minus range (-16 to -80 HU) (Cornell 1977; Laster 1977). Calcification of the epidermoid is generally an inconstant feature of epi-

Table 7-4 Features Useful in CT Identification of Various Types of Neoplasm*

Tumor	Initial density	Frequency calcification	Edema	Enhancement pattern	Age group	Location	Other findings
Extraaxial							
Meningioma	↑	20%	+1	+3 H	A	Dural attachment	Occasional hemorrhage
Pinealblastoma	↑	Rare	0	+3 H	P	Post-3d ventricle	Irregular margin
Choroid plexus papilloma	↑	Rare	0	+3 H	P	Ventricular system	Occasional hemorrhage
Choroid plexus carcinoma	↑	Rare	0	+3 H	P	Ventricular system	Irregular margin
Colloid cyst	↑	0	0	0/+1 H	A	Anterior 3d ventricle	
Germinoma	↑/↔	Rare	0	+3 H	A	Suprasellar, pineal	
Pituitary adenoma	↔/↑	< 5%	0	+3 H	A	Sella	Rare hemorrhage
Neuroma	↔/↑	0	+1	+3 H	A	Cerebellopontine angle	Occasionally cystic
Pinealcytoma	↔	Frequent	0	+2 H	P	Post-3d ventricle	
Craniopharyngioma	↔/↓	30/80%	0	+2 M/R	A/P	Suprasellar	Some cystic
Teratoma	↓	Frequent	+1/0	0	P/A	Midline supratentorial	Some cystic
Dermoid	↓	Frequent	+1/0	0	P/A	Post-fossa base of skull	Some cystic
Epidermoid	↓	Frequent	+1/0	0	A	Post-fossa base of skull	Some cystic
Lipoma	↓	Rare	+1/0	0	P/A	Supratentorial midline	
Intraaxial							
Primary lymphoma	↑	0	+1	+2 H	A	Midline, deep structures	Indistinct, irregular margin
Medulloblastoma	↑	10%	+2	+2 H	P	Vermis	Irregular margin
Oligodendroglioma	↑	> 90%	+1	+2 M	A	Supratentorial	Irregular margin
Ependymoma	↔/↑	30–40%	+2	+2 H	P	4th ventricle	Irregular margin
Embryonal cell carcinoma	↑/↓	Rare	+1	+3 H	P	Pineal	
Hemangioblastoma	↔	0	+1	+3 H	A	Post-fossa	Cystic, mural nodule
Ganglioglioma	↔	> 50%	0	+1 M	A	Supratentorial	Irregular margin, hemorrhage
Neuroblastoma	↔/↓	Common	+2	+2 M	P	Supratentorial	Hemorrhage
Low-grade astrocytoma	↔/↓	< 30%	+1	0/+1 M	A	Supratentorial	Indistinct margin
High-grade astrocytoma (glioblastoma)	↔/↓	Rare	+2	+2-3 M/R	A	Supratentorial	Can be cystic, irregular margin
Brainstem glioma	↓/↔	0	0	+1/M	P	Brainstem	Indistinct margin
Cystic astrocytoma	↓	Rare	+1	+1 H	P	Post-fossa	Mural tumor nodule

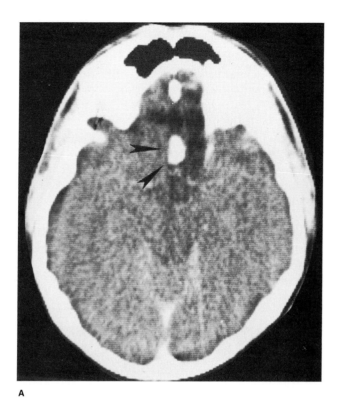

A

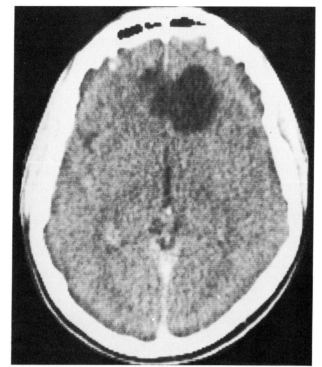

B

Figure 7-5 Epidermoid tumors. **A** and **B.** Multiple areas of hypodensity in the basal frontal area, with the crista galli anteriorly and a calcification posteriorly (arrowheads) within the tumor. Lobulated epidermoid crosses the midline. The absence of contrast enhancement of the wall and the absence of mass effect are noteworthy. **C.** A large epidermoid tumor in the cerebellopontine angle. Hypodensity and sharp margination of the lesion are noteworthy. *(Courtesy of Dr. R. A. Zimmerman.)*

◀ TABLE 7-4 KEY

Key: ↑ = Hyperdensity
     ↔ = Isodensity
     ↓ = Hypodensity
   +1 = Minimal enhancement
   +2 = Moderate enhancement
   +3 = Intense enhancement
    H = Homogeneous
    M = Mixed
    R = Ring pattern
    A = Adult: P = Pediatric
* This table was prepared by Russell A. Blinder, M.D., and S. H. Lee, M.D.

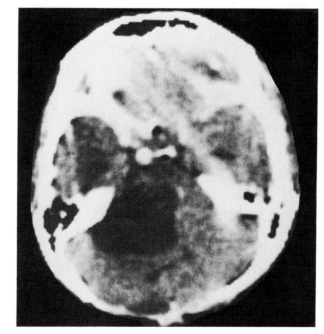

C

dermoids. However, occasional increased density (+80 to +120 HU) and mural calcification (Figs. 7-5A, 7-6) are thought to be due to calcification of the keratinized debris, with saponification to calcium salts (Fawcitt 1976; Braun 1977). The absence of enhancement on CECT is a constant finding. This reflects the structureless, avascular nature of the contents of these tumors and their thin avascular wall (Davis 1976; Chambers 1977). Cerebral arteriogram merely confirms the avascular nature of this tumor. Rare occurrence of contrast enhancement at the periphery of the lesion is considered to be a result of the surrounding vascular connective tissue and dura mater (Tadmor 1977), the presence of gliosis (Mikhael 1978), and cerebral arteries stretched around the mass (Chambers 1977). Nosaka (1979) reported that primary epidermoid carcinoma presents as an isodense or slightly increased density which enhances homogeneously throughout the lesion on CECT.

Absence of hydrocephalus, relative absence of a mass effect, and lack of surrounding edema in spite of the size and site of these lesions are noteworthy and are due to the soft consistency, the slow rate of growth, and the expansion of tumor into the available spaces (Mikhael 1978). Rupture of the capsule further reduces the mass effect. Intraventricular epidermoids may not be readily detected because their density is similar to that of CSF. They may rarely be accompanied by focal dilatation or noncommunicating hydrocephalus. Diagnosis of intraventricular epidermoid can be made following intrathecal metrizamide. The characteristic CT pattern shows the metrizamide demonstrating the tumor and occasionally filling its interstices (Fig. 7-6)—a finding diagnostic of intraventricular epidermoid. Rupture

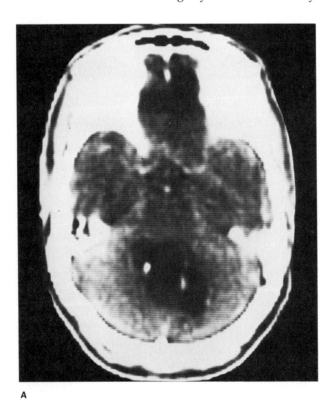
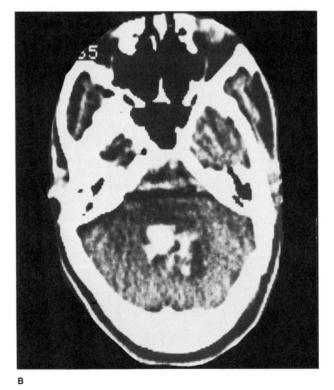

A   B

Figure 7-6 Intraventricular epidermoid.   **A.** The fourth ventricle is enlarged and deformed, with flecks of calcification within and at the periphery of the hypodense lesion. The lateral and third ventricles are normal on a higher level.   **B.** CT following intrathecal metrizamide. The metrizamide fills the interstices of the epidermoid within the fourth ventricle.

of the tumor, with escape of keratin and cholesterin into the ventricular system, allows the less dense cholesterin to float, while the heavier keratin sinks (Laster 1977). As a result, a fat–CSF level is present in the ventricles, which can be clearly detected by CT. Rupture of the tumor into the subarachnoid space may deposit cholesterin droplets in the adjoining spaces.

Early diagnosis may permit curative surgery. Satisfactory treatment consists of surgical removal of the mass with its capsule. Iatrogenic liberation of its contents into the CSF compartments during surgery can stimulate a chemical or granulomatous meningitis.

Dermoid

Dermoids occur less frequently than epidermoids and account for approximately 1 percent of all intracranial tumors. The age range includes primarily the first three decades, with only a slight female predominance. The inclusion of ectodermal and mesodermal elements at the time of closure of the neural groove leads to the development of sebaceous, apocrine, and adipose tissue within the tumor. These buttery contents fill in between hairs, and toothy calcifications are also found in the dermoid. It is the demonstration of hair, skin, and fat elements that distinguishes dermoids from epidermoids. Calcifications are also more frequent in dermoids. A stratified squamous epithelium lines the inside of the tumor.

Dermoids occur throughout the posterior fossa and at the base of the brain, near the midline. On skull radiographs, dermoids may be seen as radiolucent masses, occasionally with peripheral calcifications (Gross 1945; Lee 1977). On angiography an avascular mass is usually found. CT demonstrates the low-density masses ranging from -20 to 120 HU (Amendola 1978; Handa 1979) (Fig. 7-7). This fat density actually represents secretions of seba-

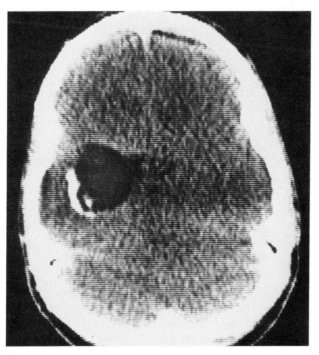
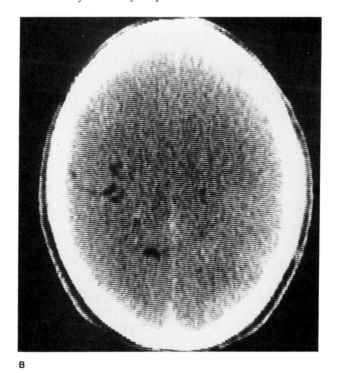

A   **B**

Figure 7-7 Dermoid tumor in the temporal lobe. **A.** Temporal-lobe hypodense mass (-70 HU) with mural calcification. Soft-tissue mass within the cavity is faintly visible. **B.** Multiple small fat densities (lipomatosis) are noted in the sylvian cisterns and convexity sulci.

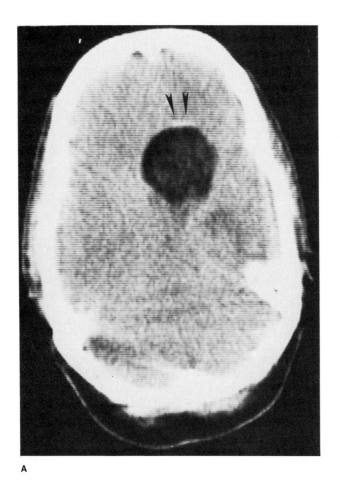

A

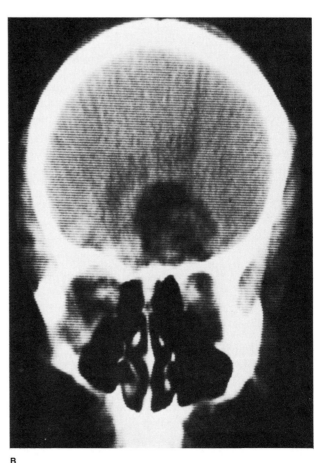

B

Figure 7-8 Dermoid containing a hair ball. **A.** A large, hypodense, round lesion (−80 HU) with minimal mural calcification (arrowheads) and a soft-tissue mass inside which turned out at surgery to be a hair ball. **B.** Coronal view shows a large soft-tissue mass within. *(Lee 1977.)*

ceous glands and desquamated degenerated epithelium. In vitro the fluid in the cyst has been noted to measure −80 HU (Handa 1979). Incomplete mural calcification may be visible at the periphery of the cavity (Figs. 7-7A, 7-8), and at an appropriate setting of center and window levels, a matted hair ball inside the cavity can also be visualized (Lee 1977) (Fig. 7-8). Contrast enhancement of the capsule is extremely unusual. The mass effect is usually slight when compared to the size of the lesion.

Spontaneous or iatrogenic rupture of dermoids may result in egress of the contents into the ventricles and subarachnoid spaces, causing a granulo-matous meningitis with marked foreign-body giant cell reaction due to irritant cholesterin from keratin breakdown; CT clearly demonstrates an intraventricular fat-fluid level (Zimmerman 1979a) (Fig. 7-9) or freely movable fatty material in the ventircles (Fawcitt 1976; Laster 1977) and in the subarachnoid cisterns (Fig. 7-7) (Laster 1977; Amendola 1978). Hydrocephalus may follow the intraventricular rupture of the cyst (Fig. 7-9), leading to death from severe chemical meningitis. As with epidermoids, surgery should include removal of tumor contents and capsule, since incomplete removal of the capsule may lead to recurrence of the tumor.

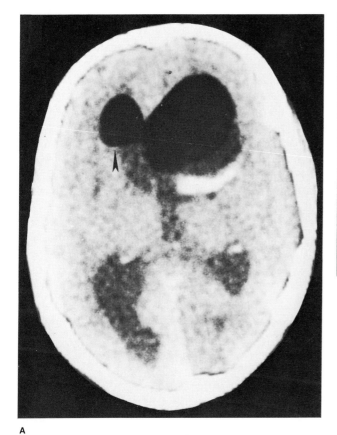

A

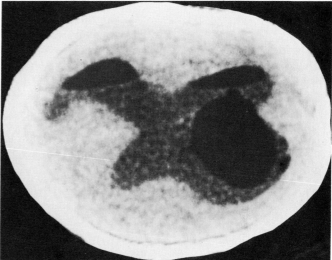

B

Figure 7-9 Frontal dermoid with intraventricular rupture. **A.** Axial CT in supine position demonstrates a large fat-containing mass projecting into the right frontal horn of the lateral ventricle. Calcification is present in the inferior wall of the mass. A fat-CSF level is present in the left frontal horn (arrowhead). **B.** Right lateral decubitus axial CT demonstrates multiple fat-CSF levels in the left lateral ventricle. Hydrocephalus and the right frontal dermoid are well visualized. *(Zimmerman 1979a.)*

Lipoma

Intracranial lipomas are rare tumors, evidently of developmental origin, implicating both the leptomeninges and subjacent neural tissue by inclusion of the mesodermal germ layer early in gestation. About 50 percent of all lipomas are asymptomatic. They are commonly found at or near the midsagittal plane, most frequently in the corpus callosum and occasionally in the cerebellopontine angle and quadrigeminal plate cisterns. Other sites of involvement are the base of the cerebrum, brainstem, roots of the cranial nerves, ventral aspect of the diencephalon, choroid plexus of the lateral ventricles, and dorsal aspect of the midbrain. Some lipomas include elements other than fat, notably calcification, and are associated with dysraphism, such as hypertelorism, myelomeningocele, agenesis of the cerebel-

lar vermis, and cranium bifidum (Zettner 1960; Kushnet 1978).

Lipoma of the corpus callosum is associated with agenesis of the corpus callosum in about 50 percent of cases (Zettner 1960). Plain skull radiographs shows curvilinear mural calcifications in the genu of the corpus callosum with radiolucency within the lipoma. Symmetrical separation of the anterior portions of the frontal horns and bodies of the lateral ventricles, with elevation of the third ventricle, has been described on ventriculography and pneumoencephalography. Cerebral angiography demonstrates dilated anterior cerebral arteries that are incorporated within the lipoma. All these findings can be clearly depicted on CT (Chapter 4). The diagnosis on CT is made by the characteristic appearance of an area of low density consistent with fat (−100 HU). Except for lipomas involving the corpus callosum, mural calcification is infrequent. Lipomas in other locations can be easily diagnosed by CT (Figs. 7-7B, 7-10), obviating invasive investigative procedures. Absence of contrast enhancement is characteristic, as with epidermoid. Surgical mortality for lipoma of the corpus callosum is reported to be as high as 65 percent (Patel 1965). Occasionally hydrocephalus is an associated finding, for which surgical relief may be indicated.

Teratoma

The occurrence rate for this tumor is about 0.5 percent but in patients under 15 years of age can be as high as 2 percent. It presents slightly more frequently in males and involves the first two decades of life. Elements of all three germ layers are incorporated early into the neural tube, so that bone, cartilage, teeth, hair, fat, and sebum may all be present at the same time. Calcification generates from the developing dentine and enamel portions of the teeth. The term *teratoid* is employed for forms of teratoma in which derivatives of all three germinal layers are not clearly identified.

The pineal body is chiefly affected (42 percent). Midline locations, such as the pituitary and third ventricle (16 percent), come next, followed by the posterior fossa (11 percent). The remaining 31 percent are widely distributed intracranially (Russell 1977). Clinical presentation depends upon the expanding pressure and infiltration of the surrounding structures, such as the pituitary gland, hypothalamus, optic chiasm and tracts, inferior and superior colliculi, and medial geniculate body. Cer-

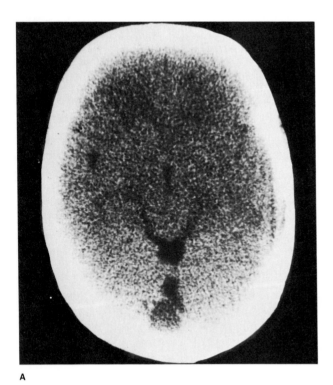

A

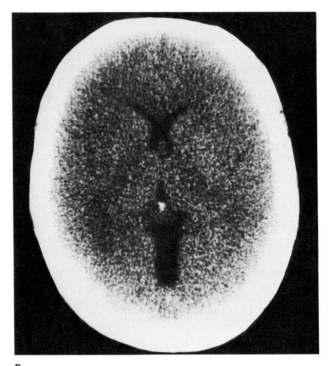

B

Figure 7-10 Lipoma in the quadrigeminal and superior vermian cisterns. **A.** Well-demarcated areas of fat density in the quadrigeminal cistern with no mass effect to the midbrain or cerebellum. **B.** Superior extension into the superior vermian cistern and the vein of Galen cistern is shown. Sharp margination, homogeneous fat density, and conformation to the adjacent structure with no mass effect and no contrast enhancement are characteristic CT findings.

ebellar signs, due to downward pressure against the tentorium, and hydrocephalus may also be present (Camins 1978).

A few cases of teratomas diagnosed by CT are reported in the literature (Gawler 1979; McCormack 1978; Zimmerman 1979a, 1980b). The areas of mixed density on CT are characterized by fat, soft tissue, and hair, as well as osseous and tooth elements. Spontaneous rupture of the tumor into the ventricles results in fat–CSF interfaces, as with epidermoid and dermoid tumors. The preponderant location in the pineal region and presence of osseous structures help to make a CT diagnosis.

Atypical teratoma (germinoma) is the most common form of growth at the site of the pineal body. The tumor may present either simultaneously or sequentially in the anterior and posterior third ventricular region. Frequently the point of origin is difficult to establish. The tumor may grow by direct continuity or by metastasis from the primary site (Camins 1978). NCCT demonstrates a density equal to or slightly higher than the normal brain, whereas CECT exhibits intense homogeneous enhancement (Takeuchi 1978; Neuwelt 1979; Naidich 1976; Zimmerman 1980b). The tumor is usually rounded, with well-defined margins (Fig. 7-11). Frequently an irregular, indistinct margin suggesting infiltration into the adjacent brain and along the ventricular wall is noted. Complete and rapid disappearance of the tumor following irradiation is usual in germinomas. Differential diagnosis from other pineal tumors, such as pinealblastoma, pinealcytoma, embryonal carcinoma, and other glial tumors in the pineal region, may be difficult on the basis of the tissue density and enhancement characteristics alone. There are no consistent CT criteria for an accurate histologic diagnosis or for predicting the benign or malignant character of a pineal region tumor (Futrell 1981), although tumors arising from the pineal cells (pinealblastoma and pinealcytoma) appear to have a much greater tendency to calcify than do germ cells (Fig. 7-12) (Zimmerman 1980b).

The role of positive-contrast ventriculography or pneumoencephalography in detecting small lesions in the sella and pineal regions is minimized, especially with utilization of a high-resolution scanner

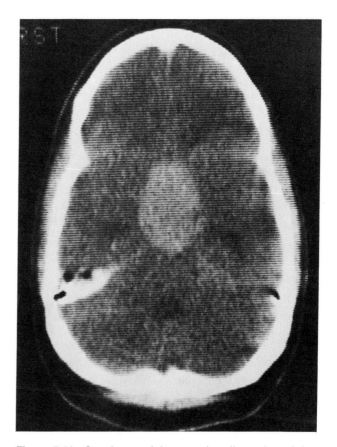

Figure 7-11 Germinoma. A large oval, well-marginated, homogeneously enhancing lesion in the region of the anterior third ventricle. The suprasellar cistern and the anterior third ventricle are obscured by the tumor. NCCT (not shown) demonstrated an isodense lesion without calcification and a normal sella turcica.

with diverse rearrangement ability in different planes. However, the exact identification of intra- versus extraaxial lesions in the sellar and pineal regions may still require ventriculography or CT cisternography with positive contrast material.

Gliomas

Gliomas are the most common primary brain tumors. The incidence in larger series varies from 30 to 60 percent of all intracranial neoplasms, but most investigators would accept 45 percent as a represen-

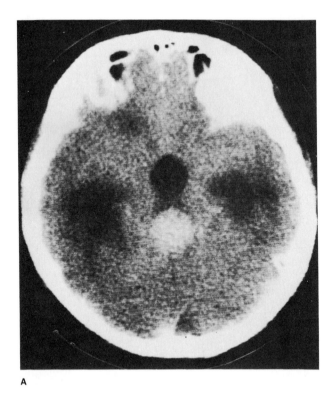

A

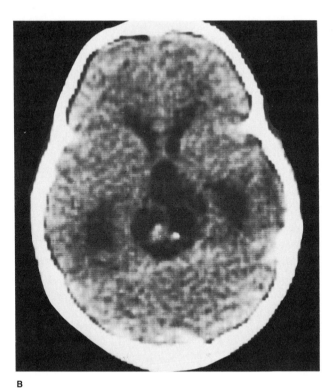

B

Figure 7-12 Pineal tumors. **A.** Pinealcytoma: a round, well-circumscribed lesion at the site of the pineal gland with intense homogeneous contrast enhancement. No calcification is present. Dilated anterior third and lateral ventricles (temporal horns) are evident, as well as obliteration of adjacent cisterns. **B.** Teratoma: a large tumor of mixed density in the pineal region. Calcifications and lipid contents are evident. *(Courtesy of Dr. R. A. Zimmerman.)*

tative figure (Russell 1977). Preponderant occurrence in childhood and in males is well known (Bodian 1953; Penman 1954). In dealing with gliomas as with other tumors, it is highly desirable to know preoperatively the type and grade of tumor so that the appropriate management strategy can be established and an adequate patient treatment plan initiated (Oi 1979).

Astrocytoma

As a group, astrocytomas make up 30 to 35 percent of all gliomas. The low-grade types have been classified by the predominant cell form, but cellular composition and biologic behavior may vary to a considerable degree according to site. Microscopically there are various histologic types such as fibrillary, protoplasmic, gemistocytic, and anaplastic forms. Macroscopically all these types have a firm, gray, granular appearance (Russell 1977).

The majority of low-grade astrocytomas (grades I and II) present on NCCT as irregular, nonhomogeneous low-density lesions (20 HU), less well demarcated than the high-grade tumors (Fig. 7-13). Occasionally, however, low-grade astrocytomas may be relatively well defined, low-density lesions which are regular in shape (Fig. 7-14). Calcification is sometimes present, probably in more cases than the reported incidence of 13 percent on plain skull roentgenograms (Gilbertson 1956). Edema around the lesion is slight or absent (Tchang 1977). Some

Figure 7-14 Low-grade astrocytomas (grade II). **A.** NCCT ▶ shows a fairly well marginated, hypodense lesion in the right frontal lobe with no mass effect on the frontal horn. **B.** CECT shows minimal contrast enhancement within the lesion (arrowheads). Cerebral angiogram (not shown) demonstrates slight tumor blush. At surgery, a solid low-grade astrocytoma was found.

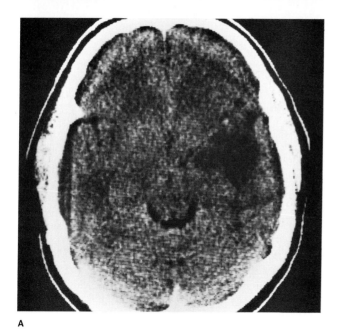

A

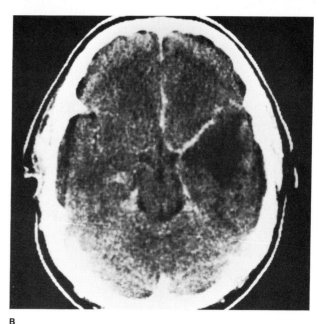

B

Figure 7-13 Low-grade astrocytoma presenting as a cystic lesion. **A.** A poorly marginated mass in the temporal lobe shows nonhomogeneous hypodensity suggestive of a cystic lesion. **B.** CECT shows no apparent contrast enhancement at the periphery of or within the tumor. The central area of hypodensity, at surgery, revealed a solid tumor, not a cyst. Differentiation between the solid and cystic components of a tumor may be difficult on the basis of CT appearance alone.

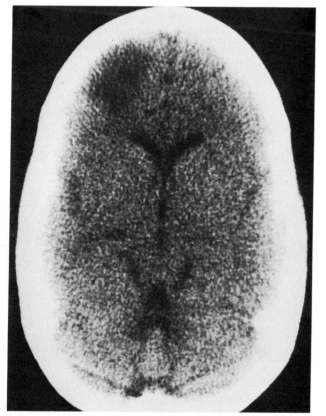

A

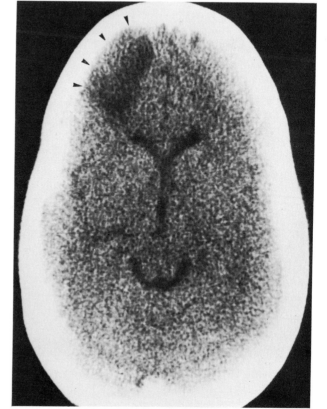

B

low-grade tumors may contain isodense areas, making it difficult to distinguish the periphery from the surrounding edema or brain. These CT findings are not unexpected, since gliomas, in general, are not encapsulated and are poorly demarcated from the surrounding parenchyma, particularly in the low-grade gliomas, on histologic examination. The low density on CT usually represents a cystic component (Fig. 7-15), but infrequently, the solid tumor also may present as a low-density lesion, as in microcystic astrocytoma (Fig. 7-13). The distinction between the two may be difficult to make on the basis of CT alone. On CECT, 45 to 50 percent of low-grade astrocytomas enhance, with a wide range of absorption values (Oi 1979). Grade I tumors generally show minimal enhancement (Steinhoff 1978) (Fig. 7-14) or no enhancement at all (Tans 1978) (Fig. 7-13). Steinhoff (1977) reported contrast enhancement in grade II neoplasms in as many as 89 percent of cases and ring enchancement in 26 percent.

High-grade astrocytomas (grades III and IV) on NCCT show nonhomogeneous moderately decreased (Fig. 7-16), mixed, or rarely increased (Fig. 7-17) densities. The low-density area usually measures 16 to 18 HU when cystic and 21 to 24 HU when necrotic. Occasionally, differentiation between cystic and necrotic components may not be possible because of the minimal CT number differ-

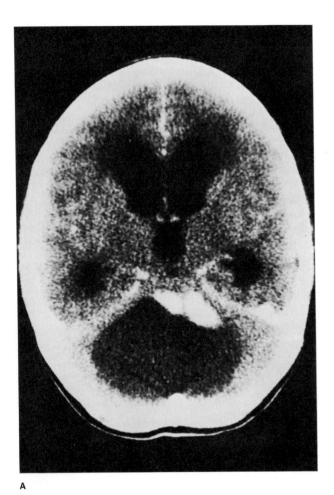

A

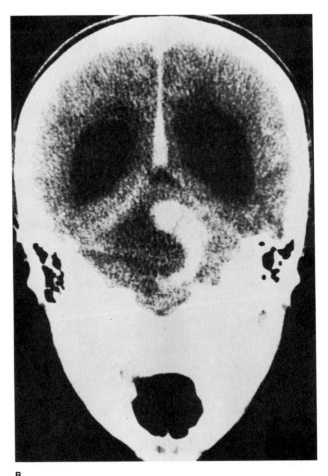

B

Figure 7-15   Cerebellar cystic astrocytoma. Axial **(A)** and coronal **(B)** CECT show a large cerebellar cystic astrocytoma with mural tumor nodules. The remainder of the cyst wall, devoid of tumor tissue, shows no contrast enhancement.

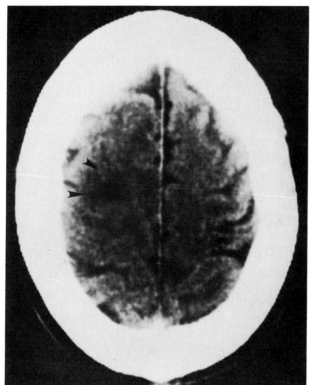

A

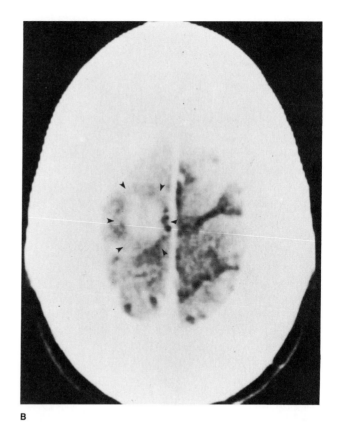

B

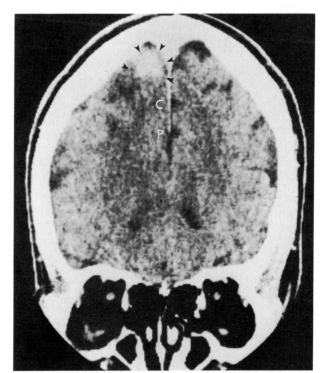

C

Figure 7-16 High-grade astrocytoma: hypodensity with nodular contrast enhancement. **A.** NCCT shows a focal area of hypodensity in the frontoparietal white matter (arrowheads). Effacement of convexity cortical sulci reflects mass effect. **B.** CECT displays a nodular enhancement in the superior border of the tumor (arrowheads). **C.** Coronal CECT exhibits nodular contrast enhancement in the cortex, with irregular hypodense areas underneath indicating deep white-matter involvement. Note effacement of ipsilateral pericallosal (*P*) and cingulate (*C*) sulci.

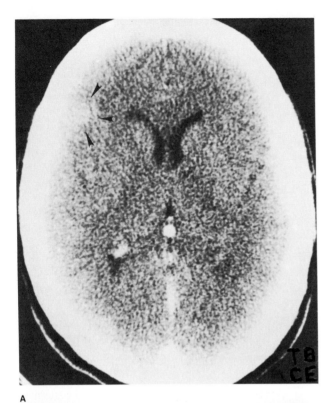

A

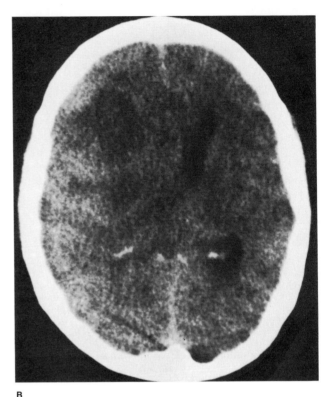

B

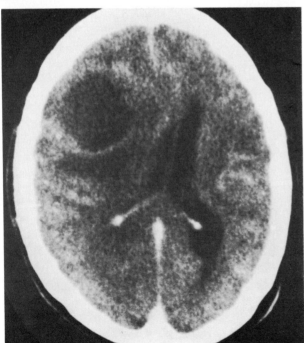

C

Figure 7-17 High-grade (grade IV) astrocytoma with necrosis. **A.** CECT shows slightly hyperdense area in the frontal lobe (arrowheads). **B.** Three months later, NCCT displays a large mixed-density lesion in the frontal lobe. The wall is partly hyperdense and irregular. Marked shift and compression of the ipsilateral ventricle is present. **C.** CECT demonstrates a ringlike, irregularly enhancing wall of varying thickness at the periphery of the tumor. The central hypodense area represents necrosis. Minimal surrounding edema is present in the white matter.

ences between the two, although morphologically, tumor cysts show a relatively thin enhancing rim and very smooth inner margins (Fig. 7-15), while central tumor necrosis exhibits irregular inner margins and relatively thick walls (Fig. 7-17). It has been reported (Afra 1980) that on delayed CECT, intracystic contrast fluid levels may be demonstrated in cystic centers but not in necrotic centers.

Tans (1978) described three types of CECT appearance of astrocytomas: (1) the annular (ring) type, characterized by an irregular wall of varying thickness with a central area of necrosis; (2) the nodular type, marked by the presence of one or more rounded nodules with fairly sharp margins and of homogeneous contrast enhancement; (3) the mixed type, showing patches of increased density distributed irregularly in a low-density lesion. Most high-grade astrocytomas are of the nodular type, with irregular, indistinct margins (Fig. 7-16). Nodular-appearing tumors usually show the most enhancement and are the most vascular. Although the degree of contrast enhancement correlates well with the amount of vascularity on histologic studies (Tans 1978), there is less correlation on angiograms. In the annular type, a faintly visible ring of isodensity or slightly increased density may surround the tumor, demarcating it from edema (Fig. 7-17). The amount of edema tends to increase with the grade of malignancy, as do ventricular distortion and mass effect. Thomson (1976) suggests that lesions showing patterns of less homogeneity or low density are more likely to be rapidly growing tumors of high malignancy; slow-growing tumors are represented by a higher-density pattern, especially one which is homogeneous.

Tans and Jongh (1978) reported that in 98 percent of astrocytomas the lesions were detected and in 93 percent were recognized as tumors. The specific diagnosis of astrocytoma was correctly made in 68 percent, and the grade of tumor was correct in 78 percent. Only one false negative was seen, and no false positives. According to Kendall (1979), a correct diagnosis was possible in 87.3 percent of 314 supratentorial gliomas, but 1.5 percent were not detected on CT; 6.5 percent were false negatives and 6.5 percent false positives (more significant in patient management). The wrong diagnoses were hemangioma, metastasis, infection, infarction, hemorrhage, and vascular malformation. All these should be considered in the differential diagnosis of gliomas.

Glioblastoma Multiforme

Glioblastoma is rare in persons under the age of 30, and its peak incidence is at about 50 years of age, with males predominating. It constitutes 50 percent of all gliomas. Average survival after surgery is 12 months (Reeves 1979). The white matter is usually affected, with the common sites being in the frontal lobes. More than one lobe may be involved. If the corpus callosum is implicated, a butterfly pattern in coronal section is seen where the mass links both hemispheres. Next in order of frequency are the temporal lobe and basal ganglia. A well-circumscribed mass may penetrate the cortex and invade the leptomeninges and dura. The tumor very often has a creamy-yellow center of necrosis with a variegated surface and contains small cysts. Rapidly growing glioblastomas may be demarcated from the surrounding brain parenchyma like the high-grade astrocytoma. A clear histologic distinction between glioblastoma and high-grade astrocytoma may not always be possible—a fact that compounds the difficulty of CT differentiation between them. Even in cases with definite histologic diagnosis, CT differentiation can be extremely difficult.

On NCCT, glioblastoma density may present as increased (8.5 to 18 percent) decreased (11.8 to 27 percent), isodense (14.4 to 16.5 percent), or mixed (38.5 to 65.3 percent) (Steinhoff 1977, 1978). Mixed density is the most frequent CT appearance prior to contrast injection (Figs. 7-18, 7-19, 7-21). Calcification is not a common feature in glioblastoma.

On CECT, almost all glioblastomas—91 percent (Tchang 1977) to 100 percent (Steinhoff 1978)—show enhancement, although hypodense glioblastomas without any change after contrast injection have been reported (Tchang 1977; Steinhoff 1977). According to Steinhoff (1978), the annular type with central low density is the most frequent pattern (55 percent) (Figs. 7-18, 7-19). The annular zone of high density represents solid vascularized tumor, while the central zone of low density usually corresponds to tumor necrosis and occasionally intratumoral cyst (Fig. 7-20). The enhanced rim of a glioblastoma is usually thick (more than 5 mm) and irregular, in contrast to the usual thin, homogeneous wall of the abscess cavity. The mixed type of enhancement, the second most frequent manifestation (27 percent), is characterized by variable density zones and heterogeneous enhancement of the glioblastoma (Fig. 7-21). The pathological substrate of this type consists of solid and necrotic parts. The

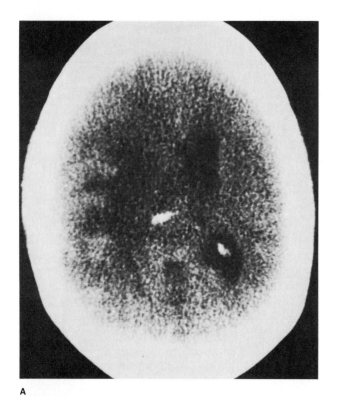

A

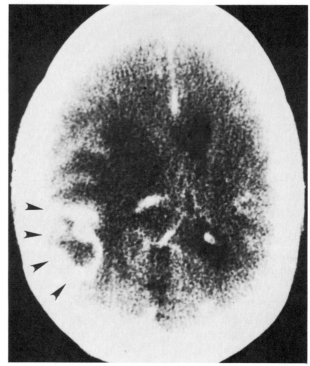

B

Figure 7-18 Glioblastoma multiforme in temporoparietal lobe. **A.** On NCCT, a poorly defined area of mixed density in the right temporoparietal lobe. Marked compression and contralateral shift of the right choroid plexus and the lateral ventricles are evident. **B.** CECT shows irregular, thick walls of the tumor (arrowheads). Central tumor necrosis and severe white-matter edema are evident. **C.** Coronal CECT displays the tumor to better advantage.

C

Figure 7-19 Glioblastoma multiforme in the temporooccipital ▶ lobe. **A** and **B.** NCCT demonstrates ventricular compression and shift of the midline structures. A large mixed-density (isodense and hypodense) area is noted in the left temporoocipital lobe. **C** and **D.** On CECT, the central necrotic area is surrounded by a thick, irregular wall of ameboid appearance. Note the involvement of the ventricular wall and extension into the choroid plexus.

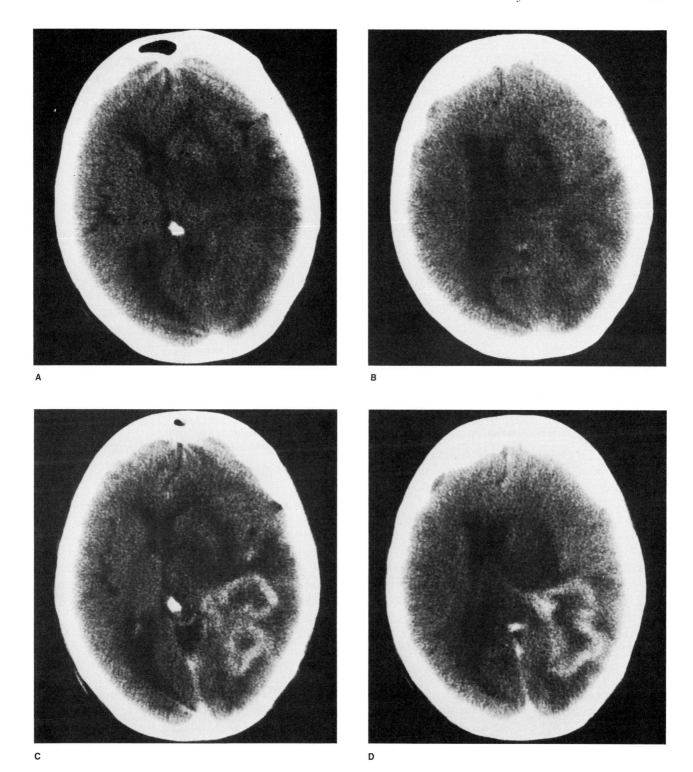

A

B

C

D

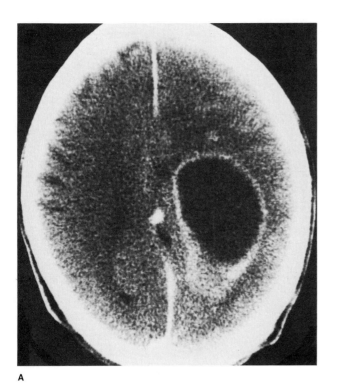
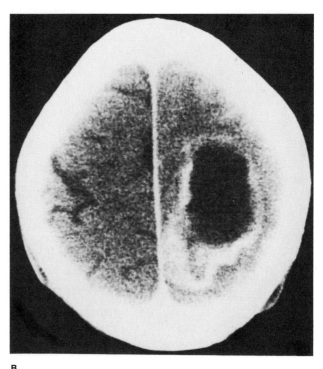

A   B

Figure 7-20   Glioblastoma with central cystic cavity.   **A.** CECT demonstrates a large oval lesion with a relatively thin enhancing rim and a large central hypodense area. Posteriorly the rim shows an irregular thick wall.   **B.** At a higher level, an irregular thick wall is well shown. Surgery revealed a large cyst of a clear yellowish fluid within the tumor.

nodular type (18 percent) represents homogeneous solid tumor, which can easily be differentiated from perifocal edema on CECT.

Perifocal edema expands in the subcortical white matter, typically exhibiting a digital configuration (Fig. 7-18). The frequency of this tumor-induced edema is 88 percent in glioblastomas (Steinhoff 1978). Grading the extent of edema was considered to be helpful: grade I when its margin has a width of 2 cm or less, grade II when it includes up to half of the hemisphere, and grade III when its larger than half of the hemisphere. In glioblastomas, edema of grades II and III predominated, but no correlation between frequency or grade of edema and specific types of intracranial neoplasms was found. However, mass effect evidenced by ventricular distortion or displacement is noted in all cases (Tchang 1977).

Oligodendroglioma

This is a relatively rare brain tumor, making up to 9 percent of all primary intracranial gliomas. Its incidence is predominantly in adult life, most frequently in the fourth and fifth decades, and it is rare in childhood and adolescence. The cerebral hemispheres, especially the frontal lobes, account for the great majority of tumors: rarely they are found in the region of the third ventricle or the cerebellum or within the spinal cord. The cerebral cortex and subcortical white matter are most affected (Russell 1977). Calcification, when present, is related to the intrinsic blood vessels: these deposits are a feature of radiologic importance and are reported to occur in 46.7 percent of cases on skull films (Kalan 1962). Slow clinical evolution is usual.

On NCCT, oligodendroglioma presents as a

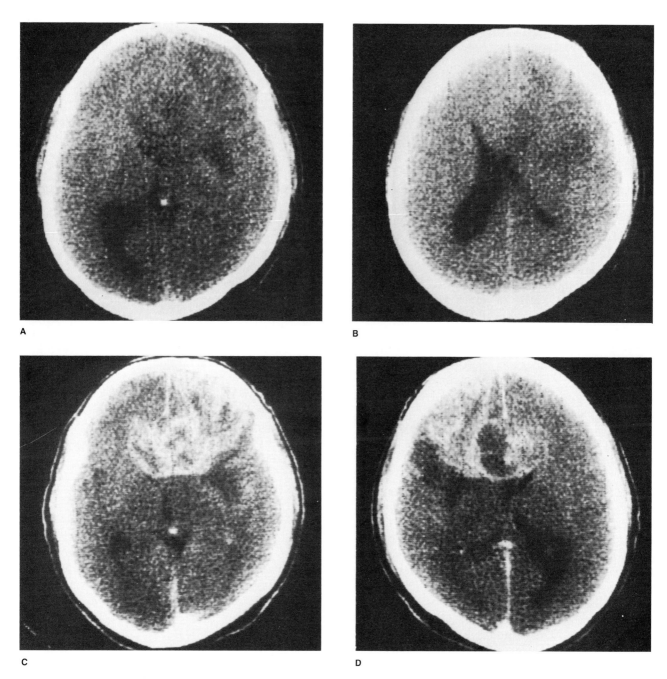

A

B

C

D

Figure 7-21 Glioblastoma multiforme involving the corpus callosum. **A** and **B.** On NCCT, a large area of mixed density (iso- and hypodensity) in the frontal lobes. Frontal horns are effaced and compressed. **C.** On CECT, a heterogeneous enhancement pattern represents solid and necrotic tumor tissues. The tumor involves the corpus callosum and extends into both frontal lobes. **D.** On CECT, at a higher level, the tumor shows a central area of necrosis, a variegated thick wall, and surrounding edema in the white matter.

hypodense lesion associated with slight to moderate mass effect and minimal surrounding edema. Intratumoral calcification on CT occurs in 91 percent of cases (Vonofakos 1979); the calcification may be located at the periphery of the lesion, in its center, or both. Segments of the peripherally located calcifications appear linear or shell-like, with incomplete ring formation, but a nodular type of calcification predominates (Vonofakos 1979) (Fig. 7-22), forming masses of considerable size. The prevalence of this characteristic calcification distinguishes oligodendrogliomas from other tumors.

On CECT thick, irregular enhancement shows at the periphery, completely defining the outer borders of the tumor with calcifications. Areas of non-enhancement within the tumor, concentric or eccentric, are frequently observed and represent foci of necrosis and cystic degeneration (Fig. 7-22). Rarely, intratumoral fluid-fluid levels indicating a cystic component are noted. Vonofakos et al. (1979) claim that all the cases with contrast enhancement and definitive evidence of a cystic component (fluid-fluid level) on CT proved to be malignant histologically. Spontaneous intratumoral hemorrhage, metastasis by way of the CSF, or remote extracranial metastasis may occur.

Choroid Plexus Papilloma

Papillomas of the choroid plexus are uncommon lesions which constitute 0.5 to 0.6 percent of all intracranial tumors and 2 percent of the glioma group. They occur usually in the first decade, with slight male predominance. The fourth, lateral, and third ventricles are affected, in that order of frequency. Choroid plexus papilloma of the fourth ventricle is commonly seen in adults, whereas in children it occurs more commonly in the lateral and third ventricles. Those tumors in the lateral ventricles show a remarkable preference for the left side (Russell 1977). Macroscopically, the tumor is readily identified as a globular mass with a round irregular surface. Occasionally it is heavily calcified and rarely undergoes ossification.

On NCCT, the tumor presents as a well-defined, smoothly marginated mass of increased density. Fo-

cal dense areas of calcification may be detected (Fig. 7-23). Local expansion of the involved ventricle and generalized hydrocephalus are common. The hydrocephalus in choroid plexus papillomas is due to overproduction of CSF and intermittent hemorrhage with blockage of the arachnoid granulations. On CECT, all these tumors enhance intensely and almost all of them homogeneously (Figs. 7-23, 7-24). Occasional demonstration of low-density areas, concentric or eccentric, within the tumor probably represents the choroid plexus itself or areas of intratumoral necrosis and infarction (Zimmerman 1979c).

Other lesions of the choroid plexus derived from the mesenchymal stromal layer are meningioma and vascular malformations such as cavernous angioma and hemangioma; those derived from the ependymal layer are carcinoma and papilloma. They present as high-density lesions prior to contrast injection and enhance homogeneously after injection. CT features such as calcification, transgression of adjacent ventricular wall and invasion of the parenchyma, absence of generalized hydrocephalus, and intratumoral hemorrhage, association with other entities—namely, neurofibromatosis and Sturge-Weber disease—are helpful in the differential diagnosis if the patient's age and sex and the clinical course are also considered.

Ganglioglioma

An uncommon brain tumor in children and young adults, the ganglioglioma occurs under the age of 30 in 60 percent of reported cases (Anderson 1942). Women are more often affected. Presenting symptoms usually relate to the location of the tumor and its protracted course. This neoplasm is most commonly found in the anterior third ventricle, less

Figure 7-22 Oligodendroglioma. **A** and **B.** NCCT shows ▶ both shell-like and nodular calcifications at the periphery of the tumor. Surrounding white matter edema is prominent. **C** and **D.** CECT shows both thick irregular peripheral (ringlike) and central homogeneous enhancement. Areas of nonenhancement represent foci of necrosis and cystic degeneration.

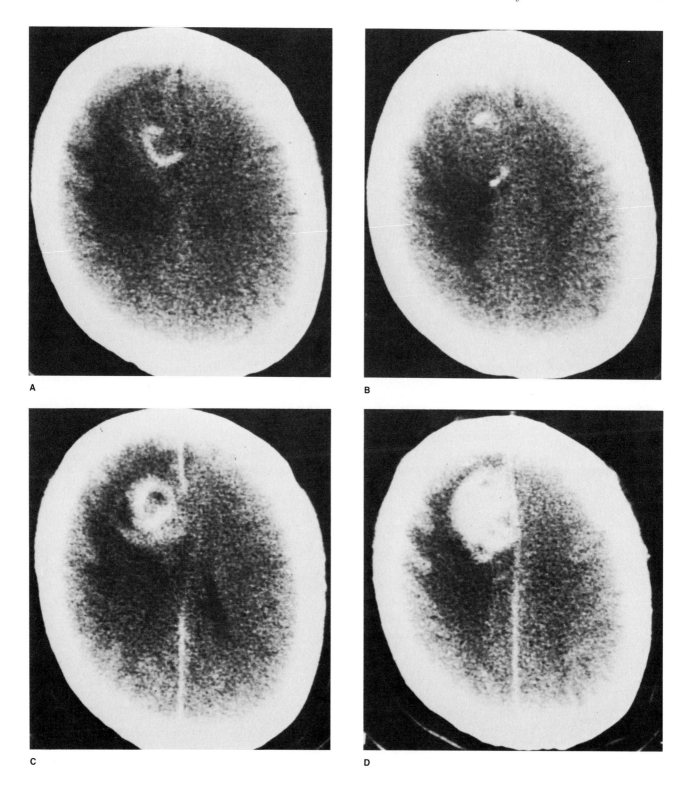

A

B

C

D

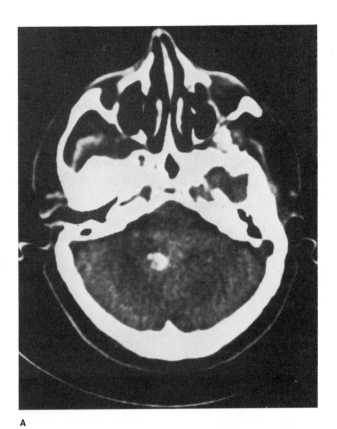

A

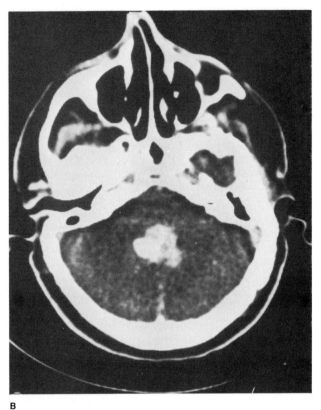

B

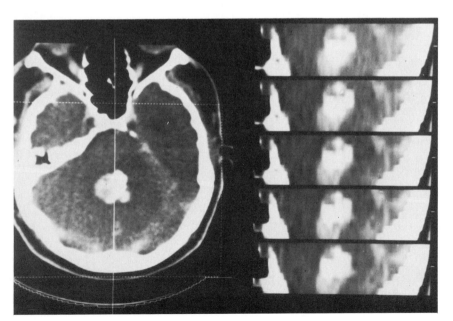

C

Figure 7-23 Choroid plexus papilloma of the fourth ventricle. **A.** NCCT: Slightly hyperdense lesion with poor demarcation is noted in the region of the fourth ventricle. Multiple calcifications are eccentrically located within the lesion. **B.** CECT: Intense contrast enhancement of the tumor manifests as a mottled appearance with sharp, irregular margins. **C.** Sagittal reformation images confirm the tumor within the fourth ventricle.

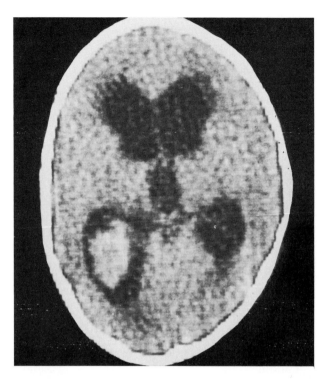

Figure 7-24 Choroid plexus papilloma of the lateral ventricle. On CECT, a large, well-demarcated tumor within the trigone of the lateral ventricle shows intense homogeneous contrast enhancement. Hydrocephalus is due to overproduction of CSF by the tumor and intermittent hemorrhage into the ventricles and subarachnoid space.

frequently in the frontal lobes, temporal lobes, and basal ganglia. No site in the central nervous system is exempt, however. The tumors are usually single masses, but a few have been multiple (Russell 1977).

Macroscopically, the lesion is small, firm, and well circumscribed, with a finely granular gray surface. It may contain one large cyst or multiple cysts. Calcified foci are frequent. Some tumors contain capillary vessels in a marked telangiectatic pattern. CT findings generally reflect the varied macroscopic appearances.

On CT, the tumor is usually well circumscribed, often isodense, but frequently hypodense with areas of increased density due to calcification. Foci of calcifications are frequent (Fig. 7-25). On CECT, single or multiple cysts with mural nodules may be seen. Contrast enhancement is observed in the ma-

jority (Fig. 7-25). Although the CT characterization is not specific, an isodense, partially calcified, contrast-enhancing tumor with or without cysts in a young patient with a prolonged clinical history should raise the question of ganglioglioma (Zimmerman 1979*b*). Histologic confirmation to establish the benign nature of the tumor is important prior to instituting any aggressive therapeutic modalities.

Colloid Cyst

This entity accounts for 0.5 to 1 percent of all intracranial tumors (Guner 1976). Very few colloid cysts are seen in infancy and childhood, with most being found in early adult life. Males and females are about equally affected. It is thought that most colloid cysts are generated from the ependymal pouches (Ariens-Kappers 1955). Mucoids or dense hyaloid material is surrounded by a smooth, spherical, fibrous wall, and the cyst is attached to the collagenous stroma of the choroid plexus. Within the third ventricle the cyst is notorious for obstructing the foramen of Monro and causing hydrocephalus, since it can grow to as much as 3 cm in size. If the mass is somewhat pendulous and movable, intermittent obstruction becomes a possibility (Guner 1976).

Common symptoms and physical findings are headache, gait disturbance, and papilledema (Little 1974). Although these tumors are benign and can be completely removed early in their course, Guner et al. (1976) report a mortality as high as 53 percent postoperatively. It is presumed that this figure is high because of the surgical approach and the complex regional anatomy.

NCCT shows a smooth, spherical or ovoid lesion of homogeneously high density (45 to 75 HU) in the anterior third ventricle in front of or behind the foramen of Monro (Fig. 7-26). Uncommonly, the lesion is isodense, and rarely, a central hypodensity within the lesion is noted (Ganti 1981). The high density on NCCT is probably due to desquamative secretory products from the cyst wall, hemosiderin, and possibly microscopic foci of calcification, although the latter are not apparent on CT. Only mild

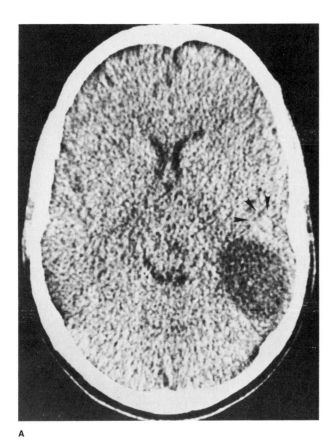

A

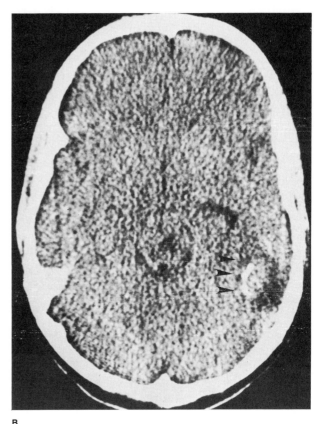

B

Figure 7-25 Ganglioglioma. A. A well-circumscribed hypodense lesion in the posterior temporal lobe contains multiple calcifications at the periphery (arrowheads). Minimal mass effect is evidenced by obliteration of the ipsilateral quadrigem-inal cistern. **B.** CECT shows minimal contrast enhancement on the medial side of the lesion where calcifications are present. Slight dilatation of the left temporal horn is due to proximal compression.

enhancement has been shown on CECT (Osborn 1977; Ganti 1981), but absence of contrast enhancement is not unusual (Fig. 7-26). The presence of blood vessels in the wall or even inside the cyst, as well as diffusion of contrast media into the cavity, may account for the enhancement. Hemorrhage is rare (Malik 1980). Although hydrocephalus, minimal to moderately severe, is present in all cases, its degree is not always proportional to the size of the cyst. In the authors' experience, the anterior portion of the third ventricle is not well visualized, and the posterior third ventricle is usually collapsed. Widening of the septum pellucidum and separation of the posteromedial aspects of the frontal horns are demonstrated in most cases on axial and coronal

sections (Ganti 1981). Intraventricular ependymoma, glioma, meningioma, choroid plexus papilloma, arteriovenous malformation, craniopharyngioma, teratomatous tumors, tuberous sclerosis, and cysticercosis should be considered in the differential diagnosis. Occasionally, metrizamide ventriculography or cisternography may be necessary to localize the lesion within the third ventricle. However, the need for additional study has greatly diminished since the recent introduction of high-resolution CT scanners with multiplanar reformation capabilities. When marked contrast enhancement is present, the possibility of aneurysm or ectatic vessels should be strongly considered and investigated by cerebral angiography (Fig. 7-27).

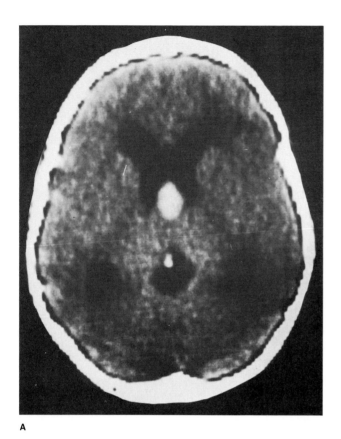

A

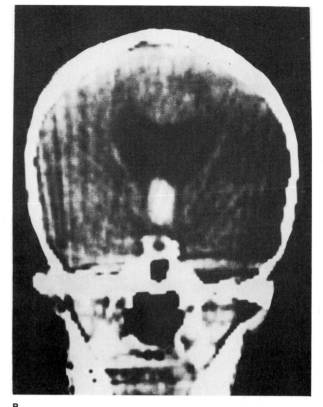

B

Figure 7-26 Colloid cyst of the third ventricle. **A.** NCCT shows an oval hyperdense lesion in the region of the third ventricle with separation of the posteromedial sides of the frontal horns. Note collapse of the posterior third ventri-cle. **B.** Coronal view confirms the tumor within the third ventricle. CECT (not shown) reveals no contrast enhancement. Noncommunicating hydrocephalus is also present.

Meningiomas

These represent 15 percent of all intracranial tumors in adults; a lower incidence of 3 to 4 percent is noted in the pediatric population. Meningiomas manifest a clear female predominance (3:2), with most tumors detected near midlife and reaching a peak in the seventh decade.

Macroscopically, meningiomas are usually spherical or globular but may be flat and platelike. They are well circumscribed, demarcated, and readily separated from the adjacent brain tissue. All meningiomas arise from meningothelial cells. Microscopically, they may be classified as syncytial, transitional, fibroblastic, angioblastic, or sarcoma-tous. The diversity of types of meningioma reflects the adaptive potential of these cells (Russell 1977).

The common sites of intracranial meningiomas are the parasagittal and lateral convexities (43 percent), sphenoid ridge (7 percent), olfactory groove (10 percent), suprasellar region (8 percent), posterior fossa (7 percent), and other rare sites (15 percent) such as the falx-tentorial junction, the intracerebral, intraorbital, and pineal regions, and the intraventricular region (Baker 1973).

CT characteristically demonstrates a rounded, sharply delineated, isodense or hyperdense tumor (16 to 35 HU) in a juxtadural location with intense homogeneous contrast enhancement. Mass effect is almost a constant CT feature of meningiomas large

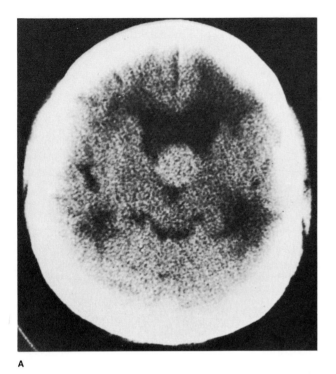

A

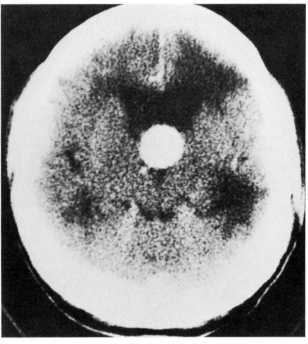

B

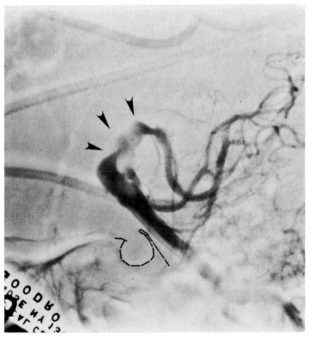

C

Figure 7-27 Basilar artery aneurysm simulating third ventricular colloid cyst. **A.** On NCCT, slightly hyperdense round lesion in the region of the anterior third ventricle. Note visualization of the posterior third ventricle, which is usually collapsed in colloid cyst. Hydrocephalus is present. Periventricular hypodensity may represent transventricular absorption. **B.** CECT shows intense homogeneous enhancement, not a characteristic feature of colloid cyst. **C.** Vertebral angiogram demonstrates a large, partially thrombosed aneurysm of the basilar artery (arrowheads) projecting into the third ventricle.

enough to obliterate CSF pathways (cisterns) or alter the shape of the ventricular system (Claveria 1977*a*). Another compressive phenomenon on CT, the inward "buckling" of the white matter, if present, helps to confirm the extraaxial location of the tumor (George 1980). In addition, other CT features, such as the broad base of the tumor abutting the dura and adjacent bone changes, hyperostotic or destructive, may be of assistance in the diagnosis of meningioma.

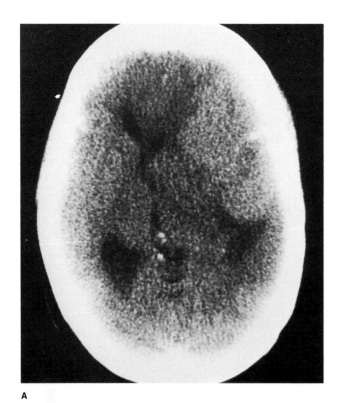

A

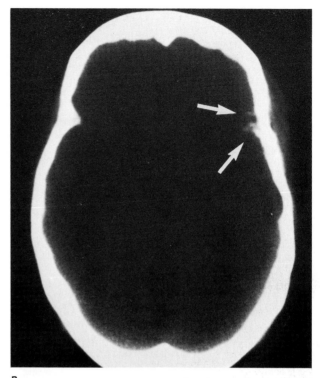

B

Figure 7-28 Pterional meningioma.   **A.** NCCT shows a large, well-demarcated, lobulated, hyperdense mass with compression and displacement of the adjacent brain tissue and the ventricle.   **B.** On bone settings, hyperostosis of the pterion, involvement of the calvarium, and extension into the scalp are well demonstrated (arrows).   **C.** CECT delineates the well-marginated, homogeneously enhancing tumor abutting the inner table of the skull.

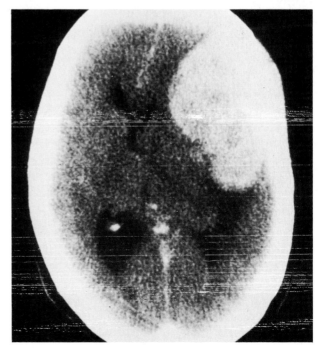

C

Hyperdensity on NCCT is attributed to the compactness of the tumor cells, the presence of psammoma bodies within the tumor, and the hypervascularity of the tumor (Fig. 7-28). Calcifications are usually punctate and may be conglomerate, peripheral, or central. They are present on CT in 20 percent of meningiomas (Claveria 1977a) (Fig. 7-29). Transitional and fibroblastic tumors are frequently seen with visible calcium aggregates (39 percent), a feature that characterizes a nonaggressive meningioma (Vassilouthis 1979; Ambrose 1975a). Isodense meningiomas on NCCT (Mani 1978; Amundsen 1978) are difficult to distinguish from the surrounding

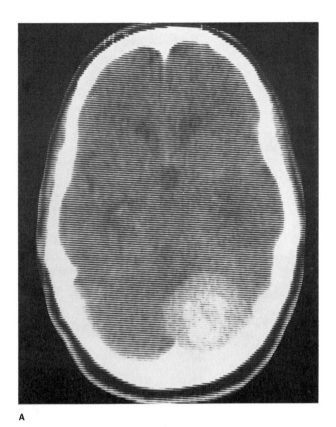

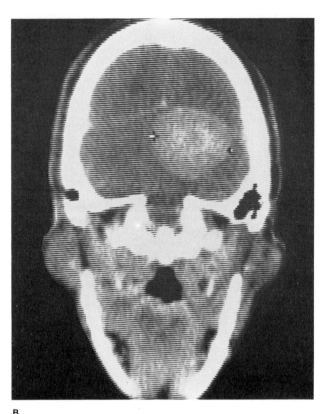

A

B

Figure 7-29 Posterior fossa meningioma with calcifications.   **A.** Axial view shows a large, well-marginated, hyperdense tumor containing multiple calcifications.   **B.** Coronal view shows tumor attachment to the tentorium cerebelli.

normal brain tissue; however, on CECT intense, persistent opacification is a usual finding. Occasionally an isodense area may represent subacute hemorrhage within the tumor. Hypodensity within the tumor on NCCT is a rare finding and may represent tumor necrosis, old hemorrhage, cystic degeneration, or lipomatous transformation (George 1980; Vassilouthis 1979). These areas of hypodensity exhibit minimal or no contrast enhancement (Fig. 7-30). Cystic formation on CT may be located centrally or peripherally within the tumor or around the tumor (peritumoral cyst) and is difficult to differentiate from the edematous brain (Rengachary 1979).

Intratumoral hemorrhage is rare and presents on CT as a focal area of high density in the acute phase (Vassilouthis 1979) (Fig. 7-31). Intratumoral hemorrhage occurs mostly in fibroblastic and meningoen-

dotheliomatous meningiomas (George 1980). Its exact mechanism is not known, although a constant association of hemorrhage with large and small thin-walled endothelial channels has been noted (Modesti 1976), and the onset of bleeding has been attributed to acute pressure changes (Vassilouthis 1979). Extremely rare coexistence of hemorrhage and necrosis within a tumor may present as a

Figure 7-31 Meningioma with intratumoral hemorrhage.   **A.** ▶ NCCT demonstrates an area of hyperdensity on the anterolateral portion of the tumor (arrowheads) with a mass effect. Increased density in the interhemispheric fissure represents subarachnoid hemorrhage.   **B.** On CECT, an eccentric intense enhancement of the posteromedial portion of the meningioma is seen. At surgery, the hyperdensity in the anterolateral portion was found to be due to hemorrhage within the tumor.

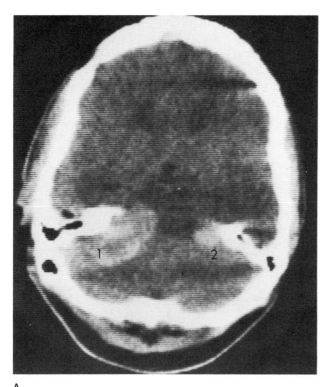

A

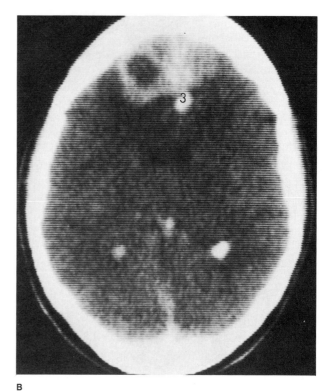

B

Figure 7-30 Coexistent acoustic neuroma, neurofibroma, and meningioma in a patient with neurofibromatosis. **A.** CECT demonstrates bilateral enhancing lesions in the cerebellopontine angles representing meningioma (1) and acoustic neuroma (2). **B.** At a higher level, a large frontal meningioma (3) with a cystic cavity is seen. *(Courtesy of William A. Buchheit, M.D., Temple University Hospital, Philadelphia, Pennsylvania.)*

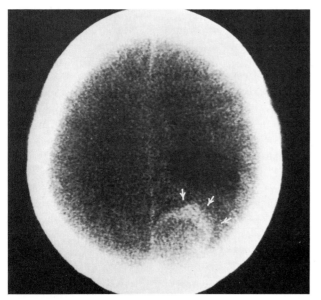

A

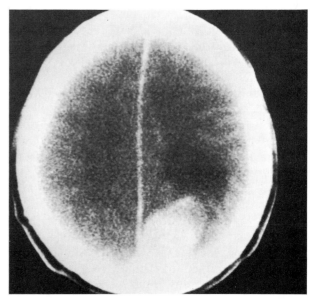

B

mixed-density lesion. Bleeding into subarachnoid or subdural spaces may rarely occur.

The consistency of meningiomas may be of surgical importance when the tumors are in close relation to vital structures. According to Kendall (1979), 90 percent of hard meningiomas, excluding those showing diffuse calcification, are hyperdense, and the other 10 percent are of the same density as brain. Of the soft meningiomas, 49 percent, excluding those showing marked cystic or necrotic changes, are hyperdense, but compared to the brain 35 percent are isodense and 16 percent are hypodense. The Kendall (1979) study, however, found no relationship between the degree of contrast enhancement and the consistency or the vascularity of the tumor as estimated by the surgeon or histologist.

CT features have been considered helpful in predicting the histology and aggressiveness of the tumor (Vassilouthis 1979). Less aggressive types such as transitional, fibroblastic, or mixed fibroblastic and transitional variants are well defined, with more or less regular shapes, and contain visible calcium aggregates. Most of the tumors (92 percent) are surrounded by edema of varying degrees, and the edema is not considered a specific feature except in the fibroblastic type, where it is almost invariably moderate. Tumor density on NCCT has not been considered specific in predicting histologic types, but a homogeneous density distribution on CECT suggests the transitional type. Marked edema, absence of visible calcium aggregates, and nonhomogeneous contrast enhancement, with nonenhancing low-density components and poorly defined irregular borders, point to aggressive or invasive characteristics, more commonly found in the angioblastic and syncytial variants.

Intraventricular meningiomas arise from either the choroid plexus or the tela choroidea. They represent 17 percent of meningiomas in children and 1.6 percent in adults. An association between intraventricular meningioma and neurofibromatosis is well known. CT demonstrates a homogeneous, well-marginated, isodense or slightly hyperdense mass in the ventricle, particularly in the region of the choroid plexus, most often within the atrium of the lateral ventricle. Intense, homogeneous contrast enhancement is almost always present on CECT, as well as ipsilateral, contralateral, or bilateral ventricular dilatation (Fig. 7-32). Differentiation from other intraventricular lesions such as papilloma, carcinoma, vascular malformation, cavernous angioma, hemangioma, and astrocytoma may be possible on the basis of age, location, density differences with contrast enhancement characteristics, and associated systemic mesenchymal abnormalities (Zimmerman 1979c).

The occurrence of multiple meningiomas is uncommon (Fig. 7-33) apart from an association with neurofibromatosis (Fig. 7-30). Association of meningioma with other types of primary neoplasm such as glioblastoma multiforme or pituitary adenoma (Brenner 1977) is probably coincidental.

Miscellaneous Tumors

Hemangioblastoma

These are histologically benign, true neoplasms of vascular structure. They constitute from 1.1 to 2.5 percent of all intracranial tumors and approximately 7 percent of posterior fossa tumors (Olivercrone 1952). They occur at any age, but young and middle-aged adults are most frequently affected. The most frequent site is the cerebellum, commonly in the paramedian hemisphere. Macroscopically, the tumor is usually well circumscribed without a capsule, and approximately 60 percent are cystic, with a mural nodule. The tumor may be associated with erythrocytosis and is the primary feature of Hippel-Landau disease (Russell 1977).

CT may demonstrate a solid, homogeneous, isodense mass with distinctive contrast enhancement after intravenous contrast injection. More characteristically, cystic tumor with solid mural nodules is demonstrated (Figs. 7-4A, 7-34). The mural nodules are enhanced homogeneously and may be solitary or multiple (Adair 1978). The central low-density areas in the cyst range from 4 to 23 HU and show

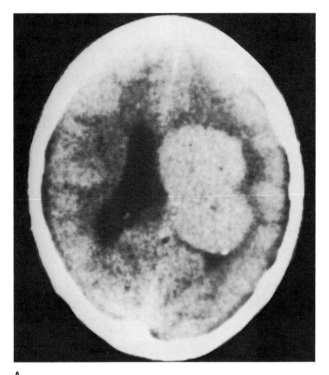

A

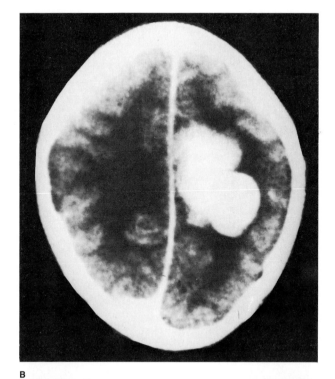

B

Figure 7-32 Intraventricular meningioma. **A.** On NCCT, a large, slightly lobulated, hyperdense tumor with clear margination is situated within the lateral ventricle. A small, calcified choroid plexus is markedly displaced posteriorly. Hydrocephalus is present. Note the absence of density changes in the adjoining brain tissue. **B.** On CECT, intense, homogeneously enhancing tumor is well demonstrated.

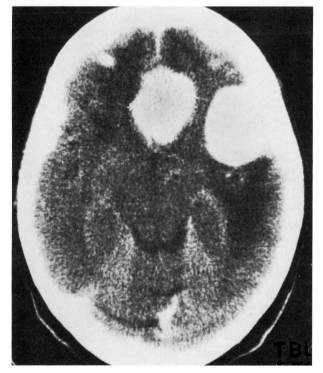

Figure 7-33 Multiple meningiomas. CECT shows two large meningiomas, one originating from the planum sphenoidale, the other from the pterion. A third one is in the frontopolar region.

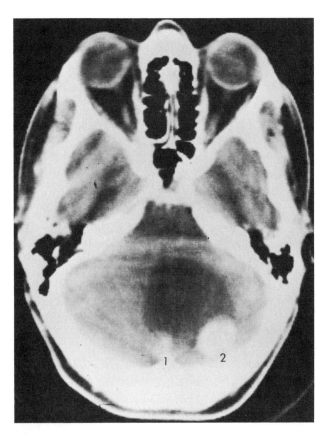

Figure 7-34 Hemangioblastoma. On CECT, a large, cystic posterior fossa tumor is noted in the left cerebellum. Two round, homogeneously enhancing tumor nodules (1, 2) are present at the posterolateral wall of the cyst. Absence of enhancement of the cyst wall itself is characteristic.

Primary Intracranial Lymphoma

Tumors of the lymphoreticular system may be primary lesions of the brain or metastatic lesions as part of generalized lymphomatous diseases. Primary malignant lymphoma of the brain is a relatively rare tumor, with incidence ranging from 0.8 percent (Jellinger 1975) to 1.5 percent (Zimmerman 1975) of all intracranial tumors.

The cells of origin of these tumors within the brain are not clearly defined; the confusion regarding cells of origin is well reflected in the literature by the multiplicity of synonyms describing this tumor, such as reticulum cell carcinoma, histiocytic lymphoma, microglioma, round cell carcinoma, lymphosarcoma, perithelial sarcoma, adventitial sarcoma, and malignant reticulohistiocytic encephalitis (Tadmor 1978; Kazner 1978).

The clinical presentation of these tumors is varied and nonspecific, and most cases run a fulminating course, with 3 to 5 months' survival after the first symptoms. This course may be altered by radiotherapy, and early diagnosis assumes major importance. Grossly, no uniform patterns of involvement by primary cerebral lymphoma are recognizable; the tumors range from solitary or multiple circumscribed nodules to diffuse infiltration or widespread distribution. A mixed pattern is rather frequent. There is a predilection for the basal ganglia, thalamus, periventricular white matter, and corpus callosum, but the tumors may occur in the cerebellar hemispheres, vermis, brainstem, and meninges as well.

On NCCT, the tumor presents usually as a homogeneous, slightly hyperdense (40 HU) area (Fig. 7-35) but occasionally as a heterogeneous area when interspersed with edema. Neither mass effect nor ventricular enlargement are conspicuous (Tadmor 1978). On CECT, there is an increase (15 HU) in density of tumor tissue, usually homogeneous and well circumscribed, separated from the surrounding edema (Fig. 7-35). The absence of a low-density center in larger lesions is distinctive (Enzmann 1979). Heterogeneous enhancement is also observed, particularly in the diffuse, infiltrating type. The tumor margins are invariably poorly defined

no contrast enhancement. The margin of a cyst, when isodense with no demonstrable contrast enhancement, represents gliosis and compressed cerebellum; areas that are hyperdense with contrast enhancement correspond to a highly vascular tumor. Rarely, central low density in a tumor suggesting a cyst may prove to be a solid tumor. Angiography not only confirms the presence of hypervascular mural nodules but also increases the detection rate for multiple lesions (Seeger 1981). Rare cases of supratentorial hemangioblastoma have been recorded (Wylie 1973; Bachmann 1978).

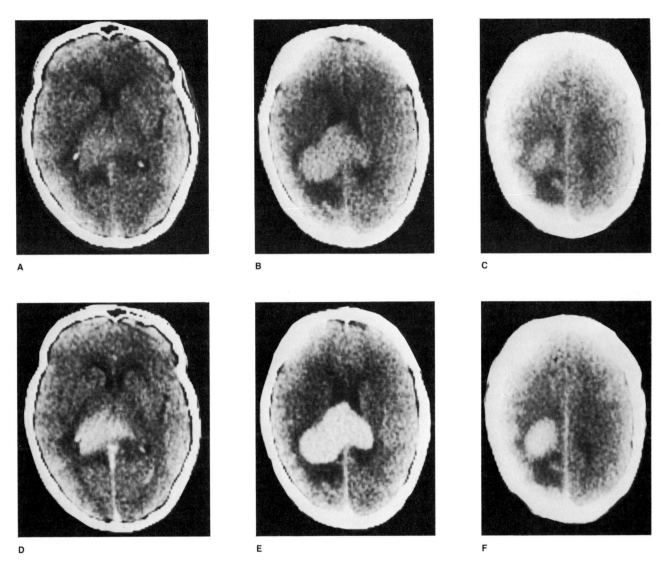

Figure 7-35 Primary malignant lymphoma. **A, B,** and **C.** On NCCT, slightly hyperdense, homogeneous, poorly marginated lesions are found in the thalamus, the splenium of the corpus callosum, and the deep parietal white matter. Note relative absence of mass effect and of hydrocephalus in spite of the extensive tumor involvement. **D, E,** and **F.** On CECT, the tu- mor shows homogeneous, intense enhancement. The margins are indistinct, particularly in the deep white matter, indicative of infiltration pattern. Multicentricity, without respect for the normal anatomic boundaries and with infiltration into the ad- joining tissue and across the midline, is characteristic.

and irregular, probably because of the characteristic perivascular and vascular infiltration pattern of the tumor cells. This was seen in 50 percent of cases and was thought to be an important diagnostic clue (Kazner 1978). Multicentricity (43 percent) and in- filtration into the adjoining tissue and across the

midline, with no respect for the normal anatomic boundaries, are frequently observed. Contrast en- hancement of the subarachnoid space due to lep- tomeningeal involvement occurs but cannot be detected on CT (Enzmann 1979). Secondary paren- chymal involvement of the brain by systemic lymphoma and by primary malignant lymphoma of the brain are indistinguishable on CT (Brant-Zawadzki 1978). Differentiation from glioma, metastasis, melanoma, meningioma, or progressive multifocal leukoencephalopathy may be difficult.

Unusual Features

HEMORRHAGE A variety of vascular changes can occur within a tumor, resulting in infarction, necrosis, and hemorrhage. Massive hemorrhage into a brain tumor may eventuate in rapidly deteriorating neurologic deficits and death. Intratumoral hemorrhage is not as rare as is usually believed. Mauersberger (1977) believes it occurs in 4 to 7 percent of all gliomas, especially in glioblastomas, medulloblastomas, and metastases. The overall incidence

detected by CT is 3.6 percent of all intracranial tumors (Zimmerman 1980a). It occurs in a variety of primary cerebral neoplasms, such as glioblastoma, chromophobe adenoma, grade I astrocytoma, medulloblastoma, central neuroblastoma, histiocytic lymphoma, oligodendroglioma, and hemangiopericytoma (Little 1979; Zimmerman 1980a; Post 1980). Less frequently, ependymoma, choroid plexus papilloma, and hemangioblastoma have been associated with intratumoral hemorrhage, and rarely, meningioma (Modesti 1976; George 1980). High-grade malignancy and extensive, abnormal vascularity have been thought to be predisposing factors. Analysis of the CT appearance of tumoral hemorrhage led Zimmerman (1980a) to classification of various patterns: central hemorrhage pattern was most commonly observed in glioblastomas and astrocytomas, and other patterns, such as solid hemorrhage and

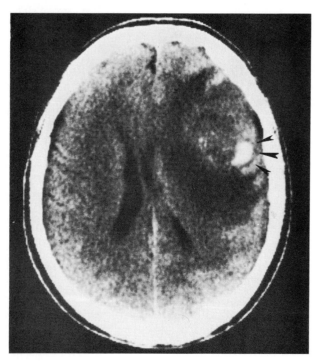
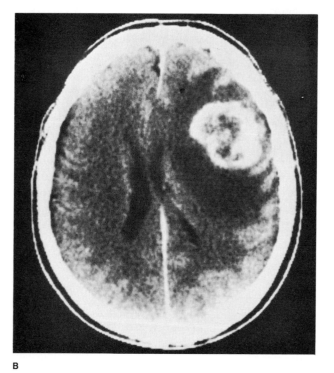

A B

Figure 7-36 Intratumoral hemorrhage in glioblastoma multiforme. **A.** NCCT demonstrates an area of hemorrhage (arrowheads) within a mixed-density tumor in the frontoparietal lobe. Note the surrounding edema. **B.** CECT shows nonhomogeneous enhancement of the entire tumor with central necrosis. The intratumoral hemorrhage is completely obscured by contrast enhancement.

hemorrhagic infarction, were most frequent in patients with metastasis. Little (1979) noted CT findings in 13 patients that include a neoplastic core (high or low density); small multifocal hemorrhage, usually at the margin of the tumor (Fig. 7-31); and surrounding, often extensive, edema (Fig. 7-36). Enhancement of tumor tissue on CECT has a peripheral distribution in proximity to the site of the hemorrhage (Fig. 7-36).

Intramural hemorrhage may dissect into the adjacent compressed and edematous brain (peritumoral hematoma) and extend through the cortex into the subarachnoid space (subarachnoid hemorrhage) (Fig. 7-31) or deep through the white matter and ependyma into the ventricle (intracerebral and intraventricular hematoma) (Mandybur 1977). Differentiation from atypical intracranial hemorrhage from various causes, such as aneurysm, vascular malformation, trauma, or hypertension, may be difficult, since most of these lesions demonstrate a mass consisting of a hematoma and concentric or eccentric contrast enhancement, almost indistinguishable from intratumoral hemorrhage. Angiography is helpful when tumor vascularity is demonstrated. The diagnosis of intratumoral hemorrhage should be considered whenever patients with certain types of tumor with a propensity for hemorrhage exhibit an intracerebral hematoma that is atypical in relation to the clinical history, age of patient, location, or CT appearance.

MULTICENTRIC TUMORS These are uncommon and account for 2.5 percent of all gliomas (Batzdorf 1963). The multicentricity is most frequently demonstrated in glioblastomas and primary malignant lymphoma, rarely in anaplastic astrocytoma. The tumors may be widely separated, occupying different lobes of the same hemisphere or opposite hemispheres. Although the diagnosis of multicentric tumors is usually obtained at autopsy because of their nonspecific clinical presentation, in vivo recognition adds significantly to the management of the patient. CT, with its high sensitivity, can easily visualize multicentric patterns such as bihemispheric involvement (Fig. 7-37) and satellite foci of a tumor (Alte-

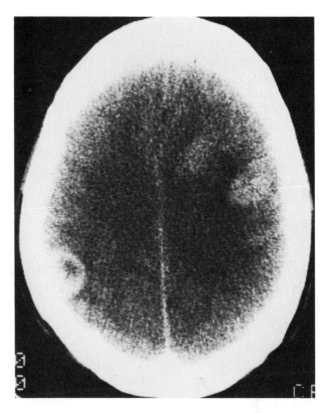

Figure 7-37 Multicentric glioblastoma multiforme. CECT demonstrates multiple enhancing lesions involving both hemispheres. Relative absence of edema is conspicuous. Differential diagnosis with metastic lesions may be extremely difficult.

mus 1977). However, differentiation from infiltrating primary tumors with microscopic or macroscopic connections as well as multiple metastatic foci may be extremely difficult on the basis of CT findings alone (Rao 1980).

CONCURRENT TUMORS The concurrence of histologically different intracranial tumors is well documented in dysgenetic syndromes such as tuberous sclerosis, Lindau's syndrome, neurocutaneous melanosis, and neurofibromatosis. Other associations of multiple tumors, such as meningioma and glioblastoma or acoustic neurinoma, or glioblastoma and sarcoma, may be coincidental. In these collision or tandem tumors, CT demonstrates multiplicity of

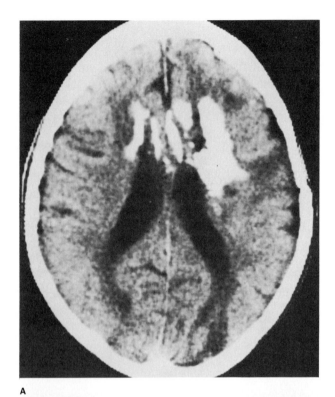

A

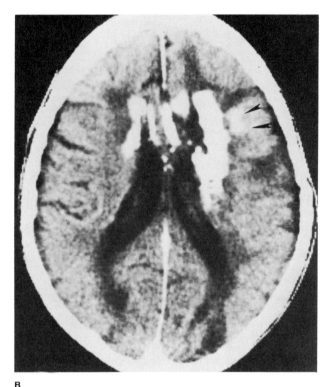

B

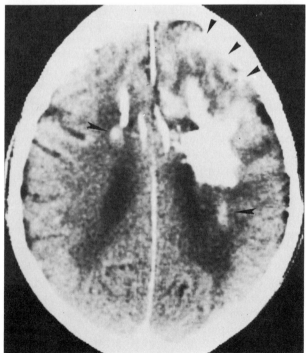

C

Figure 7-38 Mixed glioma (oligodendroglioma and astrocytoma). **A.** NCCT exhibits multiple thick, bandlike calcifications in both frontal lobes. Frontal horns are compressed. **B** and **C.** On CECT, multiple small scattered areas of contrast enhancement (arrowheads) are intermixed with calcifications. On histologic examination, mixed glioma (oligodendroglioma and astrocytoma) was found.

lesions (Fig. 7-30), but histologic diagnosis should rely on the CT characteristics and location of each tumor (Brenner 1977). The rare occurrence of mixed gliomas such as mixed oligodendroglioma and astrocytoma may render CT diagnosis difficult. Unfortunately, CT distinction between the two histologically different tumor components may not be possible, although the characteristic CT features of one tumor component may predominate (Fig. 7-38).

RAPID GROWTH OR ALTERATION   Rapid growth or morphologic alteration of gliomas may present as false negative CT scans initially, presumably because of the infiltrating nature of the lesions. They become positive 14 to 17 days later (Tenfler 1977;

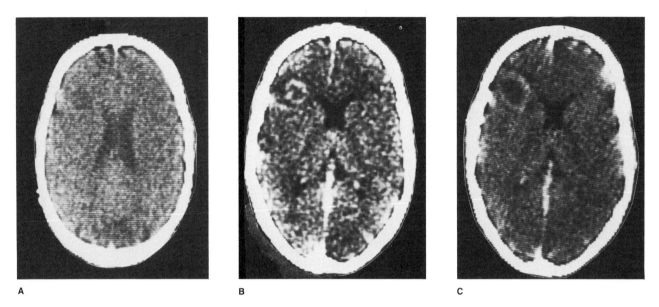

A   B   C

Figure 7-39 Rapid growth of glioma. CT at weekly intervals. Initial study **(A),** one week later **(B),** and at two weeks **(C)** demonstrate a rapidly enlarging, enhancing ring lesion proved to be a high-grade astrocytoma.

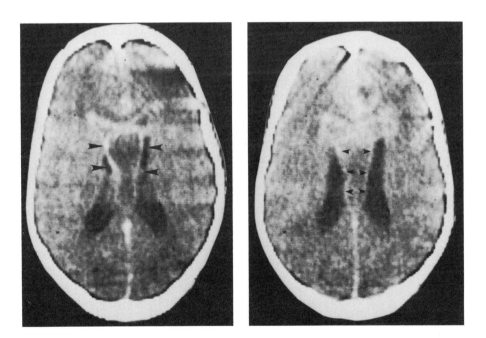

Figure 7-40 Ependymal dissemination of frontal high-grade astrocytoma. CECT exhibits the characteristic ventricular-wall enhancement associated with ependymal spread (arrowheads) to the cavum septi pellucidi, which is enlarged because of obstruction by the neoplasm.

Rao 1979) and present as mass lesions, probably because of sudden vascular changes and rapid necrosis or rapid growth of tumors (Fig. 7-39).

METASTASIS Local spread beyond the confines of a primary tumor by direct infiltration into the immediately adjacent meninges and ependymal surface is sufficiently known, although this feature bears little relation to the intrinsic malignancy of the tumor. Of greater concern is the manner in which this ependymal infiltration leads to metastasis via the CSF. Dissemination to distant points, in either the ependyma or the meninges, is noted in glioblastoma multiforme, medulloblastoma, ependy-

moma, teratoma, and pinealblastoma. These diffuse or nodular metastases via CSF pathways are easily detectable in the ependymal and subependymal layers of the ventricles on CECT (Fig. 7-40) (Osborn 1978a), but meningeal spread is difficult to detect on CT (Enzmann 1978; Pagani 1981).

Remote metastasis of a primary tumor may occur when the tumor cells obtain access to the lymphatics or to veins outside the central nervous system. Such metastasis is recorded in glioblastoma, medulloblastoma, ependymoma, and oligodendroglioma, in order of frequency. All the patients had had one or more previous operations, and this mechanical access to the hematolymphatic system must play a decisive role in the process.

Bibliography

ADAIR LB, ROPPER AH, DAVIS KR: Cerebellar hemangioblastoma: CT, angiographic and clinical condition in seven cases. *CT: J Comput Tomogr* **2**(4):281–294, 1978.

AFRA D, NORMAN D, LEVIN CA: Cysts in malignant glioma identification by CT. *J Neurosurg* **53**:821–825, 1980.

ALDERSON PO et al: Optimal utilization of computerized cranial tomography and radionuclide brain imaging. *Neurology* **26**:803–807, 1976.

ALDERSON PO, GADO MH, SIEGAL BA: CCT and RN imaging in the detection of intracranial mass lesions. *Semin Nucl Med* VII:161–174, 1977.

ALTEMUS LR, RADVANY J: Multifocal glioma visualized by contrast enhanced computed tomography: Report of a case with pathologic correlation. *J Maine Med Assoc* **68**:324–327, 1977.

AMBROSE J, GOODING MB, RICHARDSON AE: An assessment of the accuracy of computerized transverse axial scanning (EMI scanners) in the diagnosis of intracranial tumor: A review of 366 patients. *Brain* **98**:569–582, 1975a.

AMBROSE J, GOODING MB, RICHARDSON AE: Sodium iothalamate as an aid to diagnosis of intracranial lesions by computerized transverse axial scanning. *Lancet*: 669–674, 1975b.

AMENDOLA MA et al: Preoperative diagnosis of a ruptured intracranial dermoid cyst by computerized tomography: Case report. *J Neurosurg* **48**:1035–1037, 1978.

AMUNDSEN P, DUGSTAD G, SYVERTSEN AH: The reliability of computer tomography for the diagnosis and differential diagnosis of meningiomas, gliomas, and brain metastasis. *Acta Neurochirurgica* **41**:177–190, 1978.

ANDERSON FM, ADELSTEIN LJ: Ganglion cell tumor in the third ventricle. *Arch Surg* **45**:129–139, 1942.

ARIENS-KAPPERS J: The development of the paraphysis cerebri in man with comments on its relationship to the intercolumnar tubercle and its significance for the origin of cystic tumors in the third ventricle. *J Comp Neurol* **102**:425, 1955.

BAKER HL, HOUSER OW, CAMPBELL JK: National Cancer Institute Study: Evaluation of CT in the diagnosis of intracranial neoplasms: I. Overall Results. *Radiology* **136**:91–96, 1980.

BAKER AB, BAKER LH: *Clinical Neurology*. Hagerstown, Md. Harper & Row, 1973.

BACHMANN K, MARKWALDER R, SEILER RW: Supratentorial hemangioblastoma: Case report. *Acta Neurochirurgica* **44**:173–177, 1978.

BANERJEE T, KRIGMAN MR: Intracranial epidermoid tumor: discussion of four cases. *Southern Med* **7**(6): 1977.

BATZDORF U, MALMUD N: The problem of multicentric gliomas. *J Neurosurg* **20**:122–136, 1963.

BECKER D, NORMAN D, WILSON CB: Computerized tomography and pathological correlation in cystic meningiomas: Report of two cases. *J Neurosurg* **50**:103–105, 1979.

BODIAN M, LAWSON D: The intracranial neoplastic diseases of childhood. *Brit J Surg* **40**:368, 1953.

BRANT-ZAWADZKI M, ENZMANN DR: Computed tomographic brain scanning in patients with lymphoma. *Radiology* **129**:67–71, 1978.

BRAUN IE et al: Dense intracranial epidermoid tumors. *Radiology* **122**:717–719, 1977.

BRENNER TG, RAO KCVG, ROBINSON W, ITANI A: Tandem lesions: Chromophobe adenoma and meningioma. *CT: J Comput Tomogr* **1**:517–520, 1977.

BUELL U, NIENDORF HP, KAZNER E et al: CAT and cerebral serial scintigraphy in intracranial tumors: Rates of detection and tumor-type identification. (Concise communication) *J Nucl Med* **19**:476–479, 1977.

BUTLER AR, HORRI SC, KRICHEFF II, SHANNON MB, BUDZILOVICH GN: Computed tomography in astrocytomas: A statistical analysis of the parameters of malignancy and the positive contrast-enhanced CT scan. *Radiology* **129**:433–439, 1978.

CAMINS MB, TAKEUCHI J: Normotopic plus heterotopic atypical teratomas. *Child's Brain* **4**:151–160, 1978.

CHAMBERS AA et al: Cranial epidermoid tumors: Diagnosis by computed tomography. *Neurosurgery* **1**:276–280, 1977.

CLAVERIA LE, SUTTON D, TRESS BM: The radiological diagnosis of meningiomas, the impact of EMI scanning. *Brit J Radiol* **50**:15–22, 1977a.

CLAVERIA LE, KENDALL BE, DUBOULAY GH: CAT in supratentorial gliomas and metastasis, in DuBoulay GH, Moseley IF (eds): *CAT in Clinical Practice*, Heidelberg, Springer-Verlag, 1977b, p 85.

CLIFFORD JR, CONNOLLY ES, VOORHIES RM: Comparison of radionuclide scan with computer assisted tomography in diagnosis of intracranial disease. *Neurology* **26**:1119–1123, 1976.

CORNELL SH, GRAF CJ, DOLAN KD: Fat-fluid level in intracranial epidermoid cyst. *Am J Roentgenol* **128**:502–503, 1977.

DAVIS KR et al: Theoretical considerations in the use of contrast media for computed cranial tomography. *Neurosurgery* **1**:9–12, 1976a.

DAVIS KR, TAVERAS JM: Diagnosis of epidermoid tumor by computed tomography. *Radiology* **119**:347–353, 1976b.

DAVIS JM, DAVIS KR, NEWHOUSE J, PFISTER RC: Expanded high iodine dose in computed cranial tomography: A preliminary report. *Radiology* **131**:373–387, 1979.

DECK MDF, MESSINA AV, SACKETT JR: Computerized tomography in metastatic disease of the brain. *Radiology* **119**:115–120, 1976.

DORSCH JA, WADSENHEIM A: Density of intracranial masses in computed tomography. *J Belge Radiol* **61**:292–296, 1978.

ENZMANN DR et al: CT in primary reticulum cell sarcoma of the brain. *Radiology* **130**:165–170, 1979.

ENZMANN DR, TOKYE KC, HAYWARD R: CT in leptomeningeal spread of tumor. *J Comput Assist Tomogr* **2**:448–455, 1978 (abstract).

EVENS RG, JOST RG: The clinical efficacy and cost analysis of cranial computed tomography and the radionuclide brain scan. *Semin Nucl Med* **VII**:129–136, 1977.

FAWCITT RA, ISHERWOOD I: Radiodiagnosis of intracranial pearly tumors with particular reference to the value of CT. *Neuroradiology* **11**:234–242, 1976.

FUTRELL NN, OSBORNE AQ, CHESON BD: Pineal region tumors: CT–pathologic spectrum. *Am J Neuroradiol* **2**:415–420, 1981.

GADO MH, PHELPS ME, COLEMAN RE: An extravascular component of contrast enhancement in cranial computed tomography. *Radiology* **177**:589–593, and 595–597, 1975.

GANTI SR, ANTUNES JL, LOUIS KM, HILAL SK: CT in the diagnosis of colloid cysts of the third ventricle. *Radiology* **138**:385–391, 1981.

GARDEUR D, SABLAYROLLES JL, KLAUSZ R, METZGER J: Histographic studies in computed tomography of contrast enhanced cerebral and orbital tumors. *J Comput Assist Tomogr* **1**(2):231–240, 1977.

GAWLER J et al: Computer assisted tomography (EMI scanner): its place in investigation of suspected intracranial tumors. *Lancet* **2**:419–423, 1979.

GEORGE AE, RUSSELL EJ, KRICHEFF II: White matter buckling: CT sign of extra-axial intracranial mass. *Am J Neuroradiol* **1**:425–430, 1980.

GILBERTSON EL, GOODING CA: Roentgenographic signs of tumors of the brain. *Am J Roentgenol* **76**:226, 1956.

GROSS SW: Radiographic visualization of an intracranial dermoid cyst. *J Neurosurg* **2**:72–75, 1945.

GUNER M, SHAW M: Computed tomography in the diagnosis of colloid cyst. *J Neurosurg* **2**:72–75, 1976.

HANDA J, HANDA H: Radiolucent intracranial dermoid cyst, case report. *Neuroradiology* **17**:211–214, 1979.

HAYMAN LA, EVANS RA, HINCK V: Rapid high dose cranial CT: a concise review of normal anatomy. *J Comput Assist Tomogr* **3**(20):147–154, 1979.

HAYMAN LA, EVANS RA, HINCK VC: Delayed high iodine dose contrast computed tomography: cranial neoplasms. *Radiology* **136**:677–684, 1980.

HILAL SK, CHANG CH: Specificity of computed tomography in the diagnosis of supratentorial neoplasms: Consideration of metastasis and meningiomas. *Neuroradiology* **16**:537–539, 1978.

HILAL SK, CHANG CH: Sensitivity and specificity of CT in supratentorial tumors. *J Comput Assist Tomogr* **2**:511, 1978.

HUCKMAN MS: Clinical experience with the intravenous infusion of iodinated contrast material as an adjunct to CT. *Surg Neurol* **4**(3):297–318, 1975.

HUCKMAN M, ACKERMAN L: Use of automated measurements of mean density as an adjunct to computed tomography. *J Comput Assist Tomogr* **1**(1):37–42, 1977.

JELLINGER K, RADSKIEWICZ T, SLOWIK F: Primary malignant lymphomas of the central nervous system in man. *Acta Neuropath*, Suppl VI: 95–102, 1975.

KALAN C, BURROWS EH: Calcification in intracranial gliomata. *Br J Radiol* **35**:589–602, 1962.

KAZNER E, WILSKE J, STEINHOFF H, STOCHDORPH O: Computer assisted tomography in primary malignant lymphomas of the brain. *J Comput Assist Tomogr* **2**:125–134, 1978.

KENDALL B, PULLICINO P: Comparison of consistency of meningiomas and CT appearance. *Neuroradiology* **18**:173–176, 1979.

KENDALL BE: Difficulties in diagnosis of supratentorial gliomas by CAT scan. *J Neurol Neurosurg Psych* **42**:485–492, 1975.

KRAMER RA, JANETOS GP, PERLSTEIN G: An approach to contrast enhancement in computed tomography of the brain. *Radiology* **16**:641–647, 1975.

KUSHNET MW, GOLDMAN RL: Lipoma of the corpus callosum associated with a frontal bone defect. *Am J Roentgenol* **131**:517–518, 1978.

LASTER DW, MOODY DM: Epidermoid tumors with intraventricular and subarachnoid fat: Report of two cases. *Am J Roentgenol* **128**:504–507, 1977.

LATCHAW RE, GOLD LHA, TORRIJE EJ: A protocol for the use of contrast enhancement in cranial computed tomography. *Radiology* **126**:681–687, 1978*a*.

LATCHAW R, PAYNE JT, GOLD LH: Effective atomic number and electron density as measured with a computed tomography scanner: Computation and correlation with brain tumor histology. *J Comput Assist Tomogr* **2**:199–208, 1978*b*.

LATCHAW R, PAYNE JT, LOEWENSON RB: Predicting brain tumor histology: Change of effective atomic number with contrast enhancement. *Am J Neuroradiol* **1**:289–294, 1980.

LEE SH, DELGADO TE, BUCHEIT WA: Intracranial dermoid tumor: Diagnosis by computed tomography, a case report. *Neurosurgery* **1**:281–283, 1977.

LEWANDER R, BERGSTROM M, BERGVALL U: Contrast enhancement of cranial lesions in computed tomography. *Acta Radiolog* **19**:529–552, 1978.

LITTLE JR et al: Brain hemorrhage from intracranial tumor. *Stroke* **10**(3):283–288, 1979.

LITTLE JR, MACCARTY CS: Colloid cysts of the third ventricle. *J Neurosurg* **40**:230–235, 1974.

MALIK GM et al: Colloid cysts. *Surg Neurol* **13**(1):73–77, 1980.

MANCES P, BABIN E, WACKENHEIM A: Contribution of histograms to the computer tomographic study of brain tumors. *J Belge Radiol* **61**(4):297–312, 1978.

MANDYBUR TI: Intracranial hemorrhage caused by metastatic tumors. *Neurology* **27**:650–655, 1977.

MANI RL et al: Radiographic diagnosis of meningioma of the lateral ventricle. Review of 22 cases. *J Neurosurg* **49**:249–255, 1978.

MAUERSBERGER W, CUEVAS-SOLORZANO JA: Spontaneous intracerebellar hematoma during childhood caused by spongioblastoma of the fourth ventricle. *Neuropädiatrie* **8**:443–450, 1977.

MCCORMACK TJ, PLASSCHE WM, LIN SR: Ruptured teratoid tumors in the pineal region. *J Comput Assist Tomogr* **2**:499–501, 1978.

MIKHAEL MA, MATTAR AG: Intracranial pearly tumors: the role of CT, angiography and pneumoencephalography. *J Comput Assist Tomogr* **2**:421–429, 1978.

MODESTI LM, BINET EF, COLLINS GH: Meningiomas causing spontaneous intracranial hematomas. *J Neurosurg* **45**:437–441, 1976.

NAIDICH TP et al: Evaluation of sellar and parasellar masses by computed tomography. *Radiology* **120**:91–99, 1976.

NAUTA HJW et al: Xanthochromic cysts associated with meningioma. *J Neurol Neurosurg Psychiat* **42**:529–535, 1979.

NEUWELT EA et al: Malignant pineal region tumors. *J Neurosurg* **51**:597–607, 1979.

NEW PFJ, SCOTT WR, SCHNUR JA, DAVIS DR, TAVERAS TM, HOCHBERG FH: Computed tomography with the EMI scanner in the diagnosis of primary and metastatic intracranial neoplasms. *Radiology* **114**:75–87, 1975.

NORMAN D et al: Quantitative aspects of contrast enhancement in cranial computed tomography. *Radiology* **129**:683–688, 1978.

NOSAKA Y et al: Primary intracranial epidermoid carcinoma. *J Neurosurg* **50**:830–833, 1979.

OI S, WETZEL N: Gliomas in computerized axial tomography, correlation with tumor malignancy in 100 cases. *Neurosurgery (Jap)* **7**(8):759–763, 1979.

OLIVERCRONE H: The cerebellar angioreticulomas. *J Neurosurg* **9**:317–330, 1952.

OSBORN AG: Diagnosis of descending transtentorial herniation by cranial computed tomography. *Radiology* **123**:93–96, 1977.

OSBORN AG, HEASTON DK, WING SD: Diagnosis of ascending transtentorial herniation by cranial computed tomography. *Am J Roentgenol* **130**:755–760, 1978a.

OSBORN AG et al: The evaluation of ependymal and subependymal lesions by cranial computed tomography. *Radiology* **127**:397–401, 1978b.

PAGANI JJ et al: Cranial nervous system leukemia of lymphoma: CT manifestations. *Am J Neuroradiol* **2**:397–403, 1981.

PATEL AN: Lipoma of the corpus callosum: A nonsurgical entity. *NC Med J* **26**:328–335, 1965.

PAXTON R, AMBROSE J: The EMI scanner: A brief review of the first 650 patients. *Brit J Radiol* **47**:530–565, 1974.

PENDERGRASS HP, MCKUSICK KA, NEW PFJ: Relative efficacy of radionuclide imaging and computed tomography of the brain. *Radiology* **116**:363–366, 1975.

PENMAN J, SMITH MC: *Intracranial gliomata*, Spec Rep Series, No. 284, Med Res Council, HM Stationary Office, London, 1954.

POST JD, NOBLE JD, GLASER JS, SAFRAN A: Pituitary apoplexy: diagnosis by CT. *Radiology* **134**:665–670, 1980.

RAO KCVG, GOVINDAN S: CAT in rapidly growing brain tumors. *Comput Tomog* **3**:9–13, 1979.

RAO KCVG, LEVINE H, ITANI A, SAJOR E, ROBINSON W: CT findings in multicentric glioblastoma. Diagnostic-pathologic correlation. *CT: J Comput Tomogr* **4**:187–192, 1980.

REEVES GI, MARKS JE: Prognostic significance of lesion size for glioblastoma multiforme. *Radiology* **132**:469–471, 1979.

RENGACHARY S et al: Cystic lesions associated with intracranial meningiomas. *Neurosurgery* **4**:107–114, 1979.

RUSSELL DS: Meningeal tumors: a review. *J Clin Path* **3**:191, 1950.

RUSSELL DS, RUBINSTEIN LJ: Pathology of tumors of the nervous system. 4th ed., Baltimore, Williams and Wilkins, 1977.

SEEGER JF et al: CT and angiographic evaluation of hemangioblastomas. *Radiology* **138**:65–73, 1981.

SHAFFER KA, HAUGHTON VM, WILSON CR: High resolution CT of the temporal bone. *Radiology* **134**:409–414, 1980.

STEINHOFF H, AVILES C: Contrast enhancement response of intracranial neoplasms: its validity for the differential diagnosis of tumors in CT, in Lanksch W, Kazner E (eds): *Cranial Computerized Tomography*, New York, Springer-Verlag, 1976, pp 151–161.

STEINHOFF H, KAZNER E, LANKSCH W, GRUMME T, MEESE W, LANGE S, AULICH A, WENDE S: The limitations of computerized axial tomography in the detection and differential diagnosis of intracranial tumours: A study based on 1304 neoplasms, in Bories J (ed): *The Diagnostic Limitations of Computerized Axial Tomography*, New York, Springer-Verlag, 1978, pp 40–49.

STEINHOFF H et al: CT in the diagnosis and differential diagnosis of glioblastomas. *Neuroradiology* **14**:193–200, 1977.

STOVRING J: Contralateral temporal horn widening in unilateral supratentorial mass lesions: a diagnostic sign indicating tentorial herniation. *J Comput Assist Tomogr* **1**:319–323, 1977.

TADMOR R, DAVIS K, ROBERSON G, KLEINMAN G: Computed tomography in primary malignant lymphoma of the brain. *J Comput Assist Tomogr* **2**:135–140, 1978.

TADMOR R, TAVERAS JM: Computed tomography in extradural epidermoid and xanthoma. *Surg Neurol* **7**:371–375, 1977.

TAKEUCHI J, HANDA H, NAGAT I: Suprasellar germinoma. *J Neurosurg* **49**:41–48, 1978.

TAKEUCHI J et al: Neuroradiological aspects of suprasellar germinoma. *Neuroradiology* **17**:153–159, 1979.

TANS J, DE JONGH IE: Computed tomography of supratentorial astrocytoma. *Clin Neurol, Neurosurg* **80**:156–168, 1978.

TCHANG S et al: Computerized tomography as a possible aid to histological grading of supratentorial gliomas. *J Neurosurg* **46**:735–739, 1977.

TENFLER RL, PALACIOS E: False negative CT in brain tumor. *JAMA* **238**:339–340, 1977.

THOMSON JLG: Computerized axial tomography and the diagnosis of glioma: A study of 100 consecutive histologically proven cases. *Clin Radiol* **27**:431–441, 1976.

TOGLIA JU et al: Epithelial tumors of the cranium: their common nature and pathogenesis. *J Neurosurg* **23**:384–393, 1965.

VASSILOUTHIS J, AMBROSE J: Computerized tomography scanning appearance of intracranial meningiomas. *J Neurosurg* **50**:320–327, 1979.

VONOFAKOS D, HACKER H: CT histogram in the pathologic definition of supratentorial brain tumors. *Neuroradiology* **16**:552–555, 1978.

VONOFAKOS D, MARCU H, HACKER H: Oligodendrogliomas: CT patterns with emphasis on features indicating malignancy. *J Comput Assist Tomogr* **3**(6):783–788, 1979.

WENDE S et al: A German multicentric study of intracranial tumors, in duBoulay GH, Moseley IF (eds): *Computerized Axial Tomography in Clinical Practice*. Heidelberg, Springer-Verlag, 1977.

WYLIE IG, JEFFREYS RV, MACLAINE GN: Cerebral hemangioblastoma. *Br J Radiol* **46**:472–476, 1973.

ZETTNER A, NETSKY MG: Lipoma of the corpus callosum. *J Neuropathol Exp Neurol* **19**:305–319, 1960.

ZIMMERMAN HM: Malignant lymphomas of the nervous system. *Acta Neuropath,* Suppl VI: 69–74, 1975.

ZIMMERMAN RA, BILANIUK LT: Cranial computed tomography of epidermoid and congenital fatty tumors of maldevelopment origin. *J Comput Assist Tomogr* **3**(1):40–50, 1979a.

ZIMMERMAN RA, BILANIUK LT: CT of intracerebral gangliogliomas. *J Comput Assist Tomogr* **3**(1):24–29, 1979b.

ZIMMERMAN RA, BILANIUK LT: Computed tomography of choroid plexus lesions. *J Comput Assist Tomogr* **3**(2):93–102, 1979c.

ZIMMERMAN RA, BILANIUK LT: Computed tomography of acute intratumoral hemorrhage. *Radiology* **135**:355–359, 1980a.

ZIMMERMAN RA et al: CT of pineal, paraspinal and histologically related tumors. *Radiology* **137**:669–677, 1980b.

8

PRIMARY TUMORS IN CHILDREN

Charles R. Fitz

Krishna C.V.G. Rao

It is perhaps unnecessary to emphasize the obvious—that is, the changes that CT has brought about in the diagnosis and management of brain tumors in children. Before CT, children in most hospitals underwent a two- or three-stage investigative diagnostic study consisting of radionuclide brain scan, arteriogram, and/or air ventriculogram or air encephalogram. This meant one or two anesthestics for the procedure, shunting of the ventricles when hydrocephalus was present, and often a 2-day interval between procedures to recover from previous anesthesias. Most often the diagnostic route is now one-stage—computed tomography. In an academic sense this is somewhat unfortunate, in that information regarding tumor vasculature is no longer available to the surgeon; but in practical terms, the lack of such information is usually of little or no significance. In some cases angiography may still be necessary, since it is helpful for comparing vascular anatomy with CT anatomy so that normality or abnormality of the underlying brain can be predicted. Angiography is also useful in defining lesions which may mimic a neoplasm because of their location or enhancing pattern (Fig. 8-1). It has become the philosophy to recommend angiography when a tumor on CT appears unusual or has an appearance unusual for a tumor in its particular location. A brainstem tumor with considerable enhancement would be such an example.

Air encephalography or metrizamide cisternography with CT is done when a brainstem tumor is strongly suspected clinically but not seen on routine CT. It is also done when the extent of an extraaxial tumor is not clear on routine CT.

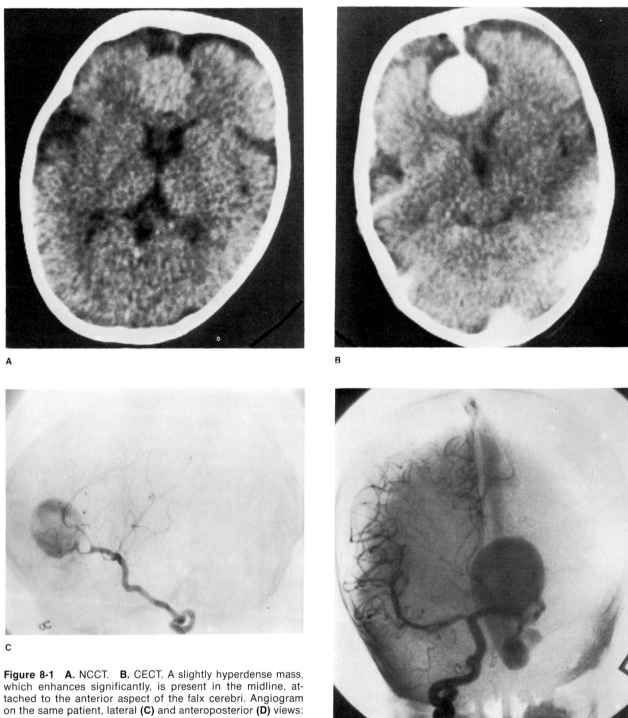

A

B

C

Figure 8-1 **A.** NCCT. **B.** CECT. A slightly hyperdense mass, which enhances significantly, is present in the midline, attached to the anterior aspect of the falx cerebri. Angiogram on the same patient, lateral **(C)** and anteroposterior **(D)** views: the enhancing mass seen on CT represents an unusual location of a vascular anomaly.

D

The skull x-ray is now a neglected part of tumor workup even in pediatric centers, but the authors believe this is an error. Relative head size is more easily recognized on skull x-ray than on CT. A child's skull responds rapidly to changes in intracranial pressure, and this part of the workup should not be neglected. The authors prefer a full skull series during the initial workup. As posttreatment follow-up CTs are done, a simple posteroanterior and lateral skull x-ray are usually obtained, not more often than every 6 months up to age 2 and once a year beyond age 2, unless some surgical procedure such as shunt replacement or decompression has been performed.

Because of the rapidity with which tumors are diagnosed with CT, shunting of hydrocephalus is less commonly needed, especially as a procedure separate from tumor exploration.

CT Technique

Even with the faster scanners, sedation still remains necessary in most children below age 5. The sedation schedule followed by the authors is given in Table 8-1. Pentobarbital is the sedative most commonly used. Usually the child will fall into a heavy sleep in 20 to 30 minutes, and this will last 20 to 30 minutes. Approximately one-third of children sedated with pentobarbital will require resedation with a smaller dose, and this will suffice in most cases. In children who require heavier sedation, such as retarded or deaf children, or in children in whom pentobarbital has previously been unsuccessful, a three-drug mixture (meperidine HCl, promethazine HCl, and chlorpromazine) is used. Valium is used only in the occasional older patient who is very nervous and needs calming rather than sedation. Use of these three medications takes care of about 98 percent of children who need sedation. Others have reported good results with rectal thiopental (White 1979).

When intravenous contrast is used, it is given in a dose of 3 ml/kg of 60% meglumine diatrizoate (282 mg/ml of iodine). Contrast is usually given in a single bolus. Specialized contrast-injection techniques such as a very rapid bolus or infusion tend to be impractical in younger children and are generally not used in infants.

Table 8-1 Sedation for CT in Children 5 Years and Younger

Drug	Initial dose	Route of administration	Supplementary dose
Pentobarbital (Nembutal)	6 mg/kg of body weight for children up to 15 kg; 5 mg/kg for children over 15 kg; maximum of 200 mg	IM 20 to 30 minutes before CT	1 to 1/2 hour later, if initial dose not effective, 2 mg/kg for children up to 15 kg, 2.5 mg/kg for children over 15 kg; maximum of 100 mg
Diazepam (Valium)	0.4 mg/kg of body weight, maximum of 12 mg	IV, slowly, 5 to 10 minutes before CT	1/2 hour later if initial dose not effective
CM3	0.1 ml/kg up to a maximum of 2 ml	IM 10 to 20 minutes before CT	No supplementary dose given
Meperidine HCl (Demerol)	25 mg/ml		
Chlorpromazine (Thorazine)	6.25 mg/ml		
Promethazine HCl (Phenergan)	6.25 mg/ml		

Metrizamide cisternography, when used, is done by lumbar injection at a dose of 2–5 ml of 170 mg/ml iodine, depending on age. The patient is usually put in a 15 to 20° Trendelenberg position for approximately 5 minutes after the injection.

CT itself is usually done in the conventional 20° semiaxial position both before and after contrast enhancement of the entire head on any initial examination. Usually the thicker 10- to 13-mm section thickness available on most equipment is sufficient, because the tumors are relatively large and easily seen through two or more slices. When symptoms are strongly in favor of a posterior fossa tumor, or other information such as calcification on the skull x-ray or positive radionuclide brain scan has already localized the lesion, the cuts before contrast enhancement are limited to the posterior fossa. The authors believe that the precontrast views are helpful in determining tumor types, though not essential for localization.

Thinner, 5-mm sections are occasionally done, especially to better see the brainstem or extraaxial lesions. Very thin sections of 1.5 to 2 mm are of limited value in children. The heat buildup of the x-ray tubes causes long delays between slices. Sick children and small children, even if sedated, usually are not able to hold still long enough to provide images that can be reconstructed in other planes without movement between slices.

Additional views are usually necessary when the extent of a tumor or parts of its intrinsic character require better definition. The most common is the clival perpendicular or Water's view (Fitz 1978a). As the slices are perpendicular to the tentorium, clivus,

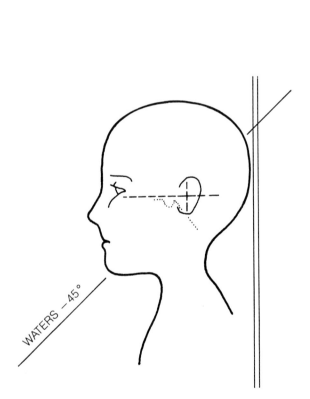

Figure 8-2 Patient positioning for clival perpendicular (Water's) view. This can be achieved by angling either the gantry or the table top, depending on the type of scanner.

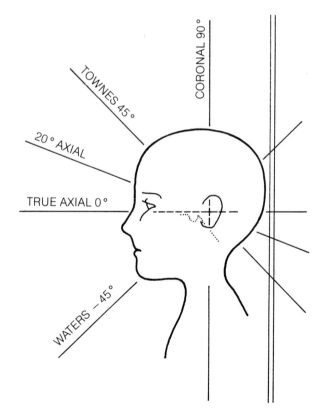

Figure 8-3 Patient positioning for Towne's view. The Towne's view can be obtained by angling the gantry and extending the patient's head backward to achieve the appropriate position.

and brainstem, they show the posterior fossa in what may be considered its coronal projection. The clival perpendicular view is easier to obtain than the true coronal, requiring only a moderate extension of the neck and forward angulation of the gantry (Fig. 8-2).

This view is most helpful to examine the extension of a tumor into the cerebellar hemispheres, displacement of the fourth ventricle by brainstem or cerebellar tumors, or the cross-sectional size of either the fourth ventricle or the brainstem.

The clival parallel, or Towne's, view is easily obtained by flexing the patient's neck and angling the gantry back (Fig. 8-3) (Byrd 1978). Being at 90° to the clival perpendicular view, the slices are through the axis of the brainstem. This view is most helpful in visualizing the fourth ventricle and brain-

stem through their length and often shows extraaxial masses to best advantage. Both accessory views are usually done in 5-mm slices through the regions determined from the standard examination.

The incidence of primary intracranial neoplasms in children is less than that of the adult population (Wilson 1975). Metastatic tumors are also less common than in adults. In the past, infratentorial neoplasms were thought to constitute more than 50 percent of all neoplasms in children. Utilizing CT, the incidence of neoplasms in the supratentorial compartment in children is almost the same as or slightly higher than that in the adult population (Table 8-2). The change in ratio is probably due to the earlier utilization of CT as a diagnostic modality, whereas in the past, neoplasms were either missed or did not undergo diagnostic studies, because of

Table 8-2 Incidence of Intracranial Neoplasm in Pediatric Age Group (Up to 15 Years)

Type	U. of Md. Hospital (76 tumors)		Hosp. for Sick Children (269 tumors)	
	No. of cases	% of total	No. of cases	% of total
Infratentorial	30	39.5	113	42
Astrocytoma	14	18.4	46	17.1
Medulloblastoma	7	9.2	39	14.5
Ependymoma	5	6.7	16	5.9
Miscellaneous	4	5.3	12	4.5
Supratentorial	46	60	156	58
Gliomas	18*	23.7	41	15.2
Neuroblastoma	4	5.3	3	1.1
Craniopharyngioma	6	7.9	23	8.5
Teratoma/pinealoma/ ectopic pinealoma	6	7.9	13	4.8
Ganglioglioma/cytoma	4	5.3	12†	4.5
Ependymoma	3	3.9	1	0.4
Choroid plexus papilloma/ carcinoma	2	2.6	3	1.1
Optic nerve glioma			22‡	8.2
Miscellaneous	3	3.9	38§	14.1

* Includes three optic nerve gliomas, two giant cell astrocytomas.
† Includes three cases of hamartoma.
‡ Includes eleven cases of intraorbital optic nerve glioma.
§ Includes four cases of lipoma, pituitary adenoma, and meningioma; eight cases of leukemia; two schwannomas of the fifth nerve; seven meningeal neoplasms; and eight other neoplasms without specific histologic findings.

their invasive nature, until late in the course of the disease. The histological characteristics of neoplasms in children are also different from those in adults. In general, tumors such as meningiomas and pituitary adenomas are less common in children. Certain cell types of tumors, however, have a greater predilection for the younger age group—e.g., neuroblastoma, hypothalamic and optic glioma, and rhabdomyosarcoma.

Certain tumors, such as neuroblastoma, are more often found in the supratentorial compartment. Similarly, choroid plexus papilloma or its malignant version, choroid plexus carcinoma, should be suspected when an enhancing mass is encountered in the trigone of the lateral ventricle in a child, whereas such a mass is more likely to be a meningioma when encountered in the older population.

A few tumors, such as craniopharyngioma, appear to have two peaks, the majority of these neoplasms being encountered either in children under 15 years or in adults beyond their fifth decade.

Although the CT appearance may not be dissimilar in neoplasms common to both the pediatric and the adult population, a combination of the CT appearance, the tumor location, the age of the patient, and attenuation characteristics (Probst 1979) provides a reasonable diagnostic clue to the type of tumor.

For descriptive purposes, neoplasms in the pediatric population are grouped in this chapter into the following major regional categories: (1) infratentorial, or posterior fossa, neoplasms; and (2) supratentorial neoplasms.

INFRATENTORIAL TUMORS

Incidence

The overall incidence of supratentorial and infratentorial tumors in children remains similar to the proportions described earlier by Harwood-Nash and Fitz (1976). Since 1976, 113 children with primary benign and malignant tumors in the posterior fossa have been examined at the Hospital for Sick Children. These represent 42 percent of all intracranial tumors found on CT. Biopsy confirmation was available for the majority of the infratentorial tumors, except when their location precluded securing adequate tissue samples. These were primarily brainstem gliomas. At the University of Maryland Hospital, posterior fossa tumors represented 40 percent of 76 cases reported. Overall, some shifts were noted in the major categories of infratentorial neoplasms, compared to the larger series, primarily before CT, that was reported by Harwood-Nash and Fitz in 1976. Ten percent of the infratentorial tumors were in children under 2 years of age. This probably reflects earlier diagnosis because of CT (Tadmor 1980). Some shift in tumor cell type was also noted, with medulloblastoma making up 35 percent of all posterior fossa tumors (Table 8-3).

Types of Tumor

Medulloblastoma

With CT, medulloblastomas have shown a slight "stretching" of age incidence, with 16 percent of the patients being less than 2 years of age and 49 percent 8 years of age or older; of the latter, nearly 50 percent were 12 years or older (Table 8-4). Medulloblastomas, though having a generally characteristic appearance (Zimmerman 1977), tend to have more variable CT findings than other posterior fossa tumors. The usual location of medulloblastoma is in the midline. Most often it is smoothly ovoid or spherical in shape. It tends to be slightly greater in density than the surrounding cerebellum and has a rim of edema (Fig. 8-4). In the authors' experience, medulloblastomas have always shown enhancement on CECT, although rare instances have been reported in which enhancement has not been found (Woodrow 1981). The density of the contrast enhancement is usually uniform throughout its extent, though the contrast enhancement is not always homogeneous. Small "cystic" areas are visible in about 10 percent of cases. On pathologic study, these represent true cysts rather than regions of necrosis within the neoplasm.

Table 8-3   Incidence of Posterior Fossa Tumors in Children

	Number of cases		Percent of posterior fossa tumors	
Histologic type	*Hospital for Sick Children*	*U. of Md. Hospital*	*Hospital for Sick Children*	*U. of Md. Hospital*
Astrocytoma	46	14	41	47
Medulloblastoma	39	7	35	23
Ependymoma	16	5	14	17
Miscellaneous	12	4	10	13

Table 8-4   Posterior Fossa Tumors Diagnosed by CT at Hospital for Sick Children

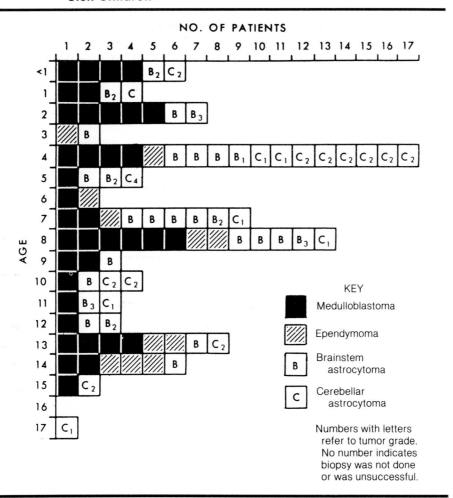

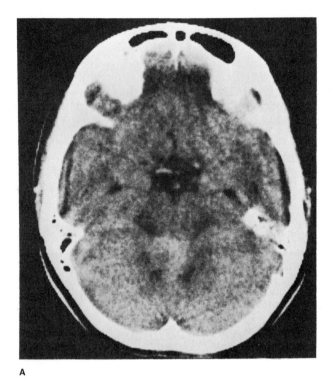
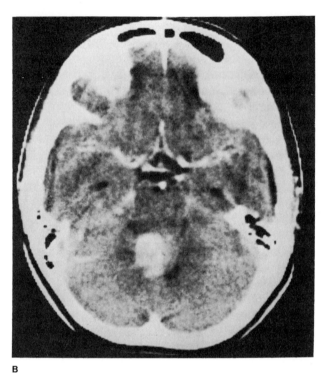

A

B

Figure 8-4 Medulloblastoma in an 11-year-old. **A.** NCCT: The centrally located vermian tumor is slightly denser than the cerebellum and has a rim of decreased density surrounding it. **B.** CECT: There is enhancement throughout nearly all of the tumor. The enhancement is relatively homogeneous.

Calcification within the neoplasm can be detected by CT in 10 percent of medulloblastomas. The calcification is usually small and homogeneous, eccentric in location, and rarely visible on skull x-ray. Hemorrhage within the tumor is also unusual, and the small punctate calcifications may be mistaken for hemorrhages (Fig. 8-5).

As the tumor is most commonly located in the vermis, the fourth ventricle is usually compressed and displaced anterosuperiorly. Moderate to severe hydrocephalus is common.

Medulloblastoma with unusual CT patterns has more often been noted in children over 8 years old. Perhaps because of its invasive quality, medulloblastoma is more likely to be mistaken for a brainstem or hemispheric astrocytoma than other tumors and more likely to be uncharacteristic in appearance, with features such as a large cyst (Fig. 8-6), an irregular, lumpy border, or an eccentric location

(Fig. 8-7). Very rarely, enlargement of the fourth ventricle, typical of ependymoma, may be seen.

Ependymoma

Ependymomas are mostly seen in older children: in the series analyzed in Table 8-4, 7 out of 11 were 8 years of age or more, and only 1 was under 4. This also is slightly different from the larger series (Harwood-Nash 1976).

Ependymomas, because they arise in the wall or, particularly, the floor of the fourth ventricle, are often nearly identical to medulloblastoma (Fig. 8-8), though sometimes visibly more inferior in location and closer to the foramen magnum. One characteristic that is nearly diagnostic but occurs in only about 10 percent of cases is the desmoplastic extension of the tumor through the fourth-ventricle foramina down over the medulla and upper cervical

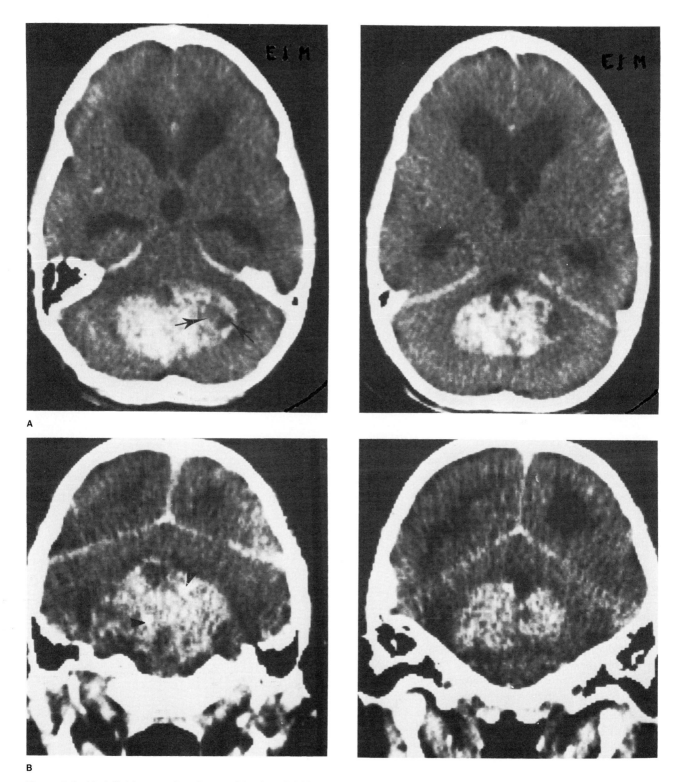

Figure 8-5 Medulloblastoma in a 9-year-old. **A.** Axial CT. **B.** Coronal CT. The enhancing tumor surrounds the fourth ventricle. It consists of regions of calcification (arrowheads), as well as unusual necrotic or cystic components (arrows).

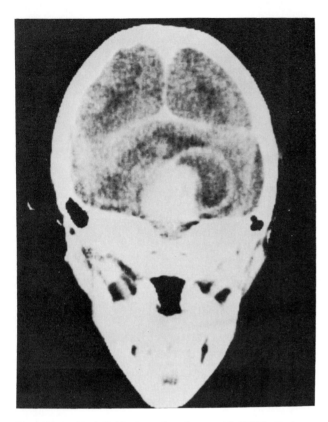

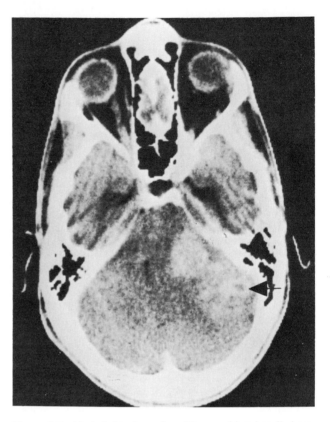

Figure 8-6 Medulloblastoma in a 2-year-old. CECT, clival perpendicular view, shows large central, enhancing, solid portion of tumor and large cyst with enhancing rim extending into right cerebellar hemisphere.

Figure 8-7 Medulloblastoma in a 13-year-old, primarily hemispheric in location and with irregular borders. Small cyst (arrow), confirmed at surgery, also visible.

cord (Fig. 8-9). On ventriculography and pneumoencephalography before CT, it was noted that this tumor very often allowed or caused the fourth ventricle to enlarge and surround it as though the tumor were invaginating a balloon. This appearance is less visible on CT but, when noted, is usually a sign of ependymoma (Fig. 8-10). Ependymoma typically has the highest incidence of calcification among posterior fossa tumors (36%); however, since they are less common in occurrence than astrocytoma and medulloblastoma, it cannot be said that a calcified posterior fossa tumor is most likely to be an ependymoma. The calcification is somewhat characteristic and is more likely to be punctate and distributed throughout much or several portions of the tumor, as compared with other posterior fossa masses (Fig. 8-10).

The tumor is of variable density before contrast enhancement, but the density tends to be equal to or slightly greater than that of the surrounding cerebellum (Figs. 8-8, 8-10). As in medulloblastomas, a ring of edema is fairly common. Contrast enhancement is present in all tumors, tending to be some-

Figure 8-9 (Opposite, left) Ependymoma in a 4-year-old. ▶ CECT slice through C2 level shows several calcified and enhancing lesions in the spinal canal from extension of an ependymoma out of the fourth ventricle.

Figure 8-10 (Opposite, right) Ependymoma, same patient ▶ as Fig. 8-9. NCCT shows multiple punctate calcifications scattered throughout the tumor. The tumor has invaginated the fourth ventricle, which surrounds much of it like a horseshoe.

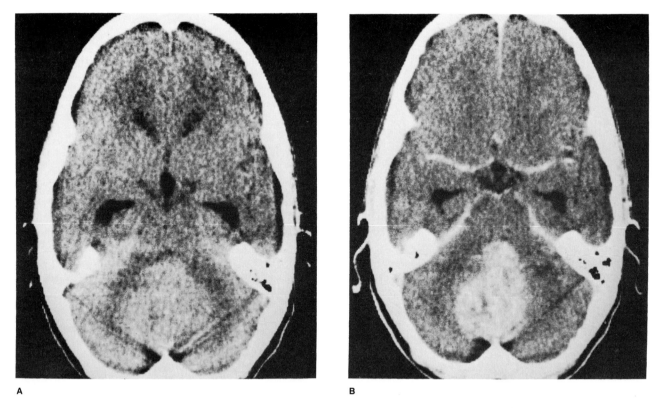

Figure 8-8 Ependymoma in a 14-year-old. **A.** NCCT shows rim of edema in large ependymoma and density equal to or just greater than surrounding cerebellum. **B.** On CECT, much of the tumor shows a blush of uniform density. Irregular, nonenhancing, central areas of necrosis are visible.

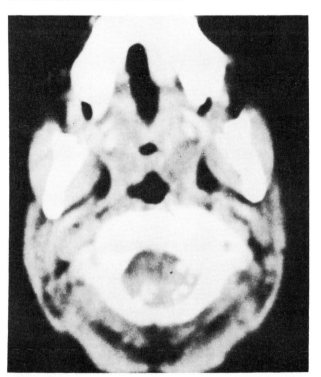

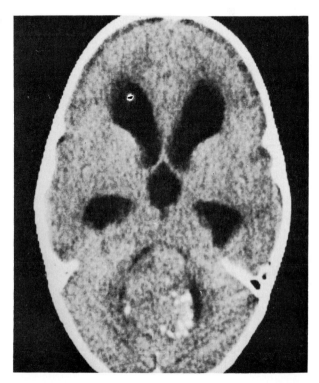

what nonhomogeneous in both area and density. Moderate hydrocephalus is common in ependymoma.

Cerebellar Astrocytoma

Astrocytoma is the most common tumor in the posterior fossa. Variable in age incidence, with a sharp peak at 4 years (Table 8-4), the tumor shows several relatively common characteristics. It is more often cystic than other posterior fossa tumors, and the cysts are frequently large and single. Whether the tumor is solid or cystic, the solid portion is typically lower in density than the surrounding cerebellum (Fig. 8-11). The cyst is of higher density than the CSF but may be difficult to distinguish from surrounding edema if the cyst wall does not show contrast enhancement.

Contrast enhancement of the solid portion and cyst wall of the cerebellar astrocytomas is variable. Particularly in the lower-grade tumors, only a portion of the solid part of the tumor may enhance (Fig. 8-12). The enhancement is frequently nonhomogeneous, with small cysts or necrotic areas of tumor within the enhancing portion of the mass. This is particularly true in those tumors without large peripheral cysts. The tumor may or may not show contrast enhancement in the cyst wall. This is most often the case in grade 1 cystic tumors (Naidich 1977*b*). Enhancement of the cyst wall and tumor nodularity is often present in malignant glioma and astrocytoma of grade 2 and over (Fig. 8-13) (Zimmerman 1978*a*). It is generally thought that enhancement of the cyst wall indicates that the wall is made of tumor cells (Goi 1963). It has also been noted that delayed scanning will show leakage or

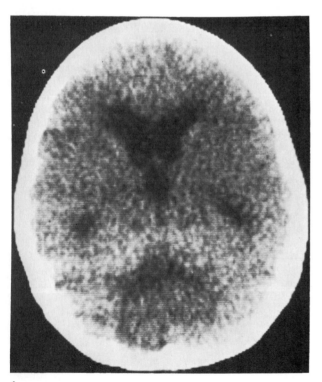
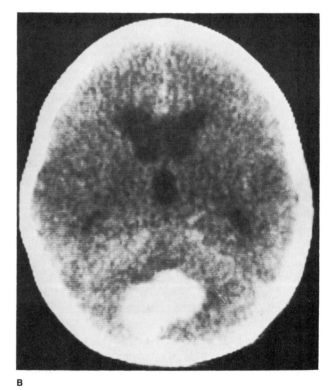

A   **B**

Figure 8-11 Astrocystoma, grade II, in a 9-year-old. **A.** NCCT slice shows large solid tumor of lower density than surrounding cerebelllum. A thin anterior rim of edema, possibly averaged with the fourth ventricle, is visible. **B.** CECT shows fairly homogeneous enhancement throughout the tumor.

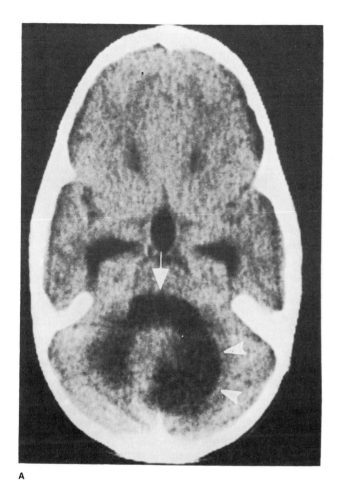

A

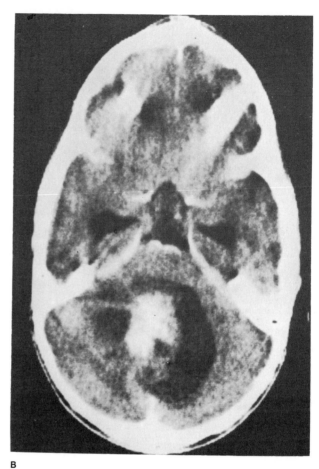

B

Figure 8-12 Astrocystoma, grade I, in a 4-year-old. **A.** NCCT shows central solid tumor surrounded by clearly marginated cyst on the left (arrowheads), dilated fourth ventricle anteriorly (arrow), and further cysts or edema posteriorly and to the right. **B.** CECT shows enhancement of only a part of the solid portion of the tumor. No enhancement of the cyst wall is identified.

excretion of contrast into the cyst itself (Kingsley 1977). Although enhancing tumor nodules are the rule in the cystic tumor, they may occasionally be too small to be seen at CT.

Calcification is less common in astrocytomas (14 percent). No characteristic features of the calcification can be described. Although the tumor often appears to be centrally located on CT, the larger tumors in particular are more likely than other posterior fossa tumors to involve one of the cerebellar hemispheres and cause some lateral displacement of the fourth ventricle. Moderate or severe hydrocephalus is the rule with cerebellar astrocytomas.

Brainstem Tumor

This is a difficult group to analyze, since in many cases biopsy proof is not available for confirmation, although biopsy may have been attempted and the location is at least visually confirmed. In the Table 8-4 series, the ages of the patients with confirmed and with unconfirmed tumors were not significantly different.

Brainstem tumors are the most homogeneous in appearance of all the posterior fossa masses. They are typically of low density throughout (Fig. 8-14). Cysts are relatively uncommon. Contrast enhance-

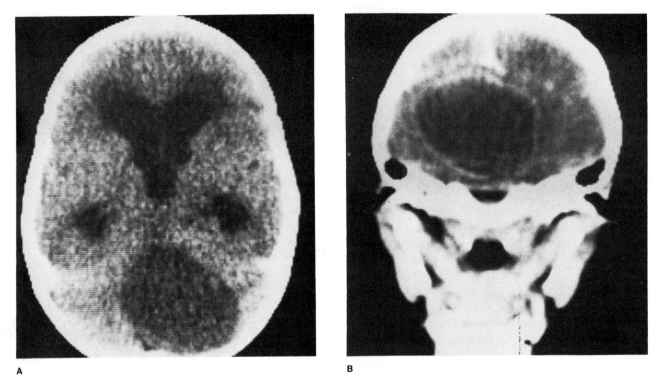

Figure 8-13 Astrocytoma, grade II, in a 5-year-old. **A.** NCCT shows a large cystic tumor with no visible nodule. **B.** CECT best shows the enhancement of the cyst wall in the clival perpendicular projection.

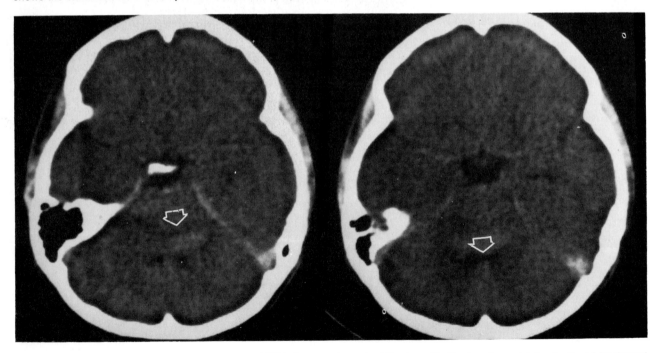

Figure 8-14 Brainstem glioma in an 8-year-old. CECT shows enlarged midbrain, with the fourth ventricle displaced backward. The floor of the fourth ventricle has a convex appearance (arrow).

ment is usually not present but does occur in the less-frequent eccentric tumors that protrude and grow into the cerebellum (Fig. 8-15). Contrast enhancement is not a reliable indicator of tumor grade (Fig. 8-16). As brainstem gliomas are usually slow-growing, the fourth ventricle and aqueduct are usually stretched over the tumor and remain open (Fig. 8-17). Hydrocephalus is uncommon in brainstem tumors. R. D. Zimmerman et al. (1980) described a method which can be used to measure the subtle anteroposterior displacement of the fourth ventricle on axial CT. The reliability of these measurements depends on precise positioning of the patient's head in relation to the x-ray beam. If a brainstem glioma is eccentric, the lateral recess of the fourth ventricle on the ispilateral side will be displaced backward

(Hayman 1979). On the other hand, in symmetrically enlarged brainstem gliomas, not only may both lateral recesses be spread apart, but the floor of the fourth ventricle is convex backward. Very rarely, thin-section CT, following intrathecal metrizamide, or even polytomography, may be necessary to define the subtle deformation of the fourth ventricle, as well as the changes in the aqueduct and the circummesencephalic cisterns.

Acoustic Neuroma

In children and adolescents, most acoustic neuromas are associated with neurofibromatosis (Jacoby 1980). Because of this association, the tumor is relatively large compared with that usually seen in

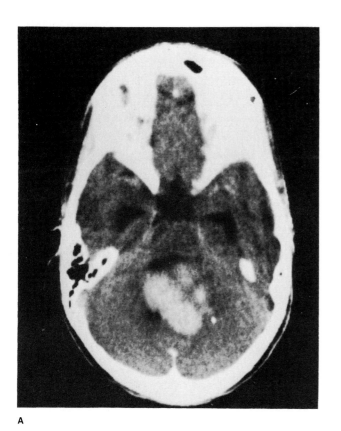

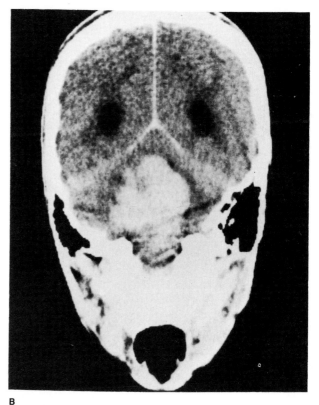

A   **B**

Figure 8-15 Brainstem glioma in an 8-year-old. **A.** CECT shows enhancing, irregular tumor with low-density area anteriorly that resembles fourth ventricle, mimicking a primary cerebellar tumor. **B.** Clival perpendicular (Waters') view shows the full extent of the tumor from brainstem to near the tentorium, with eccentric growth out into the left hemisphere.

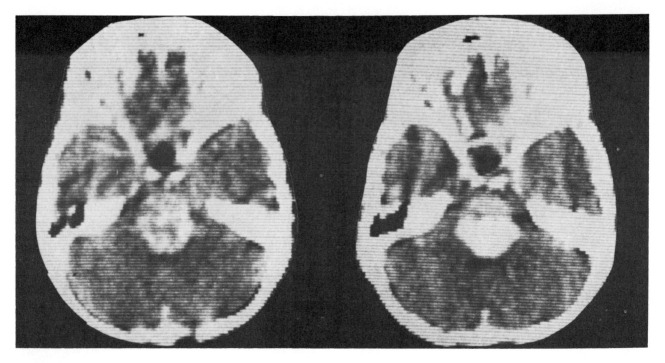

Figure 8-16 Brainstem glioma in an 11-year-old. CT following radiation therapy, shows significant enhancement in a biopsy-proven low-grade glioma.

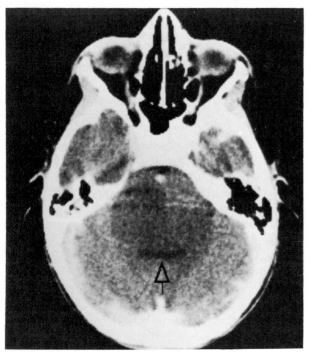

A

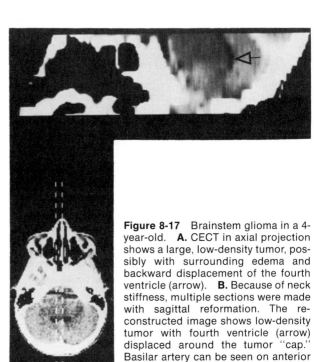

B

Figure 8-17 Brainstem glioma in a 4-year-old. **A.** CECT in axial projection shows a large, low-density tumor, possibly with surrounding edema and backward displacement of the fourth ventricle (arrow). **B.** Because of neck stiffness, multiple sections were made with sagittal reformation. The reconstructed image shows low-density tumor with fourth ventricle (arrow) displaced around the tumor "cap." Basilar artery can be seen on anterior surface of tumor.

adults. A mild contrast enhancement of the rim of the entire mass (Fig. 8-18) and an enlarged internal auditory canal are present in all cases. Bilateral acoustic neuromas may be seen in neurofibromatosis. The other CT findings are detailed extensively elsewhere (Chapter 10).

Miscellaneous Tumors

HEMANGIOBLASTOMA   Hemangioblastoma is rare in children below 15 years. On CT the tumor is visible as a cyst with a small nodule visible at its periphery (Fig. 8-19). The diagnosis is best made by angiography, which shows the extremely vascular nodule to advantage. Angiography is recommended as a confirmatory examination when this tumor is suspected on CT. The CT finding of a small enhancing nodule within a large cyst is characteristic, though solid tumors also occur (Naidich 1977*b*) (see Chapter

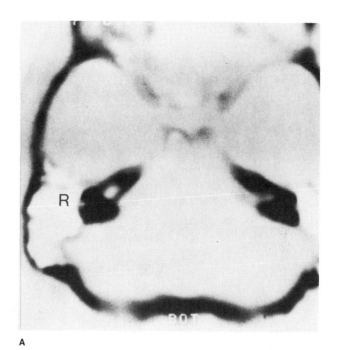

A

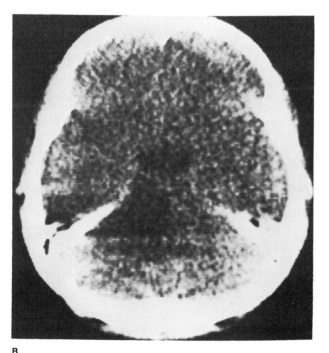

B

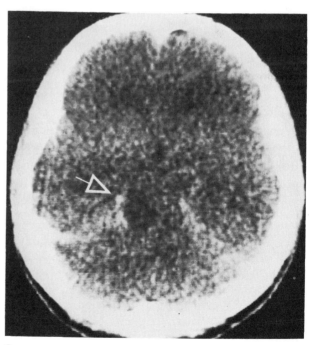

C

Figure 8-18   Acoustic neuroma in a 15-year-old. **A.** CT section through petrous bone shows enlarged right internal auditory canal (reverse gray scale).   **B.** Higher section without enhancement shows low-density tumor and surrounding edema.   **C.** CECT shows a small rim of enhancement (arrow) adjacent to tentorium along tumor border.

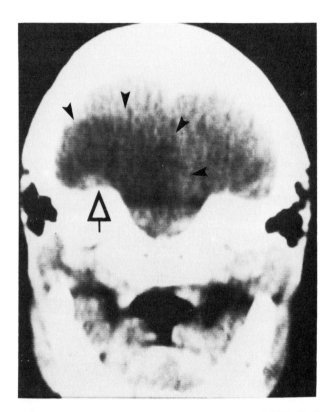

Figure 8-19 Hemangioblastoma in an 8-year-old. CECT, clival perpendicular view, shows tumor nodule (arrow) at skull base with large surrounding cyst.

7). A cystic astrocytoma can have a similar appearance on CT but does not show the intense vascular blush on angiography.

CAVERNOUS HEMANGIOMA Although rare, cavernous hemangioma can occur in the posterior fossa. Calcification may be present and may enhance significantly. The calcification is multifocal and quite dense. This may be a significant diagnostic finding (Fig. 8-20), although noncalcified cavernous hemangiomas have also been described (Tera 1979). Diagnostic distinction from other posterior fossa lesions on the basis of CT alone is difficult (see Chapter 14).

GANGLIOGLIOMA The CT appearance is often similar to a low-grade tumor related to other gliomas. Calcification may occasionally be present within the

tumor. The tumor shows some surrounding edema and slight diffuse contrast enhancement (Fig. 8-21) (see Chapter 7).

RHABDOSARCOMA Although frequently arising in the middle ear, rhabdosarcoma uncommonly invades the posterior fossa. Zimmerman et al. (1978*b*) reported one case of posterior fossa subarachnoid seeding, and one case presenting with an extraaxial posterior fossa mass, bone erosion, and lateral nasopharyngeal mass (Fig. 8-22) has been seen at the Hospital for Sick Children. Homogeneous enhancement of both intracranial and extracranial portions of rhabdosarcomas is common. Extension into the posterior fossa is not common, even among rhabdosarcomas originating in the middle ear.

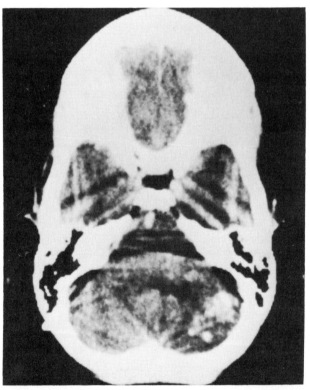

Figure 8-20 Cavernous hemangioma in a 17-year-old. CT shows calcified left cerebellar hemispheric mass that does not enhance. No displacement of the fourth ventricle is present. Lesions also were present in the frontal lobe and thalamus. The child had been misdiagnosed as having a malignant tumor by pneumoencephalogram 8 years earlier at another hospital.

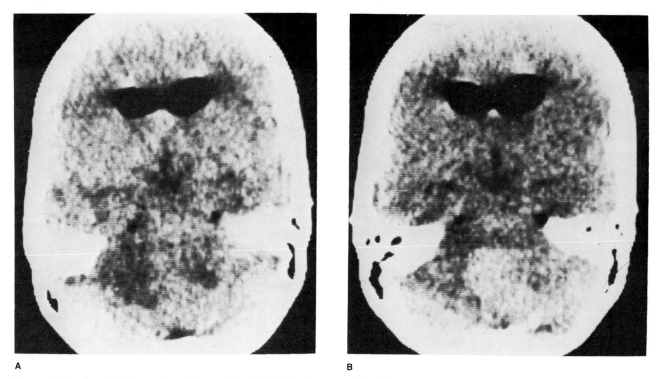

Figure 8-21 Ganglioglioma in a 14-year-old. NCCT **(A)** shows poorly defined posterior fossa mass with irregular low-density regions of tumor and central isodense portion which shows low grade and nonspecific contrast enhancement **(B).** Air is in ventricles from previous pneumoencephalogram.

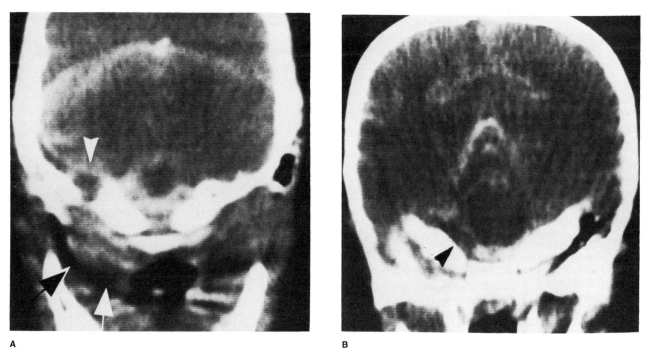

Figure 8-22 Rhabdosarcoma in a 6-year-old. **A.** Clival perpendicular view with intrathecal metrizamide shows pharyngeal mass (arrows), erosion of medial petrous bone, and extradural posterior fossa extension of tumor (arrowhead). **B.** Same examination at the dorsum shows forward extension of extradural tumor beneath brainstem on the right side (arrowhead).

CHORDOMA Chordomas typically occur in older children. Combined erosion and reactive thickening of the clivus is seen on CT. The tumor mass is visible as an enhancing extradural mass over the clivus (Fig. 8-23) and is often calcified. The extracranial component of the tumor is variable but can be quite extensive. CT following intrathecal metrizamide, along with reformatted images, is helpful in defining the intraspinal extension of chordoma.

Postoperative Examination

Following operation and x-ray treatment of tumors, those showing recurrence as well as residual tumor undergo morphologic changes. No matter what the pretreatment type, they are more likely to be cystic after treatment. This is probably related to the radiation therapy. Residual tumors may be present and unchanged for two or three years, then quickly undergo growth for no apparent reason.

SUPRATENTORIAL TUMORS

For purposes of comparison between different histological grades of tumor, the CT findings are discussed on a regional basis. Neoplasms that have no significant differences from the adult variety are mentioned only in passing.

Sellar and Parasellar Tumors

Lesions around the sella account for 20 percent of all intracranial neoplasms in children (Wilson 1975; Harwood-Nash 1976). One of the most common neoplasms encountered in the pediatric age group in this region is craniopharyngioma. Other less common neoplasms in this age group include hypothalamic glioma, optic chiasm and nerve glioma, hypothalamic histiocytosis, hypothalamic hamartoma, arachnoid cyst, and ectopic pinealoma (teratoma, germinoma, embryonal carcinoma, and the rare choriocarcinoma).

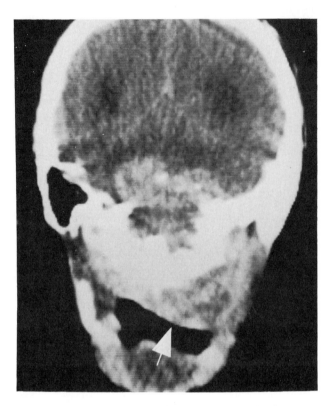

Figure 8-23 Chordoma. CECT, clival perpendicular view: Large recurrent chordoma shows clival erosion and enhanced and calcified bilobed mass extending up from the clivus and a large pharyngeal extension (arrow).

Even after the availability of CT, numerous authors indicated the need for positive contrast CT studies or pneumoencephalography to define the presence and location of the lesion within the suprasellar cistern (Strand 1978; Reich 1976; Kishore 1980; Volbe 1978). In most cases, CT not only is diagnostic but shows the extent of the lesion. In occasional cases, CT following intrathecal metrizamide with axial and coronal sections obviates the need for other invasive studies.

Craniopharyngioma

This is a relatively common tumor in the pediatric age group, accounting for about 7 percent of all intracranial neoplasms and more than 50 percent of all sellar and parasellar neoplasms (Harwood-Nash 1976). Most often the tumor is suprasellar in location, although in less than 10 percent of children it may be totally intrasellar (Rao 1977). Craniopharyngiomas in children tend to have calcific components either within the tumor or around its rim: calcification is seen in nearly 80 percent of cases, especially by computed tomography.

Cystic components within the tumor are more common in children than in adults, as is enhancement of the tumor on CECT. An isodense, nonenhancing craniopharyngioma is more common in the adult population.

In the majority of craniopharyngiomas, CT demonstrates a calcified mass located in the suprasellar region. The calcification may be along the periphery of the tumor, as in purely cystic forms of craniopharyngioma (Fig. 8-24), or may be present within

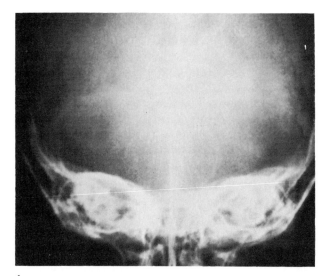

A

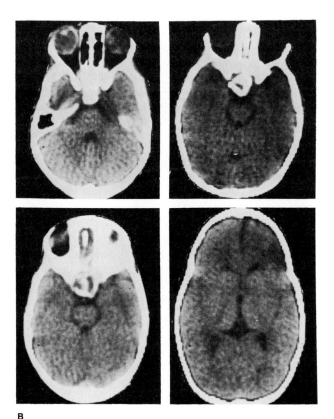

B

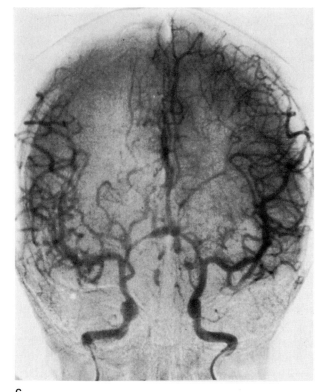

C

Figure 8-24 Craniopharyngioma in a 2-year-old. **A.** Curvilinear calcification around the rim of tumor identified on skull x-ray. **B.** CT demonstrating calcified mass in the suprasellar cistern. This pattern of calcification is characteristic of craniopharyngioma. **C.** Angiogram (superimposed) anteroposterior view demonstrating the characteristic angiographic appearance of sellar mass with suprasellar extension.

(Continued on p. 316.)

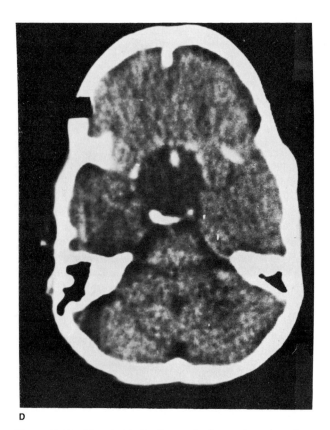
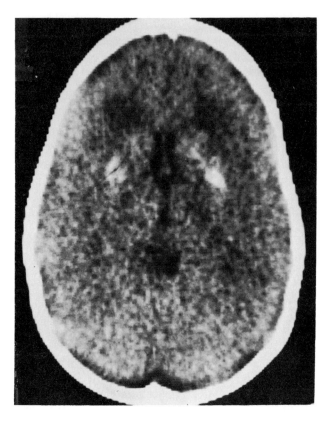

D

Figure 8-24 *(Cont.)* **D.** Cystic craniopharyngioma in a 4-year-old: large cystic craniopharyngioma with marginal calcification. A catheter tip is noted, used for intermittent drainage. In a slightly higher section, calcification of the basal ganglia secondary to radiation therapy is present.

the tumor as discrete masses (Fig. 8-25). CECT will usually show a variegated pattern, depending on the nature of the calcification as well as cystic components within the tumor. Nonhomogeneous enhancement is thus a common finding, the hypodense regions probably representing cysts containing a mixture of keratin and cholesterol debris. Occasionally the neoplasm is isodense and enhances significantly (Fig. 8-26). In these cases, differentiation from a chromophobe adenoma or even a giant aneurysm may become difficult. Rarely, the tumor may be massive, occupying a large portion of the intracranial compartment (Fig. 8-27) (Lipper 1981), or may be totally within the third ventricle (Fitz 1978*b*). Craniopharyngioma, or its variant the Rathke's cleft cyst, occasionally may be hypodense (Fig. 8-28) and when small has been missed on routine CT examination (Volbe 1978; Eisenberg 1976).

Coronal CT, either by reformation or in the direct coronal mode, helps in defining the superoinferior limit of the neoplasm and its relation to the sellar and hypothalamic areas. Metrizamide CT cisternography, in both axial and coronal planes, is occasionally necessary to define the neoplasm and its relation to adjacent structures.

Other neoplasms in this area which should be differentiated from craniopharyngioma include optic chiasm glioma, hamartoma of the tuber cinereum, hypothalamic glioma, pituitary adenoma, aneurysm, and arachnoid cyst.

Diagnostic characteristics are the presence of calcifications, usually ringlike; nonhomogeneous enhancement; and the location of the mass. Angiography may be needed if intense homogeneous enhancement and clinical presentation suggest a giant aneurysm (Kokoris 1980) or before surgery.

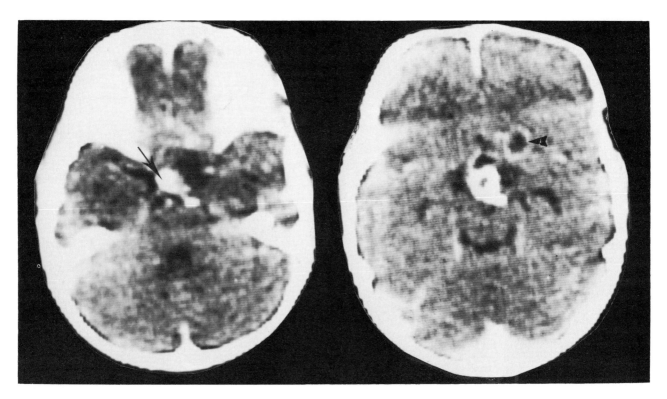

Figure 8-25 Craniopharyngioma in a 12-year-old. The tumor shows areas of calcification (arrow), ring enhancement (arrowhead), and a hypodense area.

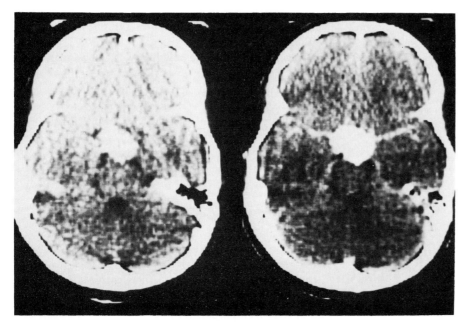

Figure 8-26 Craniopharyngioma in a young adult. A homogeneous, dense, enhancing suprasellar craniopharyngioma. This is the least common enhancement pattern in craniopharyngioma.

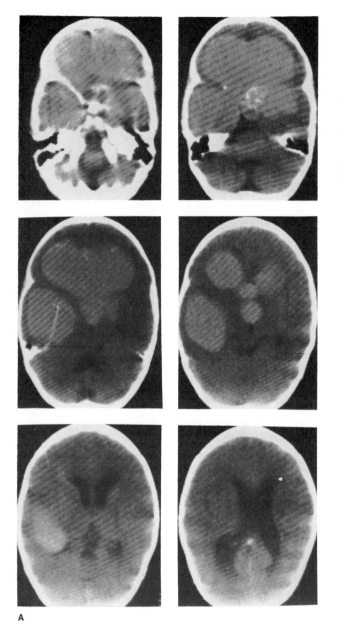

A

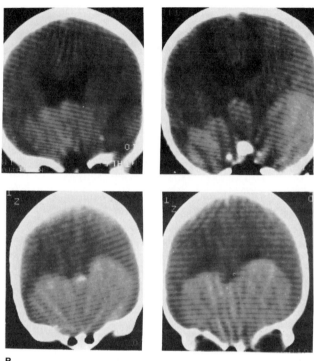

B

Figure 8-27 Craniopharyngioma Axial **(A)** and coronal enhanced CT **(B)** demonstrating a massive craniopharyngioma extending into both temporal regions, besides its suprasellar extension.

of glial cells. Hamartomas can occur anywhere, but when located in the hypothalamic region they are usually close to the tuber cinereum. The presenting clinical history usually includes diabetes insipidus. The tumor is slightly more common in males than in females. The CT characteristics are nonspecific (Fig. 8-29). The mass if large will usually obliterate the suprasellar cistern. Enhancement characteristics are variable, but the majority do not enhance (Lin 1978). The hamartoma may also be multiple (Fig. 8-30). Differentiation from solitary hypothalamic histiocytosis (Miller 1980) by CT may be difficult.

Hamartoma

Hamartomas are rare neoplasms which are not true tumors (Lin 1978; Mori 1981). They are congenital heterotopic collections of tissue located in normal or abnormal locations. The tissue usually consists

Ectopic Pinealoma

Tumors with histological characteristics similar to those in the pineal region occur in the parasellar region, predominantly in the suprasellar cistern. Their CT appearance and enhancement character-

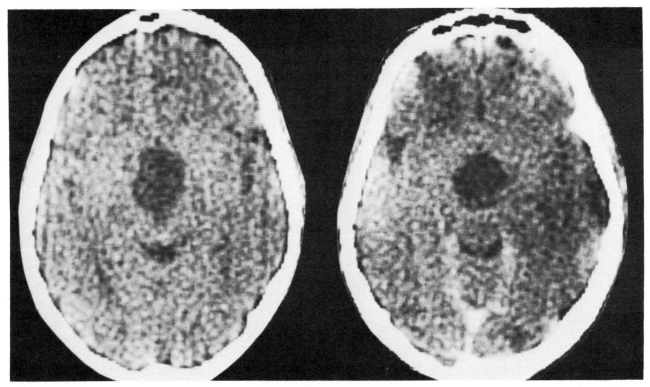

Figure 8-28 Nonenhancing, low-density, suprasellar cystic craniopharyngioma.

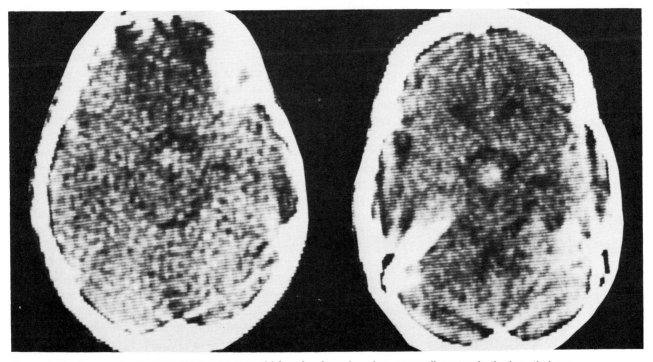

Figure 8-29 Suprasellar hamartoma in a 14-year-old female. An enhancing suprasellar mass in the hypothalamus.

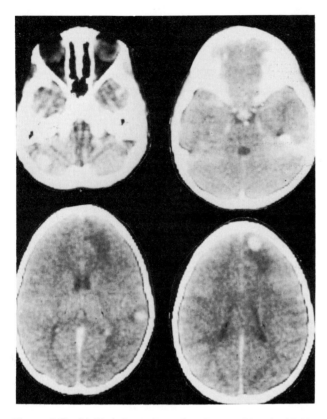

Figure 8-30 Multiple hamartoma in a 5-year-old male. Multiple enhancing lesions, proved at biopsy to be hamartomas, in a child presenting with diabetes insipidus.

istics are similar to histologically different neoplasms in the pineal region. Embryonal carcinoma and endodermal sinus tumors in the suprasellar hypothalamic region do not demonstrate calcification, unlike those in the pineal region. Primary choriocarcinoma is a rare form of embryonal carcinoma, usually presenting as an isodense mass with intense enhancement. Hemorrhage within this tumor is common (Fig. 8-31). Differentiation from other suprasellar masses may require further diagnostic studies.

Optic Nerve Glioma

Glioma of the optic nerve can be focal, involving either the intraorbital segment of the nerve or the intracranial component. Or the tumor may be diffuse and involve the intraorbital as well as the intracranial component of the optic nerve. The CT features of intraorbital optic nerve glioma and its intracranial extension have been dealt with elsewhere (Chapter 3). Optic glioma is most often seen in children. Since the majority of the neoplasms are low-grade gliomas, on NCCT they appear as isodense masses obliterating the suprasellar cistern. If the glioma involves the intracranial component of the optic nerve, asymmetry of the anterior aspect of the "pentagonal" suprasellar cistern provides a clue to the presence of the optic or perioptic neoplasm (Naidich 1976). On the other hand, in large and bulky chiasmatic gliomas, dilatation of the basal and sylvian cisterns has been noted (Savoiardo 1981). The mechanism is presumed to be similar to projection of extraaxial masses into the cisterns. Enhancement of the glioma is variable but often intense (Fig. 8-32); however, it may occasionally be minimal. Evaluation of the total extent and spread of the neoplasm requires thin CT sections in the axial as well as the coronal plane. Occasionally, in spite of these additional methods of CT examination, differentiation of the enhancing mass from such other suprasellar neoplasms as hypothalamic glioma with extension to the chiasm and optic tract may be difficult. CT following intrathecal metrizamide, angiography, and pneumoencephalography may become necessary (Fig. 8-33).

These additional studies may still be indicated, in the absence of appropriate clinical findings, to define other suprasellar masses discussed in this chapter as well as other less common masses in children, such as pituitary adenoma and giant internal carotid aneurysm. In childhood pituitary adenomas, the sella is often enlarged in association with an enhancing intrasellar mass. In one large series, pituitary adenomas in patients under 20 years of age were most often in females, the majority presenting with delayed puberty (Richmond 1978). In the presence of clinical findings and an enhancing sellar mass, pituitary adenoma should be considered (see Chapter 10). Since calcification rarely occurs in optic gliomas, differentiation from craniopharyngioma may occasionally be difficult.

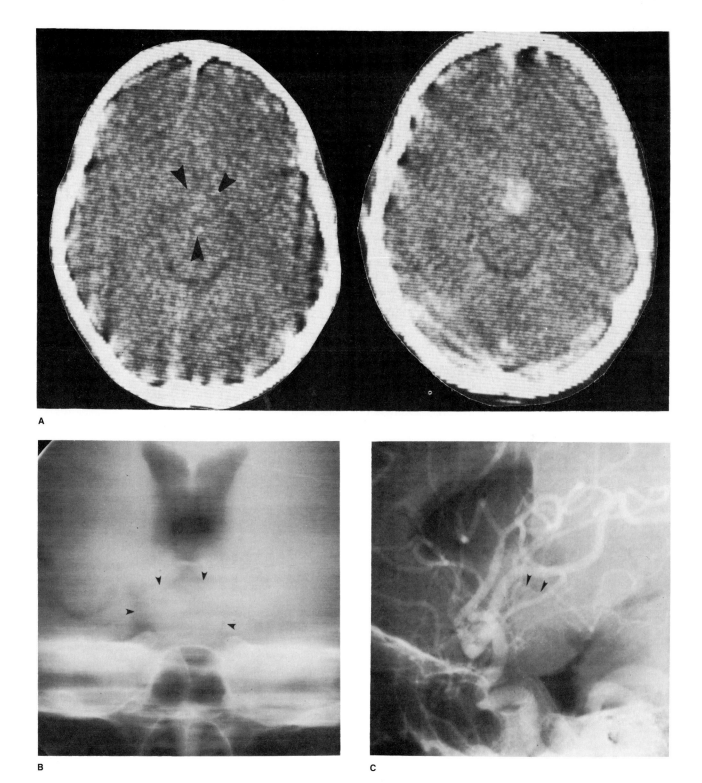

Figure 8-31 Primary suprasellar choriocarcinoma. **A.** Because the suprasellar cistern cannot be seen, an isodense hypothalamic mass is suspected. Avascular mass is disclosed in A-P polytomogram made during air study **(B)** and in lateral-view angiogram **(C).**

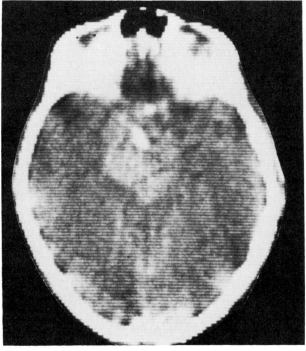

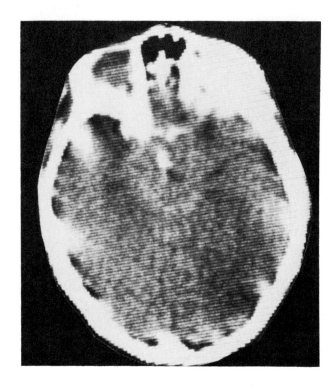

D

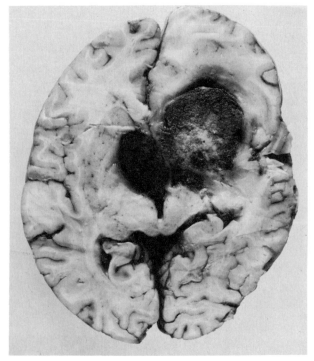

Figure 8-31 *(Cont.)* **D.** Same patient, showing the rapid increase in volume of the tumor prior to death. **E.** Brain section from autopsy showing intraparenchymal extension of the hypothalamic primary choriocarcinoma.

Arachnoid Cyst

Congenital arachnoid cysts are commonly seen in the temporal region and in the posterior fossa as extraaxial cysts. Other less common locations of arachnoid cysts are the suprasellar and prepontine regions, the quadrigeminal and circummesencephalic cisterns, and the interhemispheric fissure, as well as the region adjacent to the lateral ventricles.

Suprasellar arachnoid cysts may occasionally be missed on routine CT studies. They produce a characteristic appearance of focal ballooning of the anterior third ventricle on axial CT (Fig. 8-34). Diagnosis can be suspected on the basis of the CT appearance and confirmed by CT following intrathecal metrizamide (Anderson 1979; Lee 1979;

E

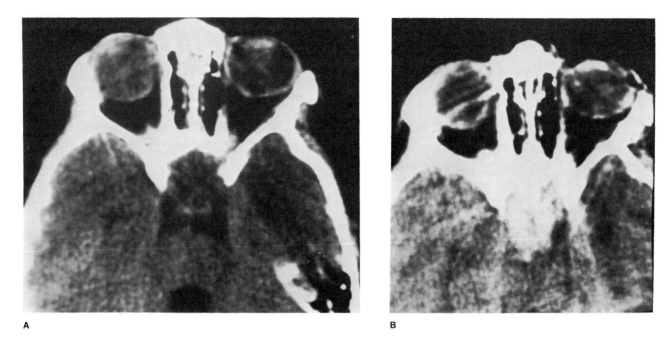

A   B

Figure 8-32 Optic nerve glioma. **A.** NCCT: A soft-tissue mass is noted in the suprasellar region (arrow). **B.** Enhancement of the chiasmatic glioma is noted on CECT. (Courtesy of Dr. R. A. Zimmerman.)

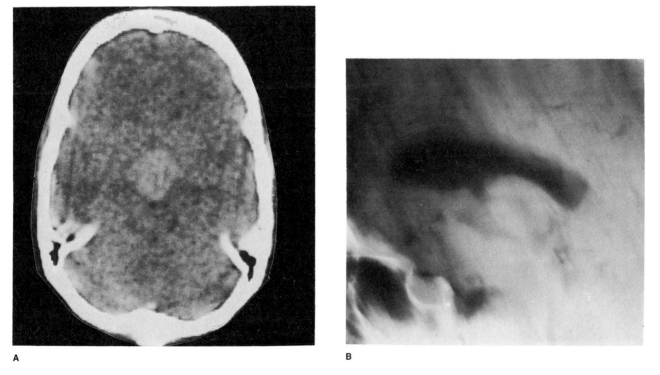

A   B

Figure 8-33 Optic nerve glioma in a 17-year-old. **A.** CT, axial plane, demonstrates an enhancing mass in the suprasellar/hypothalamic region, avascular on angiography. **B.** Polytomography following air studies precisely defines the mass and its relation to the adjacent structures.

(Continued on p. 324)

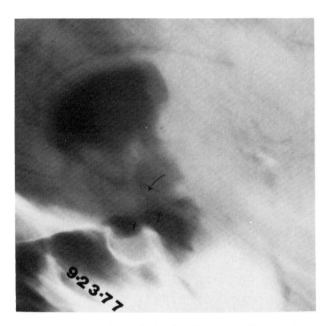

Figure 8-33 *(Cont.)* **C.** Reduction in size of the neoplasm following radiation therapy.

Leo 1979). The extent of the cyst can be precisely defined by axial and coronal CT. Large suprasellar arachnoid cysts invaginate the third ventricle and, in some cases, appear to be intraventricular.

Tumors of the Pineal Region

Tumors of the "pineal region" have in the past commonly been identified as *pinealomas*, whatever their histologic character. Similar tumors occurring in the anterior aspect of the third ventricle, within the suprasellar cistern, have been termed *ectopic pinealomas*. Pineal tumors have been classified according to their behavior, clinical presentation, and histological characteristics (Russell 1977) into true pineal neoplasms and neoplasms of other cellular origin.

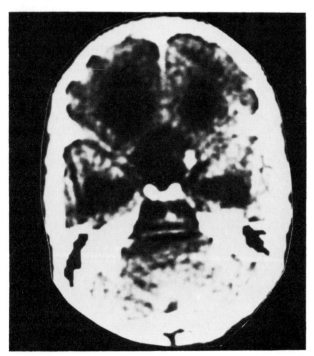

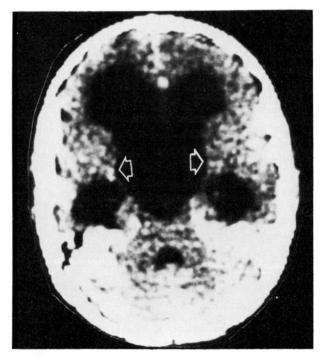

Figure 8-34   Suprasellar arachnoid cyst. The massive dilatation of the lateral and third ventricles with normal appearance of the fourth ventricle mimics the CT appearance of aqueduct stenosis. Lateral bowing of the third ventricle (arrows) was secondary to a large suprasellar arachnoid cyst confirmed by ventriculography.

Pineal and ectopic pineal tumors represent less than 1 percent of all intracranial tumors, although in the series summarized in Table 8-2 they represented 5 to 8 percent of all pediatric-age neoplasms.

In the pineal region, the greatest likelihood of confusion occurs in differentiating the various types of pineal neoplasms from those arising in regions adjacent to the pineal gland, such as astrocytoma involving the splenium of the corpus callosum or the tectum of the midbrain.

Since certain histological types of pineal tumors are radiosensitive (germinoma, pinealcytoma, embryonal cell carcinoma), not only precise localization of the neoplasm but its histological typing by the use of CT have been attempted (Zimmerman 1980b; Futrell 1981; Messina 1978). Pursuit of these ends requires evaluation of the CT findings by pre- and post-contrast studies. Occasionally, even with thin-section as well as direct coronal or sagittal and coronal multiplanar reformation to localize the origin of the tumor, angiography for tumor stain and vascular pattern may be necessary. The most frequent tumors of the pineal region are the germinoma and the teratoma. They occur in older children (over 15) in the second decade and are more frequent in males. Tumors of the pineal cell origin, however—pinealcytoma and pinealblastoma—have no significant sex predilection although they are slightly more common in females. Their biological and clinical features, besides such CT findings as calcification, presence or absence of hemorrhages, and cysts, are helpful in arriving at a CT diagnosis and appropriate treatment. The CT characteristics of the major pineal tumors are briefly discussed below.

Germinomas are teratomatous tumors commonly seen in males. On NCCT they appear as hyperdense or isodense masses, usually deforming and encroaching on the posterior aspect of the third ventricle. Punctate calcification within the mass is usually apparent. In the absence of calcification, obliteration of the quadrigeminal cistern, as well as deformity of the posterior aspect of the third ventricle, should be looked for, since the tumor commonly infiltrates the adjacent tissues (Fig. 8-35). Often, depending on the size of the tumor, there is noncommunicating hydrocephalus. On CECT, intense enhancement of the neoplasm occurs. Occasionally these tumors have two components, one in the pineal region and the other an ectopic component in the anterior third ventricular region.

Teratoma in the pineal region usually appears as a hypodense mass (Fig. 8-36). Calcification within the mass and occasionally other formed elements may be present (Zimmerman 1980b). Minimal enhancement is the rule. In the absence of formed elements such as a tooth or the like, CT differentiation from other lesions in this region, such as epidermoid tumor or quadrigeminal plate arachnoid cyst, may be difficult. Spontaneous rupture of this variety of neoplasm into the ventricular system or the subarachnoid cisterns has also been documented (Goshhajra 1979; McCormack 1978). Malignant degeneration of the tumor is associated with significant contrast enhancement.

Embryonal cell carcinoma, as well as endodermal sinus, or "yolk sac," carcinoma, are tumors found both in the pineal region and in the suprasellar region (Zimmerman 1980b; Rao 1979). On NCCT they may be hypodense or slightly hyperdense (Fig. 8-37). Calcification has been described in these neoplasms when located in the pineal region (Zimmerman 1980b). They are prone to hemorrhage within the neoplasm. Intense enhancement of the tumors is characteristic, although rarely they may not enhance.

The pinealblastoma has an appearance almost like that of the embryonal cell carcinoma. Calcification within or surrounding the neoplasm is rare. Pinealcytoma, on the other hand, is associated with dense calcification with mild to moderate enhancement on CECT (Fig. 8-38). In spite of the above features, histological diagnosis on the basis of CT alone is extremely difficult. Spread of tumors along the ependymal surface of the ventricles can be seen not only with dysgerminoma (Osborn 1978) but also with pinealblastoma, choriocarcinoma, and teratocarcinoma. CT plays an important role after surgery or radiation therapy.

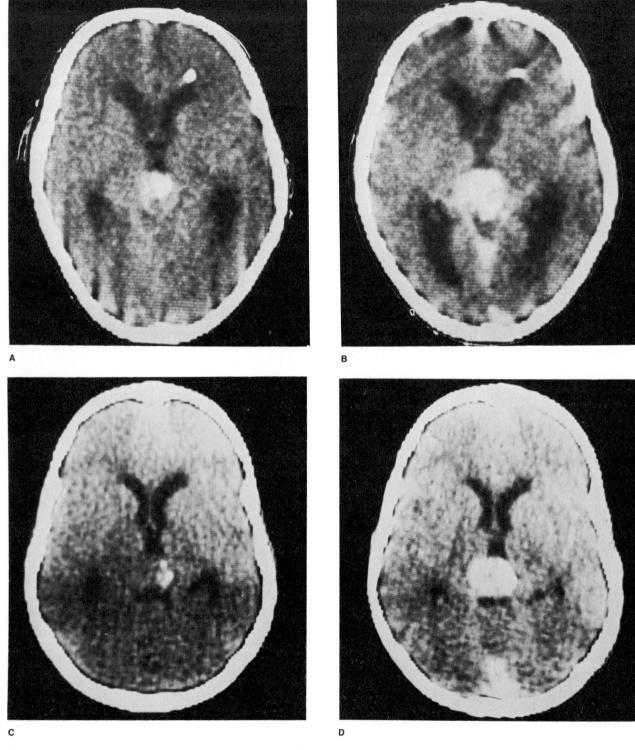

Figure 8-35 Pineal germinoma. **A.** A dense pineal calcification associated with a soft-tissue mass, indenting the posterior aspect of the third ventricle, is present on NCCT. **B.** On CECT the mass enhances and has ill-defined margins. A shunt catheter tip is noted in the frontal horn. Precontrast CT **(C)** and postcontrast CT **(D)** in another patient. The calcified component is eccentric in location. There is intense enhancement of the neoplasm, with sharply defined margins.

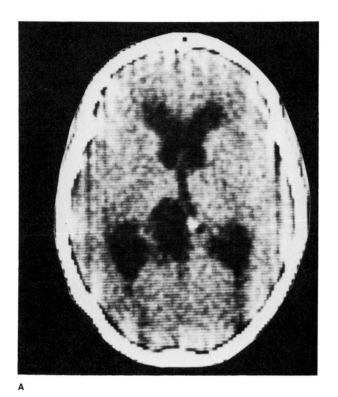 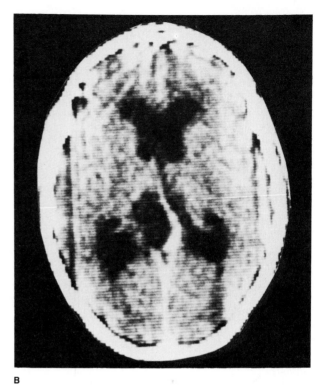

A   B

Figure 8-36 Pineal tumor: teratoma. Precontrast CT **(A)** and postcontrast CT **(B):** A nonenhancing mass with density similar to that of CSF is present. The mass indents the posterior aspect of the third ventricle, with slight displacement of the pineal calcification.

Ependymal and Intraventricular Tumors

Neoplasms derived from the ependyma include (1) ependymoma, (2) choroid plexus papilloma and its malignant version, choroid plexus carcinoma, and (3) heterotopias and cysts extending into the parenchyma or within the ventricle, the walls of the cyst being lined by ependymal cells. Parenchymal neoplasms may spread along the ependymal surface. These neoplasms may be primary or secondary and may project into the ventricular cavity due to their location and proximity to the ventricular spaces. In the majority of cases, CT in the axial and coronal plane following contrast enhancement will delineate the exact site of origin of these neoplasms and their extent. From the clinical history, the enhancing pattern, and the location of the neoplasm, the nature of the tumor can often be predicted. Angiography is helpful not only in the evaluation of tumor vascularity and the tumor's histological characteristics but in excluding vascular lesions extending along the ependymal surface (Coin 1977). A majority of neoplasms arising from the ependymal surface or from its derivatives result in hydrocephalus. Thus in children below 5 years, the presenting feature is progressive enlargement of the head size (not rapid). In children over 10 years of age the presenting feature is constant or intermittent headache. Cranial-nerve involvement and ataxia are late findings. Tumors involving the ependyma and its derivatives in general are rare.

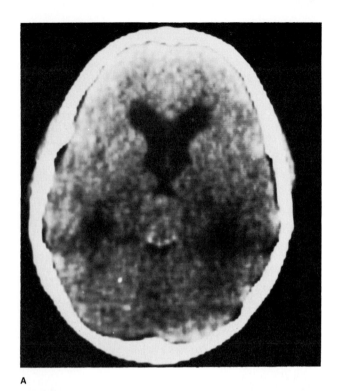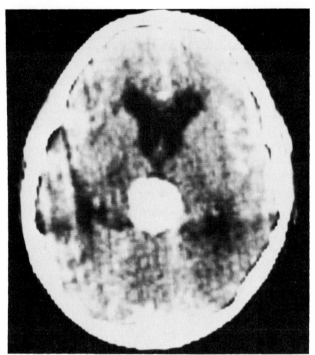

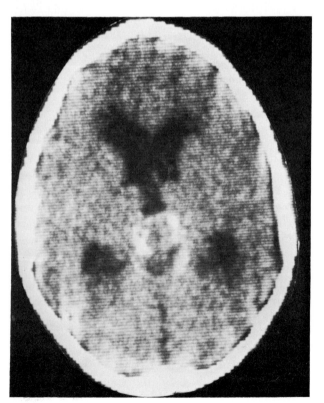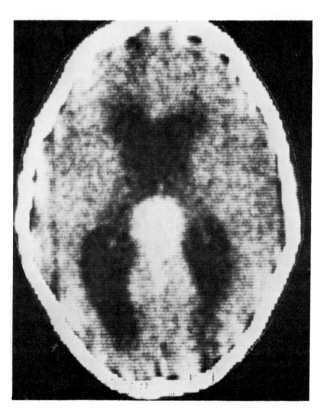

A

B

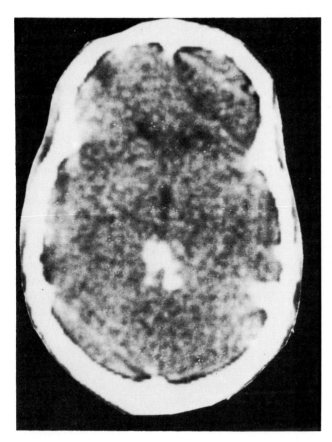 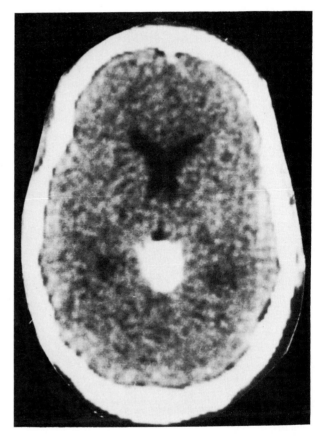

Figure 8-38 Pineal tumor: pinealcytoma. A densely calcified pineal tumor with minimal enhancement and avascularity on angiography. Not biopsy-proven but treated by radiation therapy.

Choroid Plexus Papilloma

Choroid plexus papillomas are rare neoplasms making up less than 2 percent of all intracranial neoplasms in children (Table 8-2). Unlike the adult form, which occurs within the fourth ventricle, the papillomas in the pediatric age group (1 to 12 years) are more common in the lateral ventricle and rarely the third ventricle. In the lateral ventricle location,

◀ **Figure 8-37** Pineal tumor: embryonal cell carcinoma. **A.** Pre- and postcontrast CT demonstrates minimal calcification with intense enhancement of the tumor. **B.** Another patient showing peripheral calcification and intense enhancement of the tumor, a common feature of malignant pineal tumors.

the tumor is more often seen in the left lateral ventricle than the right. The majority of benign choroid plexus papillomas are detected in children around the age of 2 years. The tumor manifests as prominence of the glomus of the choroid plexus, located in the trigone of the lateral ventricle and having a frondlike appearance. Calcification may be detected within the mass. The hydrocephalus associated with this neoplasm cannot be explained on the basis of obstruction of the CSF pathway, although a large mass in the trigone can result in entrapment of the ipsilateral temporal horn (Fig. 8-39). The hydrocephalus has been attributed to a variety of factors: (1) elevated intraventricular pulse pressure, (2) diffuse spread along the meninges, (3) decreased CSF absorption by arachnoid granulations from frequent

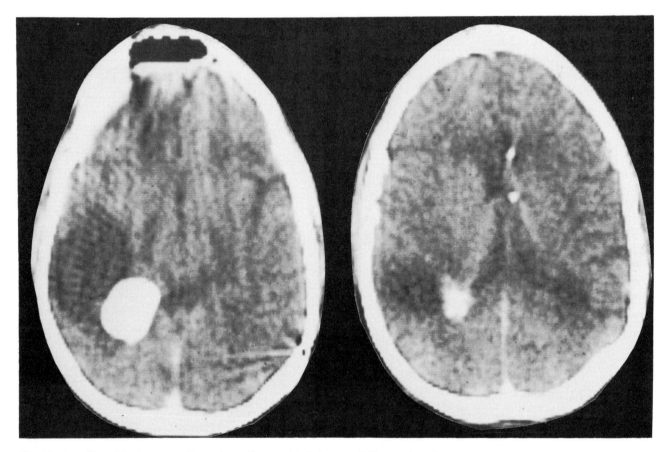

Figure 8-39 Choroid plexus papilloma in a 12-year-old. A large calcified, enhancing mass representing a benign papilloma involving the glomus of the left lateral ventricle. Hydrocephalus controlled by ventricular shunting. Note entrapment of the ipsilateral temporal horn with dilatation.

occult bleeding, and (4) increased CSF production. The fact that the hydrocephalus disappears after removal of these neoplasms indicates that the last factor is probably the most important mechanism. On NCCT the tumor is seen as a mass of slight hyperdensity compared to the rest of the parenchyma, due partly to the tumor vascularity and partly to the tumor's location within the CSF space. It enhances significantly on CECT.

Hydrocephalus with an enlarged, enhancing choroid plexus in a child with enlarging head is characteristic of choroid plexus papilloma. On angiography, choroid plexus papillomas are noted to be characteristically fed by the choroidal arteries. Intense vascular stain is a frequent finding.

Choroid Plexus Carcinoma

Choroid plexus carcinoma is the malignant form of the papilloma. The malignancy of the tumor can be suspected from the extension of the tumor beyond the confines of the ependymal barrier into the cerebral parenchyma. These neoplasms are less common than choroid plexus papilloma. Like the benign form, the choroid plexus carcinoma is associated with massive hydrocephalus. On NCCT the lesion can be seen, within the ventricle as well as extending into the parenchyma, as an isodense to slightly hyperdense mass (Fig. 8-40). Intense enhancement on CECT is a common feature.

Since a parenchymal extension or component is

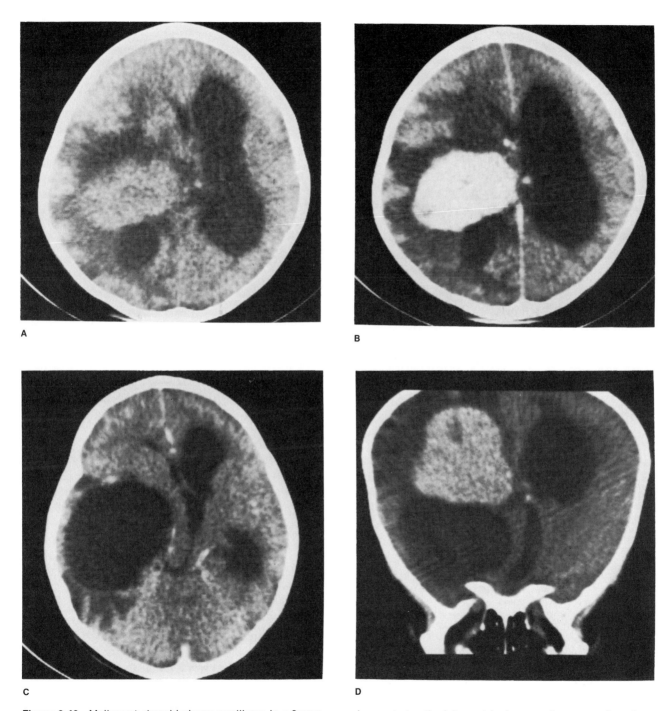

Figure 8-40 Malignant choroid plexus papilloma in a 2-year-old. Axial CT demonstrates a hyperdense mass in the lateral ventricle **(A)** with intense enhancement on CECT **(B)** associated with trapped temporal horn **(C). D.** Coronal CECT demonstrates the intraventricular as well as parenchymal extension of the neoplasm. The combination of communicating hydrocephalus and an enhancing intraventricular mass with parenchymal extension indicates a choroid plexus carcinoma. (*Continued on p. 332.*)

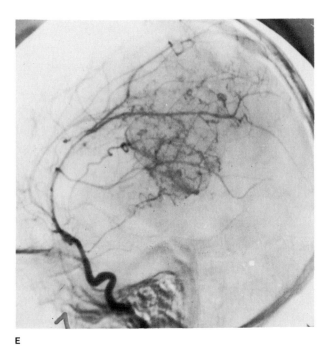

E

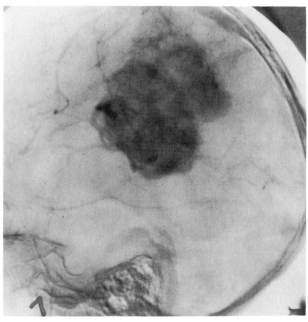

F

Figure 8-40 *(Cont.)*   Arterial **(E)** and capillary **(F)** phases of the angiogram indicating the vascular feeders and intense tumor stain.

common in choroid plexus carcinoma, it may have to be differentiated from other neoplasms such as ependymoma, glioblastoma, and meningioma or, rarely, vascular anomalies.

Glioblastomas and vascular anomalies within the ventricles are rare in children. It is not unusual for even an experienced neuropathologist to call this tumor ependymoma, since the choroid plexus is derived from ependymal cells. However, the CT and the angiographic characteristics are usually helpful in differentiating the two neoplasms.

The choroid plexus carcinoma is always associated with hydrocephalus, which extends distal to the location of the neoplasm. The tumor mass has frondlike projections, almost like a "ball of spaghetti," with areas of hypodensity within it, most often representing old focal hemorrhages or necrosis. These are highly vascular on angiography, although rarely the neoplasm can be avascular (Zimmerman 1979*b*).

Ependymoma

In children, ependymomas are most common in the posterior fossa but can arise from the walls of the third and lateral ventricles and the adjacent white matter. Supratentorial ependymomas often arise from cell rests adjacent to or farther from the ventricular wall. They are common at sites where the ventricles are sharply angled, and posterior to the occipital horns (Swartz 1982). The trigone of the lateral ventricle appears to be a common site (Shuman 1975; Swartz 1982). In the few cases the author has seen, the ependymomas were located in the region of the foramen of Monro (Fig. 8-41). Supratentorial ependymoma is often seen in children or in young adults between the ages of 15 and 25 years.

On NCCT, the tumor is isodense or slightly hyperdense. Punctate calcification within the neoplasm is common, as is enhancement of the neo-

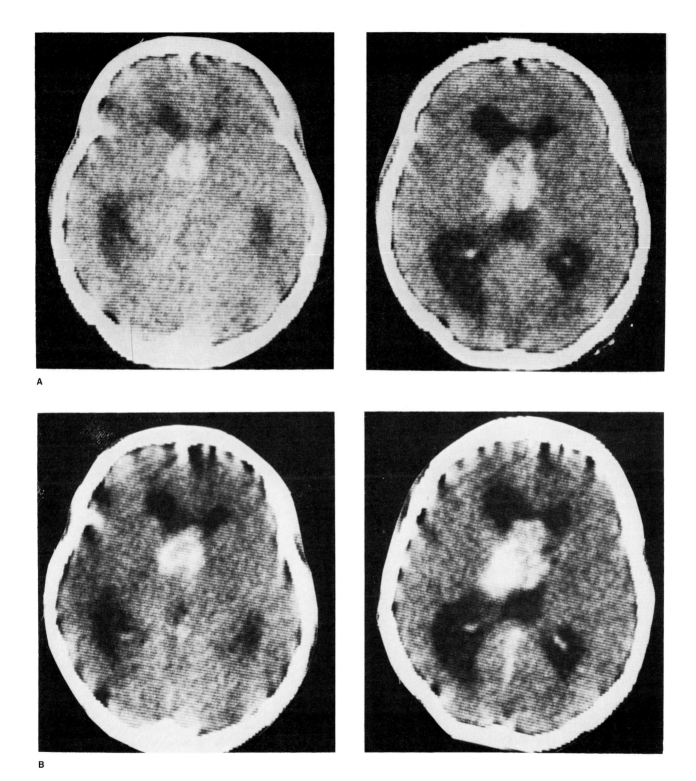

Figure 8-41 Intraventricular ependymoma. **A.** Precontrast CT shows a mass in the region of the anterior third ventricle, with dense calcification. **B.** Postcontrast CT shows some enhancement of the neoplasm, proven to be an ependymoma at surgery.

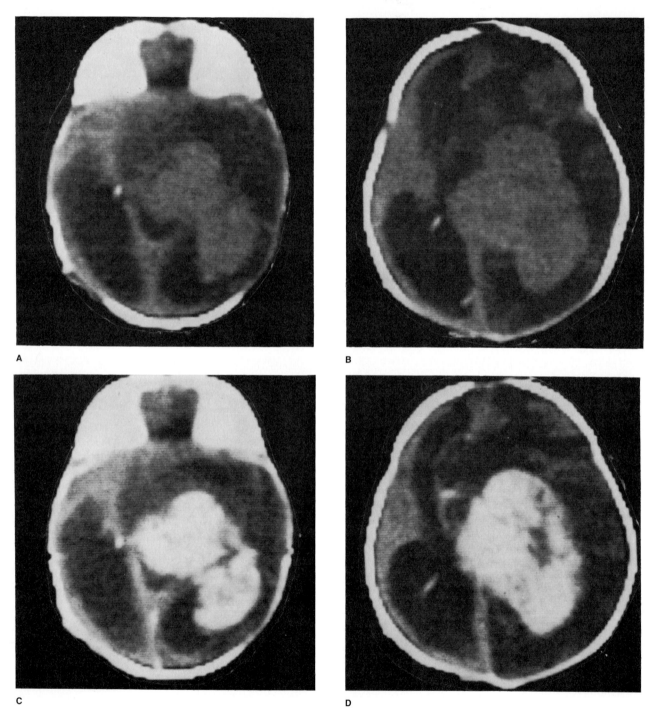

A

B

C

D

Figure 8-42 Ependymoblastoma. **A, B.** NCCT: Marked enlargement and distortion of the ventricles from an isodense mass. **C, D.** Intense enhancement is noted. The mass arose primarily from the ependymal surface of the lateral ventricle, extending into the ventricle at autopsy.

plasm following CECT. The enhancement, unlike that in choroid plexus carcinoma, is nonhomogeneous to homogeneous. When the tumor arises from the ependymal wall of the ventricles, obstructive hydrocephalus beyond it is common. Ependymoma can be differentiated from choroid plexus carcinoma by the CT characteristics and by angiography.

Ependymoblastoma is a malignant form of ependymal tumor in which the tumor grows rapidly; spread by meningeal seeding is common. The growth of the tumor can be so rapid as to involve the whole ventricular system, almost forming a cast of the ventricle (Fig. 8-42). Although a histological diagnosis cannot be made by CT, this CT finding is associated with a high mortality.

Hamartomas of tuberous sclerosis or other heterotopias along the ependymal surface do not enhance unless malignant transformation takes place.

Subependymal Giant Cell Astrocytoma

This neoplasm is most often seen in children with tuberous sclerosis. It is due to malignant transformation of hamartoma. The astrocytoma is most often located in the region of the foramen of Monro (Fig. 8-43). On NCCT, other hamartomas may be noted along the ependymal wall of the ventricles. Many subependymal, as well as parenchymal, hamartomas show calcification. In the presence of these findings, the CT diagnosis is specific for this neoplasm.

Parenchymal Tumors

Astrocytoma

Astrocytoma is the most common primary neoplasm in the pediatric age group as it is in the adult

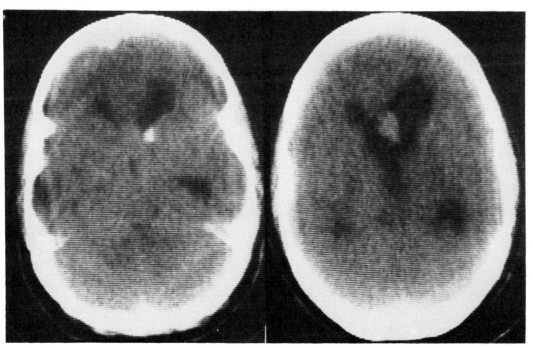

A

Figure 8-43 Subependymal giant cell astrocytoma.   **A.** NCCT shows a soft-tissue mass in the region of the foramen of Monro, with calcification of the ependymal hamartoma.   (*Continued on p. 336.*)

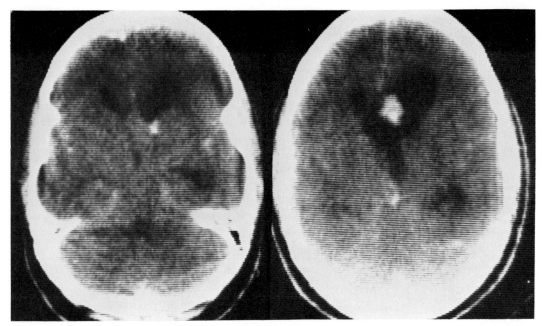

B

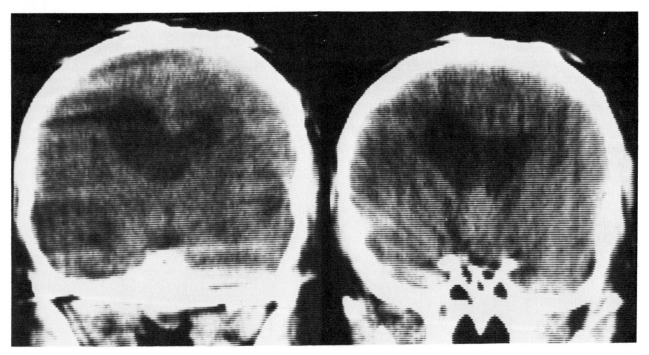

C

Figure 8-43 *(Cont.)* **B.** CECT shows the enhancing tumor causing unilateral obstruction of the left lateral ventricle. **C.** Coronal CT helps in better localization of the mass.

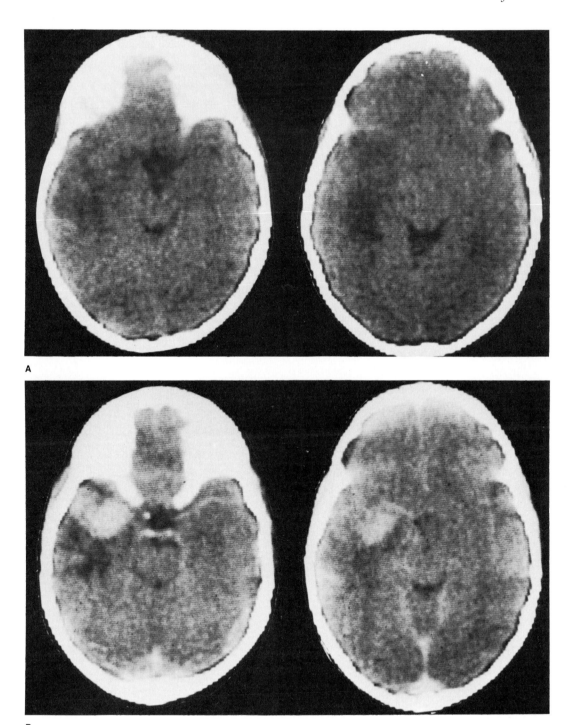

A

B

Figure 8-44 Low-grade astrocytoma. Precontrast CT **(A)** and postcontrast CT **(B)** of a low-grade glioma. The relatively low volume of edema (low density) compared to the enhancing mass (tumor) is noted.

population. Among the pediatric age group, supratentorial astrocytomas are more common in older children. Unlike astrocytomas in the posterior fossa, which are usually cystic and carry a better prognosis, the supratentorial astrocytomas behave as in adults. The CT findings are also similar to those in the adult population. Low-grade astrocytomas (grades I and II) appear hypodense or isodense and may not show significant enhancement on CECT (Fig. 8-44). Higher-grade astrocytomas (grades III and IV) will show either homogeneous enhancement or a ring pattern and are often associated with peritumoral edema. When the glioma has the appearance of a ring with a smooth outer and inner wall, which may happen occasionally, differentiation from an abscess may be difficult. Most often a nodular component or an irregular, shaggy inner wall is seen in gliomas (Fig. 8-45). The other CT features are similar to those described for adults (Chapter 7).

Neuroblastoma

Primary cerebral neuroblastoma is a relatively rare tumor. Unlike extracranial neuroblastoma with intracranial metastasis, which is common in the younger age group, primary neuroblastoma is more common in older children and adolescents. The neoplasm is often seen in the cerebrum (Chambers 1981; Zimmerman 1980a) but not in any specific location. Neuroblastoma appears to be slightly more frequent in females (Zimmerman 1980a; Chambers 1981).

On NCCT, the neoplasm appears as a hypodense or isodense mass (Fig. 8-46). Focal areas of hyperdensity are often present, most often representing calcification or hemorrhages. The calcification can be punctate or occasionally dense and large (Chambers 1981). On CECT, varying degrees of enhancement ranging from a ring pattern to homogeneous enhancement, with areas of pathological

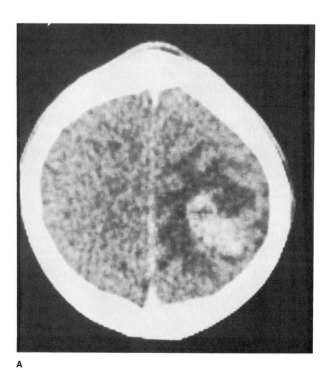

A

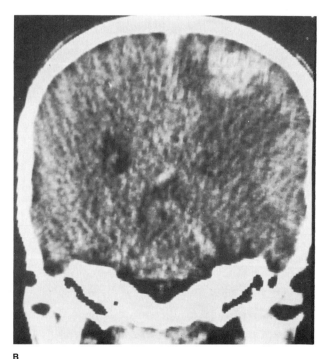

B

Figure 8-45   Glioblastoma in a 4-year-old. Postcontrast axial CT **(A)** and coronal CT **(B)** in high-grade astrocytoma. Note the volume of edema relative to the tumor volume and the intense enhancement of the neoplasm.

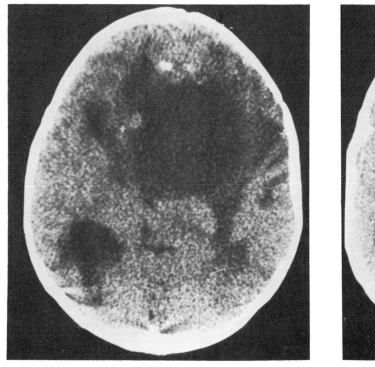

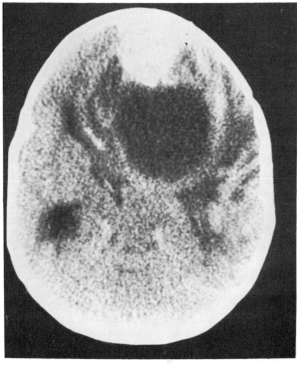

A

B

Figure 8-46   Neuroblastoma.   **A.** A large, low-density mass with regions of different degrees of hyperdensity representing calcification is present on NCCT.   **B.** CECT shows marked enhancement of the hyperdense component of the tumor, demarcating its cystic from its solid component.

cysts or necrosis, are usual. Peritumoral edema is also a common feature.

These CT findings are helpful in differentiating this neoplasm from astrocytoma, either benign or malignant. The diagnosis of neuroblastoma should be considered when calcification as well as hemorrhages with associated cystic areas are seen in a parenchymal neoplasm.

Ganglioglioma

Gangliogliomas are relatively benign parenchymal neoplasms most commonly encountered in the younger age group; 60 percent of the tumors have been reported in persons under the age of 30 years (Russell 1977).

The tumor consists of mature ganglion cells and glial tissue. Depending on the predominant cell type, the tumor has been classified as ganglioglioma (astrocytes predominant) or ganglioneuroma (ganglion cells predominant). In the series reported by Zimmerman (1979*a*), gangliogliomas constituted 14 percent of supratentorial tumors in the pediatric age group. The neoplasm is most common in the cerebral parenchyma, often in the region of the anterior third ventricle. It is usually solid, although cyst formation and calcification within it are not uncommon. The tumor appears on CT as an isodense mass with some enhancement. Punctate calcifications within the tumor are often seen (see Chapter 7).

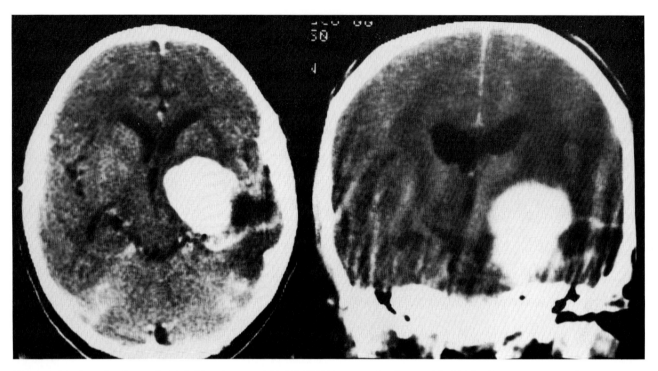

Figure 8-47 Ganglioglioma. Axial (left) and coronal (right) CECT images of a 9-year-old girl. The homogeneous enhancement with minimal surrounding edema is unusual for this tumor. Its location may suggest a meningioma.

Bibliography

ANDERSON FM, SEGALL HD, CATON WL: Use of computerized tomography scanning in supratentorial arachnoid cyst. *J Neurosurg* **50**:33, 1979.

BYRD SE, HARWOOD-NASH DC, FITZ CR, BARRY JF, ROGOVITZ DM: Two projection computed tomography: Axial and Towne projection. *Radiology* **128**:512, 1978.

CHAMBERS EF, TURSKI PA, SOBEL D, WASA W, NEWTON TH: Radiologic characteristics of primary cerebral neuroblastomas. *Radiology* **139**:101–106, 1981.

COIN CG, COIN JW, GLOVER MB: Vascular tumors of the choroid plexus: Diagnosis by computed tomography. *J Comput Assist Tomogr* **1**:146–148, 1977.

EISENBERG HM, SARWAR M, SCHOCHET S: Symptomatic Rathke's cleft cysts. *J Neurosurg* **45**:585–588, 1976.

FITZ CR, HARWOOD-NASH DC, CHUANG SH, RESJO IM: The clival-perpendicular or modified Waters' view in computed tomography. *Neuroradiology* **16**:15–16, 1978a.

FITZ CR, WORTZMAN G, HARWOOD-NASH DC, HOLGATE RC, BARRY JF, BOLDT DW: Computed tomography in craniopharyngioma. *Radiology* **127**:687–691, 1978b.

FUTRELL NN, OSBORNE AG, CHESON BD: Pineal region of tumors: CT—pathological spectrum. *Am J Neuroradiol* **2**:415–420, 1981.

GOI A: Cerebellar astrocytomas in childhood. *Am J Dis Child* **106**:21–24, 1963.

GOSHHAJRA K, BHAGAI-NAINI P, HAHN HS: Spontaneous rupture of a pineal teratoma. *Neuroradiology* **17**:215–217, 1979.

HARWOOD-NASH DC, FITZ CR: *Neuroradiology in Infants and Children.* St. Louis, The C.V. Mosby Company, 1976.

HAYMAN LA; EVANS RA; HINCK VC: Choroid plexus of the fourth ventricle: Useful CT landmark. *Am J Roentgenol* **133**:285–290, 1979.

HORTON BC, RUBENSTEIN LC: Primary cerebral neuroblastoma: Clinicopathological study in 35 cases. *Brain* **99**:735–756, 1976.

JACOBY CG, GO RT, BERAN RA: Cranial CT of neurofibromatosis. *Am J Neuroradiol* **1**:311–315, 1980.

KINGSLEY D, KENDALL BE: Dependent layering of contrast medium in cystic astrocytomas. *Neuroradiology* **14**:107–110, 1977.

KISHORE PRS, RAO KCVG, WILLIAMS JP, VINES FS: The limitations of computerized tomographic diagnosis of intracranial midline cysts. *Surg Neurol* **14**:417–431, 1980.

KOKORIS N, ROTHMAN LM, WOLINTZ AH: CT and angiography in the diagnosis of suprasellar mass lesions. *Am J Ophthalmol* **89**:278–283, 1980.

LEE BCP: Intracranial cysts. *Radiology* **130**:667–674, 1979.

LEO JS, PINTO RS, HULVAT GF, EPSTEIN F, KRICHEFF II: Computed tomography of arachnoid cysts. *Radiology* **130**:675–680, 1979.

LIN SR, BRYSON MM, GOBIEN RP, FITZ CR, LEE YY: Radiologic findings of hamartomas of the tuber cinereum and hypothalamus. *Radiology* **127**:697–703, 1978.

LIPPER MH, RAD FF, KISHORE PRS, WARD JD: Craniopharyngioma: Unusual computed tomographic presentation. *Neurosurgery* **9**:76–78, 1981.

MCCORMACK TJ, PLASSCHE WM, LIN SR: Ruptured teratoid tumor in the pineal region. *J Comput Assist Tomogr* **2**:499–501, 1978.

MESSINA AV, POTTS DG, SIGEL RM: Computed tomography evaluation of the posterior third ventricle. *Radiology* **119**:581–592, 1978.

MILLER JH, PENA AM, SEGALL HD: Radiological investigation of sellar region masses in children. *Radiology* **134**:81, 1980.

MORI K, HANDA H, TAKEUCHI J, HARAKITA J, NAKANO Y: Hypothalamic hamartoma. *J Comput Assist Tomogr* **5**:519–521, 1981.

NAIDICH TP: Infratentorial masses, in Norman D, Korobkin M, Newton T (eds): *Computed Tomography.* St. Louis, The C.V. Mosby Company, 1977a, pp 231–242.

NAIDICH TP, LIN JP, LEEDS NP, PUDLOWSKI RM, NAIDICH JB: Primary tumors and other masses of the cerebellum and fourth ventricle: Differential diagnosis by computed tomography. *Neuroradiology* **14**:153–174, 1977b.

NAIDICH TP, PINTO RS, KUSHNER MJ, LIN JP, KRICHEFF II, LEEDS NE, CHASE NE: Evaluation of sellar and parasellar masses by computed tomography. *Radiology* **120**:91, 1976.

OSBORN AG, DAINES JH, WING SK: The evaluation of ependymal and subependymal lesions by cranial computed tomography. *Radiology* **127**:397–401, 1978.

PROBST FP, LILIEQUIST: Assessment of posterior fossa tumors in infants and children by means of computed tomography. *Neuroradiology* **18**:9–18, 1979.

RAO KCVG, GOVINDAN S: Intracranial choriocarcinoma. *J Comput Assist Tomogr* **3**:400–404, 1979.

RAO KCVG, HARWOOD-NASH DC; FITZ CR: Neurodiagnostic studies in craniopharyngiomas in children. *Rev Interam Radiol* **2**:149–159, 1977.

REICH NE, ZELCH JV, ALFIDI RJ: Computed tomography in the detection of juxtasellar lesions. *Radiology* **118**:333–335, 1976.

RICHMOND IL, WILSON CB: Pituitary disorders in childhood and adolescence. *J Neurosurg* **49**:163–168, 1978.

RUSH JL, KUSSKE JA, DeFOE DR, PRIBRAM HW: Intraventricular craniopharyngioma. *Neurology* **25**:1094–1096, 1975.

RUSSELL DS, RUBINSTEIN LJ: *Pathology of Tumors of the Nervous System*, 4th ed. Baltimore, Williams & Wilkins, 1977.

SAVOIARDO M; HARWOOD-NASH DC; TADMORE R; SCOTTI G; MUSGRAVE M: Gliomas of the intracranial anterior optic pathways in children: the role of computed tomography, angiography, pneumoencephalography and radionuclide brain scanning. *Radiology* **138**:601–610, 1981.

SCHULLER DE, LAWRENCE TL, NEWTON WA: Childhood rhabdomyosarcomas of the head and neck. *Arch Otolaryngol* **105**:689–694, 1979.

SHUMAN RM; ALVORD EC JR; LEECH RW: The biology of childhood ependymomas. *Arch Neurol* **32**:731–739, 1975.

STRAND RD, BAKER RA, IDAHOSA JO, ARKINS TJ: Metrizamide ventriculography and computed tomography in lesions about the third ventricle. *Radiology* **128**:405–410, 1978.

SWARTZ JD; ZIMMERMAN RA; BILANIUK LT: Computed tomography of intracranial ependymomas. *Radiology* **143**:97–101, 1982.

TADMOR R, HARWOOD-NASH DC, SAVOIARDO M, SCOTTI G, MUSGRAVE M, FITZ CR, CHUANG S: Brain tumors in the first two years of life: CT diagnosis. *Am J Neuroradiol* **1**:411–418, 1980.

TAKEUCHI J, HANDA H, OTSUKA S: Neuroradiological aspects of suprasellar germinomas. *Neuroradiology* **17**:153–159, 1979.

TERA H, HORI T, MATSUTANI M, OKEDA R: Detection of cryptic vascular malformations by computed tomography. *J Neurosurg* **51**:546–551, 1979.

VOLBE BT, FOLEY KM, HOWIESON J: Normal CAT scan in craniopharyngioma. *Ann Neurol* **3**:87, 1978.

WHITE TJ, SIEGLE RL, BURCKART GJ, RAMEY DR: Rectal thiopental for sedation of children for computed tomography. *J Comput Assist Tomogr* **3**:286–288, 1979.

WILSON CB: Diagnosis and surgical treatment of childhood brain tumors. *Cancer* **35** (suppl):950–956, 1975.

WOODROW PK, GAJARAWALA J, PINCK RL: Computed tomographic documentation of a non-enhancing posterior fossa medulloblastoma: An uncommon presentation. *CT: J Comput Tomogr* **5**:41–43, 1981.

ZIMMERMAN RA, BILANIUK LT, PAHLAJANI H: Spectrum of medulloblastomas as demonstrated by computed tomography. *Radiology* **126**:137–147, 1977.

ZIMMERMAN RA, BILANIUK LT, BRUNO L, ROSENSTOCK J: Computed tomography of cerebellar astrocytoma. *Am J Roentgenol* **130**:929–933, 1978a.

ZIMMERMAN RA, BILANIUK LT, RAMEY RB, LITTMAN P: Computed tomography of pediatric craniofacial sarcoma. *CT: J Comput Tomogr* **2**:113–121, 1978b.

ZIMMERMAN RA, BILANIUK LT: Computed tomography of intracerebral gangliogliomas. *CT: J Comput Tomogr* **3**:24–30, 1979a.

ZIMMERMAN RA, BILANIUK LT: Computed tomography of choroid plexus lesions. *CT: J Comput Tomogr* **3**:93–103, 1979b.

ZIMMERMAN RA, BILANIUK LT: CT of primary and secondary craniocerebral neuroblastoma. *Am J Neuroradiol* **1**:431–434, 1980*a*.

ZIMMERMAN RA, BILANIUK LT, WOOD JH, BRUCE DA, SCHULTZ A: Computed tomography of pineal, parapineal and histologically related tumors. *Radiology* **137**:669–677, 1980*b*.

ZIMMERMAN RD, RUSSELL EJ, LEEDS NE: Axial CT recognition of anteroposterior displacement of fourth ventricle. *Am J Neuroradiol* **1**:65–70, 1980.

9

INTRACRANIAL TUMORS: METASTATIC

Krishna C.V.G. Rao

J. Powell Williams

AN OVERVIEW

Cancer is the second-leading cause of death in the United States, with 690,000 new cases a year and over 1000 deaths a day (Silverberg 1977). Extensive amounts of money are spent in the detection, palliation, and cure of cancer. Twenty percent of patients who die of systemic cancer harbor intracranial metastases (Posner 1978; Aronson 1964). These figures suggest that more patients present with intracranial metastatic disease than primary glioma, although in clinical practice, metastatic disease, when compared with all brain tumors, as reported in different series (Black 1979; VanEck 1965), constitutes only 7 to 17 percent of the brain tumors seen. This probably reflects selection of clinical material in the different series. In a recent National Cancer Institute study (Baker 1980; Potts 1980) dealing with an evaluation of CT in the diagnosis of intracranial neoplasms, metastatic brain disease accounted for nearly 31 percent (343/1071 patients) of the intracranial lesions by CT.

An important feature of CT in the diagnosis of intracranial metastases is its ability to detect small metastatic foci, especially with the present high-resolution, thin-section CT. To a certain degree the myth of the high incidence of solitary metastases seen in clinical practice as opposed to pathological studies is being resolved by better scanner resolution. Even with the sensitivity of present-generation scanners, a fair number of metastases less than 5 mm in diameter, especially in certain areas of the brain parenchyma, may remain undetected.

The authors believe that with the escalating cost of health care, CT will play an important role in the detection and management of patients with systemic cancer as well as intracranial metastases. In a study of patients with lung cancer who were neurologically intact, nearly 5 percent had asymptomatic intracranial metastases. These patients were treated on an outpatient basis by irradiation therapy, resulting in significant savings in hospital costs as well as patient morbidity (Butler 1979). Although this study included only a small number of patients, its impact on health-care costs as well as patient management is an important consideration. More such management protocols should be forthcoming in the near future, especially with escalating health-care costs. Computed tomography will play an important role in the management and care of these patients.

Metastases to the cranial vault and intracranial contents can occur from any primary source (Table 9-1). The most common primary sites or types with metastases to the brain, in order of frequency, are lung, breast, kidney, and melanoma. Less common are metastases from the gastrointestinal tract (predominantly the colon), thyroid, ovary, and prostate (Ranshoff 1975), and rarely from the pancreas and from sarcomas. In a few series nearly 50 percent of the patients presented with CNS findings as the first manifestation of their malignancy (VanEck 1965; Simionescue 1960; Vieth 1965). However, most patients with intracranial metastases have known primary sites of cancer. This information is extremely helpful in the CT diagnosis. In the authors' own series of 482 metastases detected by CT, 14 percent presented with neurological symptoms without a known primary site of cancer. The probable histologic type was suggested from the CT study and subsequently confirmed by other diagnostic studies. In 4 percent the primary source was not found after extensive diagnostic work-up of the patient, but the histologic type of the metastatic lesion was confirmed by biopsy of the intracranial lesion. Metastases may involve the cranial vault as well as the intracranial contents. Parenchymal metastases, apart from the calvarium and leptomeningeal carcinomatosis, may be solitary or multiple.

The incidence of solitary metastasis detected by various diagnostic modalities is reported to be between 50 and 55 percent (Black 1979; Walker 1973), although in autopsy series the incidence is between 25 and 40 percent (Walker, 1973; Posner 1978). In the authors' own series, the examinations were done on an EMI 1005 head scanner and Pfizer 0450 body scanner (first- and fourth-generation scanners). The overall incidence of solitary metastasis was 43 percent (Table 9-2). A subsequent analysis

Table 9-1   Primary Origin of Intracranial Metastatic Tumors

Organ System	University of Maryland series	Posner's series (1980)	Paiella's series (1976)	National Cancer Institute study (1980)
Lungs	156	61	55	129
Breast	69	33	26	44
Digestive tract	16	6	16	14
Kidney	8	11	14	4
Bladder	3	-	1	-
Genital tract	6	3	7	-
Skin and mucous membrane	1	0	4	-
Thyroid	2	0	1	-
Other	-	57	45	24
Unknown primary	-	-	-	37
Multiple primary	-	-	-	7

Table 9-2   Frequency of Solitary versus Multiple Intracranial Metastasis

	Solitary, %	Multiple, %
University of Maryland*	38	62
Posner (1980) 225 patients	47	53
Chason (1963) Autopsy series	14	86

* Based on CT-pathological correlation.

of metastatic intracranial deposits studied on the fourth-generation (Pfizer 0450) scanner demonstrated a lower incidence of solitary metastatic deposits, 38 percent. These findings suggest that with improvement in technology and utilization of higher amounts of contrast (Hayman 1980), the incidence of solitary metastasis will be closer to the results of pathological studies.

CLINICAL AND PATHOLOGICAL FINDINGS

The clinical presentation in the majority of intracranial metastatic brain tumors is due to the mass effect. These include headache, nausea, vomiting, ataxia, and papilledema (Russcalleda 1978). These findings are due to metastatic foci, either single or multiple, in the brain parenchyma, leptomeninges, or adjacent calvarium. Occasionally, the clinical presentation will be acute in onset like that of a patient with an infarct or intracerebral hemorrhage. In these patients, a careful history usually reveals episodes of headaches and transient neurological changes prior to the acute episode. Rarely, patients with intracranial metastases may present with a finding of dementia. Absence of focal neurological findings may be as high as 5 to 12 percent (Butler 1979; Jacobs 1977). Although intracranial metastases may occur in any age group, their highest incidence is between the fourth and seventh decade (Vieth 1965). Intracranial metastases, although less common, can also be seen in children. In one large series, postmortem studies demonstrated an incidence of 6 percent in 273 children (Vannucci 1974).

Brain metastases are often circumscribed. Central necrosis is fairly common. A few of them may have discernible calcification (Potts 1964). Parenchymal metastases are most often seen at the junction of the gray and white matter. Edema forms a significant component of the mass seen, even with small metastases. There have been very few reports dealing with the ultrastructural alteration in the brain parenchyma secondary to intracranial metastases, although absence of the tight junctions in the

blood vessels of the tumor has been noted (Hirano 1972; Long 1970). Suffice it to say that the vascular architecture within the metastatic deposit is often similar to the cellular-vascular architecture in the primary cancer. Ultrastructural alteration in the form of fenestrated vessels has been reported with metastatic hypernephroma (Hirano 1975; Hirano 1972). Similar changes probably occur in other types of metastases, although no detailed analysis of the vascular anatomy in different types of cerebral metastases is available. The presence of the metastatic deposit within the brain parenchyma probably causes an alteration in the blood-brain barrier associated with varying degrees of edema, as manifested by enchancement on CT scan. The different amounts of edema with different cell types of tumor probably reflect a specific tissue response. The edema seen on CT in different types of intracranial metastases, in association with the enhancement pattern, may thus help indicate the histological cell type.

In an analysis of 482 metastases in the authors' series, where histological proof was available in 294 cases (Tables 9-3, 9-4), metastatic tumors which

Table 9-3 Frequency of Pathological Confirmation of Source of Intracranial Metastases

Site of tissue	No. of cases	Adeno-	Oat-cell	Squa-mous	Mela-noma	Other
Primary + intracranial	98	38	23	21	8	12
Primary only	182	67	36	36	24	15*
Intracranial only	14	4	3	3	1	3†
TOTAL	294	109	62	60	33	30

* Based on 294 of the 482 cases for which pathological confirmation was available from either surgical specimen or autopsy.
† The 15 patients in this category included patients with metastatic tumors which did not fall in the above histological group. Three patients had bladder cancer, three renal cell carcinoma, two thyroid metastasis and one squamous cell carcinoma.
‡ The three patients in this group included two with multicentric glioma and one with coccidioidomycosis.

Table 9-4   Cellular Differentiation from the Various Organs*

Site (or type)	No. of cases	Adeno-	Oat-cell	Squa-mous	Undiffer-entiated
Lungs	156	55	58	37	6
Breast	69	47	-	14	8
Melanoma	33	-	-	-	-
Digestive tract	16	9	-	-	7
Kidney	8	3	-	-	5
Genitourinary tract	3	-	-	-	-
Reproductive system	6	3	-	-	3
Thyroid	2	-	-	-	2
Skin	1	-	-	-	1

* Based on 294 proved cases in authors' series. Categorization was done on the basis of maximum cell population.

were relatively less vascular demonstrated the maximum amount of edema. This was further confirmed in proven intracranial metastases from different cell types of lung carcinomas. Analysis of the amount of edema on CT shows that usually adenocarcinoma has the maximum surrounding edema, with oat cell carcinoma next and squamous cell carcinoma having the least edema. It has also been noted that edema may increase dramatically coincident with central necrosis in a tumor. The tumors with the poorest blood supply are probably earliest to develop central necrosis. Potts et al. (1980), however, in their analysis of metastatic tumors, did not find this to be a useful feature in analysis of different types of metastases.

THE ROLE OF NEURODIAGNOSTIC STUDY

The detection of intracranial metastases as well as their management has been revolutionized by the availability of CT. There has been a dramatic decrease in the demand for other diagnostic modalities except in unusual circumstances (Table 9-5). *Plain skull views* in metastatic work-up are indicated only when there is suspicion of calvarial metastases on CT, to demonstrate the location of the lesion visualized by CT as well as to search for other smaller calvarial metastatic foci, particularly if they are osteoblastic.

Radionuclide brain scan is rarely indicated with the CT scanner resolution presently available. The complementary role of CT and radionuclide scanning had been the subject of a series of reports in the early days of CT (Gawler 1974; Gado 1975; New 1975; Pendergrass 1975; Bradfield 1977; Fordham 1977). In these reports, although all agreed on the superiority of CT in detecting intracranial pathology, radionuclide scan was felt to be slightly superior to CT in the detection of metastases which were less than 1 cm in size located in the posterior fossa. Factors which decreased the sensitivity of CT studies in these early reports were related to the fixed matrix (80×80 or 160×160) and slice thickness available in the earlier CT scanner as well as the amount of contrast utilized in those studies. Comparative studies (Table 9-6) made by different authors support the present role of CT as the primary modality of examination for intracranial neoplasms, including metastatic disease. Buell (1978) stated that CT was superior to radionuclide scanning in the detection of intracranial neoplasms: the detection

Table 9-5   Frequency of Neurodiagnostic Studies—University of Maryland Hospital

Type of study	1975	1980	Change, %
Skull radiography (neuro-related)	740	323	− 56
Radionuclide brain scan	1590	236	− 84
Cerebral angiography	479	421	− 12
Pneumoencephalogram	87	2	− 97
Cranial computed tomogram	1953	5027	+ 257

Table 9-6 Comparison of Radionuclide Brain Scan and Cranial CT

	CT/RN both +	CT + RN −	CT − RN +	CT − RN −
NCI study (Potts et al. 1980), 225 patients	174	43	1	7
Bradfeld et al. (1977) 47 patients	44	44		
Pendergrass et al. (1975) 22 patients*	19	3		
Univ. of Maryland Hosp. series 187 patients†	161	23	1	2

* Only patients with metastases were used for comparison.
† Only patients who had both CT and radionuclide brain scans are included in this table.

rate (sensitivity) was 99 percent for CT and 91 percent for radionuclide brain scanning. In this series, it was also possible to correctly identify tumor type (specificity) in 76 percent of neoplasms by CT as against 69 percent by radionuclide scanning.

Radionuclide scanning has a place in the evaluation of patients with cranial or intracranial metastases, primarily in the group of patients who have a definite history of prior allergic reaction to intravenous contrast medium as well as a few patients in whom motion is a problem. The radionuclide study may also be useful for localizing the tumor on the patient's scalp before craniotomy.

Cerebral angiography is rarely necessary for evaluation of intracranial parenchymal metastases, but there are some situations in which it is helpful. As an example, when a solitary hemorrhagic lesion is seen on noncontrast CT (NCCT) which appears to accentuate further on contrast-enhanced CT (CECT), in the absence of a known systemic cancer the lesion may be difficult to differentiate from other intracranial pathologic processes such as ruptured vascular malformation, primary intracranial glioma, or abscess. Cerebral angiography is also occasionally helpful in differentiating a primary glioma from

a solitary metastasis, but more often it is performed to provide a map of the arteries and superficial veins relative to the neoplasm when surgery is contemplated.

Pneumoencephalography has no place in the evaluation of intracranial metastases.

Computed tomography is today most often the initial study performed when evaluating for intracranial metastases. With the improvement in technology, as well as use of increased amounts of contrast material, the detection rate of metastatic lesions by CT has improved significantly. Most centers have evolved various protocols for CT studies, with guidelines for contrast enhancement (Latchaw 1978b; Kramer 1975). The necessity of NCCT in evaluation of intracranial pathology has been the subject of a few reports (Butler 1978; Latchaw 1977). Elimination of NCCT may result in decreasing the radiation dose to the patient. However, the authors believe that eliminating NCCT may cause the examiners to miss fresh hemorrhage or calcification of a tumor when masked by contrast enhancement. These findings can occasionally be of clinical importance. NCCT followed by CECT may help characterize the tumor histologically and provide the optimum mode of study in screening patients for metastases in the initial work-up. However, for practical purposes, procurement of CECT only in patients with a known primary tumor may suffice in the management of the patient. Occasionally, thin sections (2 to 5 mm) following a high dose of contrast are necessary to demonstrate multiplicity of metastatic lesions (Fig. 9-1), especially when the decision as to the treatment modality of both the primary and intracranial metastases depends on the CT findings.

CT DIAGNOSIS

Calvarial Metastases

The incidence of metastatic involvement of the cranial vault or base is approximately 5 percent (Willis 1973). Calvarial metastases may present as lytic or blastic lesions, although most commonly there is an

Figure 9-1 A. *Left:* Contrast-enhanced CT. Initial CT following 42 g iodine and using 13 mm section thickness demonstrates a single enhancing lesion. *Right:* Following 56 g iodine and using 5 mm section thickness, the enhancing lesion is well visualized. **B.** On this examination, other lesions are also present.

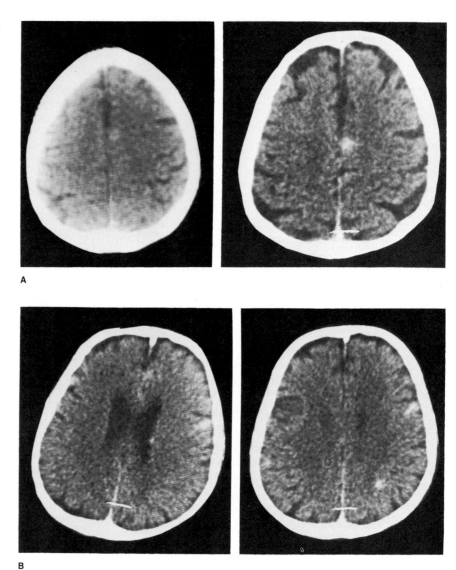

A

B

admixture. The result may be expansion of the inner and outer table, causing compression of the brain parenchyma (Fig. 9-2). When the involvement is predominantly of the inner table, with extension over the surface of the dura or invasion through the dura, determination of a purely epidural or subdural component is difficult (Fig. 9-3). The most common primary cancers associated with calvarial

or dural metastases, in the authors' experience as well as those reported in the literature (Naheedy 1980, Deck 1980), are those of the prostate, breast, lung, and kidney. The metastatic lesion may have a crescentic or biconvex appearance. The shape of the lesion is not helpful in distinguishing an epidural from a subdural metastasis (Fig. 9-4). Bony changes can be missed if CT is viewed with a nar-

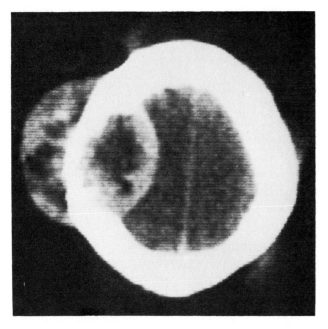

Figure 9-2 Metastases from renal carcinoma involving the calvarium, with expansion of the inner and outer table of the skull.

row window setting. To demonstrate the calvarial lesions, visualization at a very wide window setting is best (Fig. 9-5).

Lytic lesions, particularly in the region of the vertex, may be missed on CT, and coronal views are necessary for best evaluation. Becker (1978) determined that lesions less than 4 mm in diameter may not be detected by CT because of partial-volume averaging. However, with thinner sections and higher kVp this resolution can be improved. In metastatic involvement of the base of the skull, sella, and sphenoid sinus, CT in axial and coronal planes provides better demonstration of the destructive lesion than conventional radiographs (Fig. 9-6).

Epidural and Subdural Metastases

Fifteen percent of metastatic foci in the cranial vault or base of the skull extend into the epidural or subdural space (Naheedy 1980). Distinction of subdural or epidural extension from calvarial metastases by CT is difficult (Naheedy 1980; Chirathivat

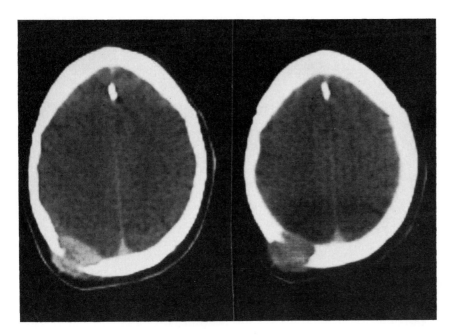

Figure 9-3 Metastases from adenocarcinoma of the kidney involving the calvarium, with epidural extension.

Figure 9-4 A. Epidural metastases from adenocarcinoma of the breast. The enhancing dura is well defined. At a wider window setting, the destructive process involving the calvarium is well defined. **B.** Another patient with subdural metastases. Lack of inner table involvement excludes epidural metastases.

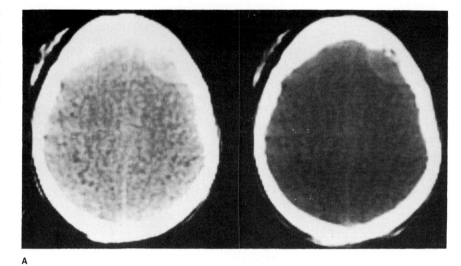

A

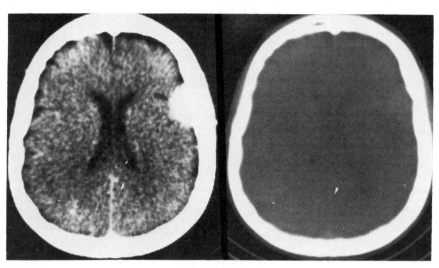

B

Figure 9-5 Axial CT in a patient with adenocarcinoma of the lung. Extensive calvarial involvement is visualized, with epidural extension.

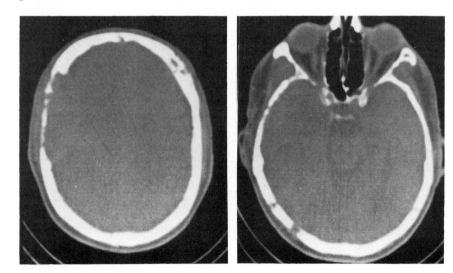

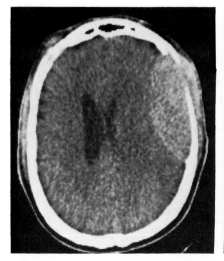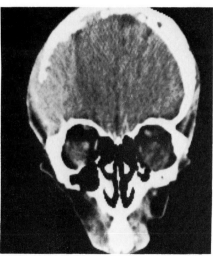

Figure 9-6 Axial and coronal CT are useful in demonstrating the total extent of the disease, as in this patient.

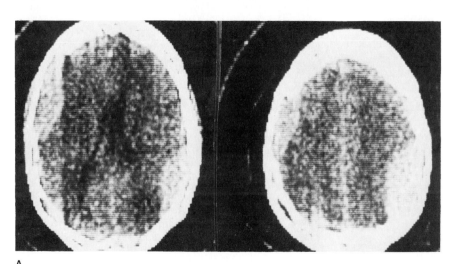

A

Figure 9-7 **(A)** Noncontrast and **(B)** contrast-enhanced CT in a patient with diffuse osteoblastic metastases and associated epidural metastases bilaterally mimicking subdural hematoma. Enhancement of the metastases differentiates them from hematoma.

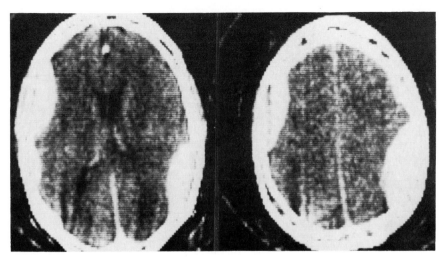

B

1980). Subdural or epidural extension of calvarial metastases is diagnosed on the basis of an irregular, moth-eaten appearance of the inner table of the skull in association with a crescent-shaped adjacent lesion, which most often shows enhancement on CECT. Differentiation of subdural metastasis from a subdural hematoma may be difficult, especially in the absence of a known systemic primary cancer. Homogeneous enhancement of the lesion is, however, highly suggestive of subdural metastasis rather than subdural hematoma (Fig. 9-7).

Intracerebral Metastases

CT has revolutionized diagnostic accuracy in intracerebral metastatic disease. It permits an earlier evaluation of patients with primary systemic cancer, providing better localization and more accurate estimation of the number or extent of metastatic deposits, with the least amount of patient morbidity.

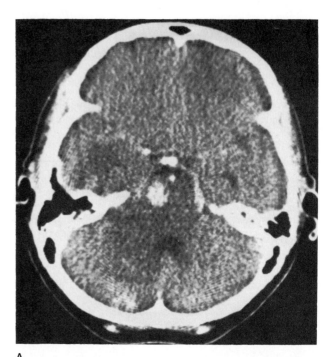

A

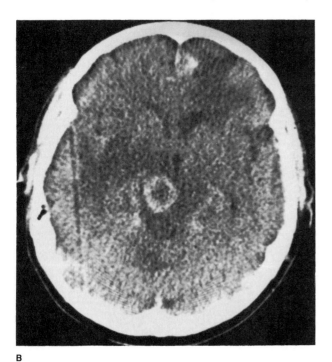

B

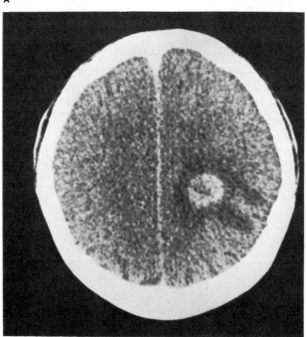

C

Figure 9-8 CECT in a patient with multiple metastatic deposits, some with necrotic centers. Extension of the edema at the gray/white-matter junction has the appearance of fingerlike projections.

On NCCT, metastatic deposits are delineated by change in tissue density and by brain edema. The extent of brain edema is variable but commonly exceeds the tumor volume. Edema is commonly seen involving the white matter, with fingerlike projections into the gray matter, which tends to be spared (Fig. 9-8). The edema may be hemispherical and may be associated with only a single small enhancing lesion on CECT. At other times, when many metastatic deposits are present on CECT, the NCCT may appear completely normal (Fig. 9-9).

The metastatic deposits on NCCT may be hypodense, hyperdense, or similar in density to normal brain tissue. These appearances are related to a variety of factors such as cellular density, tumor neovascularity, and degree of necrosis. Metastases from lung, breast, kidney, and colon and those from lymphoma tend to be hypodense or isodense (Deck 1980). In the authors' experience, metastatic lymphoma appeared to be isodense or hyperdense. Hyperdensity on NCCT is commonly due to a dense cellular structure, and these metastases appear slightly denser than normal brain tissue but certainly less dense than when there is hemorrhage or calcification, either within or adjacent to the tumor.

It is not uncommon for hemorrhage to occur in metastases (Fig. 9-10), as in some primary gliomas of the brain; 3.7 percent of all gliomas show intra-

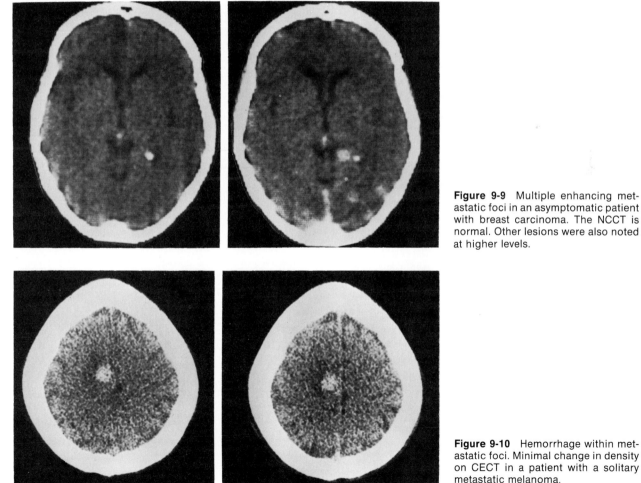

Figure 9-9 Multiple enhancing metastatic foci in an asymptomatic patient with breast carcinoma. The NCCT is normal. Other lesions were also noted at higher levels.

Figure 9-10 Hemorrhage within metastatic foci. Minimal change in density on CECT in a patient with a solitary metastatic melanoma.

tumoral or adjacent hematoma (Olderberg 1933). Although similar data are not available for intracerebral metastases, the detection rate by CT of hemorrhage within tumors, primary or metastatic, is probably high (Little 1979).

Among metastatic tumors, intratumoral hemorrhage is most commonly seen with melanoma and choriocarcinoma and less commonly with hypernephroma and lung carcinoma (Deck 1976; Gildersleeve 1977; Solis 1977; Mandybur 1977; Enzmann 1978b; Little 1979). A variety of factors have been implicated to explain hemorrhage within metastatic tumors. Conditions such as hypertension, coagulopathy, and extreme tumor vascularity are predisposing factors. Chemotherapy and radiation therapy may also produce hemorrhage within tumors.

Hemorrhage may be associated with rapid increase in size of a metastatic focus or may be from adjacent damaged brain tissue (Mandybur 1977). Hemorrhage may be the first sign of a previously unsuspected metastatic tumor or other neoplasm (Weisberg 1977). Diagnosis of hemorrhage within a metastatic tumor by CT depends on the time interval between the episode and CT examination, as well as other factors such as location of the hematoma and amount of surrounding edema. Contrast enhancement may or may not be helpful, since hemorrhagic infarcts, unlike solid hematomas, may demonstrate some degree of enhancement, like a neoplasm with hemorrhage. Contrast enhancement may obscure hemorrhage or calcification in tumors, and a preliminary unenhanced scan is important in the diagnosis.

Unlike hemorrhage, calcification within a metastatic tumor is rare, except in metastatic osteogenic sarcoma (Danziger 1979). However, 5 to 6 percent of metastatic brain tumors tend to show calcific densities within the lesion (Potts 1964). The calcification is usually discrete and scattered rather than homogeneous and often occurs following radiation therapy.

ENHANCEMENT PATTERN IN METASTASES

Contrast enhancement of metastatic tumors, as in other enhancing lesions, is presumed to be due to the tumor vascularity and blood-brain or blood-tumor barrier defects (Lewander 1978). Most metastatic neoplasms demonstrate enhancement, although the degree of enhancement is variable. In a study in which both CT and radionuclide scans were performed, only one metastatic neoplasm

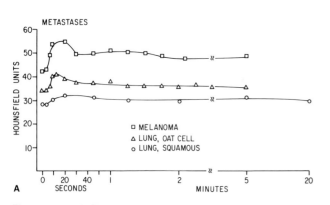

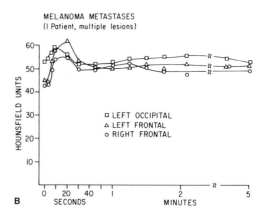

Figure 9-11   A. Time curves of density numbers in three different types of intracranial metastasis. Apart from the initial phase, no change in density is seen with increase in time. The curves also demonstrate the difference in density numbers between the different types of metastasis.   **B.** Time/density curve in multiple melanoma. No change seen in the curves in spite of the different size and location of the melanoma deposits. *(Courtesy of Dr. S.D. Wing, University of Utah.)*

failed to enhance on CT (Bradfield 1977). The degree of enhancement depends on such factors as the initial density of the lesion (on NCCT), the volume of contrast material administered, the elapsed time between contrast infusion and CT study, and the influence of therapeutic drugs, mainly steroids, although radiation and chemotherapy may both cause changes in density and enhancement characteristics. Apart from these general factors, the degree of enhancement in different metastatic tumors depends also on the cellular structure and vascularity. Intracranial metastasis from choriocarcinoma, melanoma, thyroid tumors, and occasionally hypernephroma demonstrates the maximum degree of enhancement. This probably is related to the highly vascular nature of the metastasis. Although enhancement in metastatic melanoma has been reported in 82 percent of lesions (Enzmann 1978*b*) and reflects the authors' own findings, others have reported low incidence of enhancement of melanoma metastases (Deck 1980; Solis 1977).

Metastatic foci which are relatively denser on NCCT enhance less on CECT than lesions which are hypodense on NCCT (Hilal 1978). The authors' experience in evaluating intracranial metastases indicates that squamous cell metastases which are relatively denser on NCCT demonstrate the least degree of enhancement; in increasing order of enhancement come adenocarcinoma, oat-cell carcinoma, melanoma, and choriocarcinoma. Similar findings based on time/density curves have also been shown by others (Wing 1980) (Fig. 9-11). The pattern of enhancement is nonspecific, appearing as ring enhancement or as solid density. Purely gyral enhancement, as seen in infarction or occasionally infiltrating gliomas, is rarely seen with metastases.

Metastatic lesions in general have a relatively larger low-density area, probably representing edema, when compared with the size of the enhancing component. Presence of multiple enhancing lesions is highly suggestive of metastatic disease in a patient known to have extracranial primary cancer. However, in the presence of multiple enhancing lesions and absence of a known primary cancer, multicentric or multifocal glioma (Fig. 9-12), as well as abscesses and rarely meningioma should be considered (Rao 1980).

Histological specificity has been attempted, utilizing the commonly seen denominators such as degree of enhancement, relative volume of edema in relation to the enhancing lesion, and density of the lesion on NCCT (Rao 1979). The following features were noted in metastases of different histologic type:

1. In metastatic melanoma (Fig. 9-13), the lesions were denser than the adjacent parenchyma, with minimal edema. Hemorrhage was seen in nearly 30 percent of cases. There was significant enhancement on CECT.
2. Oat-cell carcinoma (Fig. 9-14) demonstrated lesions isodense with or slightly denser than normal brain parenchyma. Most oat-cell metastases showed significant enhancement, with mild to moderate surrounding hypodensity. Although these tumors are histologically prone to central necrosis, a central low-density area in oat-cell carcinoma was less commonly seen.
3. The typical metastatic adenocarcinoma (Fig. 9-15) was usually isodense with or minimally denser than normal brain parenchyma. Edema was more prominent and usually greater than the volume of the enhancing lesion. Ring pattern was a common feature seen in 62 percent of the cases.
4. Squamous-cell metastases (Fig. 9-16) were associated with large low-density areas. Nonhomogeneous enhancement was a common feature. The degree of enhancement was less when compared with other cell types of metastases.
5. Metastatic lymphoma (Fig. 9-17) involving the brain are similar to primary lymphoma. Differentiation from glioma can be difficult (Kazner 1978). These metastases tended to have ill-defined margins with homogeneous enhancement. Periventricular spread of tumor was common (DuBois 1978), although other types of metastasis may also present with homogeneous periventricular enhancement.

Figure 9-12 Multiple enhancing lesions suggestive of metastatic disease, which was subsequently proved to be multicentric glioma.

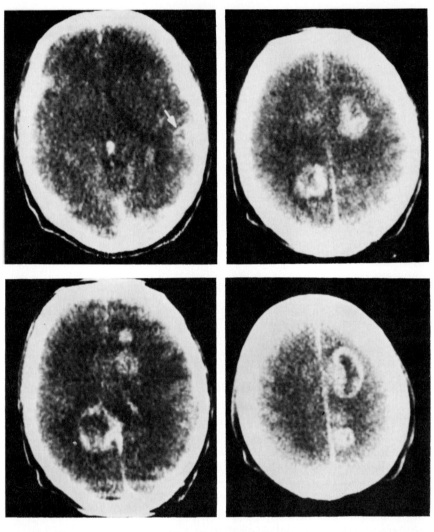

Figure 9-13 Metastatic melanoma. Slightly denser lesion than adjacent parenchyma on NCCT, which enhances significantly on CECT. The amount of edema is minimal.

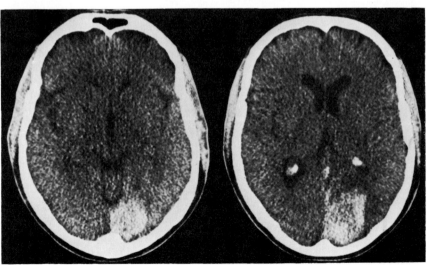

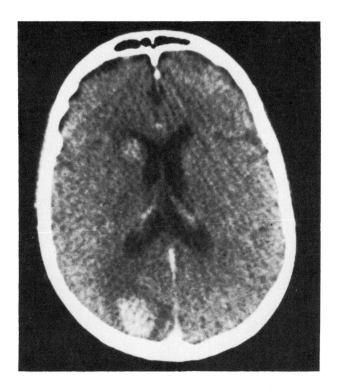

Figure 9-14 Metastasis in a patient with proven oat-cell carcinoma of the lung. The hypodense area, which most often represents edema relative to the enhancing component, is small.

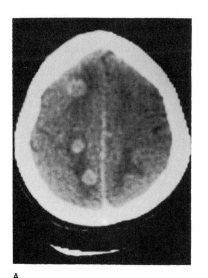

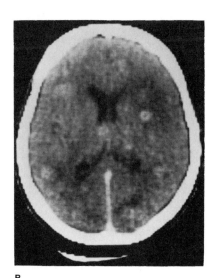

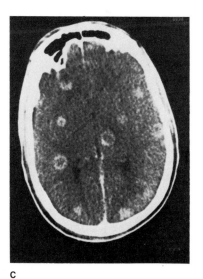

A

B

C

Figure 9-15 Metastatic adenocarcinoma: three examples. **A.** Typical appearance: NCCT demonstrates an isodense or slightly denser area surrounded by a large hypodensity. A ring lesion is seen on CECT. **B.** Another patient with adenocarcinoma of the colon demonstrates multiple enhancing ring lesion. The ratio of edema (low density) relative to the enhancing metastases is less. **C.** Metastatic adenocarcinoma in a patient treated with steroids. Note the lack of edema around the multiple enhancing ring lesions.

Figure 9-16 Metastatic squamous cell carcinoma. A solitary minimally enhancing lesion with significant edema is present. A ring lesion or non-homogeneous enhancement is not uncommon.

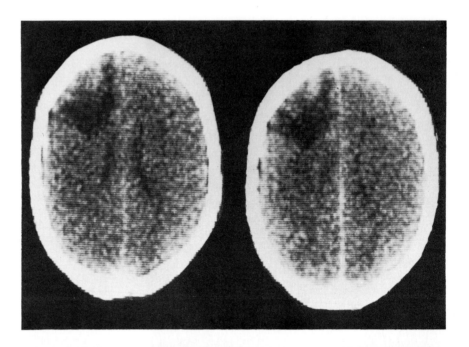

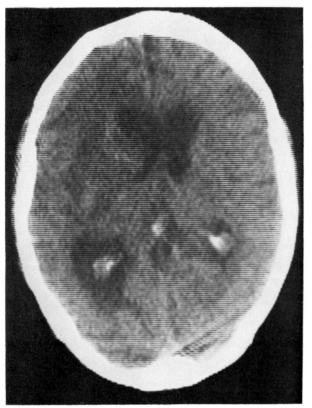

A

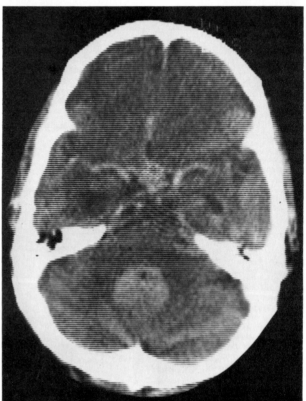

B

MENINGEAL CARCINOMATOSIS

Meningeal carcinomatosis is due to infiltration of the basal cisterns and leptomeninges. On CECT, intense enhancement of gyri and basal cisterns has been described (Enzmann 1978*a*). Enhancement was seen more commonly in patients with melanoma (100 percent) and carcinoma (44 percent) than in those with leukemia and lymphoma (3 percent), although these tumors are more prone to spread along the leptomeningeal surface. Presence of this type of enhancement pattern on CECT is highly suggestive of leptomeningeal carcinomatosis (Fig. 9-18), although only a minority of patients with positive CSF cytology demonstrate this finding. Hydrocephalus was seen in only 11 percent of patients,

but rapid increase in size of ventricles on serial CT is almost pathognomonic of leptomeningeal carcinomatosis (Fig. 9-18).

DIFFERENTIAL DIAGNOSIS

An attempt has been made to define the CT pattern in metastatic disease, with some criteria relating to specific histological patterns. A variety of intracranial processes may mimic metastases, including primary brain tumors, meningiomas, infarcts, and abscesses. Other less common entities which may be confused with intracerebral metastases include multiple sclerosis, drug-induced leukoencephalopathy, multifocal leukoencephalopathy, and radiation necrosis.

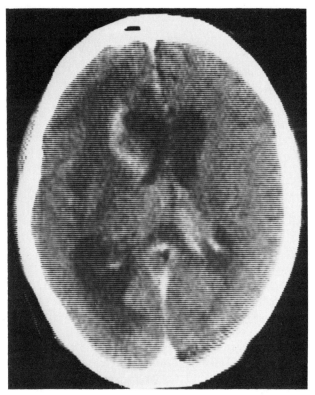

C

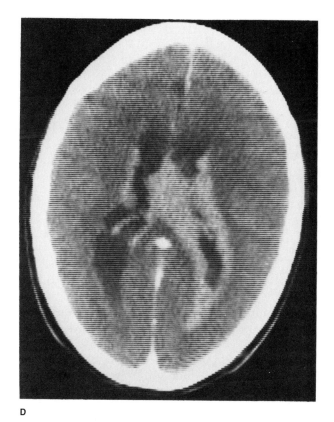

D

Figure 9-17 Metastatic lymphoma. Homogeneous periventricular spread of tumor. Similar spread may also be seen in primary glioma or other types of metastases. **A.** NCCT. **B, C, D.** CECT.

Figure 9-18   **A.** CECT in a patient with proven leptomeningeal carcinomatosis. There is significant enhancement of the subarachnoid cisterns. The ventricles are not enlarged.   **B.** CECT in the same patient 3 weeks later. Apart from enhancement of the subarachnoid cisterns, there is enlargement of the ventricular system, indicating communicating hydrocephalus. *(Courtesy of Dr. A.J. Kumar, Johns Hopkins Hospital.)*

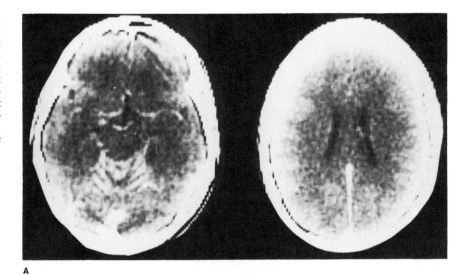

A

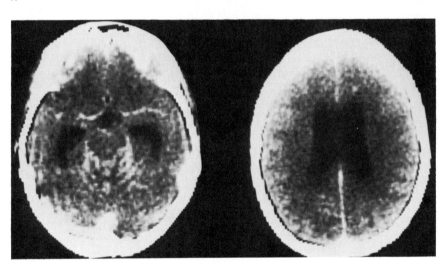

B

In multiple sclerosis, during the active phase, enhancing lesions with surrounding low density may be seen on CECT (Fig. 9-19) (Cala 1976; Aita 1978; Allen 1978; Sears 1978). They usually disappear spontaneously in a few weeks, unlike metastases, and occur only during an acute exacerbation.

In drug-induced leukoencephalopathy, focal or generalized areas of low density are present. They usually do not show any enhancement. Some amount of ventricular enlargement is a common feature. Differentiation from leptomeningeal carcinomatosis may occasionally be difficult.

Progressive multifocal leukoencephalopathy is commonly seen in patients who have been treated by chemotherapy for systemic cancer and subjected to immunosuppression. Areas of decreased density on CT are common. Most often these are located periventricularly in the frontal or occipital area and are symmetrical. Differentiation from cerebral metastasis is based on the location of these low-density areas and by lack of enhancement (Lane 1978; Norman 1978). Diagnosis of progressive multifocal leukoencephalopathy is by brain biopsy and viral culture.

RADIATION NECROSIS

Occasionally in the past prophylactic radiation to the brain was utilized as part of the treatment of systemic cancer. Radiation-induced necrosis of the brain may present as a mass lesion (Fig. 9-20). On CT such lesions are usually hypodense, with some contrast enhancement and surrounding edema (Mikhael 1978). Differentiation from primary or metastatic tumor or abscess by CT alone is difficult (Danziger 1979).

CT FOLLOWING TREATMENT MODALITIES

Following various therapeutic modalities, CT provides an innocuous method of evaluating their efficacy. The edema-reducing effect of steroids and

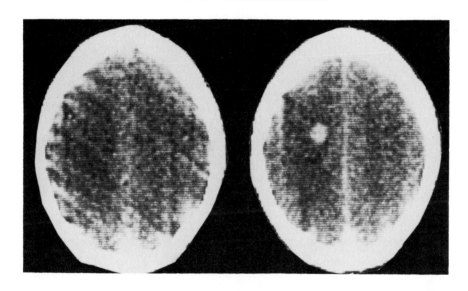

Figure 9-19 Patient with multiple sclerosis. An enhancing lesion is present with surrounding edema, which is nonspecific and may be seen in a variety of lesions. *(Courtesy of Dr. P.R.S. Kishore, Medical College of Virginia.)*

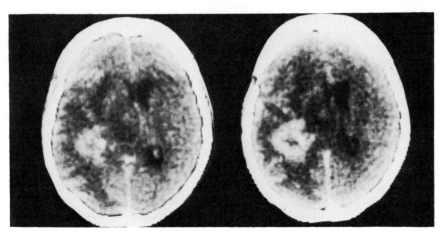

Figure 9-20 Postradiation necrosis. The enhancing ring lesion with surrounding edema could represent either primary or metastatic tumor. Mass proved at autopsy to represent postradiation necrosis with sarcomatous changes in a patient who had had surgery for solitary metastasis.

the dramatic clinical response to them are well known. Steroids may also decrease the degree of enhancement within the metastasis and occasionally may mask metastatic foci. This effect of corticosteroid has been shown both on CT and on radionuclide brain scan (Crocker 1976).

Serial CT studies are also useful in determining the response to various chemotherapeutic agents and radiation therapy (Hyman 1978; Kretzchmar 1978). Most chemotherapeutic agents have not had significant impact in metastatic brain tumors. On the other hand, dramatic response can be observed following radiation therapy, especially in oat-cell carcinoma (Fig. 9-21). Unfortunately, the metastases

Figure 9-21 CECT in a patient with metastases from oat-cell carcinoma. **A.** Preradiation. **B.** Postradiation. Demonstrates role of CT in evaluating intracranial metastasis.

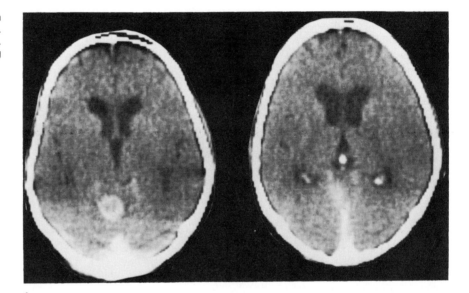

A

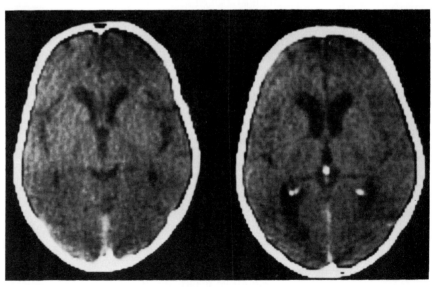

B

reappear with both modalities, eventually exceeding their original size. Treatment may increase the density of tumors on NCCT or decrease the density by producing necrosis. Enhancement characteristics may be altered as with steroids.

Delayed effects of radiation therapy include postradiation cerebral atrophy, which may be suggested by CT when there is an increase in the size of the ventricles and sulci. Other complications have been discussed earlier.

SUMMARY

CT in metastatic disease has resulted in the following benefits: (1) earlier evaluation of patients suspected of having intracranial metastases; (2) better determination of the number, size, and location of metastatic foci; (3) noninvasive follow-up of the various treatment modalities; and (4) occasional suggestion of possible primary site or sites when not already known.

Bibliography

ARONSON SM, GARCIA JH, AARONSON BE: Metastatic neoplasms of the brain: Their frequency in relation to age. *Cancer* **17**:558–563, 1964.

AITA JF, BENNETT DR, ANDERSON RE, ZITER F: Cranial CT appearance of acute multiple sclerosis. *Neurology* **28**:251–255, 1978.

ALLEN JC, THALER HT, DECK MDF, ROTHENBERG DA: Leukoencephalopathy following high-dose intravenous methotrexate chemotherapy: Quantitative assessment of white matter attenuation using computed tomography. *Neuroradiology* **16**:46–64, 1978.

BAKER HI, HOUSER OW, CAMPBELL JK: National Cancer Institute study: Evaluation of computed tomography in diagnosis of intracranial neoplasms. *Radiology* **136**:91–96, 1980.

BECKER H, NORMAN D, BOYD DP, HATTNER RS, NEWTON TH: Computed tomography in detecting calvarial metastases: A comparison with skull radiography and radionuclide scanning. *Neuroradiology* **16**:504–505, 1978.

BLACK P: Brain metastasis: Current status and recommended guidelines for management. *Neurosurgery* **5**(5):617–631, 1979.

DUBOULAY GH, RADUE EW: Comparison of computerized tomography with other neuroradiological methods: A plea for a different kind of analysis. *Neuroradiology* **16**:474–476, 1978.

BRADFIELD PA, PASSALAQUE AM, BRAUNSTEIN P, RAGHAUENDRA BN, LEEDS NE, KRICHEFF II: A comparison of radionuclide scanning and computed tomography in metastatic lesions of the brain. *J Comput Asst Tomogr* **1**:315–318, 1977.

BRISMAR J, STROMBLAD LG, SALFORD LG: Impact of CT in neurosurgical management of intracranial tumors. *Neuroradiology* **16**:506–509, 1978.

BUELL U, NIENDORF HP, STEINHOFF H: Validity of serial scintigraphy with 97m Tc-Pertechnetate in comparison with computerized tomography, in Lauksch W, Kazner E (eds): *Cranial Computerized Tomography.* New York, Springer-Verlag 1976, pp 177–182.

BUELL U, NIENDORF HP, KAZNER E, LAUKSCH W, WILSKE J, STEINHOFF H, GAHR H: Computerized transaxial tomography and cerebral serial scintigraphy in intracranial tumors—Rates of detection and tumor type identification: Concise communication. *J Nucl Med* **19**:476–479, 1978.

BUTLER AR, KRICHEFF II: Noncontrast CT scanning: Limited value in suspected brain tumors. *Radiology* **126**:689–693, 1978.

BUTLER AR, LEO JS, LIN JP, BOYD AD, KRICHEFF II: The value of routine cranial computed tomography in neurologically intact patients with primary carcinoma of the lung. *Radiology* **131**:399–401, 1979.

CALA IA, MASTAGLIA FL: Computerized axial tomography in multiple sclerosis. *Lancet* **1**:689, 1976.

CHASON JL, WALTER FB, LANDERS JW: Metastatic carcinoma in the central nervous system and dorsal root ganglia. A prospective study. *Cancer* **16**:781–787, 1963.

CHIRATHIVAT S, POST MJD: CT demonstration of dural metastases in neuroblastoma. *J Comput Assist Tomogr* **4** (3): 316–319, 1980.

CONSTANT P: Cerebral metastases—A study of computed tomography. *Comput Tomogr* **1**:84–94, 1977.

CROCKER EF, ZIMMERMAN RA, PHELPS ME, KUHL DE: The effect of steroids on the extra-vascular distribution of radiographic contrast material and technetium pertechnetate in brain tumors as determined by computed tomography. *Radiology* **119**:471–476, 1976.

DANZIGER J, WALLACE S, HANDEL SF, DESANTOS LA: Metastatic osteogenic sarcoma of the brain. *Cancer* **43**:707–710, 1979.

DECK MDF, MESSINA AV, SACKETT JF: Computed tomography in metastatic disease of the brain. *Radiology* **119**:115–120, 1976.

DECK MDF: Computed tomography of metastatic disease of the brain, in Weiss L, Gilbert H, Posner J (eds): *Workshop on Brain Metastasis*, Memorial Sloan-Kettering Cancer Center, 1978. Boston, Hall, 1980.

DICHIRO G, BROOKS RM, KESSLER GS, JOHNSTON EA, HERDT JR, SHERIDAN WT: Tissue signatures from dual energy computed tomography. *Radiology* **124**:99–107, 1977.

DUBAL L, WIGGLE U: Tomochemistry of the brain. *J Comput Assist Tomogr* **1**(3):300–307, 1977.

DUBOIS PJ, MARTINE AJ, MYEROWITZ RL, ROSENBAUM AE: Subependymal and leptomeningeal spread of systemic malignant lymphoma demonstrated by cranial computed tomography. *J Comput Assist Tomogr* **2**:218–221, 1978.

ELKE M et al: The diagnosis of intracranial metastases: The efficiency of CT and scintigraphy in patients investigated by both methods, in Lanksch W, Kazner E (eds): *Cranial Computerized Tomography*. New York, Springer-Verlag, 1976, pp 171–176.

ENZMANN DR, KRICORIAN J, YORKE C, HAYWOOD R: Computed tomography in leptomeningeal spread of tumor. *J Comput Assist Tomogr* **2**:448–455, 1978*a*.

ENZMANN DR, KRAMER R, NORMAN, D, POLLOCK J: Malignant melanoma metastatic to the central nervous system. *Radiology* **127**:177–180, 1978*b*.

FORDHAM E: The complementary role of computerized axial tomography and radionuclide imaging of the brain. *Semin Nucl Med* **7**(2): 137–159, 1977.

GADO MH, PHELPS ME: The peripheral zone of increased density in cranial computed tomography. *Radiology* **117**: 71–74, 1975.

GAWLER J, DUBOULAY GH, BUELL JWD: Computer assisted tomography (EMI scanner): Its place in investigation of suspected intracranial tumors. *Lancet* **2**:419–423, 1974.

GILDERSLEEVE N, KOO AH, MCDONALD CJ: Metastatic tumor presenting as intracerebral hemorrhage: Report of 6 cases examined by computed tomography. *Radiology* **124**:109–112, 1977.

GREITZ T: Computer tomography for diagnosis of intracranial tumors compared with other neuroradiolographic procedures. *Acta Radiol* [Suppl] (Stockh) **346**:14–20, 1975.

HAYMAN LA, EVANS RA, HINCK VC: Delayed high iodine dose contrast computed tomography: Cranial neoplasms. *Radiology* **136**:677–684, 1980.

HILAL SK, CHANG CH: Specificity of computed tomography in the diagnosis of supratentorial neoplasms. *Neuroradiology* **16**:537–539, 1978.

HIRANO A, MATSUI T: Vascular structures in brain tumors. *Human Pathol* **6**:611–621, 1975.

HIRANO A, ZIMMERMAN HM: Fenestrated blood vessels in a metastatic renal carcinoma in the brain. *Lab Invest* **26**(4):465–468, 1972.

HUCKMAN MS, ACKERMAN LV: Use of automated measurements of mean density as an adjunct to computed tomography. *J Comput Assist Tomogr* **1**(10):37–42, 1977.

HYMAN RA, LORING MI, LIEBESKIND AL, NAIDICH JB, STEIN HL: Computed tomographic evaluation of therapeutically induced changes in primary and secondary brain tumors. *Neuroradiology* **14**:213–218, 1978.

JACOBS L, KINKEL WR, VINCENT RG: Silent brain metastasis from lung carcinoma determined by computerized tomography. *Arch Neurol* **34**:690–693, 1977.

KAZNER E, WILSKE J, STEINOFF H, STOCKDORPH O: Computer assisted tomography in primary malignant lymphoma of the brain. *J Comput Assist Tomogr* **2**:125–134, 1978.

KIDO DK, GOULD R, TAASTI F, DUNCAN A, SCHNUR J: Comparative sensitivity of CT scans, radiographs and radionuclide scans in detecting metastatic calvarial lesions. *Radiology* **128**:371–375, 1978.

KRAMER RA, JANETOS GP, PENDSTEIN G: An approach to contrast enhancement in computed tomography of the brain. *Radiology* **116**:641–647, 1975.

KRETZCHMAR K, AULICH A, SCHINDER E, LANGE S, GUMME T, MEESE W: The diagnostic value of CT for radiotherapy of cerebral tumors. *Neuroradiology* **14**:245–250, 1978.

LANE B, CARROLL BA, and PEDLEY TA: Computerized cranial tomography in cerebral diseases of white matter. *Neuroradiology* **28**:534–544, 1978.

LATCHAW RE, GOLD LHA, MOORE JS, PAYNE TJ: The nonspecificity of absorption coefficients in the differentiation of solid tumors and cystic lesions. *Radiology* **125**:141–144, 1977.

LATCHAW RE, PAYNE JT, GOLD LHA: Effective atomic number and electron density as measured with a computed tomography scanner: Computation and correlation with brain tumor histology. *J Comput Assist Tomogr* **2**(2):199–208, 1978*a*.

LATCHAW RE, GOLD LHA, TOURJE EJ: A protocol for the use of contrast enhancement of cranial computed tomography. *Radiology* **126**:681–687, 1978*b*.

LEWANDER R, BERGSTROM M, BEGVALL U: Contrast enhancement of cranial lesions in computed tomography. *Acta Radiol* [Diagr] (Stockh) **19**:529–552, 1978.

LITTLE JR, DIAL B, BELANGER G, CARPENTER S: Brain hemorrhage from intracranial tumor. *Stroke* **10**(3):283–288, 1979.

LONG DM: Capillary ultrastructure in human metastatic brain tumors. *J Neurosurg* **32**:127–144, 1970.

MANDYBUR TI: Intracranial hemorrhage caused by metastatic tumors. *Neurology* **27**:650–655, 1977.

METZGER J, GARDEUR O, NACHANAKIAN A, MILLARD JC: Comparison des tomodensitometre, cinegammagraphique et angiographique dousé les diagnostics topographique et histologique préoperatives des 300 tumors intracraniennes sustentorielles. *Neuroradiology* **16**:495–498, 1978.

MARSHALL WH, EASTER W, ZATZ LM: Analysis of the dense lesion at computed tomography with dual kVp scans. *Radiology* **124**:87–89, 1977.

MESSINA AV: Cranial computed tomography. *Arch Neurol* **34**:602–607, 1977.

MIKHAEL MA: Radiation necrosis of the brain: Correlation between computed tomography pathology and distribution. *J Comput Assist Tomogr* **2**:71–80, 1978.

NAHEEDY MH, KIDO DK, O'REILLY GV: Computed tomography evaluation of subdural and epidural metastases. *J Comput Assist Tomogr* **4**(3):311–315, 1980.

NEW PFJ et al: Computed tomography with the EMI scanner in the diagnosis of primary and metastatic intracranial neoplasms. *Radiology* **114**:75–87, 1975.

NORMAN D, STEVENS EA, WING SD, LEVINE V, NEWTON TH: Quantitative aspects of contrast enhancement in cranial computed tomography. *Radiology* **129**:683–688, 1978.

OLDERBERG E: The hemorrhage into glioma: A review of eight hundred and thirty-two consecutive verified cases of glioma. *Arch Neurol Psychiatry* **30**:1061–1073, 1933.

PAILLAS JE; PELLET W: Brain metastases, in Vinken PJ and Bryn GW (eds): *Handbook of Clinical Neurology*, vol. 18. New York, American Elsevier Publishing Co., 1976, pp 201–232.

PENDERGRASS HP, MCKUSICK KA, NEW PFJ, POTSAID MS: Relative efficacy of radionuclide imaging and computed tomography of the brain. *Radiology* **116**:363–366, 1975.

PEYLAN-RAMU N, POPLACK DG, BLIE LC, HERDT GR, VERMESS D, DECHIRO G: Computer assisted tomography in methotrexate encephalopathy. *J Comput Assist Tomogr* **1**(2):216–221, 1977.

PEYLAND-RAMU N: Abnormal CT scans of the brain in asymptomatic children with acute lymphocytic leukemia after prophylactic treatment of the central nervous system with radiation and intrathecal chemotherapy. *N Engl J Med* **293**:815–818, 1978.

POSNER J.B: Brain metastases: A clinician's view, in Weiss L, Gilbert H, and Posner JB (eds): *Brain Metastases*, Boston, G.K. Hall, 1980.

POSNER JB: Diagnosis and treatment of metastases to the brain. *Clin Bull* **4**:47–57, 1974.

POSNER JB, CHERNIK NL: Intracranial metastases from systemic cancer. *Adv Neurol* **19**:575–587, 1978.

POTCHEN EJ: Radiologic approaches to the diagnosis of cerebral metastases. *Int J Radiat Oncol* **2**(1–2):173–178, 1977.

POTTS DG, SVARE GT: Calcification in intracranial metastases. *Am J Roentgenol* **92**:1249–1251, 1964.

POTTS DG, ABBOTT GF, VONSNEIDEN JV: National Cancer Institute Study: Evaluation of computed tomography in diagnosis of intracranial neoplasms: III. Metastatic tumors. *Radiology* **136**:657–664, 1980.

RANSHOFF J: Surgical management of metastatic tumors. *Semin Oncol* **2**:21–27, 1975.

RAO KCVG, KUMAR AJ, FOUAD G: Computed tomography in metastatic disease. Paper presented at 65th Annual Meeting of the Radiological Society of North America, November 1979.

RAO, KCVG, LEVINE H, SAJORE, ITANI, A, WALKER, R: CT in multicentric glioma: Radiological-pathological correlation. *CT: J Comput Tomogr* **4**(3):187–192, September 1980.

ROTHE R, FISHER K: Comparison between computerized tomography and conventional contrast medium methods in the diagnosis of brain tumors, in Lanksche W, Kazner E (eds): *Cranial Computerized Tomography*. New York, Springer-Verlag, 1976, 183–187.

RUSSCALLEDA J: Clinical symptomatology and computerized tomography in brain metastases. *Comput Tomogr* **2**(2):69–77, 1978.

SEARS ES, TINDALL RSA, ZARNOW H: Active multiple sclerosis: Enhanced computerized tomographic imaging of lesions and effects of corticosteroids. *Arch Neurol* **35**:426–436, 1978.

SILVERBERG E: Cancer statistics 1977. *CA* **27**:26–41, 1977.

SIMIONESCUE MD: Metastatic tumors of the brain: A follow-up study of 195 patients with neurosurgical considerations. *J Neurosurg* **17**:361–373, 1960.

SOLIS OJ, DAVIS KR, ADAIR LB, ROBERTSON AR, KLEINMAN G: Intracerebral metastatic melanoma—CT evaluation. *Comput Tomogr* **1**:135–143, 1977.

STEINHOFF H, KAZNER E, LAUKSCH W, GRUMME T, MEESE W, LANGE S, AULICH A, WENDE S: The limitation of computerized axial tomography in the detection and differential diagnosis of intracranial tumors: A study based on 1304 neoplasms, in Bories J (ed): *Diagnostic Limitations of Computerized Axial Tomography*. New York, Springer-Verlag, 1978.

SYLVESTER AH, DUGSTAD G, AMUNDSEN P: Computerized tomography in brain tumors correlated to histology, angiography, gas encephalography, in Lanksch W, Kazner E (eds): *Computerized Cranial Tomography*. New York, Springer-Verlag, 1978, pp 167–170.

VANECK JHM, GO KG, EBELS EJ: Metastatic tumors of the brain. *Neurol Neurochir* **68**:443–462, 1965.

VANNUCCI RC, BATEN M: Cerebral metastatic disease in childhood. *Neurology* **24**:981–985, 1974.

VIETH RG, ODOM GL: Intracranial metastases and their neurosurgical treatment. *J Neurosurg* **23**:375–383, 1965.

WALKER MD: Brain and peripheral nervous system tumors, in Holland JF, Frei E (eds): *Cancer Medicine*. Philadelphia, Lea & Febiger, 1973.

WEISBERG LA, NICE CN: Intercranial tumors simulating the presentation of cerebrovascular syndromes. *JAMA* **63**:517, 1977.

WENDLING LR: Computed tomography of intracerebral leukemic masses. *Am J Roentgenol* **132**(2):217–220, 1979.

WILLIS RA: *The Spread of Tumors in the Human Body*, 3d ed. London, Butterworth, 1973.

WING DS, ANDERSON RE, OSOBORN, AG: Cranial computed angiotomography. Paper presented at the Radiological Society of North America, Dallas, November 18, 1980.

ZIMMERMAN RA, BILANIUK LT: Computed tomography of acute intratumoral hemorrhage. *Radiology* **135**:355–359, 1980.

10

THE BASE OF THE SKULL

Harvey L. Levine

Jonathan Kleefield

Krishna C.V.G. Rao

The skull base is one of the most difficult and demanding areas to evaluate. A complex bony and nervous system anatomy is concentrated in a relatively narrow cross section of the head. Furthermore, below the skull base lie the paranasal sinuses, nasopharynx, orbits, and cervical structures, which may be involved by skull base lesions and from which some lesions may arise and extend into the skull base. The difficulty is further compounded by the proximity of critical neural structures to the skull base (hypothalamus, optic system, and brainstem), making precise anatomic definition of pathology of paramount importance. The cranial nerves course along and through the skull base en route to their innervations; arteries and veins for the brain and its coverings pass along and through the skull base as well. These structures may become involved in skull base pathology, and pathologic processes arising in them can involve the skull base and contiguous areas.

Until recently, bone abnormalities of the skull base have been evaluated by plain radiography and tomography (preferably pluridirectional). Evaluation of the intracranial soft-tissue mass component of skull base lesions has required demonstration of vascular displacements or tumor vasculature by cerebral arteriography and, in many cases, pneumoencephalography or positive-contrast cisternography. Extracranial soft-tissue extensions of masses often remained a mystery.

The advent of computed, or computerized, tomographic (CT) scanning revolutionized the approach to these lesions. With advancing CT technology, both bone and soft-tissue abnormalities can be demonstrated and evaluated exquisitely. In a relatively short time, specific approaches to evaluation of specific areas and lesions have developed.

Because of the multitude and complexity of the abnormalities involving the skull base, a regional approach to specific areas is employed. A separate section on generalized diseases which may also affect the skull base (metastases, systemic bone diseases, etc.) is presented first to avoid unnecessary repetition in each section. For the same reason, lesions which can involve various areas of the skull base are considered in detail in the section in which the region where they are most prevalent or important is discussed. They are discussed briefly in other sections only with respect to unusual features or differential diagnostic problems.

TECHNICAL ASPECTS

The technical aspects of CT scanning in general are considered in Chapter 1. Specific principles and procedures which apply particularly to the skull base are enumerated briefly below; there is further elaboration as various anatomic areas are considered in detail.

Bone Evaluation

Scanning with new-generation scanners provides a very satisfactory tomographic evaluation of bone, especially with the use of thin sections. As with conventional tomography, the scan plane should be at right angles to the area of bone to be evaluated. Only in this manner can the distinction between erosion and destruction be made reliably and bone expansion demonstrated. Widened windows are necessary for bone evaluation; evaluation is markedly improved in systems providing region-of-interest (ROI) reconstruction (selection of a focal area of interest of the scan section in which pixels smaller than usual are used, permitting true magnification).

Soft-Tissue Mass Evaluation

For full outline of a mass, scanning in at least two right-angle dimensions is needed. Direct coronal and axial scanning is possible on body scan units and is the usual method for accomplishing this goal. Reconstruction programs permitting axial scanning with reformatting of images into coronal, sagittal, and various oblique projections are available on new units. Because of the need to restrict radiation dosage, the higher the resolution desired in the reconstructed plane, the thinner the original axial sections must be; therefore, very high resolution reconstructions are limited to only striplike portions of the skull (e.g., the base, the orbits, and the lateral ventricles) (Fig. 10-1).

If the soft-tissue mass does not enhance sufficiently with contrast to permit adequate delineation, a double dose of contrast (80 g of iodine) may produce adequate enhancement. Delayed scanning (1 hour after injection of conventional or double-dose contrast) will also be helpful in more slowly enhancing lesions. If these measures are not adequate, the mass may be outlined by scanning with contrast added to the cerebrospinal fluid via lumbar injection; this may be negative-contrast (air) or positive-contrast (currently metrizamide, a nonionic, water-soluble, iodinated contrast). By increasing the contrast of the subarachnoid spaces, lesions may be outlined and communicating cystic spaces filled (Drayer 1977a, b). This method is of great value either when no lesion is demonstrated and there is still strong clinical suspicion or when bone erosion or destruction is seen but no soft-tissue mass is revealed by intravenous contrast.

Determination that a mass is extradural requires demonstration that the subarachnoid space is displaced away from the bone of the skull base. Tangential projections are necessary to make this evaluation; intrathecal contrast may be necessary to permit more adequate visualization of the subarachnoid spaces. Determination that a mass is intraaxial, or intradural but extraaxial, requires reevaluation of the subarachnoid spaces. An intradural, extraaxial mass displaces the brain away from the skull base, thus widening the subarachnoid space in that area.

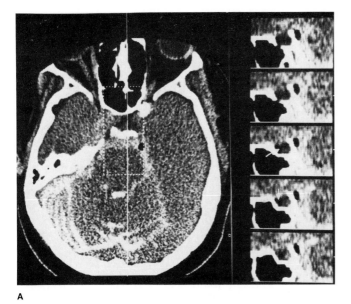

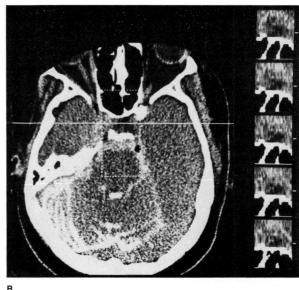

A   B

Figure 10-1 CT images of a patient with pituitary microadenoma. Study was done following intrathecal metrizamide. **A.** Sagittal reformatted images centered on the white line and passing through the sella. Note the hypodense tumor anteriorly (white arrow in the reformatted image) within the sella. Metrizamide is present in the prepontine cistern, excluding the possibility of an "empty" sella. **B.** Coronal reformatted image centered along the white line.

Furthermore, the mass can be seen to be outlined by cerebrospinal fluid, especially if opacified. Again, tangential projections are necessary.

Metallic dental fillings produce artifacts which can seriously degrade images on direct coronal scanning, especially those at and anterior to the level of the sella. Alteration of the angle to which the head is extended, or the tilt of the scanning gantry, causes the metallic densities to shift with respect to the area of interest, permitting satisfactory scans in many cases. Digital localization, available on newer scanners, or lateral skull radiography may be used to plan the scan angle, or the angle may be altered during the scanning procedure. Coronal reformation of axial scans also circumvents this problem.

GENERALIZED DISEASES AFFECTING THE SKULL BASE

Metastatic Disease

Metastases may affect any area of bone of the skull base or may involve soft-tissue structures close to or within the base (e.g., pituitary, hypothalamus, cerebellopontine angle structures). Bone involvement may be purely destructive, producing lytic areas with poorly defined margins, or may produce an osteoblastic reaction, which is typical of metastatic prostatic carcinoma and can be seen with metastatic breast carcinoma, but is far less common in other forms of metastatic disease. With metastases to structures along the skull base, bone involvement may be either present or absent. Following intravenous contrast enhancement, the soft-tissue component is usually well visualized (Fig. 10-2).

Myeloma

On CT scanning, multiple myeloma resembles osteolytic metastatic disease to bone. Because of the risk of renal failure, intravenous contrast is seldom used for improved visualization of the soft-tissue component. "Solitary" myeloma (plasmacytoma) may occasionally be seen in the skull base; intravenous contrast injection results in prominent enhancement of these lesions. On CT scanning, such

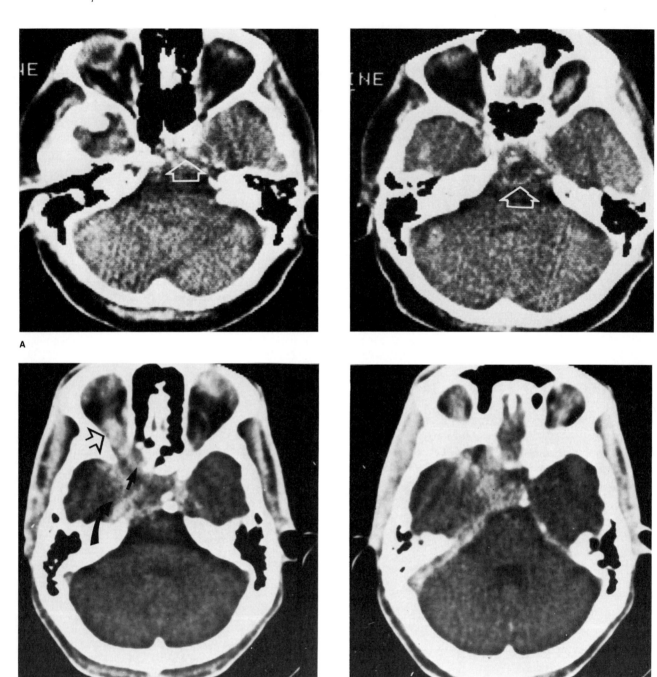

A

B

Figure 10-2 Metastatic disease.   **A.** Two nonenhanced scan sections demonstrating destruction of the dorsum (arrow). **B.** An enhancing metastatic lesion to the sella (curved arrow). There is destruction of the right side of the tuberculum and planum (arrow). The dorsum is destroyed in this case also.

Extension into the orbit is present (clear arrow).   **C.** (*Opposite*) A metastatic lesion (large arrow) producing destruction in the right middle cranial fossa. The foramen ovale, present on the left side (arrowhead), is not seen on the right.

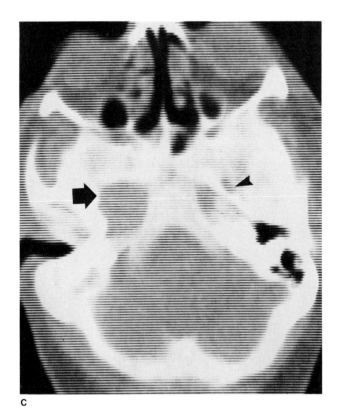

c

an isolated destructive lesion is not distinguishable from metastatic disease with an unknown primary malignancy.

Histiocytosis X

This group of diseases, the proliferative reticuloses, are characterized by granulomatous proliferation of reticulum cells in one or more portions of the reticuloendothelial system; they may involve the bones, lymph nodes, spleen, liver, thymus, lungs, and skin (Caffey 1972). Letterer-Siwe disease (non-lipid reticulosis) occurs early in life, shows extensive visceral involvement which overshadows the accompanying bone lesions, and is rapidly progressive and usually fatal. Hand-Schüller-Christian disease (lipid reticulosis) occurs in older children, adolescents, and young adults; the skeletal lesions

predominate and the visceral involvement is more focal. The course is more protracted. Eosinophilic granuloma is the most focal and mildest of the three types. It commonly presents as a single bone lesion, but there may be more than one bone lesion or bone lesions plus visceral involvement (such as lung and mediastinum).

The skull lesions are radiologically the same in all forms of histiocytosis X (Caffey 1972); they are purely lytic, typically with beveled edges because of differential involvement of the inner and outer tables. The lesions typically have lobulated, scalloped borders. A bony sequestrum may be present within the lytic area. With healing either spontaneously or after treatment, a faint zone of mild sclerosis may be seen about the lesion. These findings are easily recognized in the skull vault but are seen with more difficulty in the skull base, where (especially in the temporal bone) the lesion may appear to have very indistinct margins resembling metastatic disease. The patient's age and the absence of a known primary malignancy are useful differential diagnostic points. Computed tomographic scanning demonstrates the same features as plain radiographs but shows beveling more clearly and the bony sequestrum more frequently in calvarial lesions (Mitnick 1980). The incidence of sequestrum formation in skull base lesions is not known. An extraosseous soft-tissue mass may be demonstrated in association with the lytic area. Contrast enhancement may be seen within and about the periphery of the lesion (Mitnick 1980).

Granulomas

Granulomas may be due to a known, specific infectious agent (tuberculosis, fungus, or lues) or may be noninfectious (sarcoid, nonspecific, or foreign-body). The granulomas are mass lesions which typically show prominent enhancement following intravenous contrast injection. The enhancement tends to be homogeneous with sarcoid granulomas (Kendall 1978), but necrosis may cause a central hypodensity in the infectious granulomas (Whelan 1981). Calcification may be present. Bone erosion may occur; that due to sarcoid granulomas tends to have no surrounding sclerosis, while that due to infection may show some reactive sclerosis. Meningeal enhancement may be seen with sarcoid granulomas as well as the infectious granulomas due to meningeal involvement. Meningeal involvement may also produce hydrocephalus due to impairment of cerebrospinal fluid flow. As meningeal enhancement is related to the activity of the inflammatory process, it may not always be present in cases with hydrocephalus.

Arteriography may show arterial narrowings, areas of dilatation or aneurysm formation, or arterial occlusions. These may be focal, in the location of a granuloma, or more generalized with meningeal involvement. The findings are due to reaction to contiguous inflammation, vessel wall invasion by inflammation, or fibrotic constriction due to scarring.

Osteomyelitis

Osteomyelitis may involve the skull base through extension of sinusitis (frontal, ethmoid, or sphenoid), otitis media and mastoiditis, or nasopharyngeal infection; hematogenous infection is rare. The bone change depends on the site of origin, the acuteness or chronicity of infection, and the infectious agent involved. Lesions secondary to sinusitis or mastoiditis show evidence of inflammation in the primary site with bone destruction at the site of extension. Acute pyogenic osteomyelitis may produce purely osteolytic changes with little sclerosis; more chronic disease leads to varying degrees of sclerosis and bone production. Tuberculous, fungal, and luetic skull base infections may produce lytic or sclerotic changes. Congenital lues may produce mainly diffuse lytic disease in young children but bone sclerosis and thickening in older children and young adults. Lytic areas have poorly defined margins; sequestra may be present. Pyogenic osteomyelitis may perforate the bone involved, leading to epidural or subdural empyema, meningitis, or brain abscess. Tuberculous, luetic, and fungal disease may lead to meningitis or the formation of focal granulomatous masses. Venous and dural sinus thrombosis may occur.

Primary Bone Tumors

Primary bone tumors, with the exception of osteoma, are rare; CT experience is limited to date. In general, CT evaluation of bone changes will parallel descriptions of plain radiographic and tomographic findings, except that CT is superior in demonstrating calcification because of superior contrast resolution. Furthermore, CT is far more capable of demonstrating the extraosseous soft-tissue masses associated with tumors and in evaluating the effects of such masses on intra- and extracranial structures. Contrast enhancement should prove useful in such determinations.

Benign Tumors

Osteomas may arise in the calvarium, sinuses, or skull base. They are generally of the dense, cortical type but may be of the less dense, cancellous variety. Although they tend to be very slow growing or static lesions, some progressively expand to encroach on the intracranial space and can, on occasion, be life-threatening. Those within the sinuses can obstruct the sinus ostia, leading to recurrent infections and/or mucocele formation. Computed tomographic diagnosis and evaluation of extent is usually easy (Fig. 10-3).

The benign "brown tumors" of hyperparathyroidism and malignant giant cell tumors are histologically indistinguishable and can be expected to show similar changes on CT of skull base lesions. Clinical and radiologic evidence of hyperparathyroidism should be sought whenever a skull lesion is diagnosed as a giant cell tumor on pathological grounds.

Malignant Tumors

Chondromas and chondrosarcomas are discussed in detail in the section on the middle cranial fossa. Osteoblastomas, chondroblastomas, and giant cell tumors may also involve the skull base. We have no experience with the CT appearance of these lesions as yet. Osteogenic sarcomas and fibrosarcomas may arise in the skull base. To date we have no CT experience with such lesions.

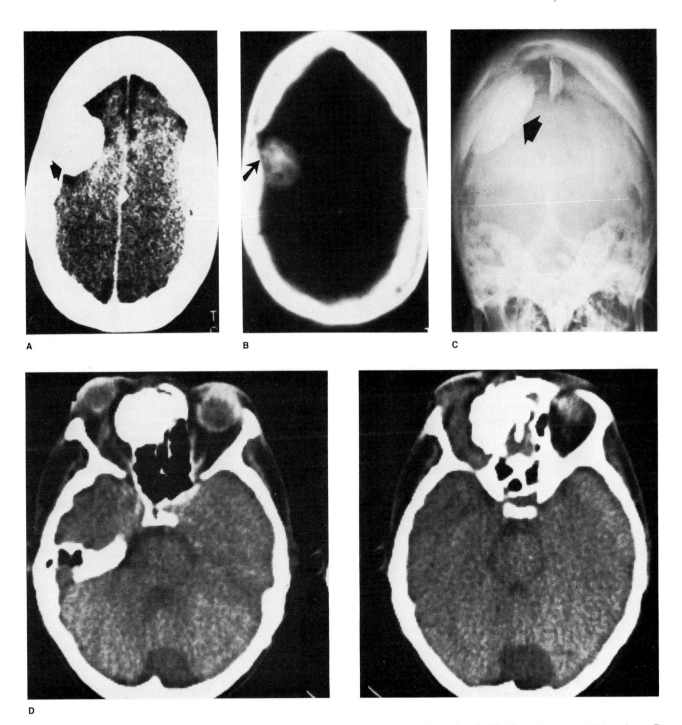

Figure 10-3 Osteoma. **A.** A large osteoma (arrow) projecting from the inner table of the skull in the anterior parietal region. **B.** The attachment of the osteoma to the inner table of the calvarium is better appreciated at a wide CT window setting. **C.** Correlation with a plain radiograph. **D.** CT of another patient with an osteoma involving the ethmoid sinus and extending into the orbit.

(Continued on p. 378.)

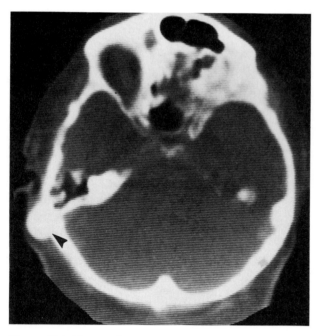

Figure 10-3 (*Cont.*) **E.** Another case of a benign osteoma involving the mastoid bone.

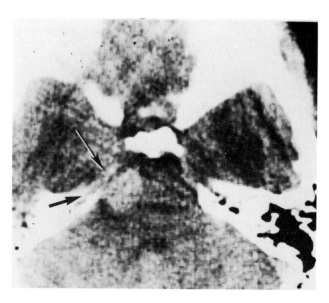

Figure 10-4   The soft-tissue mass of a reticulum cell sarcoma (arrows) arising in the region of the petrous apex. While this resembles a trigeminal neuroma, it proved to be a reticulum cell sarcoma on pathological examination.

Ewing's sarcoma, a malignant primary bone tumor of young people (rarely occurring in patients over 30 years of age), and reticulum cell sarcoma, a malignant primary or secondary bone tumor of all age groups, have essentially identical appearance on CT or conventional radiography (Fig. 10-4). These sarcomas produce irregular bone destruction but can cause reactive new bone formation within the lytic area and provoke periosteal new bone formation. A soft-tissue mass may be demonstrated.

Paget's Disease

Paget's disease is a disorder of unknown cause which may involve a portion of one bone, portions of several bones, or much of the skeleton (particularly the axial skeleton). Initially there is bone destruction, which is followed by an intermediate stage of combined destruction and repair and finally a sclerotic (or quiescent) stage. During the destructive and mixed stages marked bone thickening occurs; the bone is still soft in these stages and sus-

ceptible to fracture or deformity. When the skull base is involved, there is usually concomitant involvement of at least a portion of the vault. Basilar invagination (due to bone softening) is common. This can result in brainstem compression at the level of the foramen magnum. Furthermore, the combination of bone thickening (narrowing of the foramen magnum region) and basilar invagination may cause impaired outflow of cerebrospinal fluid from the fourth ventricle, leading to hydrocephalus. Finally, the bone thickening can cause encroachment on neural foramina and fissures, the optic canal, or the internal auditory canal, causing cranial nerve compression and dysfunction. Computed tomographic scanning is quite useful in the evaluation of the complications of this disorder (Fig. 10-5).

Fibrous Dysplasia

Fibrous dysplasia is a disorder of unknown cause which results in filling and expansion of medullary cavities of bone by fibrous tissue which undergoes

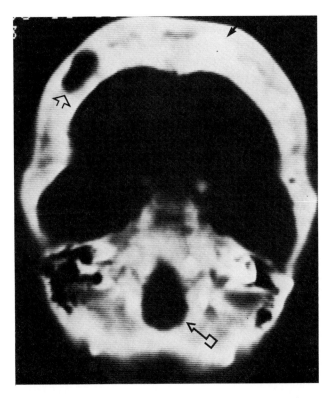

Figure 10-5 Extensive Paget's disease with marked bony thickening. There are areas of sclerosis (black arrow), as well as lytic areas (clear arrow). Because of the bony thickening, the foramen magnum is narrowed (boxed clear arrow).

and a rather homogeneously dense appearance (Fig. 10-6). Encroachment on neural foramina and fissures may cause cranial nerve dysfunction. Basilar invagination may develop because the thickened bone is weaker than normal bone. Extensive involvement of the skull may, on occasion, resemble the appearance of Paget's disease. Focal areas of sclerosis with varying degrees of bone thickening may be present, requiring differentiation from meningioma en plaque (a plaquelike form of meningioma producing hyperostosis in the bone it spreads along) and osteoblastic metastatic disease. Occasionally the distinction may not be possible on the basis of appearance alone. The bone thickening of fibrous dysplasia tends to be smoother and more extensive than that of meningioma en plaque. Osteoblastic metastases tend to be more focal than fibrous dysplasia involvement, and other clinical and/or radiologic evidence of the disease is often present. Fibrous dysplasia of the skull base commonly involves adjacent facial bones and encroaches on sinuses and orbits.

Hyperparathyroidism

This is a systemic bone disorder due to parathormone overproduction. It may be primary (due to parathyroid hyperplasia or tumor) or secondary (due to renal disease, rickets, or calcium insufficiency). Bone changes include generalized deossification, subperiosteal bone resorption, and focal destructive lesions (brown tumors). Skull changes consist of generalized demineralization, indistinctness of cortical bone, and focal areas of bone destruction representing brown tumors. The brown tumors, which are histologically indistinguishable from giant cell tumors, can become necrotic, resulting in cyst formation. Soft-tissue calcification, which is far more common with secondary hyperparathyroidism, leads to calcification of the vessel walls, the falx, and the tentorium. Skull base involvement can result in basilar invagination; a brown tumor produces a lytic lesion with poorly defined edges. The diagnosis of giant cell tumor of the skull should prompt laboratory evaluation for possible hyperparathyroidism.

varying degrees (from none to marked) of osseous metaplasia. The radiologic appearance depends on the degree of ossification which has occurred. Cyst-like lesions, bone expansion with lesions of "ground glass" appearance, and densely sclerotic areas may be seen. The lesion may involve a single bone (monostotic type) or multiple bones (polyostotic). In the polyostotic type, Albright's syndrome may be present, with a tendency for lesions to be unilateral, ipsilateral café au lait spots and for endocrine dysfunction which produces precocious puberty in females. In the skull, calvarial involvement tends to show more "cystic" changes or combined "cystic" and sclerotic changes with bone thickening. Cystic expansions tend to spare the inner table, which shows only minimal expansion. In the skull base the appearance is sclerotic, with bone thickening

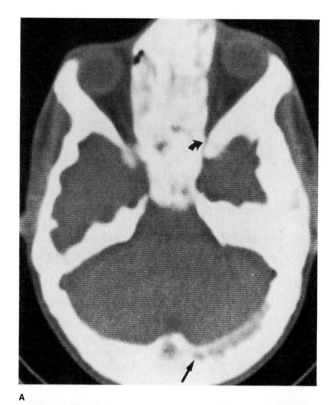

A

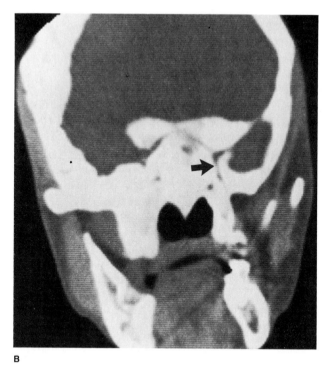

B

Figure 10-6 Fibrous dysplasia with extensive involvement producing marked bony thickening. Here, as in Paget's disease, there are areas of increased as well as decreased density. **A.** A zone of decreased density is seen in the occipital region (arrow). There is also narrowing of the optic canal (curved arrow). **B.** This coronal section shows marked narrowing of the superior orbital fissure (arrow). **C.** A marked bony overgrowth encroaches upon the nasal cavity (arrows).

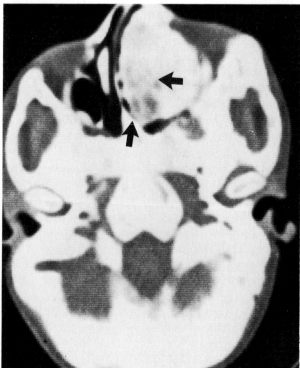

C

Bone Dysplasias

These represent disorders of bone growth and development. They are diagnosed by clinical findings and conventional radiography. Computed tomographic scanning can be quite useful, however, in demonstrating alterations of foramina and fissures, encroachment on neural structures, and development of hydrocephalus due to compromise of cerebrospinal fluid flow. Only features related to the skull are discussed.

Cleidocranial Dysostosis

This is a hereditary disorder characterized by delayed or defective ossification (Rubin 1964). There is delayed ossification of the skull, with fontanels remaining open and the sutures appearing wide into adolescence; intersutural (Wormian) bones are present. The paranasal sinuses are hypoplastic. Basilar impression may be present.

Osteogenesis Imperfecta

This hereditary disorder of collagen production affects bones, sclerae, skin, ligaments, tendons, fascia, and the inner ear (Rubin 1964). Both the inner and outer tables of the skull are thin and the diploe porous. The sutures may remain evident into adult life, and Wormian bones may be seen. There may be basilar invagination. Involvement of the petrous portion of the temporal bone may produce a clinical and radiologic picture resembling otosclerosis, although the bone changes are more extensive in osteogenesis imperfecta.

Achondroplasia

This is a hereditary disorder of endochondral bone formation (Rubin 1964) that affects the skull base (formed largely by endochondral bone production) while sparing the calvarium. The skull base is small because the calvarium compensatorily expands to accommodate brain growth. The foramen magnum is small, and basilar invagination may be present (Fig. 10-7); hydrocephalus may develop as a result of impaired cerebrospinal fluid flow.

Osteopetrosis

This is an inherited disorder in which impaired resorption of primitive chondroosteoid tissue interferes with replacement of cartilage by normal bone (Rubin 1964). The bones are dense, brittle, and more easily fractured than normal bone. The skull base is involved, but the calvarium is involved to a lesser degree in the less severe cases. Increased bone density and thickening of the skull base are seen with narrowing of fissures and foramina; cranial nerve dysfunction may result.

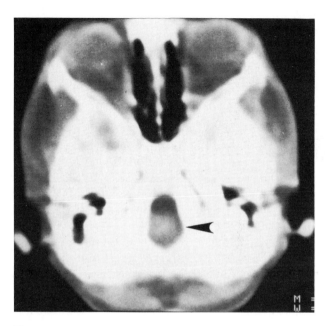

Figure 10-7 Achondroplasia. CT through the base of the skull of a 12-year-old child. The foramen magnum (arrowhead) is narrow and elongated in an anteroposterior direction.

Pyknodysostosis

This hereditary disorder shows features of both cleidocranial dysostosis and osteopetrosis. The skeletal bones are dense, the fontanels and sutures remain open, and the skull base is dense.

Progressive Diaphyseal Dysplasia (Engelmann's Disease)

This is a familial disorder, commencing in childhood (Rubin 1964) and characterized by symmetrical, sclerotic expansion of the midshaft of long bones, progressing toward both ends. The skull may be involved—the base more commonly than the vault. Sclerosis with varying degrees of thickening causes the skull base to become dense. Cranial nerve dysfunction is unusual.

Pyle's Disease

This hereditary disorder is characterized by flaring of the ends of long bones, phalanges, clavicles, and ribs. The skull may be involved to varying degrees. In mild cases there is mild skull base thickening and sclerosis of the vault. In severe cases the face is also involved and there is massive thickening of the base, with impaired pneumatization of sinuses and mastoids, encroachment on foramina and fissures, and narrowing of internal and external auditory canals.

Chronic Idiopathic Hyperphosphatasia (Juvenile Paget's Disease)

This is a familial disorder characterized by excessive osteoid and elevated serum phosphatase. Widening of the diploic space and patches of sclerosis are seen in the skull. The skull base is involved, and foraminal encroachment can occur. Onset is early in life. Chronic hyperphosphatemia tarda shows similar skull changes but begins in adolescence.

ANTERIOR CRANIAL FOSSA

Anatomy

The floor of the anterior fossa is formed by the orbital plates of the frontal bone, the cribriform plate of the ethmoid bone, and the body and lesser wings of the sphenoid bone. The posterior margin of the anterior fossa includes the lesser wings of the sphenoid bone and the limbus sphenoidalis. Foramina of interest include those within the cribriform plate for passage of the olfactory nerve fibers as well as the anterior and posterior ethmoidal foramina, through which course ethmoidal vessels and nerves. The frontal crest and crista galli, to which the dura of the falx cerebri is attached, lie within the median sagittal plane from anterior to posterior; the olfactory grooves lie on either side of the crista galli. Behind the crista galli and olfactory grooves is the planum sphenoidale, and the orbital plates and lesser sphenoid wings are located laterally.

CT Technique

Computed tomographic scanning carried out in both the axial and coronal planes will satisfactorily image both the contents and the bony floor of the anterior fossa. Coronal sections will be roughly perpendicular to the floor of the fossa, permitting optimal evaluation of bone as well as the best definition of intra- and extracranial extension of lesions. Sagittal reconstructions may be useful in some instances, but the combination of the two scan planes at right angles is usually ample in this area. Artifacts due to metallic dental fillings may obscure detail; visualization may be improved by changing the angle of the scan slightly or by the use of different filter functions available on some of the newer scanners. Coronal reformation of axial scans also circumvents this problem.

Pathology

Meningioma

These are the most common lesions to involve the floor of the anterior cranial fossa. They may arise from any portion of the floor; common sites include the planum sphenoidale and cribriform plate (midline masses) and the orbital roof (eccentric location). The characteristic bone changes due to the tumor and the extension of tumor into sinuses or orbits are best demonstrated on coronal scans. Involvement of the roof of the sphenoid or ethmoid sinus can cause a cerebrospinal fluid fistula due to bone destruction. The characteristic findings in meningioma are described in detail elsewhere.

Paranasal Sinus Disease

Lesions of the sinuses, both benign and malignant, may extend (through the roof of the ethmoid or the posterior wall of the frontal sinus) to involve the anterior fossa. Furthermore, nasal lesions may extend upward to involve the ethmoid sinuses and from there, the anterior fossa (Fig. 10-10). In most cases involvement of the other walls of the sinus will indicate the true origin of the lesion, but occasionally the distinction between a sinus lesion extending intracranially and an intracranial lesion (such as a meningioma) extending into the sinuses may be difficult. The bony walls of the sinus involved may show expansion, erosion, or destruction in locations other than the interface with the cranial lesion (Fig. 10-8). Arteriography can show the typical vascular supply and tumor vasculature of a meningioma or the largely cerebral arterial supply and venous drainage of an exophytic glioma eroding the roof of a sinus and producing reactive fluid formation. Conversely, displacement of intracranial vasculature can aid in identifying an extracranial mass extending intracranially. Sinus infection can extend intracranially, resulting in meningitis, subdural or epidural empyema, or brain abscess (Fig. 10-9).

Olfactory Neuroblastoma

These rather rare tumors arise in the olfactory mucosa. Three types are recognized: esthesioneuroepithelioma, esthesioneurocytoma, and esthesioneuroblastoma, in order of decreasing differentiation (Manelfe 1978). They occur in all age groups, peaking in the second to fourth decade. The tumor mass occupies the upper part of the nasal cavity and extends to involve the ethmoid and maxillary sinuses. Bone destruction is not uncommon, involving the sinus walls and cribriform plate (Fig. 10-10). Intracranial extension occurs in 20 percent of cases. The bone destruction is well seen on CT; occasionally

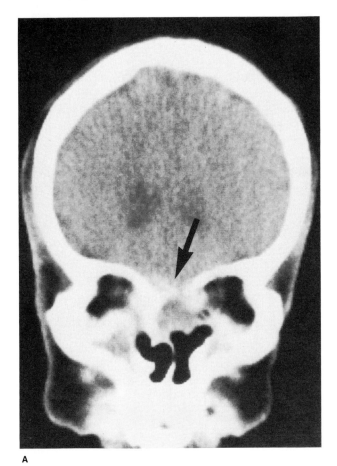

A

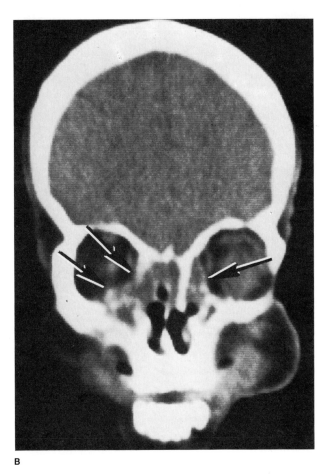

B

Figure 10-8 Carcinoma of the ethmoid sinuses. **A.** A coronal section showing destruction of the roof of the ethmoid sinuses with extension of an enhancing soft-tissue mass into the anterior cranial fossa (arrow). **B.** A coronal section with bone window settings showing opacification of the ethmoid sinuses and bone destruction of the lateral walls of the ethmoid sinuses as well as the medial portion of the floor of the orbit (arrows).

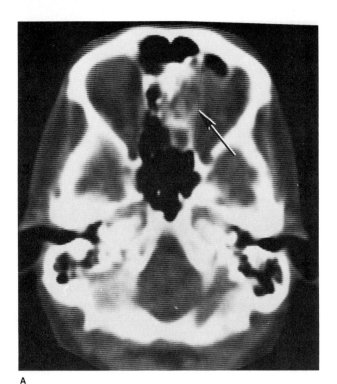

A

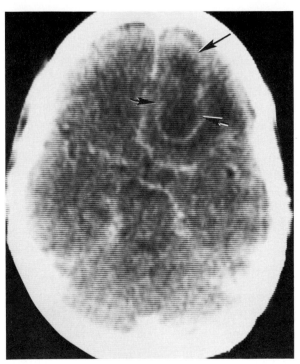

B

Figure 10-9 Frontal lobe abscess resulting from extension of infection from the ethmoid sinus. **A.** Opacified right ethmoid air cells with indistinctness of the bony walls of the sinus (arrow). **B.** The frontal lobe abscess (arrow) shows ring enhancement with surrounding edema.

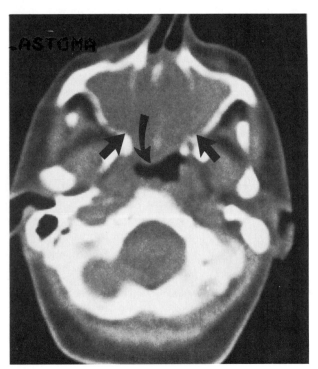

A

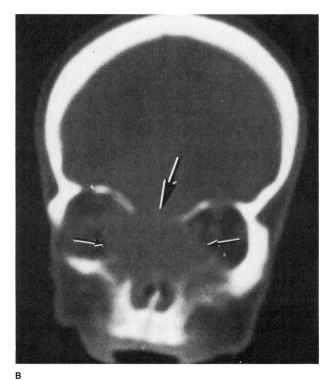

B

calcification may be detected. Some authors have noted contrast enhancement regularly (Manelfe 1978), while others have found enhancement infrequent (Burke 1980; Rosengren 1979). In our experience, the intracranial component has regularly shown prominent enhancement.

Other Lesions

Chronic pressure caused by long-standing frontal intracranial masses may result in focal bone thinning and erosion. Chronic pulsation of the dilated vessels from arteriovenous malformations against the floor of the anterior fossa can cause focal bone erosion.

MIDDLE CRANIAL FOSSA

Anatomy

The middle fossa is bounded anteriorly by the greater and lesser wings of the sphenoid bone and the anterior clinoid process; laterally, by the squamous portion of the temporal bone, the sphenoid angle of the parietal bone, and the greater wing of the sphenoid bone; and posteriorly, by the petrous portion of the temporal bone and dorsum sellae. Medially, it ends at the carotid sulcus in the sphenoid bone (Fig. 10-11). It provides a cavity which contains the anterior portion of the temporal lobe. There are several bone landmarks of note in the middle cranial fossa (Fig. 10-11).

◀ **Figure 10-10** An olfactory neuroblastoma. **A.** Axial section with bone window showing an extensive mass which opacifies the nasal cavity and both maxillary antra (arrows). There is destruction of the medial walls of maxillary antra. The soft tissue mass encroaches upon the nasopharyngeal cavity (curved arrow). **B.** A coronal section with bone window showing marked destruction of the lateral walls (small arrows) and roof (large arrow) of the ethmoid sinuses.

Superior Orbital Fissure

This is a cleft between the greater and lesser wings of the sphenoid bone communicating between the orbit and the middle fossa. Cranial nerves III, IV, VI, and the first division of cranial nerve V; filaments from the cavernous plexus of the sympathetic nervous system; the orbital branch of the middle meningeal artery; the recurrent branch from the lacrimal artery to the dura mater; and the superior ophthalmic vein course through the superior orbital fissure.

Foramen Rotundum

This canal connects the middle cranial fossa with the pterygopalatine fossa and contains the second division of cranial nerve V.

Foramen Ovale

This connects the middle fossa with the infratemporal fossa. The third division of cranial nerve V, the emissary veins between the cavernous sinus and the pterygoid venous plexus, the accessory meningeal branch of the internal maxillary artery, and the lesser superficial petrosal nerve course through the foramen ovale.

Foramen Spinosum

This structure lies just posterolateral to the foramen ovale. The middle meningeal artery and a recurrent branch from the third division of cranial nerve V course through the foramen spinosum.

Foramen Lacerum

This foramen, which in vivo is filled with fibrocartilage, lies medial to foramen ovale and is bounded anteriorly and laterally by the greater wing of the sphenoid, posteriorly by the petrous apex, and medially by the body of the sphenoid and the basioccipital bone. Piercing the fibrocartilage are the nerve of the pterygoid canal and the meningeal branch of the ascending pharyngeal artery. The internal carotid artery passes over the foramen immediately beyond its exit from the petrous carotid canal.

Figure 10-11   Bony landmarks of the middle cranial fossa.   **A.** The greater wing of the sphenoid bounding the middle fossa anteriorly (clear arrow). The petrous portion of the temporal bone demarcates the posterior limit of the middle cranial fossa (large curved arrow). The lateral aspect of the body of the sphenoid (straight arrow) forms the medial boundary. The superior orbital fissure is visible (small curved arrow).   **B.** A slightly lower CT section demonstrates the following normal structures: foramen ovale (A), foramen spinosum (B), foramen lacerum (C), clivus (D), jugular foramen (E), styloid foramen (F), infratemporal fossa (G), vomer (H), maxillary antrum (I), sphenoid sinus (J).

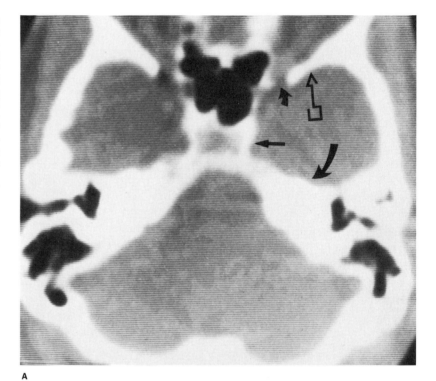

A

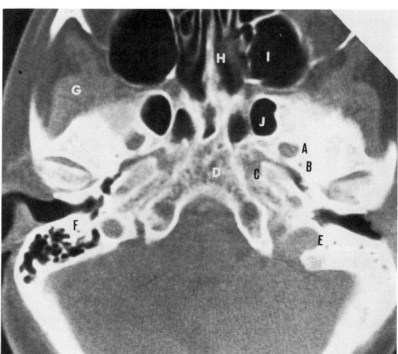

B

Pterygoid (Vidian) Canal

This canal connects the foramen lacerum with the pterygopalatine fossa, originating posteriorly in the anterior wall of the foramen lacerum and passing anteromedially in the lateral portion of the body of the sphenoid. The Vidian artery (branch of the internal maxillary) and nerve (an autonomic nerve) pass through the pterygoid canal.

Foramen of Vesalius

This structure is an inconstant foramen anteromedial to the foramen ovale through which courses a vein connecting the cavernous sinus and the pterygoid plexus.

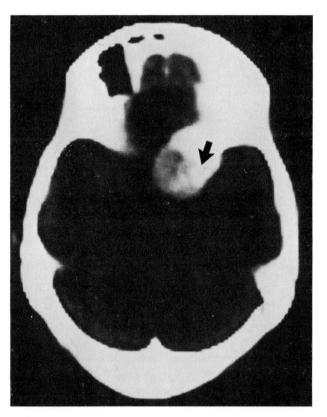

Figure 10-12 A calcified meningioma producing hyperostosis of the medial portion of the greater wing of the sphenoid and the anterior clinoid process (arrow).

CT Technique

The principles that apply to the evaluation of the skull base region in the middle cranial fossa are the same as those discussed in the section on the anterior fossa. Satisfactory visualization and evaluation of all the fissures, foramina, and canals of the middle fossa requires the newer generation scanners with high-resolution capacity, although the large foramina can be visualized on most scanners now available. Wide window settings must, of course, be used for bone evaluation.

Pathology

Meningioma

In the middle cranial fossa, these tumors arise along the greater and lesser sphenoid wings. They show the same features here as elsewhere. Bone erosion or destruction is present in some, hyperostosis with others (Fig. 10-12), and a combination in still others. Bone destruction and extracranial extension of tumor are best defined on coronal CT. Meningioma en plaque can lead to extensive hyperostosis which can result in significant narrowing of fissures, canals, and foramina with symptoms due to compression of the structures that course through these cavities. Medially located tumors can invade the cavernous sinus and may encircle and narrow the carotid siphon or the middle cerebral artery, compromising these vessels and limiting surgical treatment. Arteriography is essential in preoperative evaluation for assessment of arterial involvement; it is also useful in confirming the diagnosis by the nature of the vascularity and vascular supply.

Trigeminal Neuroma

Neurofibromas can arise in most cranial or spinal nerves of the central nervous system. In the middle cranial fossa, the trigeminal (cranial nerve V) nerve is the cranial nerve most frequently involved. Trigeminal neuromas arise from Schwann sheath cells, most commonly from the gasserian ganglion (about

50 percent of cases); these are extradural middle cranial fossa lesions (Goldberg 1980). About 25 percent of trigeminal neuromas arise from the trigeminal nerve root in the posterior fossa; these present as intradural posterior fossa lesions (Goldberg 1980). In the remaining 25 percent, the mass involves both the middle and posterior fossa, having a "dumbbell" configuration and being both intra- and extradural. Occasionally middle cranial fossa trigeminal neuromas arise on only one division of the trigeminal nerve. Furthermore, a lesion arising in the ganglion can extend along one or more divisions of the nerve.

The lesions can erode adjacent bone. The most frequent bone involvement is sharply marginated erosion of the tip of the petrous pyramid (K. F. Lee 1979). Forward extension with erosion of the floor of the middle cranial fossa is a common feature. The foramen ovale often is expanded (Fig. 10-13); further anterior extension causes the foramen rotundum and the superior orbital fissure to enlarge; this enlargement is best seen on coronal sections. There may also be erosion of the inferolateral aspect of the optic canal, the clinoids, and the side of the sella. Extension of the mass through the floor of the middle fossa into the nasopharynx can occur with larger lesions. When only one divison of the nerve is involved, enlargement of (and erosion adjacent to) the corresponding foramen will be seen. On CT, the lesion is typically isodense with brain or slightly

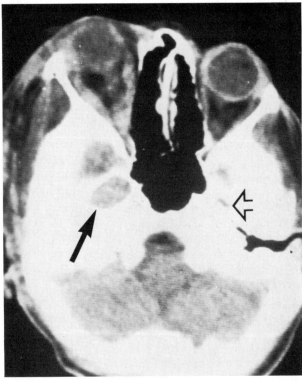

A

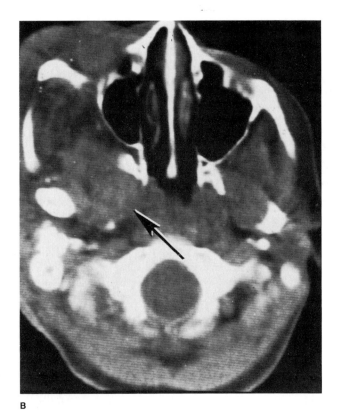

B

Figure 10-13 Three examples of trigeminal neuroma. **A.** In the first patient, there is marked expansion of the foramen ovale on the right side (dark arrow). The normal left foramen is indicated by the clear arrow. **B.** Section at a lower level shows the extracranial extension of the tumor (arrow). **C.** Visible in the second patient is a cystic trigeminal neuroma producing erosion of the right petrous apex (curved arrow). **D.** The tumor is outlined by peripheral enhancement (white arrow). **E.** In the third patient two CT sections demonstrate a large, slightly nonhomogeneously enhancing neuroma which occupies much of the middle cranial fossa (arrowhead).

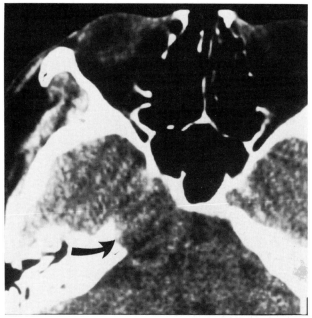

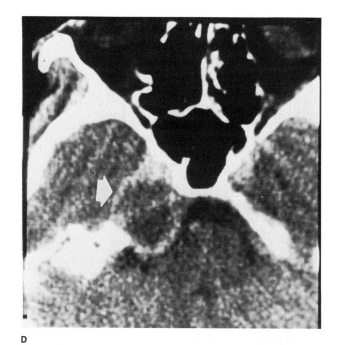

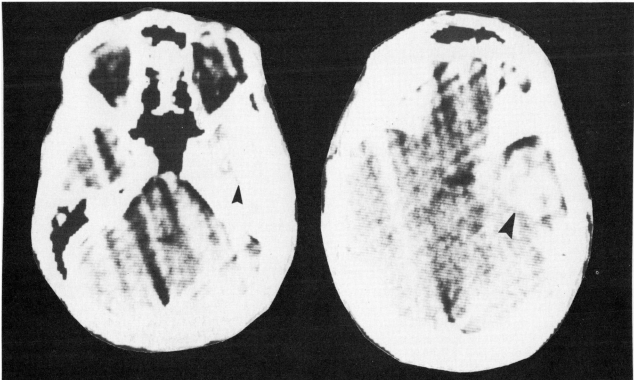

less dense, with an occasional case more dense than brain (Goldberg 1980). Nodular or curvilinear calcification may be seen (B. C. P. Lee 1979). There is typically pronounced enhancement which may be homogeneous, but cystic areas of nonenhancement may often be noted (Fig. 10-13) (Goldberg 1980; B. C. P. Lee 1979; Naidich 1976*b*); some lesions show only rim enhancement.

Long-Standing Middle Cranial Fossa Masses

Both intracerebral (temporal lobe) and extracerebral (arachnoid cyst and chronic subdural collections) can produce focal bone thinning and erosion over a period of time. If they occur early in life, when the skull is malleable, the middle cranial fossa may be expanded in comparison to the contralateral side (Fig. 10-14); there is also anterolateral displacement of the greater wing of the sphenoid and elevation of the lesser wing, with widening of the superior orbital fissure. Computed tomographic scanning shows not only the bone alterations, but the underlying pathology. Temporal lobe masses are discussed elsewhere. Obstruction of the temporal horn of the lateral ventricle with focal dilatation can contribute to the mass effect. Extraaxial fluid collections can be identified by their low density relative to the adjacent brain. With arachnoid cyst hypoplasia of the anterior portion of the temporal lobe is an associated feature and is the probable cause of the frequent straightness of the posterior margin of the cyst. Cysts show no contrast enhancement; the membranes of chronic subdural hematomas frequently enhance. Long-standing subdural hematomas may calcify.

Epidermoid Tumors

These lesions are discussed in detail in the section on the cerebellopontine angle, the location where they most commonly occur; they may be seen in the middle fossa also (Fig. 10-36). When the tumor is extradural, bone erosion with sharply defined edges, often with a thin margin of sclerosis, is frequently seen. These lesions may extend inferiorly into the nasopharynx and superiorly as an intracranial mass.

Giant Aneurysm

Giant aneurysms of the cavernous portion of the internal carotid artery may, in addition to eroding the sella and lateral aspect of the body of the sphenoid bone, cause erosion of the adjacent portion of the middle cranial fossa, depending on their size and the direction of their expansion (these lesions are discussed in Chap. 14).

Chondroma and Chondrosarcoma

Chondromas are benign, slow-growing tumors believed to arise from cartilaginous rests; these rests are located typically along the skull base (the bones of which derive from cartilage), most commonly in relation to the sphenooccipital and sphenoethmoidal synchondroses; occasionally the rests are located ectopically. Most chondromas arise in the sphenoid region, particularly in a parasellar location (Fig. 10-15), with the cerebellopontine angle next in frequency (Lee 1979). Chondromas may rarely arise in the bones of the calvarium and may even be intradural.

Chondromas may be associated with enchondromatosis of Maffucci's syndrome. Bone erosion occurs in 50 percent of chondromas; calcification, usually irregular and mottled (but sometimes stippled or even ringlike), occurs in 60 percent (Sarwar 1976). But calcification is rare in chondromas of the cerebellopontine angle region (K. F. Lee 1979; Roukkula 1964; Sarwar 1976). The incidence of these findings is similar to that in chondrosarcoma, but the bone destruction is more poorly defined. Chondromas grow very slowly and frequently do not become symptomatic for years; chondrosarcomas are also relatively slow growing, frequently leading to death as early as 5 years after the onset of symptoms (Bahr 1977). In addition to revealing the bone destruction and calcification of these lesions, CT scanning typically shows mild to moderate contrast enhancement in chondrosarcomas; in the one reported case of CT scanning with contrast in a proven chondroma, enhancement was also seen (Sarwar 1976). Chondrosarcomas are malignant cartilaginous tumors which may either result from malignant trans-

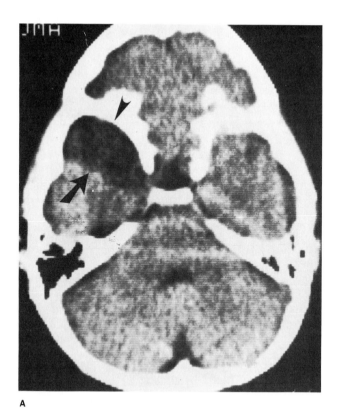

A

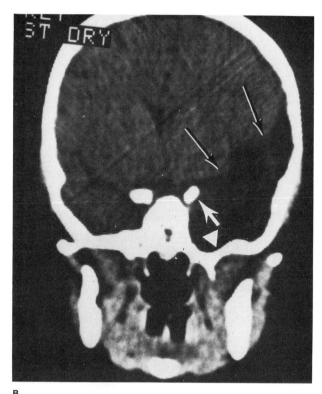

B

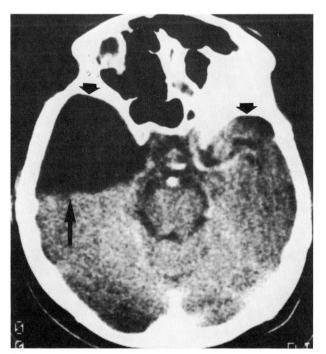

C

Figure 10-14 Middle cranial fossa arachnoid cyst. **A.** CT in axial projection shows a hypodense arachnoid cyst in the middle cranial fossa (arrow). The sphenoid wing is bowed anteriorly, without any bone destruction (arrowhead), a sign of the mass being benign and developmental in origin. **B.** Coronal projection shows the extent of the arachnoid cyst (long arrows). The anterior clinoid process is elevated (white arrow) and the floor of the middle cranial fossa is depressed (white arrowhead) compared to the normal side. **C.** In another patient the large arachnoid cyst (arrow) expands the right middle cranial fossa. There is anterior displacement of the right sphenoid wing as compared with the left (short arrows).

formation of a chondroma (Berkmen 1968), or, more commonly, originate as a malignant tumor.

Bone Dysplasia in Neurofibromatosis

This is a congenital malformation of bone which may involve various areas of the body. In the cranial region, one of the more common anomalies is or-

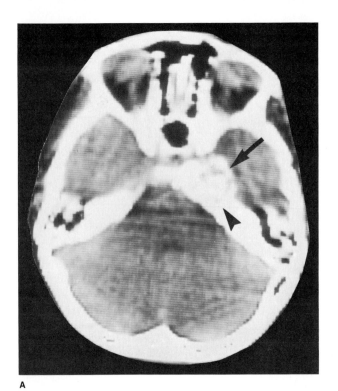

A

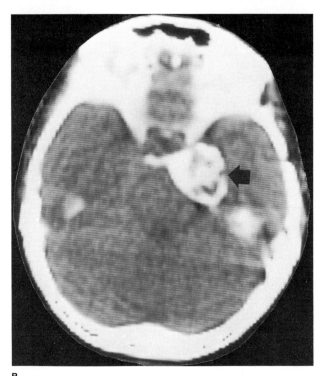

B

Figure 10-15   Chondroma in the left parasellar region.   **A.** A calcified mass is seen (arrow) to the left of the sella. There is erosion of the petrous apex (arrowhead).   **B.** A higher section shows the calcified mass (arrow) more clearly.

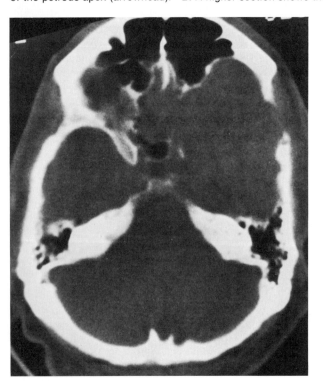

A

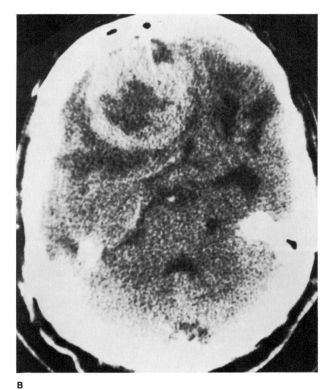

B

bital dysplasia, which involves the middle cranial fossa as well (Fig. 10-16). There is unilateral absence of a large part of the greater wing of the sphenoid and hypoplasia and elevation of the lesser wing, resulting in a markedly widened superior orbital fissure; essentially this is a large defect in the posterolateral wall of the orbit. The temporal lobe protrudes through the defect, resulting in pulsating exophthalmos. Intracranially, there is expansion of the middle cranial fossa in all directions, with the greater wing of the sphenoid displaced downward and forward (Bradac 1978); there is also tilting of the floor of the sella downward on the involved side. Although this malformation is associated with neurofibromatosis, no neurofibroma is associated with the bone defect; it is purely bone dysplasia (Kieffer 1971).

Nasopharyngeal Malignancy

Nasopharyngeal tumors can extend superiorly, invading and destroying the floor of the middle cranial fossa and obliterating its bony landmarks (Fig. 10-2C).

SELLAR REGION

Anatomy

The sella turcica (Fig. 10-17) has been described as the central depression within the sphenoid bone (Pribram 1971). The floor of the sella is the roof of the sphenoid sinus. The sella is bounded by the following structures: anteriorly, by the tuberculum sella, anterolaterally, by the anterior clinoid processes and optic struts; laterally, by the carotid sulci and the cavernous sinus; posteriorly, by the dorsum

---

◀ **Figure 10-16** CT of a patient with proptosis and known neurofibromatosis. **A.** Section through skull base demonstrates absence of the sphenoid wing on the left side extending to the calvarium. **B.** CT at a higher level in the same patient demonstrates a frontal glioblastoma on the right side.

sellae from whose superior surface project the posterior clinoid processes; and superiorly, by the diaphragma sellae.

Anterior to the tuberculum sellae is the chiasmatic sulcus, which is, in turn, distinguished from the planum sphenoidale by the limbus sphenoidale. Superior to the carotid sulci are the cavernous sinuses, which form the lateral walls of the sella and through which course the internal carotid arteries and cranial nerves III, IV, V_1, V_2, and VI. The dorsum sellae merges inferiorly with the clivus. The petrous apices approximate the lateral aspect of the base of the dorsum sellae and the posterior portion of the carotid sulci bilaterally.

Superior to the sella is the suprasellar cistern, which contains cerebrospinal fluid, the optic chiasm, the supraclinoid carotid arteries, the circle of Willis, and the infundibulum (Fig. 10-18). It is bounded anteriorly by the posterior inferior aspects of the frontal lobes and communicates anteriorly in the midline, with the interhemispheric fissure. Anterolaterally, on either side, the cistern merges with the proximal portions of the sylvian fissures. Laterally, it is bounded by the uncus of the hippocampal gyrus of the temporal lobes and posteriorly by the crural cisternal complex, consisting of the midline interpeduncular and the more lateral circummesencephalic cisterns.

CT Technique

Section Thickness

Since the maximal sellar volume is less than 1500 mm^3 (Robertson 1978), it is clear that optimal CT evaluation of the sella and adjacent structures requires meticulous scanning technique. Specifically, thin contiguous sections (newer scanners permit 1.5- to 8-mm sections) should be employed in order to avoid degraded images due to the partial volume phenomenon (New 1975). Since extremely thin sections with unchanged radiation dose yield scans with decreased contrast resolution and increased "noise" as a result of poorer counting statistics, there are two implications: (1) thin sections with

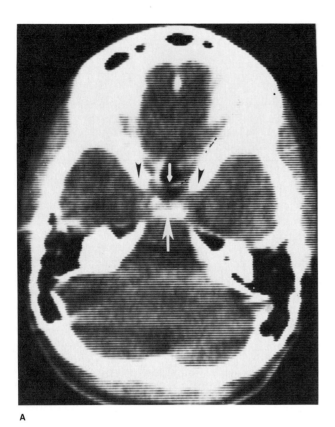

A

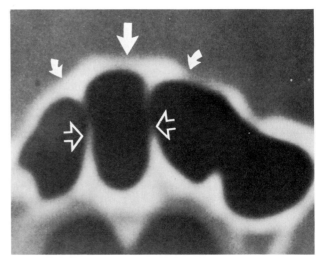

B

Figure 10-17 Normal anatomy of the sellar region. **A.** Section through the sellar inlet demonstrates the anterior clinoid process (arrowheads), tuberculum (small arrow), the upper portion of the dorsum sella with two posterior clinoids (large arrow) and the sellar cavity with the pituitary gland. **B.** Coronal CT with wide window settings to show the floor of the sella (white arrow) with the carotid sulci on either side (curved white arrows). Beneath the sellar floor is the sphenoid sinus with two septations (clear white arrows).

low dosage may be used for examinations not demanding high-contrast resolution; for example, evaluation of thickness and contour of the sellar floor on coronal CT produces images similar to those obtained by pluridirectional tomography; and (2) use of multiple thin sections with high resolution increases patient dose due to the higher dose per slice and greater scattered radiation to adjacent sections. Therefore, an ultrathin scanning protocol should be used with discretion.

If the scanner does not provide thinner slices, evaluation may be improved by overlapping scan sections. This improves the likelihood of the area of interest occupying most or all of the section thickness, thus minimizing partial volume effects. For example, if only 10-mm sections are available, the centers of each slice should be spaced 5 mm apart. This technique, of course, results in increased patient dose.

Orientation of Sections

We have found that for axial examination of the sella, sections parallel with Reid's baseline or at 25° caudal angulation to Reid's baseline are satisfactory for imaging the sella and suprasellar cistern structures (K. R. Davis 1979; Naidich 1976a). However, because of the difficulty encountered in obtaining accurate absorption values of the intrasellar pituitary gland (despite thin-section technique) as a result of partial volume averaging with the sellar floor and suprasellar cistern, coronal scanning is recommended for pituitary imaging (Syvertsen 1979). Coronal sections are superior in depicting the sellar floor, superior surface of the pituitary gland, thickness of the gland, and suprasellar extension of tumor (Figs. 10-18, 10-22). Currently these can be best obtained by direct coronal scanning with hyperextension of the patient's neck and tilting of the scan-

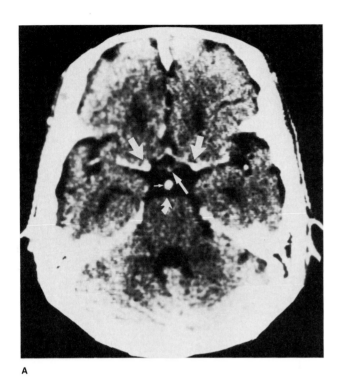

A

Figure 10-18 The suprasellar cistern following intravenous contrast. **A.** The following structures can be identified: the internal carotid artery (large white arrows), basilar artery (small white arrow), the enhancing pituitary stalk (medium-sized arrow) with the soft-tissue density on either side representing the optic nerves and the anterior aspect of the pons (curved arrow). **B.** Direct coronal CECT. The homogeneously enhanced pituitary gland has a flat superior surface (large white arrows). The anterior clinoids are visible on each side (clear white arrows). Above the anterior clinoid is the supraclinoid portion of the internal carotid artery (small white arrows). Anterior end of the third ventricle (curved white arrow). **C.** Direct coronal CT at a slightly more posterior level shows the pituitary stalk (small white arrow) extending down to the enhancing pituitary gland (curved white arrow). The infundibular recess of the third ventricle is also visible (large white arrow).

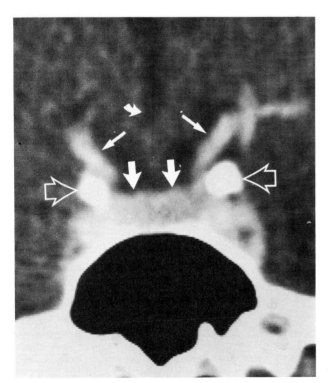

B

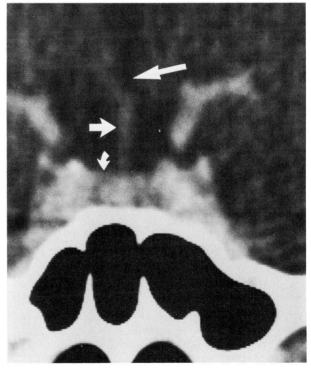

C

ning gantry or bed to approximate sections perpendicular to the skull base. Angulation is modified to exclude metallic dental fillings from the sections to avoid marked degradation by streaking artifacts from the fillings. This is most easily accomplished by digital radiographic localization available in current scanners but can be accomplished by changing the patient's position during the scanning procedure or by using a lateral skull radiograph prior to scanning. Coronal and sagittal sections may also be obtained by reformation of images from data obtained by axial scanning (Glenn 1975*a, b*) (Fig. 10-1). For satisfactory spatial resolution in the cephalocaudal axis, the original axial sections must be thin. Therefore, while scanning need be carried out in only one plane, radiation is increased because of the need for thinner sections. Reasonably good reconstructed images are available on scanners, providing 1.5- to 2-mm section thickness. The ability to evaluate lesions in the coronal or sagittal planes is of great use in both diagnosis and treatment planning.

Contrast Material

Like other intracranial neoplasms, the majority of pituitary tumors, as well as parasellar masses, may undergo contrast enhancement. Enhancement may occur secondary to extravascular accumulation of contrast material (Gado 1975*a, b*) or secondary to hypervascularity. The pituitary gland, the infundibulum, the cavernous sinuses, and the arteries of the circle of Willis enhance normally as well (Fig. 10-18).

In general, we use a 300-ml intravenous infusion of iodinated contrast providing 42 g of iodine. When necessary, an additional 150-ml bolus equivalent to 42 g of iodine is given intravenously to increase faint enhancement for better definition [Hayman 1980; J. M. Davis 1979].

Cisternography

The fluid density of the basal cisterns is well imaged by CT scanning; however, there are instances in which improved contrast resolution is needed. For example, the distinction between extension of the subarachnoid space ("empty sella") and the low density of a partially necrotic pituitary tumor (Wolpert 1979) is easily resolved by adding contrast material to the cerebrospinal fluid and determining whether it enters the enlarged sella. Poorly enhancing or nonenhancing suprasellar masses of low density may be difficult to outline because of the relatively low contrast between the fluid density of the basal cisterns and the density of the lesion; here, too, intrathecal contrast material permits improved diagnostic accuracy.

Contrast material is injected by means of lumbar puncture. Air can be used for this purpose; however, small amounts of air can be difficult to position accurately, and large volumes produce severe headache. If metrizamide (water-soluble, nonionic iodinated contrast) is used, the entire subarachnoid space can be opacified with ease. Although varying degrees of morbidity may be associated with intrathecal metrizamide administration (headache, nausea, vomiting, and rarely, seizures), the incidence is related to the total dose and the concentration delivered intracranially. Because of the high-contrast-resolution capacity of CT scanning, metrizamide can produce satisfactory opacification of the subarachnoid spaces in concentrations much lower than those needed for myelography (Greitz 1974). One method for reliable opacification (Drayer 1977*b*) is to inject 6 ml of a solution containing 190 mg of iodine per milliliter (using the dilution chart enclosed with the contrast agent) into the lumbar subarachnoid space through a 22-gauge needle with the patient on a tilting table. The patient is then tilted head down about 60° and the contrast, which has a specific gravity higher than that of cerebrospinal fluid at this concentration, flows cephalad. After 2 minutes in this position, the table is brought back to 10° head down and the patient is transferred by a stretcher to the CT table. (We have found the horizontal position satisfactory for the transfer.) The contrast material, of course, becomes diluted as it flows craniad but is still well imaged by scanning (Fig. 10-19).

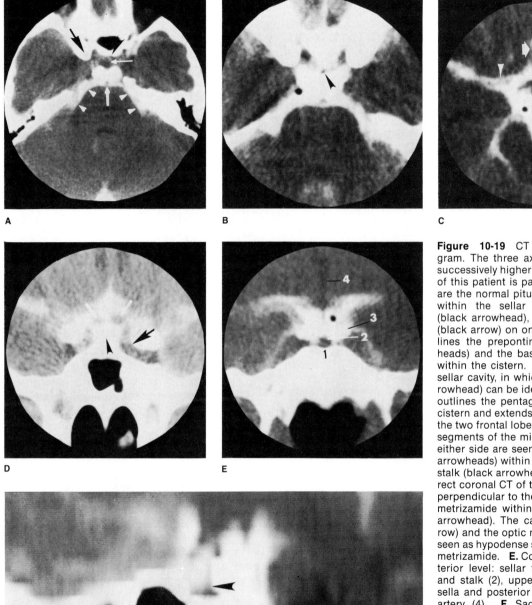

Figure 10-19 CT metrizamide cisternogram. The three axial views were made at successively higher 3-mm intervals. The sella of this patient is partially empty. **A.** Visible are the normal pituitary gland (white arrow) within the sellar cavity, the tuberculum (black arrowhead), and the anterior clinoid (black arrow) on one side. Metrizamide outlines the prepontine cistern (white arrowheads) and the basilar artery (white arrow) within the cistern. **B.** Metrizamide fills the sellar cavity, in which the pituitary stalk (arrowhead) can be identified. **C.** Metrizamide outlines the pentagonal-shaped suprasellar cistern and extends into the fissure between the two frontal lobes (white arrow). Proximal segments of the middle cerebral arteries on either side are seen as filling defects (white arrowheads) within the cistern. The pituitary stalk (black arrowhead) can be seen. **D.** Direct coronal CT of the same patient. Section perpendicular to the anterior clinoids shows metrizamide within the sellar cavity (black arrowhead). The carotid arteries (black arrow) and the optic nerves (white arrows) are seen as hypodense structures surrounded by metrizamide. **E.** Coronal CT at a slighly posterior level: sellar floor (1), pituitary gland and stalk (2), upper part of the dorsum of sella and posterior clinoids (3), and basilar artery (4). **F.** Sagittal reformatted image through the sella. The anterior part is filled with metrizamide, and the compressed pituitary gland (arrowhead) is seen posteriorly. Note the optic and infundibular recess of the third ventricle.

Pathology

The array of lesions involving the sellar region is large (Table 10-1). However, a portion of this differential diagnostic list occurs with sufficient frequency to merit discussion.

Pituitary Adenoma

Adenomas arising from the anterior lobe of the pituitary gland, are divided into nonsecreting (chromophobe) and secreting adenomas based on the presence or absence of hormone production. The former type presents clinically in one or a combination of three ways:

1. Incidental finding of sellar enlargement on skull radiograph.
2. Impaired pituitary trophic hormone production due to compression of the pituitary gland.
3. Mass effect with compression of parasellar structures.

The secreting adenomas produce syndromes as a result of trophic hormone overproduction with or without associated findings of mass effect. Syndromes include:

1. Growth hormone.
   a. Before epiphyseal closure—gigantism.
   b. After epiphyseal closure—acromegaly.
2. Prolactin.
   a. Amenorrhea and galactorrhea in females.
   b. Gynecomastia and decreased libido in males.
3. Adrenocorticotropic hormone (ACTH).
   a. Cushing's disease.

Pituitary adenomas as they increase in size typically produce sellar erosion and expansion, which may be focal or generalized. With continued growth, they extend beyond the confines of the sella as follows:

1. Laterally.
   a. Compressing or invading the cavernous sinuses, rarely encasing the carotid artery.
   b. Entering the middle cranial fossa to impinge on the temporal lobe.
2. Superiorly—directly.
   a. Entering the suprasellar cistern and compressing optic nerves or chiasm.
   b. Indenting the anterior portion of the third ventricle, rarely reaching sufficient size to obstruct the foramen of Monro and produce hydrocephalus (Taveras 1976).
3. Superiorly—anteriorly.
   a. Extending underneath or between the frontal lobes.
4. Superiorly—posteriorly.
   a. Projecting into the interpeduncular cistern and impinging on the midbrain.
5. Posteriorly.
   a. Eroding through the dorsum sellae to enter the pontine cistern, extending, on occasion, into the cerebellopontine angle cistern.
6. Anterolaterally.
   a. Rare extension through the superior orbital fissure into the orbit.
7. Inferiorly.
   a. Eroding into the sphenoid sinus and, with continued growth, even involving the pharynx.

Computed tomographic investigation of such lesions demonstrates effects of bone erosion, effects of compression of structures by the mass, and the mass itself. Pressure erosion leads to sharply marginated loss of bone in one or both anterior clinoid processes and the dorsum (Fig. 10-20). The anterior sellar wall and tuberculum show symmetrical or asymmetrical concavity with large tumors. On axial projection with wide window widths, these changes can be well appreciated. However, frequently, the earliest changes are in the sellar floor, and coronal sections are necessary for detection of early changes with mild degree of sellar expansion.

The tumors are typically homogeneously slightly hyperdense or isodense with respect to surrounding brain (Naidich 1976a). Some tumors have areas of necrosis or cyst formation producing inhomogeneity due to these areas of low density; when they involve much of the lesion, a low-density mass re-

Table 10-1   Masses of the Sellar Region

Masses arising within sella (intrasellar)
  Pituitary adenoma
  Pituitary carcinoma
  Pituitary metastasis
  Pituitary abscess
  Pituitary enlargement due to target organ (adrenal, thyroid, gonads) failure
  Myoblastoma
  Intrasellar arachnoid cyst
  Intrasellar craniopharyngioma
  Intrasellar meningioma—rare

Masses arising above sella (suprasellar)
  Craniopharyngioma
  Meningioma of tuberculum sellae or diaphragma sellae
  Optic glioma
  Aneurysm—carotid siphon or anterior communicating artery origin
  Arachnoid cyst
  Metastasis
  Granuloma
  Epidermoid
  Dermoid
  Teratoma
  Chordoma
  Germinoma (ectopic pinealoma)
  Anterior third ventricular pathology
    Markedly dilated third ventricle in hydrocephalus
    Intraventricular tumors and cysts
  Hypothalamic tumors
    Glioma
    Metastasis
    Hamartoma
    Teratoma
  Arteriovenous malformations

Middle cranial fossa masses arising lateral to sella (parasellar)
  Cavernous carotid aneurysm
  Meningioma—sphenoid wing
  Metastasis
  Trigeminal neuroma
  Granuloma
  Chondroma, osteochondroma, chondrosarcoma
  Chordoma
  Sarcoma

Anterior cranial fossa masses arising anterior to the sella

Meningioma—origin: planum sphenoidale, olfactory groove
Craniopharyngioma
Dermoid
Epidermoid
Metastasis
Osteoma
Lesions extending upward from ethmoid sinuses
  Ethmoid sinus carcinoma
  Ethmoid sinus polyposis
  Ethmoid sinus mucocele
  Inverting papilloma
  Granulomas
  Wegener's granulomatosis
  Epidermoid
  Nasal cavity lesions invading ethmoids
    Inflammatory
    Neoplastic

Clivial masses arising behind sella (retrosellar)
  Chordomas
  Meningioma—clivus origin
  Craniopharyngioma
  Basilar artery aneurysm
  Arachnoid cyst
  Chondroma
  Primary bone tumor
  Metastasis
  Exophytic brainstem glioma
  Dermoid
  Epidermoid
  Teratoma
  Granuloma

Masses arising below sella (infrasellar)
  Sphenoid sinus
    Malignancy
    Mucocele
    Polyposis
    Granulomas (infectious, sarcoid, nonspecific)
    Wegener's granulomatosis
    Epidermoid
  Primary bone tumor of sphenoid
  Chordoma
  Metastasis
  Nasopharyngeal tumor invading sphenoid
    Malignancy
    Juvenile angiofibroma

Figure 10-20 Sellar expansion due to pituitary adenoma. **A.** Moderate expansion of the sella. Medial concavity of the left anterior clinoid (arrowhead) due to erosion is noted. The tuberculum posteriorly is concave (arrows). Finally, there is marked erosion of the dorsum (clear arrow) with only a thin shell of bone remaining. **B.** Mild sellar expansion. There is asymmetrical concavity of the tuberculum (arrow). **C.** Marked asymmetrical expansion of the sella, the right side showing greater expansion than the left. The central and right portions of the dorsum are no longer visualized (solid arrow). The tuberculum posteriorly is markedly concave (clear arrow), with asymmetrical expansion.

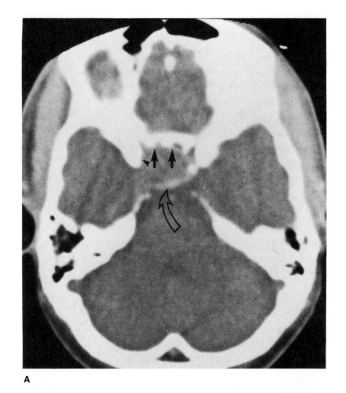

A

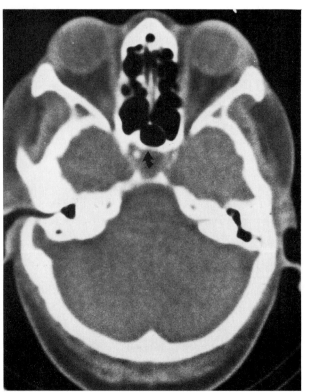

B

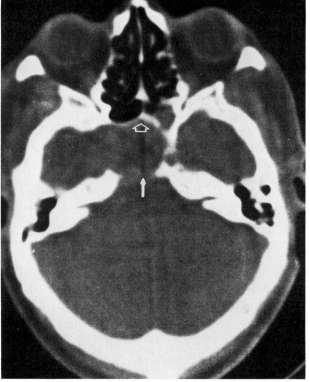

C

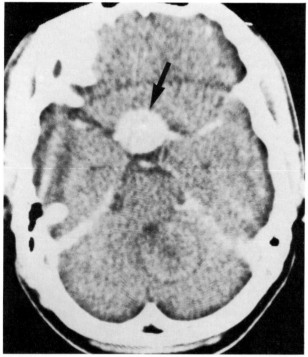

A

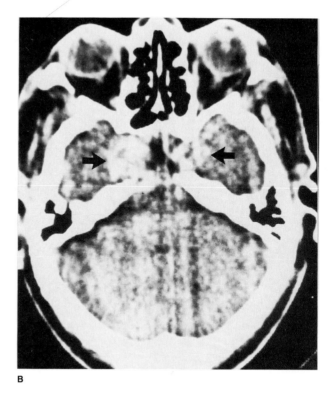

B

Figure 10-21 Pituitary adenoma following contrast injection. **A.** Homogeneously enhancing adenoma (arrow) extends into the suprasellar cistern. **B.** Pituitary adenoma extends laterally into the middle cranial fossae (arrows). **C.** A large pituitary adenoma with nonenhancing center (arrow) due to necrosis.

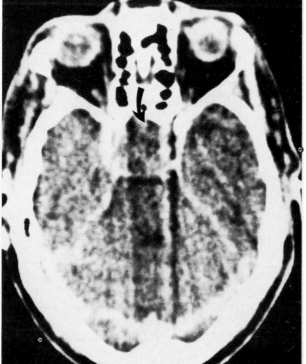

C

sults, with CT values approaching those of cerebrospinal fluid. Following intravenous contrast injection, most adenomas enhance considerably (Fig. 10-21). With lesions extending beyond the confines of the sella, the enhancement permits excellent demonstration of the mass in its entirety. Coronal scanning yields the most accurate information concerning the superior margins of the tumor (Fig. 10-22). Furthermore, when the mass is confined to the sella with only slight upward bulging, coronal scans are far superior to axial sections in demonstrating the tumor because the partial-volume effect is eliminated. Mild impingement on the third ventricle is more easily recognized in coronal sections where the indented area is seen in tangent; greater degrees of upward extension with third ventricular compression are seen on axial section (Fig. 10-23). Im-

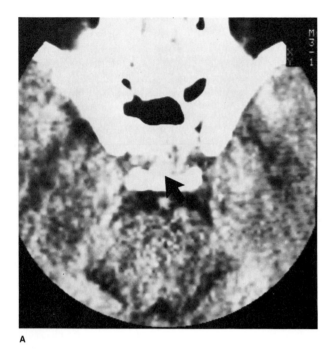
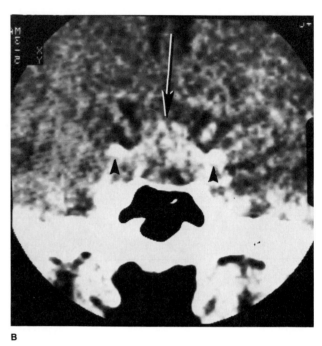

A   **B**

Figure 10-22 Suprasellar extensions of pituitary adenomas.   **A.** CT in axial view shows an enhancing tumor at the level of the sellar inlet (arrow).   **B.** CT in coronal view clearly shows suprasellar extension (arrow) above the level of the anterior clinoids (arrowheads).

pingement on the optic nerves or chiasm is also best seen on coronal section. Sagittal reformation are also quite useful in visualizing suprasellar extension and impingement on suprasellar structures. When pituitary adenomas do not enhance sufficiently for delineation of their extension, metrizamide cisternography is extremely effective in outlining the various projections of the tumor from the sella (Hall 1980) (Fig. 10-24). Again, axial, coronal, or sagittal views may be elected, depending on the area to be viewed in tangent (Fig. 10-1).

Extension of tumors into the sphenoid sinus can be demonstrated easily because of the air contrast provided by the sinus (unless the sinus is opacified by fluid or mucosal thickening as a result of sinusitis). Coronal and sagittal sections are necessary for evaluation (Fig. 10-23); if such sections are not available, conventional pluridirectional tomography is quite satisfactory. Penetration of tumors through the pharyngeal surface of the sphenoid is well demonstrated by either of these means as well (Fig. 10-23).

Calcification of pituitary tumors (Banna 1976*b*; Deery 1929; du Boulay 1962; Taveras 1976), while uncommon, occurs in either curvilinear (in the "capsule" of the adenoma) or nodular (in the tumor itself) fashion. Rarely, dense solid calcification may occur. Since these are uncommon findings, the occurrence of these tumors suggests the possibility of craniopharyngioma, meningioma, or aneurysm (more commonly calcified lesions).

When the adenomas are less than 1 cm in diameter, they are referred to as *microadenomas* (Hardy 1969). Since these are too small to produce compression of nearby structures, the clinical presentation is that of hypersecretion of the anterior lobe pituitary trophic hormones.

Until recently, it was believed that pluridirectional tomography with multiple thin sections was the method of most validity in demonstrating these lesions (Geehr 1978; Richmond 1980; Robertson 1978; Vezina 1974). Focal areas of expansion or bone thinning were considered indicative of the presence and location of the tumor. The focal changes typi-

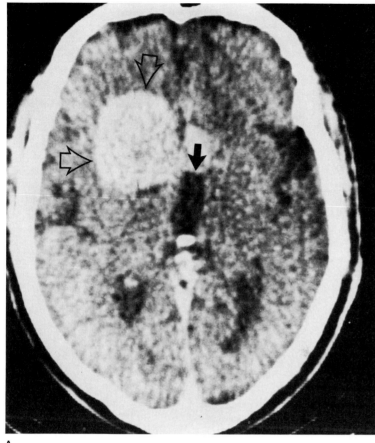

A

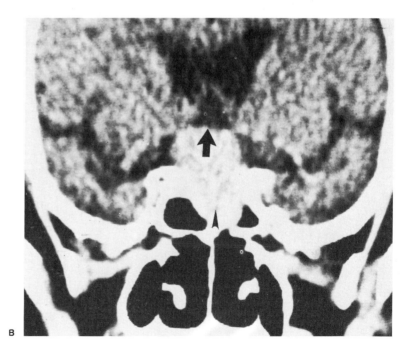

B

Figure 10-23 Supra- and infrasellar extension of pituitary adenomas. **A.** Axial CT showing massive suprasellar extension of a large pituitary adenoma (clear arrow). The tumor has a lobulated appearance and has caused indentation of the anterior margin of the third ventricle (arrow). **B.** Coronal section demonstrates the suprasellar extension of the adenoma with indentation of the anterior end of the third ventricle (arrow). (*Continued on p. 404.*)

Figure 10-23 (*Cont.*) **C.** A more posterior coronal section demonstrating not only the suprasellar extension (arrow) but also invasion of the sphenoid sinus (arrowhead).   **D.** Same section as **B** viewed at wide window settings shows the destruction of the floor of the sella and the tumor within the sphenoid sinus (arrowheads).

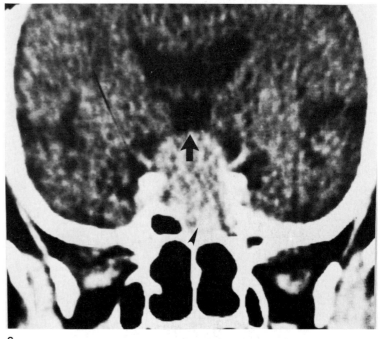

C

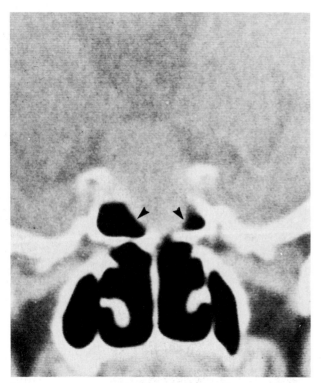

D

cally occurred on one side (producing asymmetry) and usually at the anteroinferior aspect of the sellar floor (with focal bulging or indistinctness) of the cortical bone in that area; occasional cases occurred in which the changes were posteroinferior.

Recent studies (Raji 1981; Wortzman 1980), however, have indicated that pluridirectional tomography is less reliable. A significant number of false positive and false negative as well as falsely localizing examinations were noted in these studies. Concomitantly, it has been shown that coronal thin-section CT or thin-section high-resolution axial CT with coronal and sagittal reformation provides a very reliable method of demonstrating and localizing a microadenoma. The normal height of the pituitary gland, utilizing coronal CT ranged up to 6.8 mm in females and 6.0 mm in males (Syvertsen 1979). In our own evaluation, utilizing the newer-generation scanners, the height of the normal pituitary gland has been as high as 7.8 mm in males and up to 8.0 mm in females. The lower limit was 4.0 mm. The difference in height is partly dependent on the contour of the sellar cavity. The superior

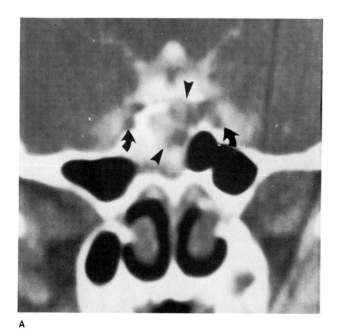

A

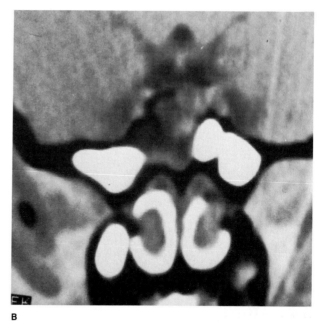

B

Figure 10-24 Pituitary adenoma associated with CSF rhinorrhea. **A.** This pituitary adenoma did not enhance sufficiently for evaluation on routine CT studies. Because of the CSF rhinorrhea, metrizamide CT cisternography was employed. The tumor is well visualized within the opacity of the contrast medium (arrowheads) and shows the upper extent of the tumor (upper arrowhead). The lower arrowhead lies within the contrast, which has entered the right sphenoid sinus, indicating the site of CSF leakage. The cavernous sinus and the carotid arteries are seen as filling defects within the contrast medium on either side of the tumor (curved arrows). **B.** Reverse image of **A** to distinguish the sellar contour from the contrast medium.

surface was flat or concave upward, and the normal gland enhanced homogeneously to about the same density as the cerebral vessels. Findings of significance in prolactin-secreting microadenomas in coronal scans are (1) increase in height above the upper limits of normal, (2) upward convexity of the superior surface of the gland, and (3) nonhomogeneous enhancement; the microadenoma typically appears as a poorly enhancing area (Fig. 10-25).

There are insufficient data to be certain of the findings in ACTH- and human growth hormone (HGH)-secreting microadenomas. They seem to enhance more than the prolactin-producing tumors, approaching the density of the pituitary gland. In such cases, gland enlargement and upward convexity become the findings of importance. Other authors (Smaltino 1980) have noted focal contrast enhancement in pituitary microadenomas of all three common types (prolactin, growth hormones, and ACTH); this occurred in about 60 percent of cases in Smaltino's series. Since the sellar floor can also be evaluated with CT, the study (on new generation scanners) will become the method of choice for complete evaluation of pituitary adenomas of all size (Rothman 1980) (Fig. 10-25). With the newer generation scanners, CT provides precise information and thus is useful in evaluating the results of various treatment modalities not available in the past. Preoperative decision whether the transsphenoidal approach or the intracranial approach can be easily made and is based on the size and direction of growth of the adenoma. CT is also useful in demonstrating the amount of residual tumor following surgery (Fig. 10-26), the results of radiation or medical therapy (Fig. 10-27), and in the long-term followup of the patient.

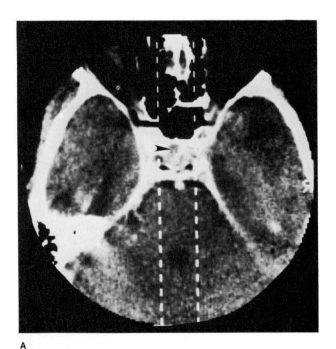

A

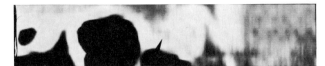

B

Figure 10-25   Pituitary microadenoma.   **A.** Axial image and **B** sagittal reformatted image of a patient with Cushing's syndrome. The adenoma (arrowhead) is seen as a slightly hypodense mass.   **C.** Axial and **D** coronal CT of another patient with an enhancing microadenoma (arrowhead).

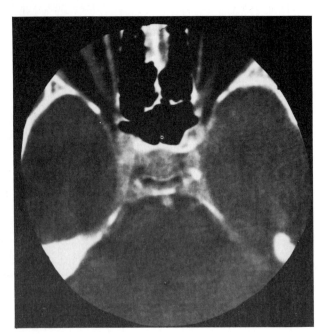

C

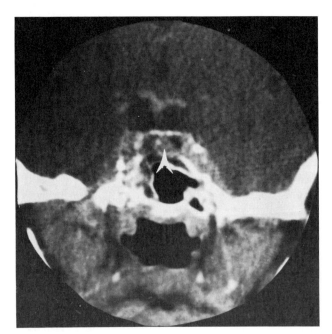

D

Figure 10-26 Residual tumor following surgery. The enhanced coronal CT shows the residual pituitary adenoma following transsphenoidal surgery (arrowhead). Note the absence of the sellar floor.

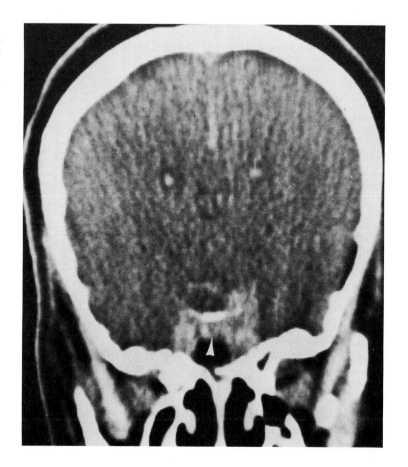

With all the above statements, a word of caution is indicated. Cerebral arteriography is currently the method for reliably detecting the following arterial abnormalities which can considerably complicate pituitary surgery:

1. Incidental associated internal carotid artery aneurysm
2. Congenital carotid abnormalities
   a. Arterial communication between the cavernous portions of the internal carotid arteries (Fig. 10-28)
   b. Intrasellar location of the cavernous portion of the internal carotid artery (Fig. 10-29)
3. Arterial encasement of the tumor
4. Intrasellar cavernous carotid aneurysm (Fig. 10-30)

Cerebral arteriography is thus considered by many surgeons to be a necessary component of preoperative evaluation for pituitary adenomas, although similar information can presently be obtained utilizing digital subtraction angiography (Fig. 10-30).

Pituitary tumors occasionally undergo infarction, either hemorrhagic or bland. In both cases the blood supply to the tumor is impaired as a result of expansion with compression at the opening of the diaphragma sellae. The patient shows evidence of a rapidly expanding sellar mass: compression of the third, fourth, and sixth cranial nerves with diplopia

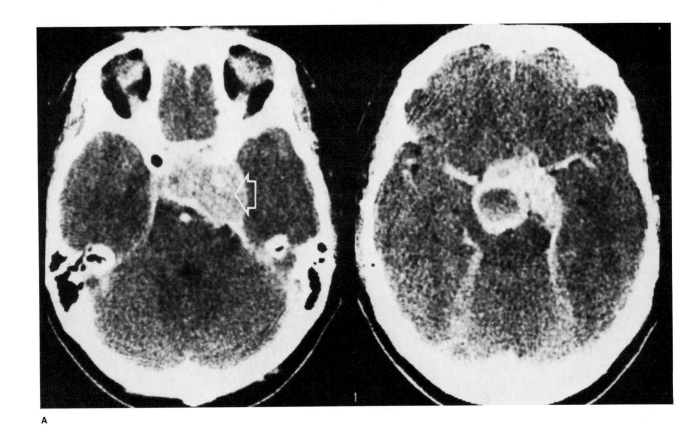

A

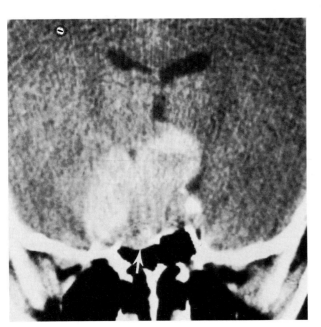

B

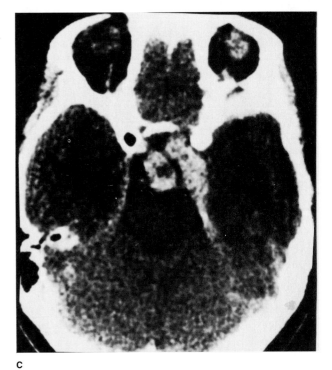

C

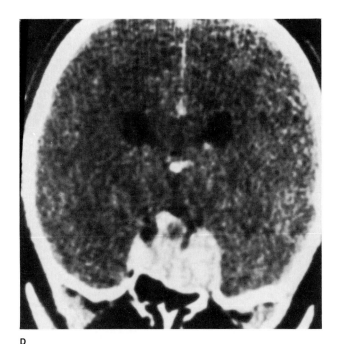

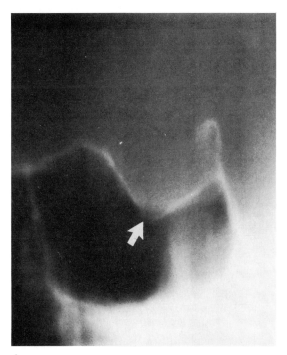

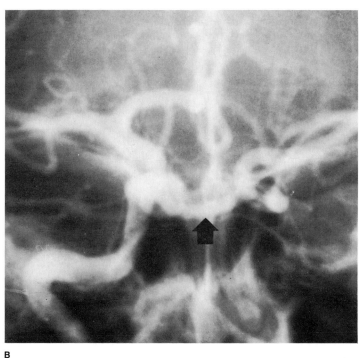

Figure 10-27 Shrinkage in size of tumor following medical therapy. **A.** Two axial sections showing the sellar and suprasellar extent of a prolactin-secreting adenoma. The tumor has extended into the cavernous sinus on one side (arrow). **B.** Coronal CT shows not only the tumor's suprasellar extent but also the erosion of the floor of the sella (arrow) by the tumor. **C** and **D.** Axial and coronal CT two weeks following Bromocryptin therapy, showing significant decrease in size of tumor.

D

A

B

Figure 10-28 Arterial anomalies. **A.** A lateral tomogram of the sella shows a small notch at the junction of the anterior wall and floor due to erosion (arrow). **B.** An anomalous communication between the cavernous portion of the two internal carotid arteries across the floor of the sella (arrow) is responsible for the focal erosion.

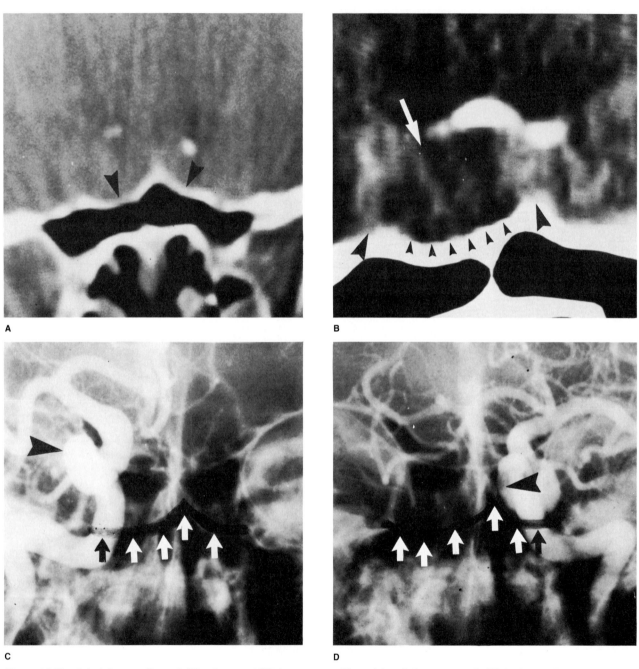

A

B

C

D

Figure 10-29   Arterial anomalies.   **A.** Direct coronal CT shows concavity of both sides of the sellar floor (arrowheads). The concavity is greater on the right than on the left.   **B.** Coronal CT following intravenous contrast demonstrates a hypodense pituitary adenoma (arrow) which fits into the concavity (small black arrowheads). The hyperdense cavernous sinus and internal carotid artery (large black arrowheads) are seen on either side of the mass.   **C.** Right internal carotid arteriogram shows lateral displacement of the posterior part of the cavernous segment of the internal carotid artery (black arrowhead). The abnormal sellar floor is indicated by the arrows. **D.** Left internal carotid arteriogram shows the intrasellar location of the artery, which conforms to the concavity on the left side of the sellar floor.

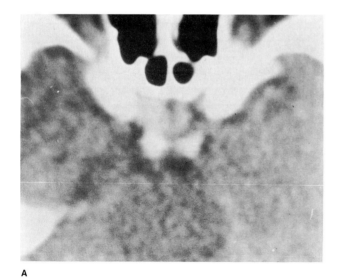

A

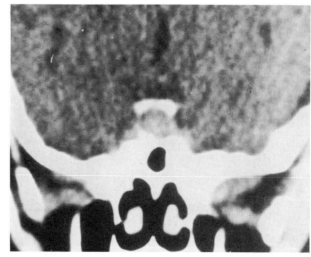

B

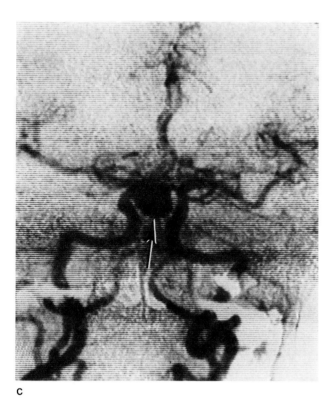

C

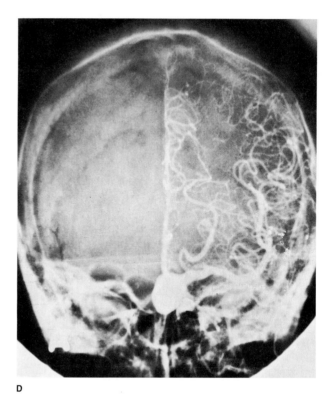

D

Figure 10-30 Arterial anomalies. **A** and **B.** Axial and coronal enhanced CT. A hyperdense mass is seen within the sella producing mild, symmetrical sellar expansion. **C.** A digital subtraction angiogram reveals that the enhancing mass seen on CT is a large intrasellar aneurysm (arrow). **D.** An internal carotid arteriogram shows similar finding, the aneurysm arising from the internal carotid artery.

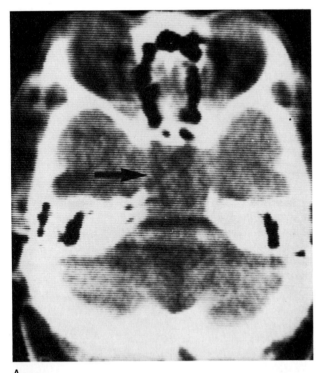

(unilateral or bilateral); optic nerve compression with rapidly decreasing visual impairment; headache; and, occasionally, signs of meningeal irritation (Banna 1976b). The CT shows evidence of a sellar mass which is either lower than brain density due to edema from infarction or shows increased density due to hemorrhage (Fig. 10-31). The syndrome of infarction or hemorrhage into a pituitary gland has been termed *pituitary apoplexy*. It is usually managed urgently to prevent permanent optic nerve damage. Some patients present at a later stage in a subacute fashion. Here the CT may show only low density in the sella with rim enhancement in a fashion similar to peripheral enhancement seen in cerebral hemorrhages and some infarcts (Post 1980). Pitui-

Figure 10-31 Two cases of pituitary apoplexy. **A.** Infarction of a large pituitary adenoma with rapid swelling. A hypodense mass is present within the markedly expanded sella (arrow). The mass is due to edema within the infarcted tumor. No enhancement was noted. **B.** Hemorrhage into a pituitary adenoma, which appears as a hyperdense mass (arrows).

A

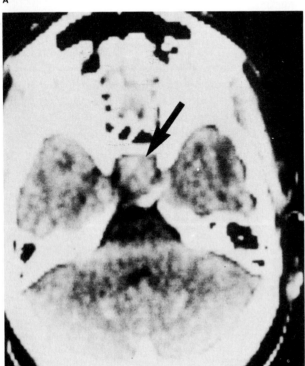

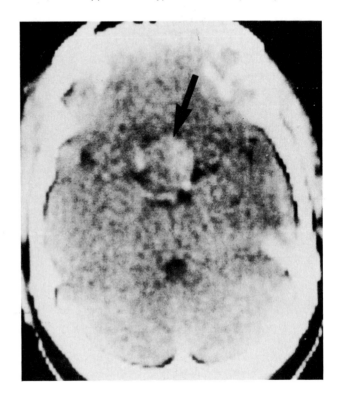

B

tary apoplexy may occur spontaneously as indicated but is known to be precipitated by radiotherapy in some instances, presumably as a result of swelling of the mass.

Pituitary Carcinoma

There are no specific CT features which distinguish pituitary carcinoma from adenoma. Local invasiveness and bone destruction per se are not evidence of malignancy (Fig. 10-25). The presence of distant metastasis is the only certain proof of malignancy.

Pituitary Metastasis

Here bone destruction with little or no expansion is the principal distinguishing feature. When there is sellar expansion, distinction from an aggressive pituitary tumor may not be possible.

Pituitary Abscess

This most commonly arises within a pituitary adenoma but can arise in an otherwise normal gland (Dominque 1977; Rudwan 1977). The infection may occur by extension of sphenoid sinusitis or by hematogeneous spread from a distant focus. The diagnosis may be suspected clinically when sellar enlargement is seen in the presence of clinical evidence of meningitis; as with abscesses elsewhere, ring or solid enhancement may be noted following intravenous contrast injection (Chap. 13).

Pituitary Enlargement Due to Target Organ Failure

This diagnosis is made on the clinical finding of adrenal, thyroid, or gonadal hypofunction in the presence of sellar enlargement with poor response to trophic hormone stimulation. Computed tomographic findings are those of sellar enlargement with a soft-tissue mass (the enlarged pituitary). In one series (Kuno 1980) the hyperplastic pituitary gland showed significant enhancement.

Myoblastoma

This is a rare benign tumor of the pituitary. It has no distinguishing radiologic or CT characteristics (Banna 1976*b*).

Empty Sella

This entity refers to sellar expansion associated with extension of the subarachnoid space into the sella (Kaufman 1968, 1973; Motara 1970; Tyrell 1978). There are "primary" and "secondary" types. The former is associated with extension of the subarachnoid space into the sella through a congenitally wide aperture (for the passage of the pituitary stalk) in the diaphragma sellae. Transmitted pulsation leads to remodeling and mild expansion of the sella; the expansion is typically symmetrical. The secondary type is associated with involution, spontaneous or following treatment, of a pituitary adenoma. In this case, the sellar enlargement is greater and often asymmetrical. An empty sella is usually an incidental finding on CT; however, patients may be symptomatic in some cases. In secondary cases, pituitary hypofunction may be present. Furthermore, the optic nerves may herniate into an empty sella and become entrapped, producing visual impairment. Finally, thinning of the sellar walls may cause cerebrospinal fluid rhinorrhea (Hall 1980; Pinto 1979*a*). In the past the diagnosis of empty sella neccesitated the use of pneumoencephalography with occasional pluridirectional tomography. Presently with CT the diagnosis can be easily made (Fig. 10-32) without resort to other studies. In occasional cases a necrotic (or partially necrotic) tumor can not be ruled out with absolute certainty (Rozario 1977). In these selected cases CT following cisternal metrizamide would help in resolving whether the hypodense region within the sella is due to the extension of subarachnoid cistern into the sella or due to a necrotic tumor (Hall 1980). The latter is preferred when coronal scanning is available because metrizamide opacifies the subarachnoid space more uniformly than does air. With newer high-resolution scanners, the pituitary gland, pituitary stalk, and

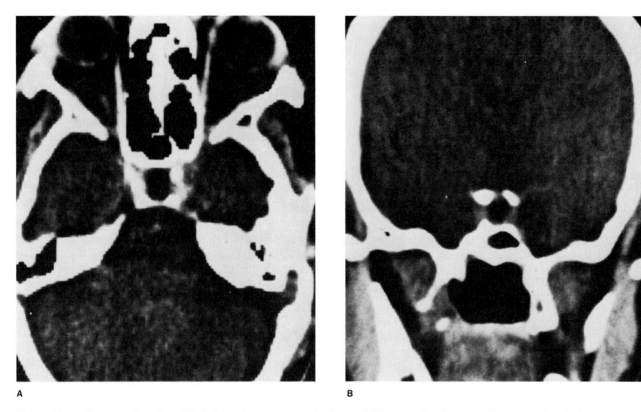

A   B

Figure 10-32 Empty sella.   **A** and **B.** Axial and direct coronal enhanced CT. Instead of the normally enhancing pituitary gland the sella has the characteristic "empty" appearance. This was an incidental finding since the patient was endocrinologically normal.

subarachnoid space can be imaged directly (especially when intrathecal contrast enhancement is used (Fig. 10-19). The presence of an empty sella does not rule out the absence of a pituitary gland tumor; if pituitary malfunction is noted, a tumor may be present in the tissue; but its location within the gland cannot be ascertained from the configuration of the gland in most cases. According to Smaltino et al. (1980), a microadenoma could be seen as a focal area of contrast enhancement within an empty sella in 6 of 10 cases.

Craniopharyngioma

This is dealt with elsewhere (Chap. 7). Briefly, these tumors are believed to arise from squamous epithelial rests (remnants of the craniopharyngeal duct,

clusters of which can occur in the infundibulum and below the diaphragma sellae). Craniopharyngiomas most commonly arise above the sella, but may originate within the sella or, very rarely, in an infrasellar location. Those arising within the sella produce sellar enlargement similar to that of pituitary tumors; in some of these cases there may be increase in the density of the sellar walls, an appearance not seen in pituitary tumors (Taveras 1976).

The tumors may be solid, cystic, or a combination of the two. Calcification is far more common in craniopharyngiomas than in pituitary tumors; it occurs in 20 percent of patients under 2 years of age, 80 percent in children over 2 years, and in 30 to 50 percent of adult patients (Banna 1976b). Calcification is shell-like in cystic lesions but may be nodular, amorphous, or cloudlike in solid lesions; mixed appearances may be seen in some lesions.

Cystic lesions (or cystic areas of solid lesions) vary in CT density from that of water to that of brain, depending on the proportions of cholesterol (low density) and other materials within the cyst; rarely cysts with density lower than that of water may be found, some showing layering of materials within the cyst, with the cholesterol lying superiorly. Solid lesions are of a density equal to or greater than that of brain tissue.

Enhancement is uncommon in cystic lesions, but peripheral enhancement may be seen in some. Solid lesions, when densely calcified, may not show recognizable enhancement; noncalcified solid areas show varying degrees of enhancement. Mixed lesions (solid and cystic) may have mixed patterns of enhancement and calcification (Fitz 1978; Miller 1980). Low-density lesions which do not enhance may require intrathecal contrast for evaluation (Fig. 10-33).

Figure 10-33 Isodense craniopharyngioma.   **A.** Axial CT demonstrates a mass in the suprasellar cistern (arrows) with a density similar to the rest of the brain parenchyma.   **B.** Two CT sections following cisternal metrizamide clearly define the tumor (arrows).

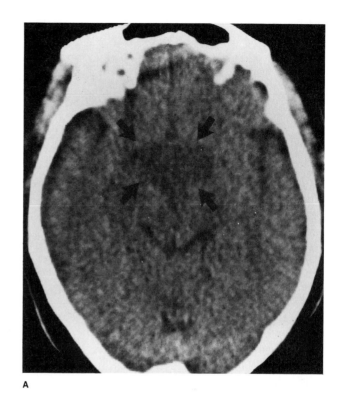

A

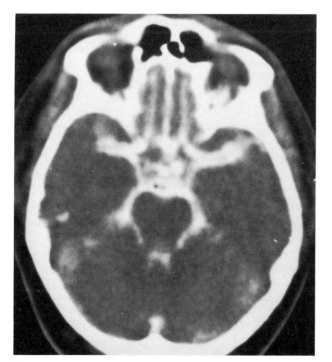

B

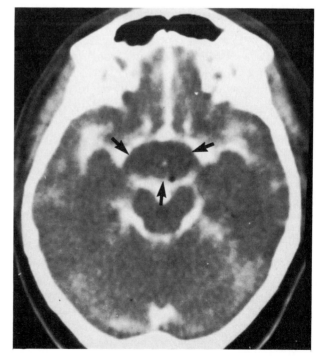

Meningioma

About 20 percent of meningiomas arise in the peri-sellar region. They show features which are typical of meningiomas in general, as described elsewhere. There are, however, some features worth mentioning. These tumors can extend into the sella and expand it. They may erode or invade bone and extend into the sinuses. In addition to producing bone changes in the planum sphenoidale, they may cause focal elevation of the planum as a result of weakening of this bone with focal expansion ("blistering") of the sphenoid sinus. Finally, the known propensity of these tumors to encase arteries makes carotid arteriography a necessity prior to surgery.

Aneurysm

This topic is thoroughly discussed in Chap. 14. Briefly, large aneurysms can present as suprasellar, suprasellar-intrasellar, intrasellar, and parasellar masses (Raymond 1978). They may be fully patent, partially thrombosed, or completely thrombosed. Completely thrombosed aneurysms are of a density equal to that of brain tissue. Some have varying degrees of peripheral, shell-like calcification. Following intravenous contrast injection, the non-thrombosed portion of the aneurysm shows dense enhancement while the thrombosed portion does not. A thin rim of enhancement about the periphery of the aneurysm is typical; this represents diffusion of contrast into the fibrous tissue wall about the aneurysm (Pinto 1979*b*). A totally thrombosed large aneurysm can mimic craniopharyngioma, whereas a fully patent aneurysm without peripheral calcification may be confused with other lesions of the sellar region which are capable of dense enhancement (meningioma, pituitary adenoma, metastasis, etc.). Arteriography resolves the issue easily in the nonthrombosed type. Clinical history of previous subarachnoid hemorrhage and the homogeneous density with a thin rim of enhancement are helpful indicators of the correct diagnosis in the thrombosed type. Bone erosion may occur when the aneurysm lies in contact with a bony area. Cavernous carotid aneurysms may erode the lateral portion of the sellar floor, the ipsilateral anterior clinoid process, the dorsum sellae, and the margins of the superior orbital fissure (widening it) (Fig. 10-34). Suprasellar aneurysms may produce erosions similar to those caused by other suprasellar lesions.

Sphenoid Sinus Mucocele

This is dealt with in detail in Chap. 3. Briefly, mucoceles of the sinuses are felt to arise secondary to obstruction of either a sinus ostium or a mucous gland (Hesselink 1979; Osborn 1979). In either case a fluid-filled, cystic, expanding lesion results which produces pressure erosion of bone with resultant thinning. The lesion progressively expands the sinus and eventually extends into adjacent areas; sphenoid sinus mucoceles may extend into the apices of one or both orbits and intracranially to present as a sellar and suprasellar mass. The decision as to the origin of such a mass can, at times, be difficult since lesions of the sellar area can extend into the sphenoid sinus. The clue of major importance on plain films and tomography is evidence of expansion of the sinus, sometimes only the presence of shell-like bone fragments at the periphery of the mass (Fig. 10-35). The sellar floor is not seen in most cases when the lesion expands into and above the sella; but a rare case of an expanded sella which mimicks the enlargement of a sellar tumor may be encountered (Osborn 1979; Simms 1970), with the mucocele entering the sella through a small defect in the sellar floor.

On CT the density of these lesions is most often equal to that of brain tissue, but a significant number can be less dense or denser (Hesselink 1979). The high-density lesions in one series were found to be infected mucoceles (pyoceles) (Hesselink 1979). Contrast enhancement does not occur without infection. The infected lesions may show a rim of enhancement (Hesselink 1979). Demarcation of the intracranial component can be difficult without intravenous contrast, which enhances the displaced dura capping the extradural mass. Metrizamide cisternography can be used for more precise definition when necessary.

Computed tomography can also show the expansile rather than invasive nature of the lesion, differentiating it from primary malignancies, metastatic disease, and chordomas.

Dermoid

This tumor, like the epidermoid, arises from inclusion of ectodermal elements during closure of the neural tube; unlike the epidermoid, a dermoid may also contain one or more mesodermal elements (hair, hair follicles, sebaceous and sweat glands, teeth, and nails) in addition to squamous epithelium. Dermoids tend to occur in the midline; epidermoids may occur either in the midline or laterally. In the sellar area, dermoids may present as suprasellar masses (similar to craniopharyngiomas) with erosion of the dorsum sellae from above and widening of the sellar opening. They are typically smooth oval or round masses of low density due to contained cholesterol debris (Lee 1979; New 1974)

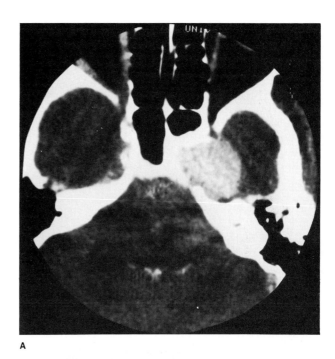

A

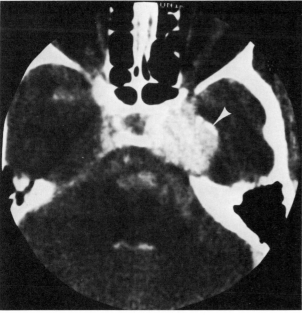

B

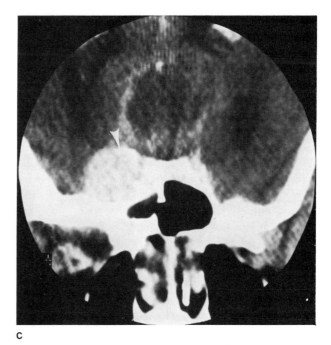

C

Figure 10-34 Cavernous carotid aneurysm: **A** and **B.** Contrast-enhanced axial CT at two different levels shows a large enhancing mass with calcification (arrowhead) along the wall of the aneurysm. The slight hyperdensity of the cisterns is due to rupture of the aneurysm. **C.** Coronal CT demonstrates the size of the aneurysm to better advantage.

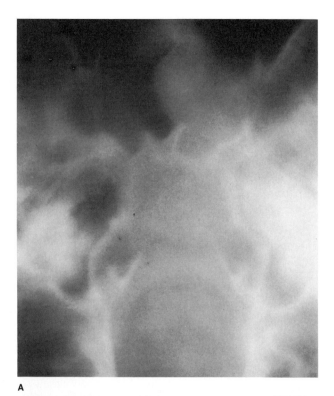

A

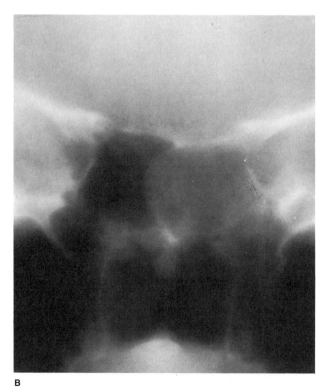

B

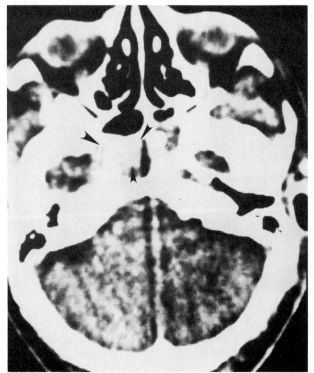

C

Figure 10-35 Sphenoid sinus mucocele. Axial **(A)** and coronal **(B)** pluridirectional tomography shows the sphenoid sinus completely opacified along its left side. The bulging septum, thinned out but not destroyed, outlines the normal right half of the sinus. **C.** Axial CT of the same patient shows the opacified right half of the sphenoid sinus (arrowheads).

but may contain elements of higher density or calcification interiorly; peripheral curvilinear calcification is common. Rarely they are uniformly calcified and dense. Contrast enhancement does not occur. There may be fat-fluid levels due to layering of the lighter cholesterol debris above the heavier fluid elements; rupture of a cyst may lead to fatty density in the subarachnoid spaces (with a fulminant chemical meningitis) and fat-fluid levels in the ventricles (Peyton 1942; Tytus 1956).

Epidermoids may occur in the suprasellar areas as well (Fig. 10-36). Their characteristics are discussed in the section on the cerebellopontine angle, where they are most common. They, too, are low-density lesions, usually less dense than surrounding brain tissue; some have peripheral or internal calcifications, and an occasional lesion is more dense than brain tissue, presumably as a result of

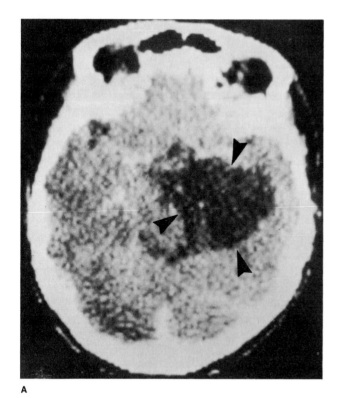

A

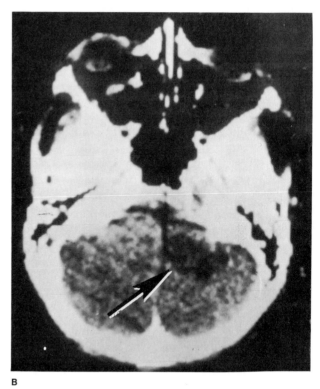

B

Figure 10-36   Epidermoid tumor. Higher **(A)** and lower **(B)** sections show a large epidermoid tumor that extends into the suprasellar area and middle cranial fossa (arrowheads) and into the cerebellopontine angle (arrow).

internal calcification. Enhancement rarely occurs, but when it does, it is peripheral, probably in the connective tissue components of the capsule. When lesions in the suprasellar cistern are of a density equal to that of cerebrospinal fluid, they will not be seen unless they expand beyond the cistern, have calcification, or show peripheral enhancement (Mikhael 1978); only intrathecal contrast will demonstrate the presence of these tumors. Computed tomography with metrizamide is an excellent method of evaluation when a suprasellar lesion is strongly suspected clinically and the scan appears normal.

Other Lesions

Optic system and hypothalamic lesions are discussed in other chapters and are not considered here. Arachnoid cysts are considered in Chap. 4. Lesions of the sphenoid, sphenoid sinus, or nasopharynx (by extension into the sphenoid) may extend superiorly to involve the sella (Fig. 10-37).

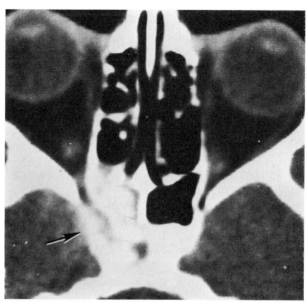

Figure 10-37   Carcinoma of the left sphenoid sinus causing opacification and destruction of the lateral wall (arrow).

THE CLIVUS

Anatomy

The clivus extends from the base of the dorsum sellae to the foramen magnum, the anterior lip of which it forms (Fig. 10-38). Its lateral boundaries are the petrooccipital fissure above and the synchondrosis between the basioccipital and exoccipital bones below. The sphenoid sinus may project into the clivus to varying degrees. From the lateral margins of the clivus inferiorly project the jugular tubercles, within which are the hypoglossal canals (Fig. 10-38B). The inferior petrosal sinuses course along the lateral margins of the clivus, running from the posterior portion of the cavernous sinus to the jugular bulbs lateral to the jugular tubercles. In sagittal section the clivus is triangular, with its base situated anterosuperiorly and its apex at the foramen magnum. The anteroinferior aspect of the clivus forms the bony roof and posterior wall of the nasopharynx. Along the posterosuperior surface of the clivus is the basilar venous plexus and the dura; behind this surface are the pons (above) and the medulla (below), separated from the clivus by the pontine and medullary cisterns.

CT Technique

In conventional axial CT, the scan sections are nearly parallel to the endocranial surface of the clivus. When indicated for accurate evaluation of bone lesions, scans perpendicular to either the endocranial or exocranial surfaces may be obtained by gantry tilt, chin elevation, or a combination of these to produce sections angulated cephalad to Reid's baseline. (This is more accurately done by either a preliminary lateral skull radiograph or digital radiographic localization when available.) Sagittal reconstructions are also useful in evaluating the intra- and extracranial extension of mass lesions in this area. Displacement of the brainstem away from the clivus is seen with extraaxial masses. Displace-

ment of the basilar artery can also be useful in making this determination. Water-soluble intrathecal contrast is of value in some instances in evaluation of extent and localization of lesions which enhance poorly. Intrathecal air can also provide reasonably good contrast in clival lesions but is less controllable and may yield incomplete information.

Pathology

Chordoma

These tumors arise from remnants of the notochord. In the cranial region, such remnants can exist in the basisphenoid and basiocciput (clivus), behind the clivus but epidural, and in the nasopharyngeal soft tissues in front of the clivus. Therefore, chordomas may arise in any of these locations; the most common origin is near the sphenooccipital synchondrosis (Banna 1976c; K. F. Lee 1979). They are soft-tissue masses with calcification (nodular, solid, flecks, reticular, or curvilinear) in 33 to 50 percent of lesions (Banna 1976c; Kendall 1977). There is a high incidence (85 to 95 percent) of adjacent bone involvement. Sometimes sequestered bone fragments add to the calcific densities in the mass. Although bone involvement is purely lytic without sclerosis, reactive sclerosis is seen in 10 percent of cases (Kendall 1977). In occasional cases bone expansion may be seen. The lesions may be midline, with symmetrical bilateral extension, or may be unilateral. Extension into the nasopharyngeal soft tissues occurs in 40 percent of cases (Banna 1976b; Kendall 1977; K. F. Lee 1979) (Fig. 10-39). Rarely chordomas may arise within the sella and expand it in the same fashion as a pituitary tumor; typically the sellar changes are erosive. On CT the lesions are slightly denser than brain and frequently demonstrate moderate enhancement with intravenous contrast (Fig. 10-39); calcification is well seen on CT. Bone erosion is typically sharply marginated, usually purely lytic, but at times shows reactive sclerosis. Since the lesions are extradural, clival lesions displace the pontine and medullary cisterns, which remain sufficiently patent in most instances

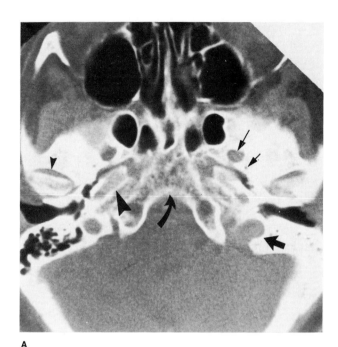

A

Figure 10-38 Posterior portion of the skull base. **A.** The curved arrow indicates the lower portion of the clivus. Visible are the left jugular foramen (large straight arrow), the foramen ovale (anterior small arrow), and foramen spinosum (posterior small arrow). Also shown is a temporomandibular joint (arrowhead). **B.** The foramen magnum (large arrow) bounded on either side by the jugular eminence (smaller arrow). The short curved arrow indicates the hypoglossal canal within the jugular eminence. Both jugular foramina are easily seen (large arrowheads). The right jugular spine is indicated by the small arrowhead. **C.** CT scan of the base of a young child's skull showing the sphenooccipital synchondrosis (arrowhead).

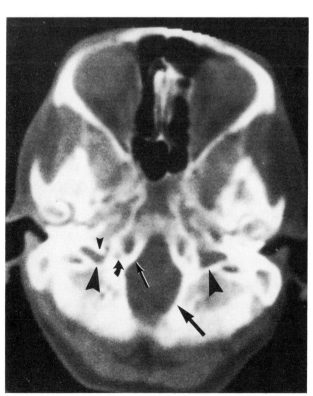

B

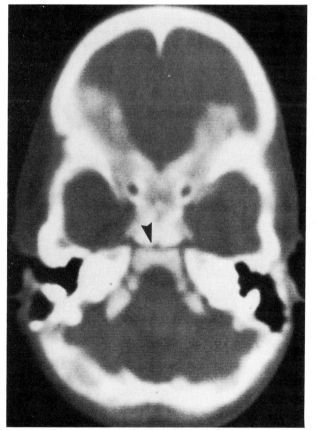

C

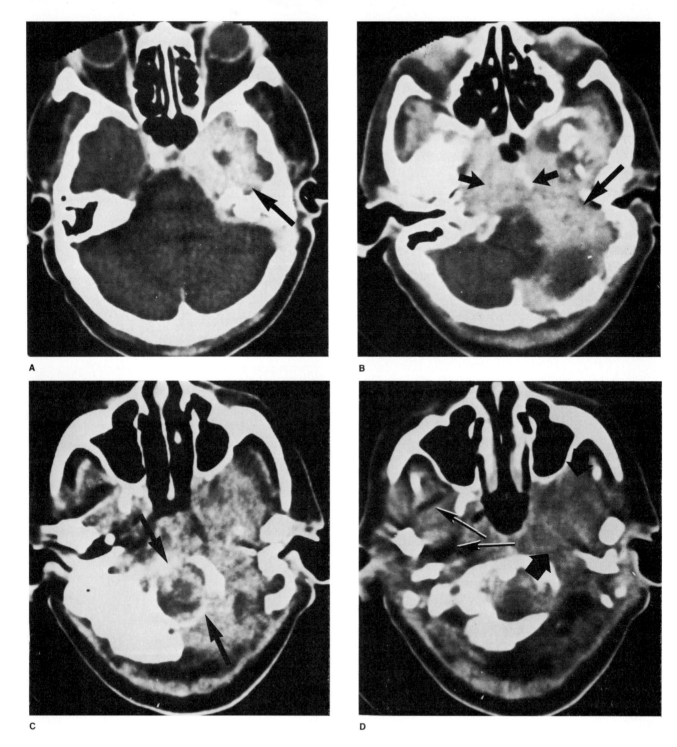

Figure 10-39 An extensive, rather massive chordoma. **A.** An enhancing mass fills the lower portion of the left middle cranial fossa (arrow). **B.** There is destruction of the entire clivus (short arrows) with only small bone fragments remaining. This is also true of the middle cranial fossa. The left petrous pyramid is also destroyed (long arrow). **C.** The foramen magnum is also involved, with two areas of destruction (arrows). **D.** A soft-tissue mass obliterates the nasopharyngeal structures (short arrows). The fat planes are totally obliterated on the left. On the right the fat planes can be seen (long arrows).

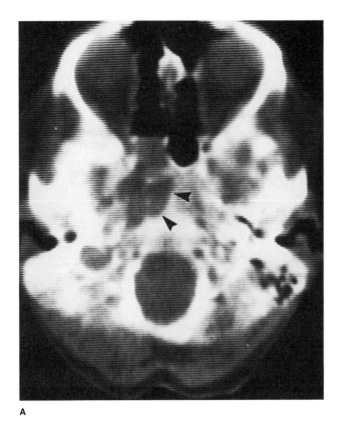

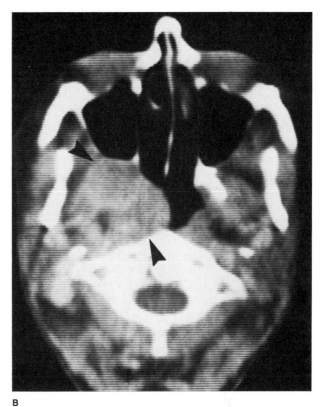

A

B

Figure 10-40 Nasopharyngeal carcinoma. **A.** Extensive destruction of the right side of the clivus (arrowheads) due to upward extension of a nasopharyngeal carcinoma. **B.** In a lower section, the infratemporal nasopharyngeal carcinoma (arrowhead) obliterates the normal muscle planes and encroaches on the nasopharyngeal airway.

to permit outlining of the extent of the mass with intrathecal positive or negative contrast. Since chordomas can encircle and narrow vessels, arteriography should be carried out prior to surgery (Kendall 1977). Nasopharyngeal carcinoma may invade the clivus and produce a picture similar to that of chordoma invading the nasopharynx (Fig. 10-40); calcification and bone sequestration, when present, are useful indicators of chordoma.

Meningiomas

These lesions show the same characteristics as described elsewhere. The bone changes and tumor characteristics may be quite suggestive of the diagnosis; however, arteriography is necessary for confirmation and as part of the preoperative evaluation.

Chondroma

These tumors have been described earlier. It should be mentioned that it may be impossible to distinguish between a chordoma and chondroma of the clivus on radiologic grounds alone, including CT (Banna 1976*b*; Sarwar 1976).

THE FORAMEN MAGNUM

Anatomy

The foramen magnum is a large orifice in the occipital bone; it is oval in shape with the long axis in the sagittal plane (Fig. 10-38). Its boundaries are the inferior edge of the clivus (basioccipital bone) anteriorly, the occipital condyles and the exoccipital portion of occipital bone laterally, and the supraoccipital portion of the occipital bone posteriorly. At birth there is an anterior synchondrosis (between the basioccipital and exoccipital portions of the occipital bone) and a posterior synchondrosis (between the exoccipital and supraoccipital portions) on each side. The anterior synchondrosis usually fuses by 3 to 4 years of age, the posterior by about 7 years (Coin 1971). Furthermore, there may be accessory ossicles in the supraoccipital bone along the posterior margin of the foramen magnum. These normal findings should not be mistaken for fractures on plain films or CT.

Through the hypoglossal canal (anterior condyloid canal), situated along the medial aspect of each occipital condyle, course the hypoglossal nerve, a meningeal branch of the ascending pharyngeal artery, and an emissary vein (Fig. 10-38). There is a depression on the exocranial surface of the occipital bone just behind each occipital condyle, the condyloid fossa; a canal, the posterior condyloid canal, is often present in the anterior margin of this fossa unilaterally or bilaterally, and an anastomotic vein connecting the sigmoid sinus and the suboccipital venous plexus passes through this canal. A variable number of emissary venous foramina close to the posterior margin of the foramen magnum may be seen in the occipital bone. The foramen magnum serves to transmit the medulla oblongata with the accompanying meninges, the dura, the accessory nerves, the vertebral arteries, the spinal arteries, occasionally a portion of the posterior inferior cerebellar arteries, and the ligaments connecting the occipital bone with the axis.

CT Technique

The foramen magnum is well imaged on axial scans, but sections perpendicular to the plane of the foramen are useful in assessment of bone involvement by tumor, superior and inferior extensions of lesions, and basilar impression and invagination. Intrathecal water-soluble positive contrast is a valuable adjunct in evaluation of masses, both intra- and extraaxially.

Pathology

Chiari Type I Malformation

This is considered in detail in Chap. 4. The cerebellar tonsils can be imaged on high-resolution CT, as can an associated enlargement of the cervical spinal cord due to hydromyelia. Furthermore, the cyst of syringomyelia of the spinal cord or medulla (syringobulbia) can be demonstrated. When the information is not conclusive, CT with intrathecal metrizamide can provide demonstration of low position of the cerebellar tonsils and spinal cord changes in syringomyelia and hydromyelia (small cord, flat cord, or enlarged cord). Delayed scanning 6 hours after intrathecal metrizamide opacifies the cyst in more than 50 percent of cases.

Brainstem Tumor

Where necessary, CT with intrathecal metrizamide can demonstrate brainstem enlargement and asymmetry. The foramen magnum may be enlarged (Williams 1969).

Foramen Magnum Meningioma and Neurofibroma

The lesions in this region show features similar to those in lesions elsewhere (Fig. 10-41). Intrathecal metrizamide is quite useful in definition of these masses when routine scanning is inadequate. Expansion of the foramen magnum may be seen (Williams 1969).

Hypoglossal Neuroma

This lesion shares the features of neuromas of other cranial nerves described elsewhere in this chapter. Moderate homogeneous contrast enhancement is typical, but cystic areas or even ring-type enhancement may be seen, as may an occasional lesion without enhancement. Diagnosis can be made on the basis of bone erosion with widening of the hypoglossal (anterior condyloid) canal and erosion of the jugular tubercle. Larger lesions may erode the adjacent jugular fossa, the occipital condyle, and the adjacent portions of the occipital bone.

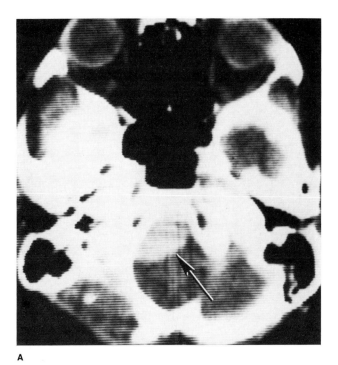
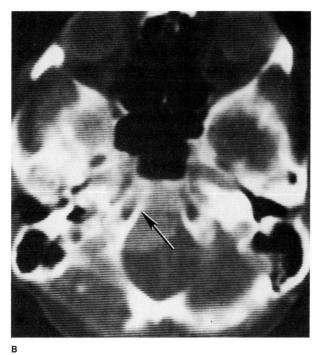

A   **B**

Figure 10-41   Meningioma of the foramen magnum.   **A.** The homogeneously enhancing tumor mass is seen within the anterior part of the foramen magnum (arrow).   **B.** Same section seen at wide window settings to show absence of erosion or hyperostosis (arrow).

Deformities of the Foramen Magnum

These may be developmental or acquired. The foramen magnum is small in achondroplasia (Coin 1971). It is also decreased in size in occipitalization of the atlas, asymmetrically when the assimilation is partial. Finally, the foramen magnum can be small because of premature closure of one or more occipital synchondroses, typically asymmetrically (Kruyff 1965). These deformities may cause neurological symptoms. Acquired narrowing of the foramen magnum can result from Paget's disease, fibrous dysplasia, and fluorosis (Coin 1971) (Fig. 10-42).

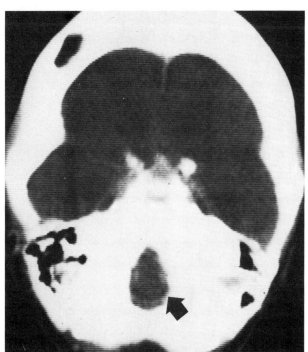

Figure 10-42   Paget's disease. Extensive bone thickening has ▶ narrowed the foramen magnum. The same may happen to the other foraminas of the skull base.

Basilar Invagination (Impression)

Basilar invagination is, by definition, invagination of the margins of the foramen magnum upward into the skull. It may be due to developmental bone anomalies involving the atlas, axis, and occiput (such as occipital condylar hypoplasia or some cases of occipitalization of the atlas) or may be secondary to systemic bone disorders, impaired ossification, bone destruction by tumor or infection, or trauma (Dolan 1977; Lee 1978). Symptoms are due to compression of the medulla, spinal cord, or cerebellum or secondary to hydrocephalus due to fourth-ventricle outlet obstruction. Furthermore, the cerebellar tonsils are frequently below the foramen magnum in basilar impression and may contribute to the symptoms of brainstem compression. Platybasia, flattening of the orientation of anterior and middle cranial fossa to one another, may coexist with basilar invagination. A variety of craniometric methods have been used to detect basilar invagination, such as Chamberlain's line, McGregor's line, Klaus' height index, Bull's angle, the bimastoid line, the digastric line, and the atlantooccipital joint angle. The first four measurements can be obtained from a lateral radiograph or on CT by use of either a digital radiographic localization mode or sagittal reformation. The latter three measurements require tomography or CT scanning in the coronal plane. On conventional axial scans, invagination of the edges of the foramen magnum can be recognized by visualization of the foramen magnum within the posterior fossa surrounded by the cerebellum (Fig. 10-43). In spite of volume averaging, the odontoid process should not project within the foramen magnum; therefore, such a finding should be viewed as indicative of basilar invagination (Lee 1978). In some cases the anterior arch and lateral masses of the atlas may project into the posterior fossa (Fig. 10-43C). When such changes are seen on axial sections, more detailed and precise evaluation may be obtained by lateral skull x-ray and by coronal and sagittal sections on which the actual upturning of the margins of the foramen can be seen.

In Paget's disease and fibrous dysplasia, bony thickening of the margins of the foramen magnum compounds the encroachment on the medulla and cervical cord. This, too, is well evaluated by CT, as is bone destruction due to tumor, infection, or histiocystosis X which may result in secondary basilar invagination.

Finally, CT can clearly demonstrate hydrocephalus.

Malignant Tumors of the Foramen Magnum

Tumors in this region, as those arising below in the spine, may compress the spinal cord and lower medulla because of the limited space provided by the foramen (Fig. 10-44).

THE JUGULAR FORAMEN

Anatomy

The jugular foramen (Fig. 10-38) is actually a short canal between the posterior fossa and the upper cervical region on each side, passing anteriorly, laterally, and inferiorly from the posterior fossa. It is situated between the lateral margin of the occipital bone and the inferior surface and inferior edge of the petrous pyramid. The jugular fossa, which forms the lateral part of the exocranial aspect of the foramen, lies below the thin bony floor of the tympanic cavity. A thin ridge of bone, the caroticojugular spine, separates the jugular foramen from the petrous carotid canal anteriorly. The jugular tubercle (with the hypoglossal canal) and the occipital

Figure 10-43 Basilar invagination. **A.** The foramen magnum (arrowhead) projects into the posterior fossa. Note the cerebellar tissue (curved arrows). **B.** Due to the upward slope of the basiocciput the foramen magnum (arrow) is still visualized in the next section, surrounded by the cerebeller hemispheres (arrowheads). **C.** In another case of severe basilar invagination the odontoid process (arrowhead) extends through the foramen magnum. **D.** Because of foreshortening, the clivus is seen along its entire length. Also visible is the anterior margin of the foramen magnum (arrow).

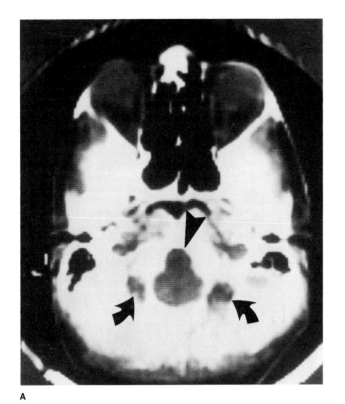

A

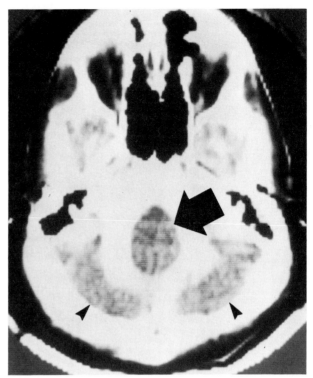

B

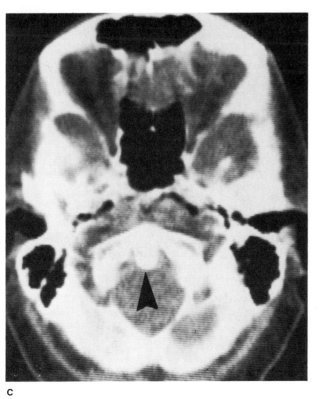

C

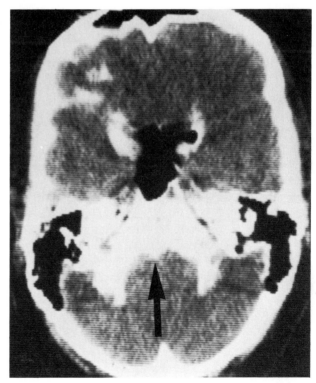

D

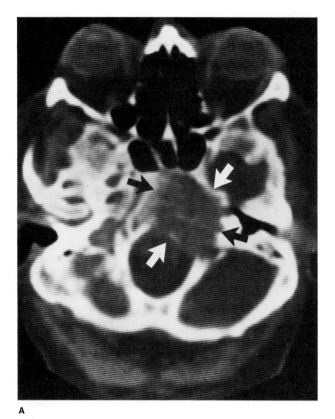
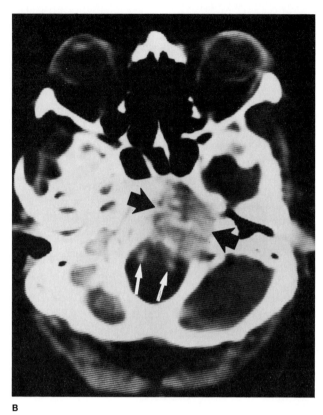

A   B

Figure 10-44 Metastatic tumor involving the foramen magnum. **A.** An extensive area of bone destruction is seen to involve the lower clivus and the anterior lip of the foramen magnum on the right side (arrows). **B.** At a normal window setting the enhancing tumor mass (black arrows) has encroached on the foramen magnum with posterior displacement of the vertebral arteries (white arrows).

condyle are located medially, the styloid process and the stylomastoid foramen are situated laterally, and the internal auditory meatus and the cerebellum are situated superiorly.

The foramen is divided into two parts by a septum (bony or fibrous). The anteromedial portion is called the *pars nervosa*, which contains the inferior petrosal sinus on its course to the internal jugular vein and the ninth cranial (glossopharyngeal) nerve. Through the posterolateral portion, the *pars vascularis*, course the tenth (vagus) and eleventh (accessory) cranial nerves, as well as the meningeal branches of the occipital and ascending pharyngeal arteries entering the cranial cavity. The internal jugular vein begins as an expansion, the jugular bulb,

in the jugular fossa and leaves the skull via the pars vascularis; it is the continuation of sigmoid sinus.

Asymmetry between the two jugular foramina is common; the sizes are related to the sizes of the transverse sinuses, which ultimately drain into the internal jugular veins. The asymmetry is related to the size of the pars vascularis. The right jugular foramen is commonly larger than the left, but this relationship is reversed in a significant number of people. To obtain quantitative assessments of such an odd-shaped structure, Di Chiro et al. (1964) developed an index of size consisting of the sum of the width of the pars nervosa, the width of the pars vascularis, and the length of the entire foramen. By use of this index, the asymmetry was found to be less than 12 mm in 95 percent of the population studied; a difference of 20 mm was considered indicative of pathologic enlargement.

CT Technique

The jugular foramina can be reasonably evaluated on conventional axial section (Fig. 10-38). Supplemental information as to the extent of tumor and bone integrity can be obtained on coronal sections. Since the axis of the foramen is at a 45° angle to the canthomeatal line, true axial views require a 45° angulation of the plane of the scan sections above that line; this can be achieved by a combination of neck flexion and gantry tilt.

Pathology

Glomus Jugulare Tumors

Glomus tumors, also called *chemodectomas* or *nonchromaffin paragangliomas*, arise from chemoreceptor cells, which are located in the glomus jugulare, middle ear, carotid body, ganglion nodosum, aortic arch, innominate artery, pulmonary artery, mediastinum, retroperitoneum, and abdominal aorta, and on lung surfaces. They may rarely be multicentric. Most are benign, but they tend to be locally invasive; a few metastasize via lymphatic and hematogenous routes. Intracranially glomus tissue is found in the adventitia of the jugular bulb, along the ninth cranial nerve, Arnold's nerve, Jacobson's nerve, and the mucosa of the cochlear promontory of the middle ear (Britton 1974; Guild 1953; Sondheimer 1971). Glomus tumors may thus arise in the tympanic cavity (glomus tympanicum) or jugular foramen (glomus jugulare).

Glomus jugulare tumors produce ill-defined bone erosion with an infiltrative appearance in spite of their benign nature. Typically there is destruction of the inferior aspect of the petrous pyramid. With posterior extension, the jugular tubercle and the hypoglossal canal may become involved, and further extension may involve the foramen magnum.

Anterior extension into the middle cranial fossa may result in extensive bone destruction. Because of the proximity of the middle ear, it is not uncommon for glomus jugulare tumors to invade that structure and present as a vascular, pulsatile soft-tissue middle-ear mass clinically. Computed tomographic demonstration of jugular foramen expansion or destruction, intra- or extracranial soft-tissue mass, and angiographic findings of jugular vein compression or invasion indicate origin in the jugular foramen; absence of these findings indicates an origin in the middle ear. Determination of the origin and extent of tumor are necessary for preoperative assessment of resectability.

Computed tomography on the new scanners is well suited for demonstration of bone destruction in these lesions (Fig. 10-45). Furthermore, these highly vascular lesions enhance well following intravenous contrast injection, permitting evaluation of the tumor mass and its extensions intracranially and extracranially into the soft tissues of the neck. Computed tomography also demonstrates displacements of intracranial structures by the mass.

Selective internal and external carotid and vertebral arteriography as well as retrograde jugular venography via catheterization or direct puncture is necessary to demonstrate the vascular supply as well as invasion or compression of the jugular vein; the lesions are highly vascular. As noted below in the section of the temporal bone, the petrous portion of the internal carotid artery may enter the middle ear aberrantly, as may the jugular bulb as a result of dehiscence of its wall; the aberrant vessel may then present clinically as a reddish pulsatile middle-ear mass resembling glomus tumors otoscopically (Britton 1974; Glasgold 1972; Potter 1974; Robin 1972). A similar presentation may be noted with petrous carotid aneurysms extending into the middle ear (Stallings 1969). Arteriography and jugular venography demonstrate well the true nature of the anomaly.

Neuromas

Neuromas of the ninth, tenth, and eleventh cranial nerves are rather uncommon lesions. They may

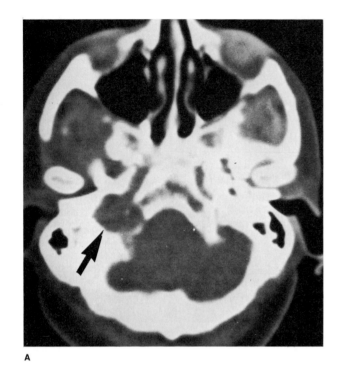

A

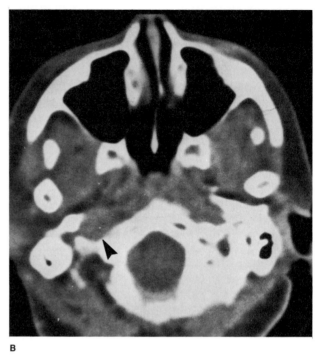

B

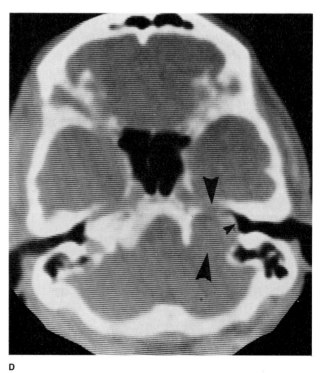

C

D

arise as isolated lesions or in patients with neuro-fibromatosis. As with neuromas elsewhere, bone erosion is sharply defined (Fig. 10-46). The jugular foramen expands rather uniformly and with sharp cortical margins; typically there is erosion of the jugular spine. When the lesions expand beyond the jugular foramen, the edge of the bony erosion remains sharp, with a thin margin of sclerosis. This finding, together with the lesser vascularity on angiography of neuromas, is important for distinction between these lesions and glomus jugulare tumors. CT characteristics are the same as those of other neuromas.

Chondroma

Chondromas have been described in the section on the middle cranial fossa. These lesions seldom calcify in the cerebellopontine angle and jugular fossa area (Roukkula 1964; Sarwar 1976), and they produce sharply marginated erosions. These findings, together with avascularity on arteriography, make differentiation of chondromas expanding the jugular foramen from neuromas impossible in many instances. They may show enhancement with intravenous contrast (Sarwar 1976).

Cholesteatoma

These lesions are discussed in detail in the section on the cerebellopontine angle. Primary cholesteatomas in the region of the jugular foramen produce, as elsewhere, sharply defined bone erosion. On CT

scanning, the nature and extent of the erosion is well seen, but the mass typically does not enhance and hence is more difficult to visualize and fully outline. Intrathecal positive or negative contrast may be necessary, especially with the smaller lesions. There may be some bony debris within the area of bone erosion. They are completely avascular on arteriography.

Large Jugular Foramen

As noted above, the jugular foramen varies considerably in size, and there is commonly asymmetry between the two sides. There can be enlargement of the pars vascularis when there is markedly increased blood flow through the jugular bulb as the result of an arteriovenous malformation. There may also be diverticulumlike extensions of the jugular bulb (and hence the jugular foramen) upward into the petrous pyramid. The walls of these extensions are sharp but may be associated with deficiency of the posterior wall of the internal auditory canal or the floor of the middle ear. On the basis of bone evaluation alone, jugular foramen expansion due to a mass should not be diagnosed merely because the pars vascularis is large, without expansion of the pars nervosa, as this portion of the jugular fossa is not subject to significant variations (see Chap. 17). Demonstration of jugular spine or caroticojugular spine erosion indicates pathologic expansion, as does indistinctness of the cortical margin of the foramen (Fig. 10-47). Opacification of the internal jugular vein and bulb (by cerebral arterial or direct internal jugular injection) may be employed to resolve questionable cases.

◀ **Figure 10-45** Glomus jugulare tumor. **A.** Enlargement of the jugular foramen (arrow) is a common finding with a mass of soft-tissue density within the foramen. **B.** The lower section shows extension of the soft-tissue mass into the jugular vein (arrowhead). **C.** CT in wide window settings in another case of glomus jugulare tumor to show enlargement of the jugular fossa (arrowheads) and involvement of the jugular tubercle. A normal tubercle and hypoglossal canal (short arrow) are visible on the opposite side. **D.** At a higher level the jugular fossa (arrowheads) is expanded with erosion of the adjacent bone. The tumor has extended into the middle ear cavity (small arrowhead).

THE TEMPORAL BONE

This area epitomizes the complexity of the skull base; the anatomy is both intricate and minute. The earlier generation CT scanners show only the grossest bony abnormalities, revealing only the larger areas of bone destruction or erosion. Newer scanners, because of improved scanner geometry and

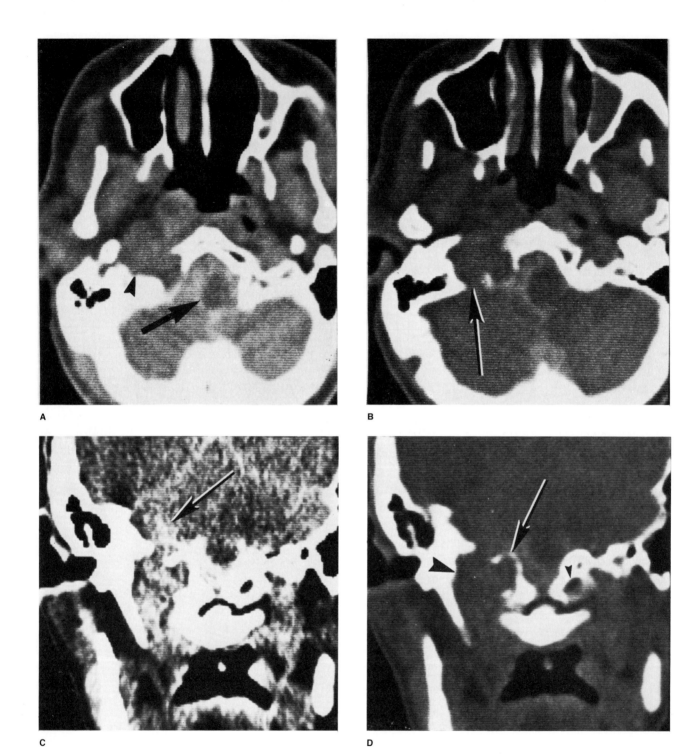

Figure 10-46 Ninth cranial nerve neuroma. CT following cisternal metrizamide. **A.** A globular soft-tissue mass (arrowhead) is seen just below the jugular foramen. The metrizamide within the cisternal space shows the brainstem displaced toward the right by the intracranial component. **B.** CT image at a slightly higher level. The jugular foramen (arrow) is enlarged. **C.** Coronal CT through the foramen shows the intracranial component of the tumor (arrow). **D.** On wide window settings the expansion of the jugular foramen (arrowhead) and erosion of the jugular tubercle (arrow) are better defined.

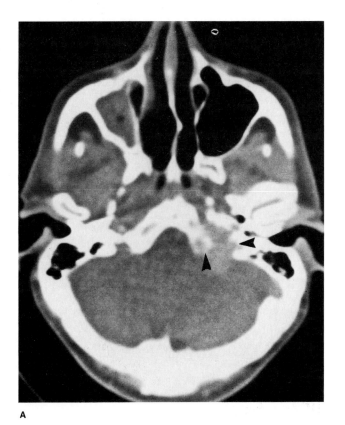

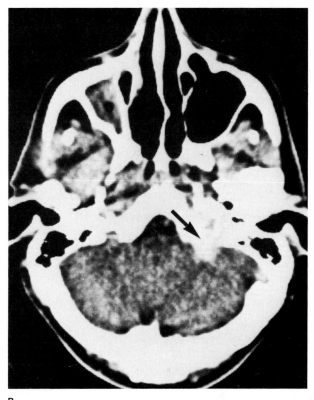

A

B

Figure 10-47 Metastatic tumor.   **A.** Metastasis resulting in destruction and expansion of the jugular foramen (arrowheads) seen with wide window setting.   **B.** The enhancing metastatic lesion (arrow) involves the jugular foramen.

new software programs (wider windows, bone correction programs, zoom reconstruction), are showing promise of rivaling or surpassing conventional pluridirectional tomography in evaluation of the temporal bone because of the inherent superior contrast resolution of the CT scanner.

CT Technique

Evaluation of the internal anatomy and pathology of the temporal bone requires high-resolution scanning with thin sections, zoom reconstruction, wide windows, and bone correction programs. As these become more widely available, CT scanning will in all likelihood become the method of choice in eval-uating the temporal bone (Fig. 10-48). As elsewhere, sections should be obtained as close to perpendicular to the plane of the structure of interest as possible in order to detect and evaluate bone changes and soft-tissue projections. As thinner sections become possible, reconstruction will be of higher resolution, permitting evaluation in any plane after scanning in the axial plane.

Anatomy

The temporal bones (Fig. 10-48) contribute to both the skull base and the inferior portion of the skull vault. Each temporal bone has five components: the petrous, tympanic, mastoid, and squamous portions and the styloid process. The squamous portion

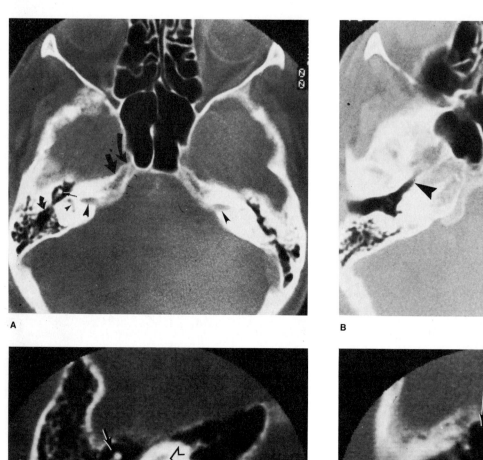

A

B

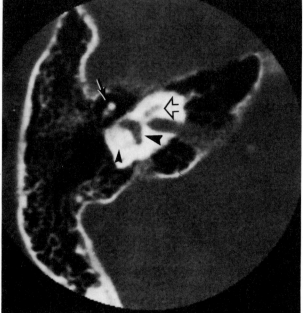

C

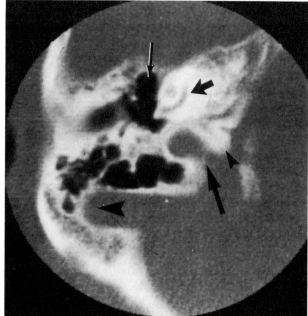

D

Figure 10-48 Temporal bone anatomy. **A.** The large curved arrow indicates the petrous apex. Next to this is the trigeminal impression (straight arrow) producing a concavity in the anterior aspect of the petrous pyramid. The ossicles of the middle ear are seen (small arrow) within the attic of the middle ear. The short curved arrow indicates the mastoid antrum, which is continuous with the attic via the aditus. The large arrowhead points to the posterior wall of the internal auditory canal. The superior semicircular canal is also seen in this section on the left (small arrowhead). **B.** On the left the ossicles are again seen within the attic (arrow). On the right the opening of the bony eustachian tube is indicated by the arrowhead. **C.** Axial CT. The ossicles are seen within the attic of the middle ear (arrow), the head of the malleus anteriorly, and the body and the short process of the incus posteriorly. The clear arrow indicates the cochlea. The vestibule is seen

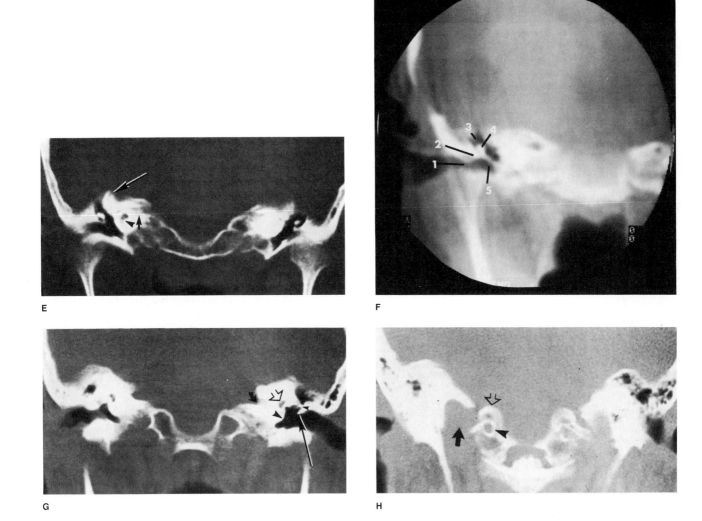

E

F

G

H

posterior to the cochlea (large arrowhead). The lateral semi-circular canal (small arrowhead) can be seen faintly. The internal auditory canal lies between the clear arrow and the large arrowhead. **D.** Visible are the cochlea (short large arrow), the jugular foramen (long large arrow), and the jugular spine (short arrowhead). The sigmoid sinus produces a groove at the posterior aspect of the mastoid portion of the temporal bone (large arrowhead). The middle ear cavity is indicated by the small highlighted arrow. **E** to **H.** Direct coronal CT from front to back. **E.** The ossicles (arrow) can be seen within the attic of the middle ear. Also seen are the internal auditory canal (small arrow), a portion of the cochlea (arrowhead), and the superior semicircular canal within the arcuate eminence

(arrow). **F.** CT through a similar level using target reconstruction showing the anatomy with better definition: bony external auditory canal (1), scutum (2), epitympanic recess (3), head of the malleus and incus (4), tympanic membrane (5). **G.** At a slightly posterior level the following landmarks can be identified: scutum (long arrow), body of the incus (small arrowhead), cochlear promontory (large arrowhead) producing a prominent bulge into the middle ear cavity, the partially visualized vestibule (clear arrow), and the posterior wall of the internal auditory canal (curved arrow) at the porus. **H.** At a more posterior level are the jugular foramen (solid arrow), the jugular eminence (clear arrow), and the hypoglossal canal within the jugular eminence.

is mainly a component of the bony calvarium, except for the small portion which contributes to the external auditory canal, and is not considered further in this section.

The petrous portion is an elongated pyramid wedged between the greater wing of the sphenoid and the basal portions of the sphenoid and occipital bones. Its base is fused to the squamous and mastoid portions of the temporal bone. Its long axis is directed anteromedially at a 45° angle with the coronal plane with a slight upward angulation. It has three surfaces (anterior, posterior, and inferior) and three ridges (superior, anterior, and posterior).

The anterior surface forms the posterior portion of the middle cranial fossa. Pertinent radiologic anatomy includes the arcuate eminence (an elevation over the superior semicircular canal) and a shallow depression for the gasserian ganglion (trigeminal impression) of the trigeminal nerve (the ganglion lying in a dural pocket, Meckel's cave, in this impression) just medial to the apex.

The posterior surface is the anterior wall of the posterior cranial fossa. A deep groove for the sigmoid sinus demarcates the lateral end of the posterior surface. Midway between this groove and the petrous apex is the internal auditory meatus (porus acusticus internus). The inferior surface, rough and irregular, contributes to the exterior of the skull base. The exocranial opening of the carotid canal presents on the inferior surface; this canal first ascends vertically and then bends to run horizontally anteromedially, opening at the petrous apex just above the foramen lacerum. It transmits the internal carotid artery intracranially. Behind the canal opening is a deep depression, the jugular fossa, in which lies the jugular bulb. This fossa, combined with the jugular notch on the adjacent occipital bone, forms the jugular foramen, through which passes the internal jugular vein. The carotid canal and jugular foramen are separated by a ridge of bone, the caroticojugular spine. Lateral to these structures is the styloid process, which is ensheathed by the vaginal process of the tympanic portion of the temporal bone. Between the styloid and the mastoid process is the stylomastoid foramen, the exocranial opening of the facial canal through which course the facial nerve and the stylomastoid artery.

Of the three petrous ridges, the superior and posterior are of particular radiologic interest. The former provides an area of attachment of the tentorium and is grooved for the superior petrosal sinus. Medially is a notch in which the trigeminal nerve lies as it crosses the petrous apex.

The posterior ridge lies adjacent to the basal portion of the occiput. Each of these bones has a sulcus on its margin, together creating a groove for the inferior petrosal sinus. Laterally it contributes to the anterior wall of the jugular foramen.

The petrous apex fits into the angle between the greater wing of the sphenoid and the basal portion of the sphenoid and occipital bones. The intracranial opening of the carotid canal is located in the petrous apex.

The tympanic portion of the temporal bone is a partial cylinder of bone lying below the squamous portion and anterior to the mastoid portion. It forms the anterior wall and the floor and inferior portion of the posterior wall of the osseous external auditory canal. (The roof and upper portion of the posterior wall are formed by the squamous portion.) The anterior wall of the external auditory canal is thus the posterior wall of the mandibular fossa. The inferior wall of the tympanic portion of the temporal bone splits laterally to form the vaginal process, enclosing the root of the styloid process.

The mastoid portion is the posterior part of the temporal bone. It fuses with the squamous portion anteriorly and lies behind the external auditory canal. Inferiorly it has a conical projection, the mastoid process, to which cervical muscles attach. Medial to the process is a deep groove, the digastric notch, to which the digastric muscle attaches. Near the posterior border of the mastoid portion is the mastoid foramen, through which courses an emissary vein from the transfer sinus. Internally the mastoid has a deep groove for the sigmoid sinus.

Having discussed the external anatomy of the temporal bone components, we shall briefly consider the internal anatomy. The external canal is composed of cartilage and membrane laterally and bone medially; it is lined by skin throughout. It has a mildly sinuous course with upward convexity. Its roof ends medially in a sharp projection of bone, the scutum, to which the superior portion of the tympanic membrane attaches. The latter two structures separate the external auditory canal from the tympanic cavity (middle ear), the lateral wall of which it constitutes. The medial wall is the lateral wall of the bony labyrinth. The middle ear includes the tympanic cavity proper and "attic" (epitympanic recess), which lies above the superior attachment of the tympanic membrane. The middle ear communicates with the mastoid antrum and mastoid air cells via the aditus. It also communicates with the nasopharynx via the eustachian tube, which begins at the anterior inferior aspect of the middle ear. This is the structure which provides the air that fills the middle ear, antrum, and mastoid cells. The middle ear and the antrum are roofed by a very thin plate of bone, the tegmen tympani, which separates them from the cranial cavity. Within the middle ear are three auditory ossicles: the malleus, the incus, and the stapes. The malleus and the incus are imaged on nearly all CT scanners to varying degrees. The stapes may be visualized only on scanners of the highest resolution. Medial to the middle ear is the inner ear (labyrinth), which consists of osseous and membranous parts. The former is of radiologic importance and consists of the cochlea, the vestibule, and the semicircular canals. These are actually spaces in the dense bone of the otic capsule, which is incorporated into the petrous bone. They are lined by periosteum and contain the structures of the membranous labyrinth. The vestibule is an ovoid cavity into which the three semicircular canals (superior, posterior, and lateral) open. The cochlea, a spinal canal with two and one-half turns, lies anterior to the vestibule. It is cone shaped with its base at the lateral end of internal auditory canal and its apex directed anterolaterally. The basal turn of the cochlea produces a bulge in the medial wall of the middle ear, the promontory.

The internal auditory canal is perpendicular to the sagittal plane. Its opening, the porus acusticus, is on the posterior surface of the petrous pyramid and, like that surface, is oblique; the anterior wall of the porus blends in with the posterior surface of the petrous pyramid and is thus ill-defined while the posterior wall is sharply defined. The lateral end of the internal auditory canal is called the *fundus*. Within the internal auditory canal runs the fa-

cial nerve, the cochlear division of the eighth nerve, the superior and inferior vestibular divisions of the eighth nerve, the internal auditory artery, and several small veins. The normal canal varies in height as follows:

1. The height at the greatest diameter is 2.0 mm minimum and 9.0 mm maximum in most series but 11.0 mm in one series; this was found in only 1 of 509 cases (Valvassori 1964).
2. The height of the porus acusticus is always less than 1 mm greater than the height at the greatest diameter; it may be as much as 3 mm less, with a minimum height of 2 mm.
3. The length of the posterior wall is 3 mm minimum and 16 mm maximum.

The heights may be equal at the point of greatest diameter and porous (straight type), narrower at the porus, and narrower at both the medial and lateral ends than at the point of greatest diameter (oval type).

The facial nerve enters the internal auditory canal at the porus acusticus and, passing through the anterior superior aspect of the canal, enters the bony facial canal. This canal runs anterolaterally above and between the cochlea and the vestibule. At the lateral wall of the attic, it curves sharply backward to run posterolaterally above the promontory and below the lateral semicircular canal. At the level of the posterior limb of the lateral semicircular canal, it turns downward and runs vertically and inferiorly in the medial wall of the middle ear to widen slightly into the stylomastoid foramen, the exit point of the facial nerve.

The carotid canal was described earlier in the section on the petrous portion of the temporal bone.

Pathology

Congenital Malformations

Congenital malformations may involve the external, the middle, and the inner ear either singly or in combination. Because of shared embryologic origins, malformations of the external and middle ear are more commonly associated with each other than with malformations of the inner ear (Frey 1971; Jensen 1974; Lapayowker 1974; Petasnick 1973). Ear malformations may be associated with facial dysplasias and a variety of systemic dysplasia syndromes.

External-ear anomalies of radiologic importance are those which narrow or occlude the external auditory canal. These vary from a simple skin web to malformation of the osseous portion of the canal, resulting in a plate of bone partially or completely obliterating the medial portion of the canal (Frey 1971; Petasnick 1973), commonly in association with ossicular malformations (Fitz 1974; Frey 1971), anomalies of the facial canal (Anson 1961; Lapayowker 1974), and varying degrees of encroachment on the middle-ear cavity. Tomography or high-resolution CT scanning is essential for evaluation of these malformations.

Middle-ear malformations typically involve the ossicles, which may show malformation, fusion, or varying degrees of aplasia (Frey 1971; Lapayowker 1974; Petasnick 1973). In addition, there may be ectopic locations of either the internal carotid artery or the jugular bulb (Britton 1974; Glasgold 1972; Potter 1974; Robin 1972). The petrous portion of the internal carotid artery lies within the carotid canal. The canal is well seen on tomography or high-resolution CT scanning, with the initial portion lying anteroinferior to the cochlea. When the canal is anomalous, its initial portion no longer appears in its normal location and the artery may extend into the middle ear, producing an appearance suggesting a glomus tumor clinically (red, pulsatile mass with tinnitus) (Potter 1974). On tomography or coronal CT there is a defect in the floor of the middle ear, the soft-tissue density of the carotid artery within the middle ear and, at times, erosion of the cochlear promontory; an arteriogram confirms the diagnosis and averts the disastrous results of surgery for suspected glomus tumor.

The jugular fossa may lie more superiorly than normal, closely approaching the middle ear; actual dehiscence of the wall of the fossa permits entry of the bulb into the middle-ear cavity (Robin 1972). The resulting reddish, pulsatile middle-ear mass may simulate a glomus tumor. Computed tomography or plain tomography may demonstrate the high position and bone dehiscence of the fossa, suggesting the diagnosis, but jugular venography definitively establishes the diagnosis and the absence of a mass expanding the jugular fossa.

Inner-ear malformations include abnormalities of the semicircular canals, most commonly the lateral canal (Jensen 1971, 1974; Petasnick 1973). The affected canal may be narrow, short and wide, incorporated into the vestibular cavity, or aplastic. Inner-ear malformations include abnormalities of the semicircular canals, the vestibule, the cochlea, and the internal auditory canal. Lateral semicircular malformation is the most common (Jensen 1971, 1974; Petasnick 1973); the canal may be narrow or short and wide, merging as a common cavity with the vestibule, or it may be aplastic. The other semicircular canals are less commonly involved. Malformation of the vestibule may be associated with semicircular canal anomalies; in addition the oval window may be hypoplastic or aplastic. Cochlear malformations include a reduced number of coils (normally there are 2.50 to 2.75), a cavity without coils, decreased lumen of coils, and aplasia. Horizontal CT scanning is quite satisfactory for evaluating the cochlea, while coronal and lateral projections are needed for evaluating the vestibule and semicircular canals. The internal auditory canal anomalies include hypoplasia and atresia.

External Auditory Canal Lesions

EXPANSILE NONAGGRESSIVE LESIONS Benign lesions such as adenoma, hemangioma, osteoma (Fig. 10-3), or multiple exostoses may present as masses within the external canal without bone involvement. Adenomas and hemangiomas may also produce slow expansion of the canal. All these lesions can obstruct the external canal, causing retention of cerumen and debris and resulting in formation of a cholesteatoma in the external canal, which can then expand and erode, a condition termed *keratosis obturans*.

AGGRESSIVE LESIONS PRODUCING ILL-DEFINED BONE DESTRUCTION These include primary malignancy, extension of adjacent malignancy, metastasis, myeloma, and inflammatory disease.

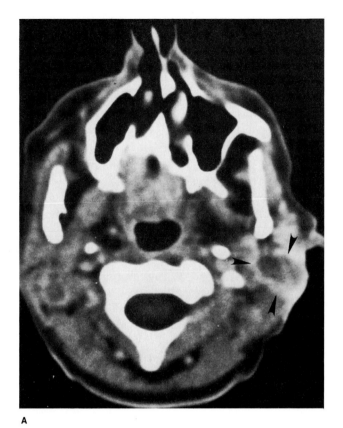

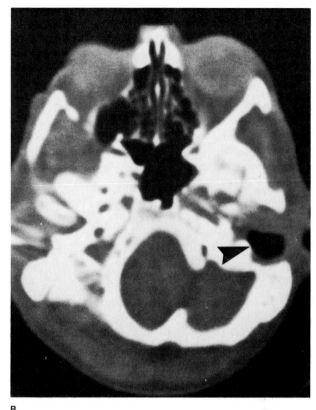

A   B

Figure 10-49   A. Abscess involving the preauricular lymph node in a patient with severe otitis externa. The periphery of the abscess enhances (arrowheads).   **B.** Same patient following drainage procedure, note air within the cavity (arrowhead).

The most common primary malignancy is squamous cell carcinoma, which occurs in a setting of chronic infection in more than 75 percent of cases (Goodwin 1980) and peaks in incidence at age 55 to 65 years. Over 50 percent of these lesions occur in the pinna of the ear, with the remainder divided between the external canal and the middle ear. Basal cell carcinoma (a less common tumor), adenocarcinoma, and melanoma (which are both rare) are not associated with chronic ear infection, although all these malignant lesions may simulate acute or subacute infection clinically.

Middle-ear inflammatory and neoplastic disease, parotid gland tumors, and preauricular lymph node metastases can extend to involve the external canal (Goodwin 1980) (Fig. 10-49).

Malignant otitis externa is typically a pseudomonas infection in elderly diabetics. These lesions produce abundant granulation tissue, irregular bone destruction, and local pain (Mendez 1979) and may extend throughout the temporal bone and break through intracranially. Anterior extension into the temporomandibular joint and posterior extension into the jugular fossa may occur, resulting in destructive changes in the locations (Mendez 1979).

Middle-Ear and Mastoid Lesions

BENIGN EROSIVE LESIONS WITH WELL-DEFINED EDGES These include secondary cholesteatoma, primary cholesteatoma (epidermoid), granuloma, facial nerve neuroma, hemangioma, eroding brain tumor, meningoencephalocele, ectopic internal carotid artery, and ectopic jugular bulb formation.

Secondary cholesteatoma   This lesion is designated "secondary" to distinguish it from the epidermoid, or primary cholesteatoma. The lesion results from ingrowth of squamous epithelium of the tympanic membrane following a perforation. Epithelial debris are deposited within the lesion, and gradual, progressive expansion occurs, leading to sharply defined bone erosion. The mastoid is poorly pneumatized and sclerotic as a result of associated chronic otitis media. There are two basic types determined by the location of the perforation, pars flaccida and pars tensa (Buckingham 1973). With the former, the cholesteatoma produces erosion of the scutum and lateral attic wall, medial displacement of the malleus and the incus, and erosion of the head of the malleus and the body of the incus. With pars tensa perforations, there is extension along the medial wall of the middle ear into the attic, displacing the malleus and incus laterally and eroding the long process of the incus. With this type of lesion there is a greater tendency for erosion of the medial wall of the attic, which can lead to a labyrinthine fistula as a result of erosion of the lateral semicircular canal. Further expansion of the cholesteatoma sac from either type of perforation leads to extension into and expansion of the antrum. Continued growth may cause involvement of the remainder of the mastoid, erosion of the sigmoid sinus plate with compression of the sinus, erosion of the tegmen tympani with intracranial extension, and medial extension, eroding the labyrinth and petrous apex. CT demonstrates the soft-tissue mass due to the cholesteatoma, and any associated inflammatory tissue and fluid, as well as any bone erosion caused by the cholesteatoma.

Primary cholesteatoma (epidermoid)   This differs from the secondary lesion in that it, like epidermoid tumors that arise elsewhere, is a congenital lesion derived from embryonic ectodermal cell rests and hence is not related to otitis media (Phelps 1980). There is a normal appearance to the tympanic membrane, and the inferior margin of the lateral attic wall (scutum) is intact. Bone erosion occurs with both primary and secondary lesions. Furthermore, primary lesions may obstruct the eustachian tube orifice in the middle ear, leading to otitis media; this situation would very closely simulate the findings in secondary cholesteatoma.

Granuloma   Chronic middle-ear infection can lead to granuloma formation. The granulomatous mass can produce bony erosion, making differentiation from cholesteatoma impossible.

Hemangioma   This rare tumor may occur as a soft-tissue mass in the middle ear, where it may erode the ossicles and walls of the tympanic cavity. Hemangiomas have no specific distinguishing features.

Facial nerve neuroma   This lesion may occur at any point along the course of the facial nerve, from the cerebellopontine angle to the stylomastoid foramen. Facial nerve neuromas are most common in the descending portion of the facial canal, where evidence of relationship to the canal establishes the diagnosis. Occasionally the portion of the nerve which runs in the medial wall of the middle ear is the site of a neuroma, leading to erosion of the canal and extension into the middle ear as an expanding, eroding soft-tissue mass.

Temporal lobe glioma   Occasionally a slow-growing temporal lobe glioma can produce pressure erosion of the tegmen tympani, leading to herniation into the middle ear. Computed tomography scanning should easily demonstrate the nature of the abnormality in such instances.

Meningoencephalocele   This type of lesion can occur either spontaneously or secondary to trauma, surgery, or bone destruction by tumor or infection. Typically the bone defect is in the tegmen tympani. Beveling of the edges of the defect inward from above and clinical evidence of cerebrospinal fluid fistula should suggest this possibility.

Ectopic location of the internal carotid artery or the jugular bulb   Lesions of this type are discussed in the sections on congenital anomalies and glomus tumors.

Surgical defect Following mastoidectomy, a large defect is seen in the mastoid; the antrum and epitympanic recess may be enlarged, and the ossicles may be removed, depending on the extent of surgery (Fig. 10-50). It may be difficult to detect recurrent disease in these patients, but certain points are useful in evaluation. Soft-tissue density within the surgical cavity after several months should be viewed with suspicion. The margins are well defined and distinct in surgical defects without superimposed disease. A sclerotic bony margin suggests recurrent cholesteatoma, as does evidence of elevation of the tegmen tympani. Herniation of brain into a mastoidectomy defect may be associated with inward-beveling of the edges of the bone dehiscence from above downward as well as soft tissue and fluid in the surgical cavity and middle ear; a cerebrospinal fluid fistula may be present.

Pseudodefects Pseudodefects may be seen radiologically. A large but otherwise normal mastoid antrum is easily recognized as such on CT scanning because of its contained air. A large sigmoid sinus should also be easily recognizable by following the sinus groove on serial sections; the intravenous contrast-enhanced scan shows increase in density within the lumen of the sinus which is equal to that in the other dural sinuses.

AGGRESSIVE LESIONS WITH POORLY DEFINED MARGINS

Inflammatory disease In acute otitis media, opacification of the middle ear occurs as a result of mucosal swelling and fluid accumulation (Fig. 10-51). This may spread into the mastoid antrum and air cells. With progression, an exudate is produced in

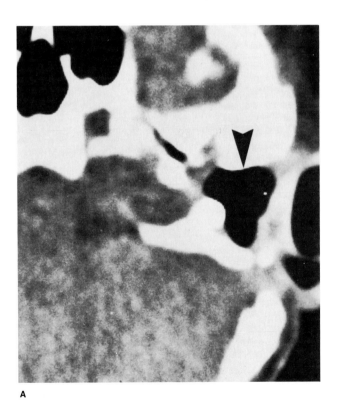
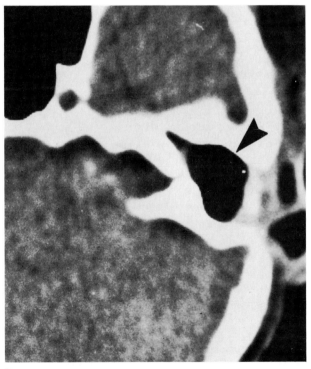

A

B

Figure 10-50 Mastoidectomy defect. **A.** Soft tissue and air within the inferior portion of the defect (arrowhead). **B.** Higher sections showing the mastoidectomy defect (arrowhead) with air within the defect and absence of mastoid air cells.

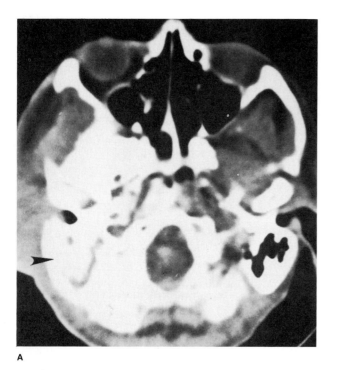

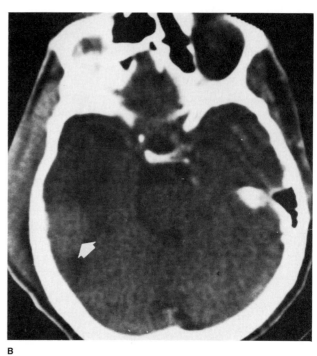

A

B

Figure 10-51   A. Suppurative otitis media in a patient with chronic middle-ear infection shows extensive soft-tissue swelling and sclerosis of the mastoid air cells (arrowhead).   **B.** At a higher level there is a focal area of cerebritis (arrow) with surrounding edema.

these areas. In the absence of treatment, or with inappropriate treatment, destruction of mastoid air cell walls develops with abscess formation. At this stage a lucent defect is seen due to the bone loss. The abscess may extend to involve the entire mastoid. At some point perforation through the mastoid cortex leads to extension subperiosteally (subperiosteal abscess) and extension into adjacent structures, including the external canal, the zygomatic root (preauricular abscess), and the cervical soft tissues (deep cervical abscess). Intracranial extension can result in sigmoid sinus thrombosis, epidural or subdural empyema, brain abscess (temporal lobe or cerebellum) (Fig. 10-52), or meningitis. Spread into other areas of the temporal bone may lead to osteomyelitis. Extension of mastoid infection to the petrous apical region may occur in the 30 percent of temporal bones in which the petrous bones are pneumatized as far as the apex. This results in apical petrositis with irregular bone destruction and epi-

dural abscess formation; clinically such patients may show the full-blown triad of Gradenigo's syndrome (otitis media, sixth cranial nerve palsy, and pain along the distribution of the trigeminal nerve). Computed tomography is well suited for demonstrating both the destructive changes in the mastoid and the intracranial and extracranial extension of infection.

Chronic or subacute middle-ear infection can lead to a granulomatous reaction. The granuloma tissue appears as a soft-tissue mass which can produce pressure erosion of middle-ear bony structures mimicking cholesteatoma.

Long-standing chronic otitis media can lead to tympanosclerosis with calcification of the inflamed mucosa of the middle ear and calcifications surrounding and fixing the ossicles. The middle ear is narrowed by the mucosal calcification. Granulomatous diseases such as tuberculosis produce changes similar to chronic otitis media (Zizmor 1974).

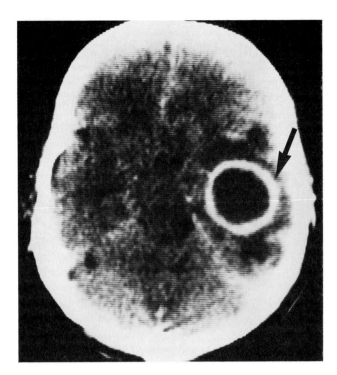

Figure 10-52 Ring enhancement in a temporal lobe abscess (arrow) secondary to severe otitis media with bone destruction. A moderate amount of edema (low density) surrounds the abscess.

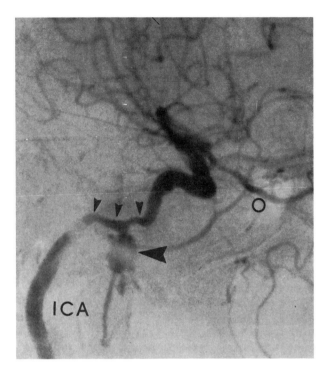

Figure 10-53 Arteriogram demonstrating arterial involvement in a case of lethal granuloma involving the petrous portion of the temporal bone. There is considerable narrowing of the internal carotid artery (ICA) within the petrous carotid canal (small arrowheads). A large pseudoaneurysm arises from the narrowed segment of the internal carotid artery and projects inferiorly (large arrowhead). The external carotid arteries had been ligated because of nasopharyngeal bleeding. There is collateral filling of branches of the external carotid artery via branches of the ophthalmic artery (O).

Wegener's granulomatosis is an autoimmune disorder with necrotizing arteritis which typically involves the nasal cavities and paranasal sinuses with erosive, destructive granulomatous masses in addition to affecting the lungs and kidneys. Occasionally it may involve the middle ear, where it produces opacification alone or concomitantly with bone destruction (Zizmor 1974).

The petrous portion of the internal carotid artery may become involved by the invasion of aggressive inflammatory or neoplastic lesions in the carotid canal. Compression or encasement may occur. Infectious disease can lead to mycotic aneurysm formation. Invasion of the arterial wall by aggressive lesions may lead to pseudoaneurysm formation (Fig. 10-53). Arteriography is necessary for evaluation when evidence of arterial compression (ischemic episodes) or aneurysm-pseudoaneurysm leakage or rupture is present.

Malignant neoplasms involving the middle ear and the mastoid These lesions may be primary, extend from adjacent areas, or be metastatic (Goodwin 1980) (Fig. 10-54). Rhabdomyosarcoma is a primary malignant tumor of the middle ear; it is a tumor of childhood, usually in children under 7 years of age. Squamous cell carcinoma (the most common primary tumor of the middle ear) and adenocarcinoma, when they involve the middle ear, are believed by some to arise deep in the external canal and extend into the middle ear through the tympanic membrane (Adams 1971; Dolan 1974). Squamous cell carcinoma typically occurs in a setting of chronic otitis

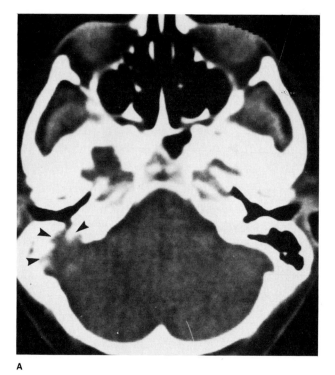

A

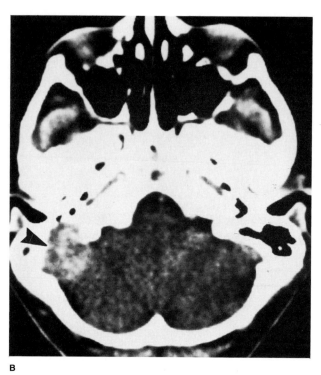

B

Figure 10-54   Metastatic tumor involving the mastoid and petrous portions of the temporal bone.   **A.** Bony defects with irregular margins (arrowheads).   **B.** Contrast enhancement demonstrating the soft tissue tumor mass within the bone defect (arrowhead).

media. Malignant lesions produce irregular bone destruction and mastoid opacification; the latter is due to fluid accumulation, secondary infection due to obstruction, or invasion by tumor. Soft-tissue density in the middle ear is due to both tumor and reactive fluid or hemorrhage only when the petrous apex is pneumatized, permitting spread of infection through the air cells.

Petrous Pyramid Lesions

This area is commonly involved by extrinsic lesions in the middle and posterior cranial fossae and the nasopharynx, in addition to the extrinsic diseases which may effect it.

WELL-DEFINED BONE CHANGES   These are produced by primary cholesteatoma (epidermoid) intrinsically and nonaggressive lesions of the cerebellopontine angle, jugular fossa (not including glomus jugulare

tumors because they commonly produce lytic changes with ill-defined edges), and middle cranial fossa extrinsically. These bone changes are discussed in other sections.

ILL-DEFINED BONE CHANGES   These are produced by inflammatory disease (petrositis or labyrinthitis), primary bone tumors, and otosclerosis intrinsically and by aggressive lesions extending from the nasopharynx, cerebellopontine angle, jugular fossa, and middle cranial fossa extrinsically.

Petrositis   This entity has been discussed in the section on middle-ear inflammatory disease; it can occur only when the petrous apex is pneumatized, permitting spread of infection through the air cells.

Bacterial labyrinthitis   Inflammation of the labyrinth of the inner ear most commonly occurs by spread from middle-ear infection, especially when there is an associated cholesteatoma or when there has been surgery. It may also arise by hematogenous spread of a distant infection or may be secondary to meningitis via the internal auditory canal or cochlear aqueduct. Clinically there is vertigo, tinnitus, nausea, and vomiting with subsequent loss of auditory and vestibular function ("dead ear"). There is bone destruction with loss of normal anatomic features of the labyrinth, leading to formation of an irregular lucent defect in its place.

Otosclerosis   This is a hereditary disorder of the labyrinth characterized by the deposition of foci of spongy bone in the labyrinthine capsule. There are two stages in the disease. Initially foci of poorly calcified spongy bone are formed in association with dissolution of mature endochondral bone, the otospongiosis phase. Subsequently, these foci mature and the spongy bone calcifies, ultimately becoming quite dense; this is the otosclerotic phase. Pathologic changes of otosclerosis may be seen at autopsy in people without history of hearing impairment. However, the bony overgrowth of this disorder leads to hearing impairment in approximately 1 percent of a white population, commencing in adolescence and eventually becoming static; bilateral disease is present in 80 percent. The foci of disease may be single or multiple and may arise in any location but occur most commonly in the region of the oval window. The cochlea may also be involved, as may the semicircular canals and the fundal end of the internal auditory canal. Involvement of the lateral wall of the labyrinth (oval window region and promontory) is termed *fenestral otosclerosis,* or *retrofenestral otosclerosis.*

Experience with high-resolution CT scanning is quite limited thus far, but this modality promises to be quite satisfactory for demonstrating both demineralization and bone overgrowth, which accompany this disease. High-resolution CT scanning may well be superior to conventional tomography in demonstrating foci or poorly calcified spongy new bone because of its inherent superior contrast resolution. Satisfactory methods for bringing the lateral wall of the labyrinth into profile, as is done with tomography, can be devised (horizontal scanning with the

head tilted away from the side examined, coronal scanning with the head extended and rotated 20° toward the side examined, and coronal scanning with 20° oblique reconstructions).

CEREBELLOPONTINE ANGLE

Anatomy

The cerebellopontine angle indicates a space bounded by the posterior surface of the petrous pyramid, lateral border of the clivus, jugular tubercle, and jugular foramen anteroinferiorly; the tentorium superiorly; the brachium pontis and the cerebellar hemisphere posterosuperiorly; and the pons medially.

The cerebellopontine angle is occupied by the cerebellopontine angle (CPA) cistern (Fig. 10-55), an extension of the basal cistern system, which com-

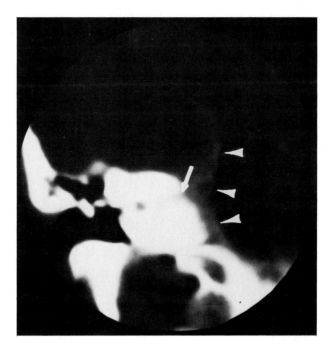

Figure 10-55 Cerebellopontine angle cistern. Coronal CT with cisternal metrizamide demarcates the cerebellopontine angle cistern (small arrowheads) from the cerebellum and brainstem. Metrizamide is also noted within the normal internal auditory canal (arrow).

municates with the pontine cistern medially and the cerebellomedullary cistern inferiorly. An extension into the internal auditory canal ensheathes the seventh and eighth cranial nerves.

The foramina of Luschka open into the CPA cisterns, and several structures course within them:

1. The sensory and motor roots of cranial nerve V exit from the lateral margin of the ventral aspect of the pons and course anterolaterally through the cistern, crossing the petrous apex to lie in Meckel's cave (described in the section on the middle fossa).
2. Cranial nerve VI leaves the lower border of the pons to pass through the cistern in a superior and anterior course, exiting it inferomedially to cranial nerve V.
3. Cranial nerves VII and VIII emerge from the brainstem just anterosuperior to the foramen of Luschka and course laterally through the cistern into the internal auditory canal.
4. Cranial nerves IX, X, and XI exit more anteriorly and inferiorly, passing into the jugular foramen.
5. The anterior inferior cerebellar artery lies within the cistern and passes close to the internal auditory canal; the internal auditory artery, which enters the canal, may arise from this vessel or directly from the basilar artery.
6. The petrosal vein crosses the cistern just above the internal auditory canal to drain into the superior petrosal sinus.

CT Technique

Routine axial scanning with and without intravenous contrast enhancement, and with a scanner providing reasonably good resolution, enables most masses larger than 1 cm in diameter to be imaged unless they are close to the CSF density of the CPA cistern. Coronal and sagittal sections can be useful in assessing extent and origin of lesions. Newer-generation scanners with "region of interest" reconstruction and thin-section capabilities are particularly useful in this area. The use of intrathecal contrast, such as air or metrizamide remarkably improves the ability to detect and evaluate smaller lesions; this method can be of great aid in determining the origin of a mass as well as its relationship to normal structures within the cistern.

Pathology

Acoustic Neuroma

This lesion, which arises from Schwann cells investing the eighth cranial nerve, constitutes 80 to 90 percent of cerebellopontine angle masses as reported in the literature. It is also the most common tumor of the inner ear. Most acoustic neuromas (at least 66 percent) arise from the vestibular division of the eighth nerve and the remainder, from the cochlear division. The superior vestibular division is the most common site of origin. About 95 percent appear to arise within the internal auditory canal and the remainder, within the cerebellopontine angle cistern just proximal to the canal; most eventually extend into the cistern to present as a mass of variable size there. For this reason acoustic neuromas are considered in this section rather than in the section on the temporal bone.

Early symptoms are due to eighth-nerve compression with sensorineural hearing loss and/or vestibular dysfunction. The seventh cranial nerve is the next impaired because of its proximity to the eighth; the fifth becomes involved only after extension of the mass into the angle and after it reaches 2.5 to 3.0 cm in diameter. Brainstem and cerebellar compression can occur with larger tumors; fourth ventricular rotation and compression can lead to hydrocephalus with the larger lesions. Inferior extension may compress the ninth and tenth cranial nerves.

Bone changes consist of erosion of the cortical bone lining the internal auditory canal (especially superiorly and posteriorly) and expansion of the canal (Hatam 1978b) (Fig. 10-56). The latter is present when any portion of the canal is 2 mm wider than the corresponding portion of the opposite canal or the posterior wall (measured from the medial wall of the vestibule to the posterior edge of the porus) is 3 mm shorter than that of the opposite

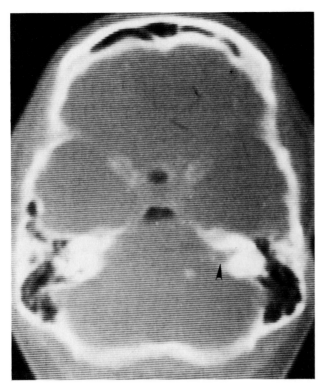

Figure 10-56 Acostic neuroma. CT at wide window settings shows the enlarged internal auditory canal of a patient with acoustic neuroma (arrow).

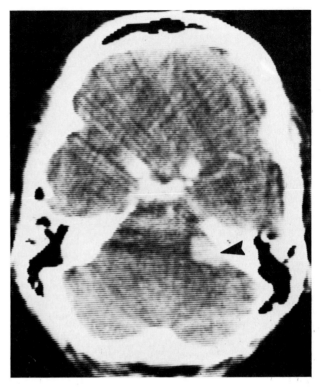

Figure 10-57 Left acoustic neuroma with homogeneous contrast enhancement (arrowhead). Note the relatively oval shape and narrow surface of contact with petrous pyramid.

side. Displacement of the crista falciformis (usually inferiorly) is diagnosed either when it is below the midway point between the roof and the floor or when it differs in position by 2 mm from that on the opposite side; this, too, indicates expansion. Asymmetry of canal size without bone erosion can occur as a result of normal variation with a large extension of the subarachnoid space into the canal. Normal internal auditory canal measurements are given in the section on the temporal bone. Furthermore, absence of evidence of expansion does not rule out the presence of a small intracanalicular lesion or one which has arisen in the cerebellopontine angle. Finally, surgical approach is dictated by tumor size and extent. For these reasons, visualization of the mass becomes the major thrust of the examination when clinical findings and/or bone evaluation indicate the likelihood of an acoustic neuroma.

CT is employed to visualize acoustic neuromas and to demonstrate their extraaxial position. Lesions over 1.5 cm in size are visualized on most scanners in use; smaller lesions can be seen with scanners capable of thin-section, high-resolution scanning. The density of these lesions is usually about equal to that of brain tissue. Following intravenous contrast injection, nearly all lesions show contrast enhancement (Fig. 10-57). Low-density areas on noncontrast scans represent cyst formation or degenerative change and are manifest as areas of nonenhancement following contrast injection (Hatam 1978a; Moller 1978a) (Fig. 10-58). Calcification occurs quite uncommonly (Moller 1978a). Most lesions are round, and some are oval; occasional tumors are lobulated.

Typically, the mass does not show a broad surface of contact with the petrous pyramid (Fig. 10-

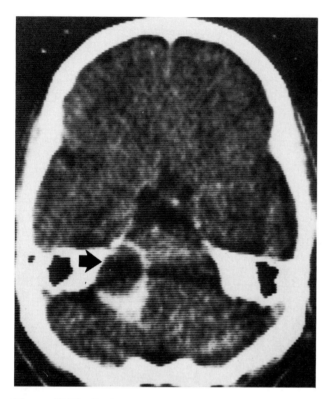

Figure 10-58 Cystic acoustic neuroma (arrow). Contrast-enhanced peripheral rim is apparent.

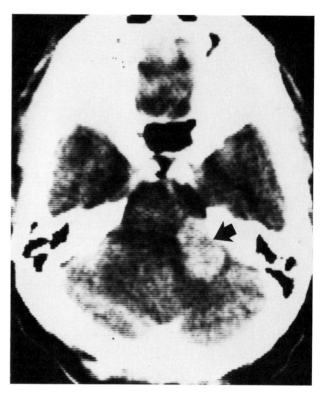

Figure 10-59 Large acoustic neuroma with narrow surface of contact with the petrous pyramid (arrow).

59), but this may be seen in as many as 20 percent (producing a false impression of a broad origin) (Moller 1978b). The tumors are usually centered at the internal auditory meatus in the anteroposterior direction; the center may be slightly posterior but not anterior, to the meatus. Although acoustic neuromas are extraaxial, they may cause edema in adjacent brain tissue.

When there are bony changes or clinical findings suggesting an acoustic neuroma and the CT scan shows no mass, intrathecal contrast examination is necessary. Until recently this was best accomplished with Pantopaque with the use of fluoroscopy, radiography, and tomography. Metrizamide with CT scanning has also proven useful in demonstrating small lesions, even purely intracanalicular tumors; demonstration of the latter requires 1- to 2-mm sections, permitting window settings sufficiently narrow for visualization of contrast within the internal

auditory canal. Recently an alternative method of opacification has been described which demands less of the scanner (Kricheff 1980; Sortland 1979). Intrathecal air injected with the patient tilted at an angle of about 45° from the horizontal (side investigated being uppermost) and the head tilted nearly 45° in the same direction causes the air to accumulate in the upper cerebellopontine angle cistern. Scanning is carried out with the patient in the decubitus position to keep the air in the appropriate cistern. Injection of 3 to 4 ml of air is sufficient for visualization of the cistern and its extension into the canal. This is excellent for detecting small lesions because of the great contrast between air and soft tissues (Fig. 10-60); wide window settings with low centering (window level) should be used (800 to 1000 HU and −300 HU, respectively). Air-enhanced CT cisternography has also been utilized for evaluating bilateral CPA masses (Lee 1981).

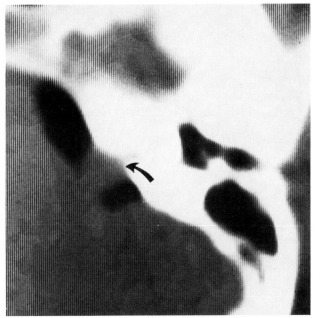

A

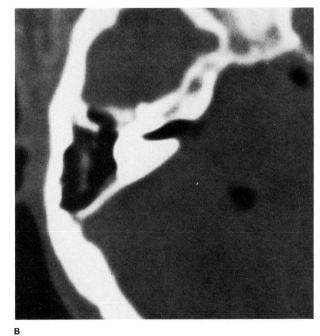

B

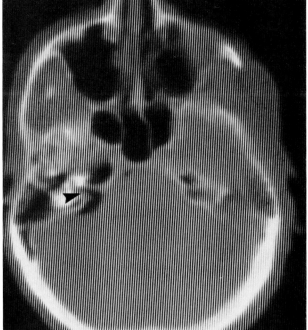

C

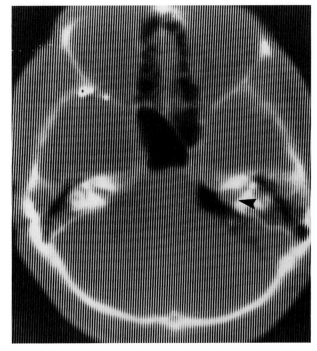

D

Figure 10-60 Air CT cisternography. **A.** The soft-tissue mass of an acoustic neuroma (arrow) is well outlined by air in the cerebellopontine angle cistern. The internal auditory canal is seen just above the arrowhead. **B.** The opposite cerebellopontine angle is normal. **C.** Normal air CT cisternogram in another case. Air has entered the internal auditory canal (arrowhead). **D.** The left side of the patient in **C.** There is expansion of the internal auditory canal (arrowhead), which is filled with soft tissue. This mass protrudes slightly into the cerebellopontine angle cistern.

The authors note that while air-contrast CT detects lesions well, it seems inferior to metrizamide in outlining the larger lesion completely and assessing its impingement on the brainstem. Our conclusion was that air-enhanced CT was the best method for detecting lesions not visualized with intravenous contrast enhancement but that metrizamide-enhanced CT may be necessary for additional information in planning surgery.

Acoustic neuromas involving the cerebellopontine angle may be sufficiently large to displace the adjacent brainstem, widening the ipsilateral cerebellopontine angle cistern and the supratentorial part of the ambient cistern. The fourth ventricle may be displaced contralaterally (sometimes posteriorly also) and rotated with lesions larger than 1 cm³ (Fig. 10-61); with very large lesions, compression may

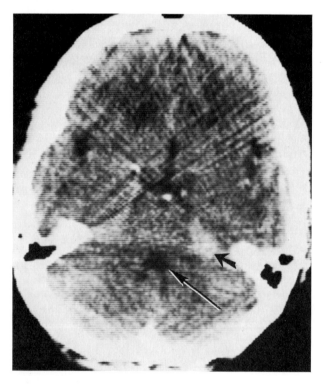

Figure 10-61 Fourth ventricular displacement by an acoustic neuroma (same patient as in Figure 10-57). The uppermost portion of the acoustic neuroma can be seen faintly with contrast enhancement (short arrow). The fourth ventricle (long arrow) has been rotated and displaced toward the right by the tumor.

prevent visualization of the fourth ventricle. Hydrocephalus may be present as a result of fourth ventricular distortion and compression.

Hamartomas and gliomas of the eighth nerve have been reported (Babin 1980; Kasantikul 1980) but are rare; the findings on CT in a reported case of glioma (Kasantikul 1980) was quite similar to those of acoustic neuroma.

Facial Nerve Neuroma

Neuromas of the facial nerve are most commonly seen in the descending portion of the nerve, where erosion of the facial canal and adjacent mastoid are seen. They may occur, however, along the entire course of the seventh nerve, which includes the cerebellopontine angle, the internal auditory canal, and the facial canal (described above in the section on anatomy of the temporal bone). Lesions in the internal auditory canal or cerebellopontine angle closely resemble the appearance of acoustic neuroma in all respects.

Trigeminal Nerve Neuroma

These tumors show characteristics identical to those of acoustic neuromas, except for enlargement of the internal auditory canal. Those which arise in the posterior fossa and are large may be indistinguishable from an acoustic neuroma arising in the cerebellopontine angle or a meningioma. Features which favor the diagnosis of trigeminal neuroma over acoustic neuroma (in addition to the clinical findings) are as follows:

1. Trigeminal neuromas commonly show a closer relationship to the tip of the petrous bone than to the internal auditory meatus.
2. Erosion of the petrous apex may be seen with trigeminal neuromas; erosion and expansion of the internal auditory canal and the porus acusticus may occur with acoustic neuromas.
3. Trigeminal neuromas may extend as far anterior as the upper clivus and the dorsum, as well as into the middle cranial fossa; acoustic neuromas normally do not.

While meningiomas may show the same location and extension as trigeminal neuromas, they show calcification and increased density more often and produce hyperostosis and ill-defined lytic changes in bone.

Neuromas of Cranial Nerves IX, X, and XI

These are considered in the section on the jugular fossa.

Meningioma

This tumor is the second most frequent cerebellopontine angle mass. Meningiomas may arise from the meninges, extending along the seventh and eighth cranial nerves, or from the meninges along the petrous pyramid. The first type may expand the internal auditory canal, the latter may produce bone changes along the petrous pyramid.

Computed tomographic examination of bone (or conventional tomography) may show (as with meningiomas that arise elsewhere) hyperostosis or ill-defined lytic changes. In those lesions arising along the seventh and eighth cranial nerves, the internal auditory canal walls and crista may show such changes; in these lesions and in those along the petrous pyramid, the pyramid itself may show such abnormalities. In contrast, acoustic neuromas produce more sharply defined expansions and erosions with sharp edges. Calcification is far more common in meningiomas; the calcification, when present, tends to be extensive, occupying much of the tumor, but occasionally may be more peripheral and shell-like (Fig. 10-62). Meningiomas tend to be denser than surrounding brain tissue; neuromas are usually of density equal to that of brain tissue. Cystic areas, large or small, may be present in both tumors, appearing as areas of lower density on nonenhanced scans and areas of nonenhancement following intravenous contrast injection. Meningiomas typically have a broad attachment along the petrous pyramid (Fig. 10-63), but acoustic neuromas may have a broad surface of contact along the petrous pyramid in about 20 percent of cases, producing a similar appearance (Moller 1978b).

The center of a meningioma is not necessarily related to the internal auditory meatus (unlike acoustic neuromas); commonly it is anterior or posterior. Anterior centering is not seen in acoustic neuromas, and posterior centering is only slight (Moller 1978b). Both tumors may extend for a considerable distance vertically, appearing at the tentorial incisura; however, the meningiomas can extend upward more anteriorly to reach the side of the upper clivus and dorsum and may enter the suprasellar cistern; acoustic neuromas show a more vertical extension and do not reach the upper clivus, dorsum, and suprasellar cistern. Meningiomas may extend sufficiently high anteriorly to displace the third ventricle contralaterally and may even enter the middle cranial fossa to present as a mass there; such extension is not seen with acoustic neuromas (Moller 1978b).

Arteriography may be of little help in differential diagnosis. Cerebellopontine angle meningiomas commonly show little or no tumor vasculature, while neuromas are more commonly seen to have both tumor vessels and "tumor staining." Meningeal vascular supply may be seen with both tumors. Early venous filling is common in neuromas but relatively uncommon with meningiomas. Both show vascular displacements characteristic of an extraaxial mass.

Epidermoids

Epidermoids, dermoids, and teratomas are developmental (congenital) tumors (see Chap. 7). Epidermoids are composed only of ectodermal elements, dermoids of ectodermal and mesodermal elements, and teratomas of elements of all three germ layers. Epidermoids and dermoids are cystic lesions. Dermoids are discussed in the section on the sellar region. Epidermoids most commonly occur in the cerebellopontine angle but also arise in the sellar region, middle cranial fossa, interhemispheric fissure, quadrigeminal region, the ventricles, and the diploe of the skull. They may be intradural or extradural.

The capsule of an epidermoid is composed of stratified squamous epithelium surrounded by vary-

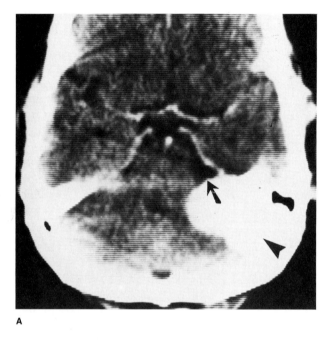

A

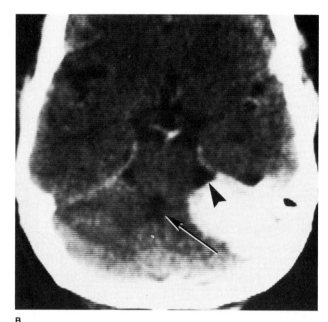

B

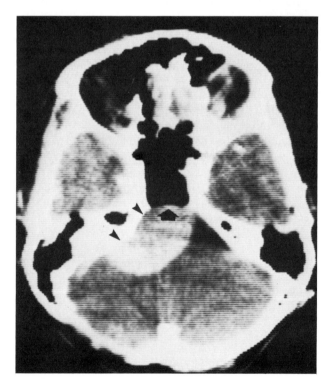

C

Figure 10-62 Meningioma. **A.** Densely enhancing tumor in the left cerebellopontine angle (arrowhead). The widening of the CPA cistern on the side of the tumor (arrow) is due to the lateral displacement of the brainstem. **B.** At a slightly higher level, the widened CPA cistern can still be seen (arrowhead). Lateral displacement of the fourth ventricle is also apparent (arrow). **C.** Coronal projection, same patient, demonstrating marked curvilinear calcification within the more peripheral portion of the tumor (arrowhead).

Figure 10-63 Meningioma showing extremely broad base of attachment along the petrous pyramid (arrowheads) and extending along the clivus (arrow).

ing amounts of connective tissue; the contents are epithelial debris and cholesterol crystals. Unlike dermoids, epidermoids commonly have a lobulated, irregular surface with numerous crevices.

CT scanning shows epidermoids to be of a density lower than that of brain tissue (Naidich 1976b), varying from slightly negative values to values just less than those of brain tissue and greater than those of cerebrospinal fluid; some are equal in density to cerebrospinal fluid. Calcification may be present in peripheral portions of the tumor; occasionally the lesions have internal calcifications, and, rarely, they are diffusely calcified and appear homogeneously dense. Contrast enhancement is not a feature of these tumors, but occasionally mild peripheral en-

hancement may be seen, presumably in connective tissue elements around the epithelial wall.

Epidermoids, as noted above, may be intradural or extradural. Extradural lesions produce well-defined erosion of bone, commonly quite extensive (Fig. 10-64). There may be a thin zone of sclerosis demarcating the periphery of the lesion, but this is not necessarily present. The contents of the lesion are as described above, with a thin rim of increased attenuation which may show contrast enhancement; this presumably represents surrounding vascular connective tissue and dura. In the cerebello-pontine angle, epidural lesions may arise in the jugular fossa region or between the dura and the remaining portions of the bone forming the floor of

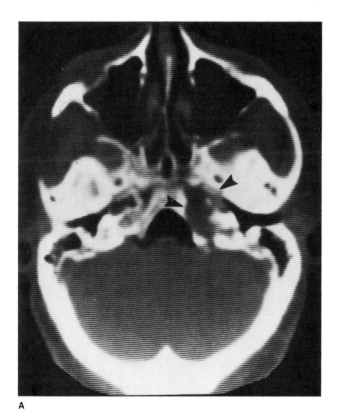

A

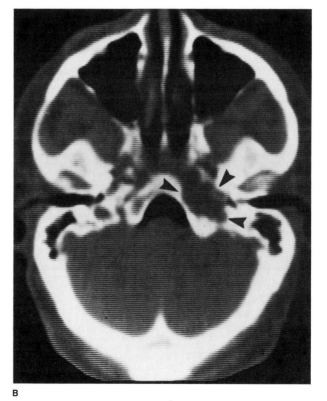

B

Figure 10-64 An extradural epidermoid with extensive bony erosion. The scans were carried out following intrathecal air injection. **A.** The lowermost section demonstrates sharply defined erosion of the inferior aspect of the petrous portion

of the temporal bone as well as the lateral aspect of the clivus (arrowheads) **B.** A slightly higher section demonstrates the bony erosion but no evidence of an extraosseous soft-tissue mass. (*Continued on page 454.*)

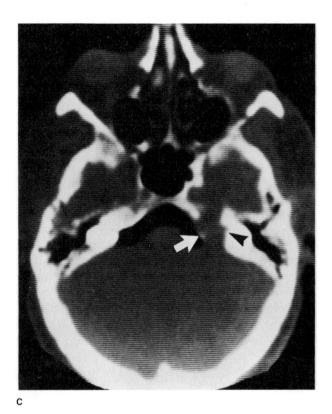

C

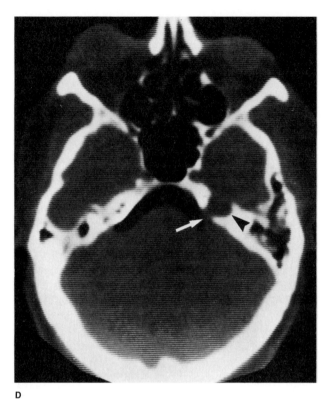

D

Figure 10-64   C. Soft-tissue mass extends into the pontine and cerebellopontine cisterns (white arrow). The arrowhead indicates the area of bone erosion.   **D.** In the uppermost sec-

tion erosion of the petrous portion of the temporal bone (arrowhead) is sharply defined. There is also a small extraosseous soft-tissue component (white arrow).

the cerebellopontine angle. Those arising within the petrous pyramid expand this structure, while those arising between it and the dura erode it from above.

Intradural lesions show a more lobulated, irregular surface in many instances, especially when outlined with intrathecal contrast. In the cerebellopontine angle, these lesions produce extraaxial mass effects similar to those described for acoustic neuromas. These lesions are very slow growing and can become very extensive. They have a tendency to envelop vessels and nerves and to insinuate themselves into cisternal spaces. For these reasons, total removal of large lesions becomes quite difficult; incomplete removal leads to recurrence.

Occasionally an epidermoid will rupture or its contents will leak into the subarachnoid space, producing a chemical meningitis. Computed tomographic scanning can demonstrate material of the

density of the cyst contents in the subarachnoid spaces and within the ventricles (Laster 1977). While the consequences of such rupture or leakage may be a fulminant and even fatal meningitis (Laster 1977; Peyton 1942; Tytus 1956), cases of essentially asymptomatic rupture have been reported. Arteriography may show an avascular mass, but encasement of arteries may be demonstrated on careful inspection (Mikhael 1978).

Differentiation between chondroma and cystic lesions of the cerebellopontine angle may be difficult. Lack of contrast enhancement, avascularity, and lobulation are useful differential features.

Other Cerebellopontine Angle Lesions

Aneurysms, arterial ectasia, and arteriovenous malformation are discussed in Chap. 14. Arachnoid cysts are discussed in Chap. 4. Chondromas and chondrosarcomas are considered in the section on the middle cranial fossa. It should be noted that calcification is quite uncommon in these lesions when they arise in the cerebellopontine angle region (K. F. Lee 1979; Minagi 1969; Roukkula 1964; Sarwar 1976). Brainstem and fourth ventricular masses may extend into the cerebellopontine angle.

Bibliography

ADAMS GL, PAPARELLA MM, FIKY FH: Primary and metastatic tumors of the temporal bone. *Laryngoscope* **81**:1273–1285, 1971.

ANSON BJ: Stapedial, capsular and labyrinthine anatomy in relation to otologic surgery. *Ann Otolaryngol* **70**:607–631, 1961.

BABIN RW, FRATKIN JD, CANCILLA PA: Hamartomas of the cerebellopontine angle and internal auditory canal. *Arch Otolaryngol* **106**:500–502, 1980.

BAHR AL, GAYLER BW: Cranial chondrosarcomas. *Radiology* **124**:151–156, 1977.

BANNA M: Pathology and clinical manifestations, in Hankinson J, Banna M (eds): *Pituitary and Parapituitary Tumors*, Philadelphia, Saunders, 1976*a*, pp 25–28.

BANNA M: Radiology, in Hankinson J, Banna M (eds): *Pituitary and Parapituitary Tumors*, Philadelphia, Saunders, 1976*b*, pp 135–149.

BERKMEN YM, BLATT ES: Cranial and intracranial cartilaginous tumors. *Clin Radiol* **19**:327–333, 1968.

BRADAC GB, SCHRAMM J, GRUMME T, SIMON RS: CT of the base of the skull. *Neuroradiology* **17**:1–5, 1978.

BRITTON BH: Glomus tympanicum and glomus jugulare. *Radiol Clin North Am* **12**:543–551, 1974.

BUCKINGHAM RA, VALVASSORI GE: Tomographic evaluation of cholesteatomas of the middle ear and mastoid. *Otolaryngol Clin North Am* **6**:363–378, 1973.

BURKE DP, GABRIELSON TO, KNACKE JE, SEEGER JF, OBERMAN HA: Radiology of olfactory neuroblastoma. *Radiology* **137**:367–372, 1980.

CAFFEY J: *Pediatric X-ray Diagnosis*, Chicago, Year Book Medical Publishers, 1972, pp 1294–1297.

COIN CG, MALKASIAN DR: Foramen magnum, in Newton TH, Potts DG (eds): *Radiology of the Skull and Brain*, vol 1. St. Louis, Mosby, 1971, pp 275–286.

DAVIS KR, NEW PFJ: Intrasellar and perisellar lesions in central nervous system, in Wolpert SM (ed): *CNS Approaches to Radiologic Diagnosis*, New York, Grune & Stratton, 1979, pp 57–81.

DAVIS JM et al: Expanded high iodine dose in computed cranial tomography: A preliminary report. *Radiology* **131**:373–380, 1979.

DEERY EM: Note on calcification in pituitary adenomas. *Endocrinology* **13**:455, 1929.

DI CHIRO G, FISHER RL, NELSON KB: The jugular foramen. *J Neurosurg* **21**:447–460, 1964.

DOLAN KD: Malignant lesions of the ear. *Radiol Clin North Am* **12**:585–600, 1974.

DOLAN KD: Cervicobasilar relationships. *Radiol Clin North Am* **15**:155–166, 1977.

DOMINQUE JN, WILSON CB: Pituitary abscesses: Report of seven cases and review of the literature. *J Neurosurg* **46**:601–608, 1977.

DRAYER BP, ROSENBAUM AE, MAROON JC, BANK WO, WOODFORD JE: Posterior fossa extracranial cyst: Diagnosis with metrizamide CT cisternography. *Am J Roentgenol* **128**:431–436, 1977(*b*).

DRAYER BP, ROSENBAUM AE, KENNERDELL JS, ROBINSON AG, BANK WO, DEEB ZL: Computed tomographic diagnosis of suprasellar masses by intrathecal enhancement. *Radiology* **125**:339–344, 1977(*a*).

DU BOIS PJ et al: Normal sellar variations in frontal tomograms. *Radiology* **131**:105–110, 1979.

DU BOULAY GH, TRICKEY SE: Calcification in chromophobe adenoma. *Br J Radiology* **35**:793–795, 1962.

FITZ CR, HARWOOD-NASH DC: Radiology of the ear in children. *Radiol Clin North Am* **12**:553–570, 1974.

FITZ CR et al: Computed tomography in craniopharyngiomas. *Radiology* **127**:687–691, 1978.

FREY KW: Malformations of the middle ear, in Jensen J, Rovsing H (eds): *Fundamentals of Ear Tomography*, Springfield, Thomas, 1971, pp 77–85.

GADO MH, PHELPS ME, COLEMAN RE: Extravascular component of contrast enhancement in cranial computed tomography, Part I: Tissue-blood ratio of contrast enhancement. *Radiology* **117**:589–594, 1975a.

GADO MH, PHELPS ME, COLEMAN RE: Extravascular component of contrast enhancement in cranial computed tomography, Part II: Contrast enhancement and the blood brain barrier. *Radiology* **117**:595–597, 1975b.

GEEHR RB, ALLEN WE III, ROTHMAN SLG, SPENCER PD: Pluridirectional tomography in the evaluation of pituitary tumor. *Am J Roentgenol* **130**:105–109, 1978.

GLASGOLD AI, HORRINGTON WD: The internal carotid artery presenting as a middle ear tumor. *Laryngoscope* **82**:2217–2221, 1972.

GLENN WV JR et al: Image generation and display techniques for CT scan data (1975 Dyke Memorial award paper). *Invest Radiol* **10**:403–416, 1975a.

GLENN WV JR et al: Further investigation and initial use of advanced CT display capability. *Invest Radiol* **10**:479–489, 1975b.

GOLDBERG R, BYRD S, WINTER J, TAKAHASHI M, JOYCE P: Varied appearance of trigeminal neuroma on CT. *Am J Roentgenol* **134**:57–60, 1980.

GOODWIN WJ, JESSE RH: Malignant neoplasms of the external auditory canal and temporal bone. *Arch Otolaryngol* **106**:675–679, 1980.

GREITZ T, HINDMARSH T: Computer assisted tomography of intracranial CSF circulation using a water soluble contrast medium. *Acta Radiol Diagn* **15**:497–507, 1974.

GUILD SR: The glomus jugulare, a nonchromaffin paraganglion in man. *Ann Otolaryngol* **62**:1045–1071, 1953.

HALL K, MC ALLISTER VL: Metrizamide cisternography in pituitary and juxtapituitary lesions. *Radiology* **134**:101–108, 1980.

HARDY J: Transphenoidal surgery of the normal and pathological pituitary. *Clin Neurosurg* **16**:185–217, 1969.

HATAM A, BERGSTROM M, MOLLER A, OLIVECRONA H: Early contrast enhancement of acoustic neuroma. *Neuroradiology* **17**:31–33, 1978a.

HATAM A, MOLLER A, OLIVECRONA H: Evaluation of the internal auditory meatus with acoustic neuromas using computed tomography. *Neuroradiology* **17**:197–200, 1978b.

HAYMAN LA, EVANS RA, HINCK VC: Delayed high iodine dose contrast computed tomography: cranial neoplasms. *Radiology* **136**:677–683, 1980.

HESSELINK JR et al: Evaluation of mucoceles of the paranasal sinuses with computed tomography. *Radiology* **133**:397–400, 1979.

JENSEN J: Malformations of the inner ear, in Jensen J, Rorsing H (eds): *Fundaments of Ear Tomography*, Springfield, Il Thomas, 1971, pp 87–93.

JENSEN J: Congenital anomalies of the inner ear. *Radiol Clin North Am* **12**:473–482, 1974.

KASANTIKUL V, PALMER JO, NETSKY MG, GLASSCOCK ME, HAYS JW: Glioma of the acoustic nerve. *Arch Otolaryngol* **106**:456–459, 1980.

KAUFMAN B: The empty sella turcica—a manifestation of the intrasellar subarachnoid space. *Radiology* **90**:931–941, 1968.

KAUFMAN B, PEARSON OH, CHAMBERLINE WB: Radiographic features of intrasellar masses and progressive asymmetrical non-tumorous enlargements of the sella turcica, the "empty sella," in Kohler PO, Ross GT (eds): *Diagnosis and Treatment of Pituitary Tumors*, Amsterdam, Excerpta Medica 1973, p 100.

KENDALL B, LEE BCP: Intracranial chordomas. *Br J Radiol* **150**:687–698, 1977.

KENDALL BE, TATLER GLU: Radiological findings in neurosarcoidosis. *Br J Radiol* **51**:81–92, 1978.

KIEFFER SA: Orbit, in Newton TH, Potts DG (eds): *Radiology of the Skull and Brain*, vol 2. St. Louis, Mosby, 1971, pp 477–478.

KRICHEFF II et al: Air CT cisternography and canalography for small acoustic neuromas. *Am J Neuroradiol* **1**:57–63, 1980.

KRUYFF E: Occipital dysplasia in infancy. *Radiology* **85**:501–505, 1965.

KUNO T, SUDO M, MOMOI T, TAKAO T, ITO M, KONISHI Y, YOSHIOKA M, SUZUKI J, NAKANO Y: Pituitary hyperplasia due to hypothyroidism. *Radiol Clin North Am* **4**:600–602, 1980.

LAPAYOWKER MS: Congenital anomalies of the middle ear. *Radiol Clin North Am* **12**:463–471, 1974.

LASTER DW, MOODY DM, MARSHALL RB: Epidermoid tumors with intraventricular and subarachnoid fat: Report of two cases. *Am J Roentgenol* **128**:504–507, 1977.

LEE BCP: Intracranial cysts. *Radiology* **130**:667–673, 1979.

LEE KF, LIN S: *Neuroradiology of Sellar and Juxtasellar Lesions*, Springfield, Thomas, 1979, pp 193–279.

LEE SH, LEWIS E, MONTOYA JH, SEELAUS JF: Bilateral cerebellopontine angle air-CT cisternography. *Am J Neuroradiol* **2**:105–106, 1981.

LEE SH, ZIMMERMAN RA, BILANIUK LT, WOO V: Computed tomographic findings in basilar invagination. *J Comput Assist Tomogr* **2**:255–266, 1978.

MANELFE C, BONAFE A, FABRE P, PESSEY J: Computed tomography in olfactory neuroblastoma: One case of esthesioneuroepithelioma and four cases of esthesioneuroblastoma. *J Comput Assist Tomogr* **2**:412–420, 1978.

MCGREGOR M: The significance of certain measurements of the skull in the diagnosis of basilar impression. *Br J Radiol* **21**:171–180, 1948.

MENDEZ G, QUENCER RM, POST MJD, STOKES NA: Malignant external otitis: A radiographic clinical correlation. *Am J Roentgenol* **132**:957–961, 1979.

MIKHAEL MA, MATTAR AG: Intracranial pearly tumors: The roles of computed tomography, angiography and pneumoencephalography. *J Comput Assist Tomogr* **2**:421–429, 1978.

MILLER JG, PENA AM, SEGALL HD: Radiological investigation of sellar region masses in children. *Radiology* **134**:81–87, 1980.

MINAGI H, NEWTON TH: Cartilaginous tumors of the base of the skull. *Radiology* **105**:308–413, 1969.

MITNICK JS, PINTO RS: Computed tomography in the diagnosis of eosinophilic granuloma. *J Comput Assist Tomogr* **4**:791–793, 1980.

MOLLER A, HATAM A, OLIVECRONA H: Diagnosis of acoustic neuroma with computed tomography. *Neuroradiology* **17**:25–30, 1978a.

MOLLER A, HATAM A, OLIVECRONA H: The differential diagnosis of pontine angle meningioma and acoustic neuroma with computed tomography. *Neuroradiology* **17**:21–23, 1978*b*.

MOTARA R, NORRELL H: Consequences of a deficient sellar diaphragm. *J Neurosurg* **32**:565–573, 1970.

NAIDICH TP, PINTO RS, KSUHNER MJ, LIN JP, KRICHEFF II, LEEDS NE, CHASE NE: Evaluation of sellar and parasellar masses by computed tomography. *Radiology* **120**:91–99, 1976*a*.

NAIDICH TP, LIN JP, LEEDS NE, KRICHEFF II, GEORGE AE, CHASE NE, PUDLOWSKI RM, PASSALAGUA A: Computed tomography in the diagnosis of extra-axial posterior fossa masses. *Radiology* **120**:333–339, 1976*b*.

NEW PFJ, SCOTT WR, SCHNUR JA, DAVIS KR, TAVERAS JM: Computerized axial tomography with the EMI scanner. *Radiology* **110**:109–123, 1974.

NEW PFJ, SCOTT W: *Computed Tomography of the Brain and Orbit (EMI Scanning)*. Baltimore, Williams & Wilkins, 1975, p 345.

OSBORN AG, JOHNSON L, ROBERTS TS: Sphenoid mucoceles with intracranial extension. *J Comput Assist Tomogr* **3**:335–338, 1979.

PETASNICK JP: Congenital malformations of the ear. *Otolaryngol Clin North Am* **6**:413–427, 1973.

PEYTON WT, BAKER AB: Epidermoid, dermoid and teratomatous tumors of the central nervous system. *Arch Neurol Psychol* **47**:890–917, 1942.

PHELPS PD, LLOYD GAS: The radiology of cholesteatoma. *Clin Radiol* **31**:501–512, 1980.

PINTO RS, HANDEL SF, SADHU VK: CT metrizamide cisternography in the recognition of intrasellar cistern. *Am J Roentgenol* **133**:320–312, 1979*a*.

PINTO RS et al: Correlation of computed tomographic, angiographic, and neuropathological changes in giant cerebral aneurysms. *Radiology* **132**:85–92, 1979*b*.

POST MJD, DAVID NJ, GLAZER JS, SAFRAN A: Pituitary apoplexy: Diagnosis by computed tomography. *Radiology* **134**:665–670, 1980.

POTTER GD, GRAHAM MD: The carotid canal. *Radiol Clin North Am* **12**:483–489, 1974.

PRIBRAM HW, DU BOULAY G: The sella turcica, in Newton TH, Potts DG (eds): *Radiology of the Skull and Brain*, vol 1, book 1. St Louis, Mosby, 1971, pp 156–405.

RAJI MR, KISHORE PRS, BECKER DP: Pituitary microadenoma: A radiological–surgical correlative study. *Radiology* **139**:95–99, 1981.

RAYMOND LA, TEW J: Large suprasellar aneurysms imitating pituitary tumor. *J Neurol Neurosurg Psychiatry* **41**:83–87, 1978.

RICHMOND IL, NEWTON TH, WILSON CB: Prolactin-secreting pituitary adenomas: Correlation of radiographic and surgical findings. *Am J Neuroradiol* **1**:13–16, 1980.

ROBERTSON WB, NEWTON TH: Radiologic assessment of pituitary microadenomas. *Am J Roentgenol* **131**:489–492, 1978.

ROBIN PE: A case of upwardly situated jugular bulb in left middle ear. *J Laryngol Otolaryngol* **86**:1241–1246, 1972.

ROSENGREN J, JING B, WALLACE S, DANZIGER J: Radiographic features of olfactory neuroblastomas. *Am J Roentgenol* **132**:945–948, 1979.

ROTHMAN SLG, GEEHR RB, KIER L, ZIMMER AE: A reasonable approach to the neuroradiology evaluation of pituitary microadenomas. Paper presented at the American Society of Neuroradiology 18th Annual Meeting, Los Angeles, California, March 1980.

ROUKKULA M: Roentgenological findings in chondromas of the pontine angle. *Acta Radiol (Diagn)* **2**:120–128, 1964.

ROZARIO R et al: Diagnosis of empty sella with CT scan. *Neuroradiology* **13**:85–88, 1977.

RUBIN P: *Dynamic Classification of Bone Dysplasias*, Chicago, Year Book Medical Publishers, 1964, pp 181–353.

RUDWAN MA: Pituitary abscess. *Neuroradiology* **12**:243–248, 1977.

SARWAR M, SWISCHUK LE, SCHECHTER MM: Intracranial chondromas. *Am J Roentgenol* **127**:973–977, 1976.

SHAFFER KA, HAUGHTON VM, WILSON CR: High resolution computed tomography of the temporal bone. *Radiology* **134**:409–414, 1980.

SIMMS NM, BROWN WE, FRENCH LA: Mucocele of the sphenoid sinus presenting as an intrasellar mass. Case report. *J Neurosurg* **32**:708–710, 1970.

SMALTINO F, BERNINI FP, MURAS I: Computed tomography for diagnosis of empty sella associated with pituitary microadenoma. *J Comput Assist Tomogr* **4**:592–599, 1980.

SONDHEIMER FK: Basal foramina and canals, in Newton TH, Potts DG (eds): *Radiology of the Skull and Brain*, vol 2. St. Louis, Mosby, 1971, pp 333–341.

SORTLAND O: Computed tomography combined with gas cisternography for the diagnosis of expanding lesions in the cerebellopontine angle. *Neuroradiology* **18**:19–22, 1979.

STALLINGS JO, MCCABE BF: Congenital middle ear aneurysm of internal carotid. *Arch Otolaryngol* **90**:65–73, 1969.

SYVERTSEN A, HAUGHTON VM, WILLIAMS AL, CUSICK JF: The computed tomographic appearance of the normal pituitary gland and pituitary microadenomas. *Radiology* **133**:385–391, 1979.

TAVERAS JM, WOOD EH: *Diagnostic Neuroradiology*, 2nd ed. Baltimore, Williams & Wilkins, 1976, p 521.

TYRELL B, WILSON CB: Pituitary syndromes in surgical endocrinology, in Friesen SR (ed): *Clinical Syndromes*, Philadelphia, Lippincott, 1978, pp 304–321.

TYTUS SJ, PENNYBACKER J: Pearly tumors in relation to the central nervous system. *J Neurol Psychol* **19**:241–259, 1956.

VALVASSORI GE, PIERCE RH: The normal internal auditory canal. *Am J Roentgenol* **92**:1232–1241, 1964.

VEZINA JL, SUTTON TJ: Prolactin-secreting pituitary microadenomas: Roentgenologic diagnosis. *Am J Roentgenol* **120**:46–54, 1974.

WHELAN MA, STERN J: Intracranial tuberculoma. *Radiology* **138**:75–81, 1981.

WILLIAMS B: The distending force in the production of "communicating syringomyelia." *Lancet* **2**:189–193, 1969.

WOLPERT SM et al: The value of computed tomography in evaluating patients with prolactinomas. *Radiology* **131**:117–119, 1979.

WORTZMAN G, HOLGATE RC, NEWCASTLE NB, BARROW GN: Abnormal sellas and pituitary adenomas in 120 post-mortem sphenoid specimens. Paper presented at American Society of Neuroradiology 18th Annual Meeting, Los Angeles, California, March 1980.

ZIZMOR J, NOYEK AM: Inflammatory diseases of the temporal bone. *Radiol Clin North Am* **12**:491–504, 1974.

11

CRANIOFACIAL TRAUMA AND CSF FISTULA

Kalyanmay Ghoshhajra

CRANIOFACIAL TRAUMA

Until recently the standard radiological examination for craniofacial injury was a plain radiograph of the skull and face followed by tomography (Taveras 1976; Fischgold 1973; Ratzen 1973). The yield of a plain radiograph in the evaluation of craniofacial trauma is very low (Masters 1980).

Cranial computed tomography (CT) is gradually replacing the standard radiological examination in patients with acute craniocerebral injuries. It replaces plain radiography of the skull, cerebral angiography, and the isotope brain scan (Ambrose 1976; New 1975; deVillasante 1976; Naidich 1977; Zimmerman 1978). The CT examination is more informative and accurate and is therefore a superior diagnostic tool.

Although skull fractures are found in 75 percent of patients with fatal head injuries (Lofstrom 1966), only a small number of patients with acute head injury demonstrate fracture on skull x-rays. CT plays a significant role in demonstrating the craniocerebral effects of trauma and, occasionally, in the identification of fractures involving the cranial vault, especially the frontal, parietal, and occipital bones.

Although a depressed or comminuted fracture may be recognized in skull roentgenograms, it often requires an additional tangential view of the skull. Computed tomography, in addition to demonstrating the depressed fracture, is helpful in demonstrating the associated extracerebral or intracerebral hemorrhage. A fracture at the base of the skull is rarely visualized in a plain film of the skull because of overlapping densities. When there is clinical and radiographic suspicion of a fracture, the bony injury is further evaluated by tomography. Pluridirectional tomography has been successful in the evaluation of craniofacial fractures (Zatzkin 1965; Fischgold 1973; Ratzen 1973). However, the tomographic examination required for the proper evaluation of these fractures is often delayed 24 to 48 h until the patient's clinical condition improves. Since serious intracranial injuries are commonly associated with craniofacial fractures, the priority of the evaluation and treatment of intracranial injuries further delays the accurate assessment of the bony injuries.

With the advent of CT, the radiographic evaluation of a patient with suspected cranial injury has been revolutionized. CT is the first choice when an intracranial injury is suspected. If a craniofacial injury is suspected, the patient is examined by plain skull film and, if necessary, pluridirectional tomography. With the availability of the newer generation of CT scanners, intracranial and craniofacial injuries can often be evaluated at the same time without

recourse to pluridirectional tomography. The high-resolution thin CT sections delineate the bony structures extremely well. The images are not only complementary but are superior to tomography. The associated soft-tissue injury and hemorrhage are often visualized better by CT. Further, utilization of CT instead of pluridirectional tomography significantly reduces the radiation dose to the patient.

Technical Aspects

Cranial vault injury can be adequately evaluated with a standard axial CT scan except in a fracture involving the vertex, in which a coronal CT section is necessary. Reformatted sagittal or coronal images may also be helpful. Although a gross fracture of the vault of the skull can easily be detected by standard axial CT scan in a normal window setting (Figs. 11-1, 11-2), the evaluation of bony injury requires adjustment of the window setting to a greater width (Fig. 11-3). At a narrow window setting, the thin

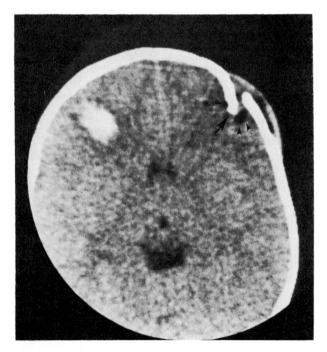

Figure 11-1 Axial CT scan through the cranial vault in a 1-year-old boy shows a depressed fracture (arrow) with presence of air (arrowheads) at the fracture site and left frontal lobe contusion.

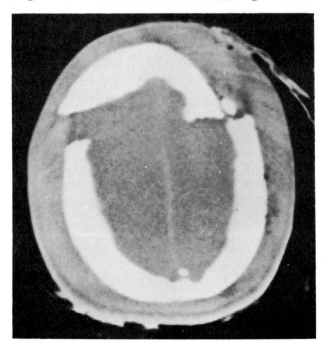

Figure 11-2 Displaced fracture of the vault of the skull. Axial CT scan through the cranial vault shows a displaced fracture involving the right frontal bone, with diffuse scalp swelling.

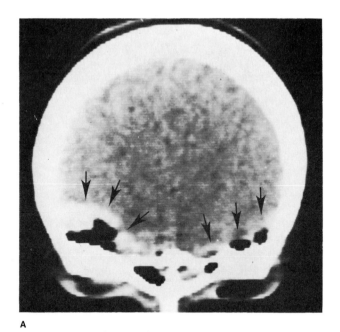

A

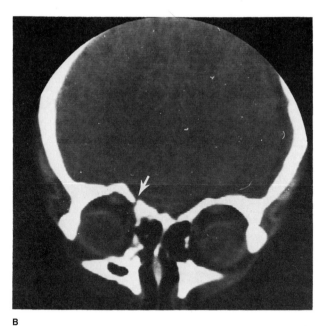

B

Figure 11-3 Fracture of the roof of the orbit. **A.** Coronal section through the anterior cranial fossa shows a bilateral subfrontal epidural collection of air and blood (arrows). **B.** At bone window, the fracture of the roof of the right orbit (arrow) is seen.

rim of an acute extracerebral hemorrhage can often blend with the adjacent skull as the same density as bone; moreover, a linear or diastatic fracture may not be seen at a normal window setting. Therefore it is imperative to examine the images at different window settings for the evaluation of intracranial hemorrhage as well as bony injury. When a fracture of the base of the skull is suspected in the axial CT scan or plain radiography of the skull, it is necessary to reexamine the patient in coronal projection using thin sections.

Anterior Cranial Fossa

Injury to the floor of the anterior cranial fossa involves the inner table of the frontal sinus, orbital roof, and cribriform plate (Figs. 11-3, 11-4, 11-5). Fractures of the planum sphenoidale may extend to the floor of the sella turcica (Figs. 11-6, 11-18). A depressed fracture of the orbital roof can compress the orbital contents. Fractures of the ethmoid sinuses, cribriform plate, and planum sphenoidale

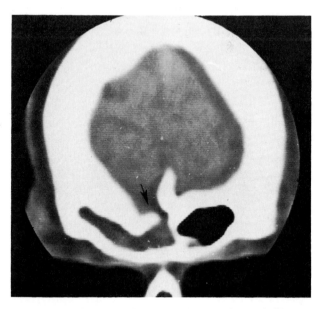

Figure 11-4 Fracture of the frontal sinus. Coronal CT scan through the anterior cranial fossa in 32-year-old man with intermittent CSF rhinorrhea following head injury 6 months earlier shows a depressed fracture (arrow) through the right anterior cranial fossa extending into the frontal sinus. Right frontal sinus is opacified with CSF.

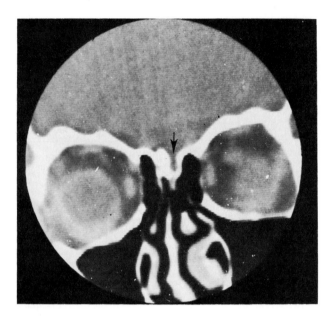

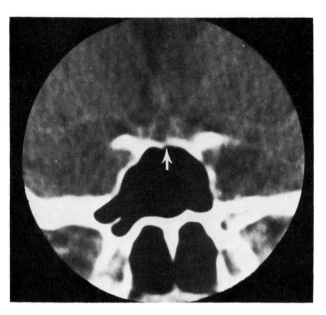

Figure 11-5   Fracture of the cribriform plate. Coronal CT scan through the anterior cranial fossa of 20-year-old woman with previous head injury and intermittent CSF rhinorrhea shows diastatic fracture of the left cribriform plate (arrow).

Figure 11-6   Fracture of the planum sphenoidale. Coronal CT scan at the level of the chiasmatic floor shows fracture of the planum sphenoidale (arrow) with slight depression. This fracture was not seen in plain skull radiography.

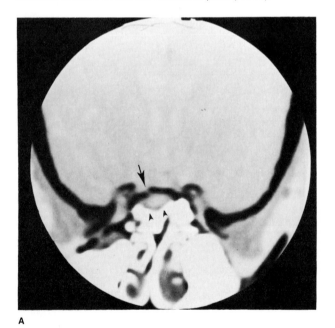

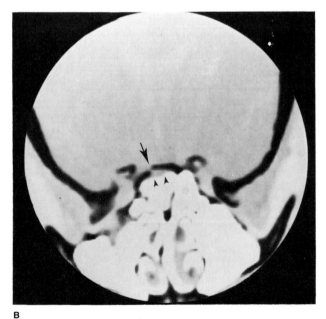

A

B

Figure 11-7   Fracture of the planum sphenoidale with herniation of subarachnoid space.   **A.** Coronal CT scan through the planum sphenoidale shows a slightly depressed fracture (arrow) on the right side of the planum sphenoidale, with herniation of subarachnoid space into the sphenoid sinus (arrowheads).   **B.** Repeat coronal CT scan after 2 months shows marked decrease in subarachnoid space herniation (arrowheads).

are often associated with recurrent cerebrospinal fluid (CSF) rhinorrhea. Ascending infection from paranasal sinuses may cause meningitis, cerebritis, and abscess formation (Zatzkin 1965; Taveras 1976; Bergeron 1971; Fischgold 1973; Ratzen 1973). If untreated, the fracture may widen, causing herniation of the subarachnoid space and brain (Figs. 11-7, 11-18, 11-20). A fracture of the cribriform plate may cause injury to the olfactory nerves, with transient or permanent loss of the sense of smell.

Middle Cranial Fossa

Fractures involving the planum sphenoidale and the floor of the sella turcica are not uncommon (Figs. 11-6, 11-7). A cribriform plate fracture may extend posteriorly to the planum sphenoidale and floor of the sella turcica (Fig. 11-18). Injury to the optic chiasma may cause visual defects (Fig. 11-6). Injury to the pituitary gland may cause panhypopituitarism or diabetes insipidus (Dublin 1976; Young 1980). Visualization of injury to the pituitary gland on CT has now been reported (Tsai 1980). CSF rhinorrhea

and leptomeningeal cyst formation through these structures are common (Figs. 11-18, 11-20). Fracture through the basisphenoid can result in involvement of the cavernous sinus and its contents. When an air-fluid level in the sphenoid sinus is seen in the axial CT or in upright or cross-table lateral skull film, further examination of the area is required with coronal CT. Cavernous sinus thrombosis may result as a delayed complication of trauma in this region. Proptosis and ophthalmoplegia are highly suggestive of carotid cavernous fistula. CT will demonstrate the fractures, prominent cavernous sinus, and ophthalmic vein. Confirmation, however, requires angiographic studies (Rao 1980).

Posterior Fossa

The temporal bone shares the boundaries of both middle and posterior cranial fossa. For convenience of description it is included in this paragraph. The most common type of fracture involving the temporal bone occurs in the petromastoid region. A fracture of the tegmen tympani may involve the

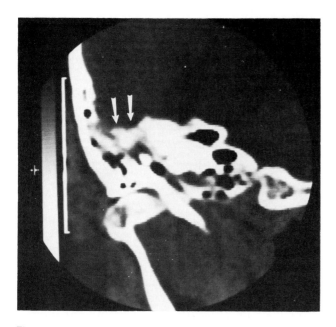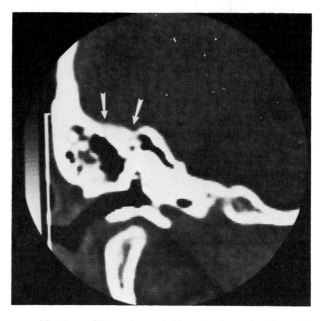

Figure 11-8 Fracture of the temporal bone. Coronal CT shows depressed fracture of the petromastoid region (arrow) with partial opacification of mastoid air cells. At surgery, the facial nerve was seen to be transected.

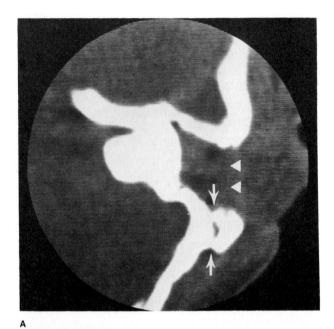

A

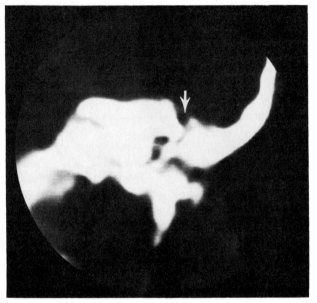

B

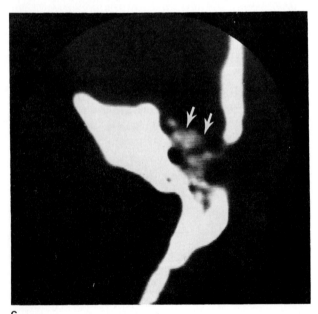

C

Figure 11-9 Fracture of the temporal bone.   **A.** Axial section through external auditory meatus shows opacification of the left external auditory canal (arrowheads), with fracture in the posterior wall (arrow).   **B.** Section through the tegmen shows a depressed fracture (arrow) extending into the middle ear.   **C.** Section through the petromastoid junction shows the depressed fracture extending inferiorly (arrow). *(Courtesy of H. Curtin, M.D., University of Pittsburgh.)*

horizontal portion of the facial canal, causing facial-nerve paralysis (Jongkees 1965). When the fracture involves the middle ear, it may cause hemotympanum and CSF otorrhea via the ruptured tympanic membrane (Figs. 11-8, 11-9). Fracture of the middle ear may result in CSF rhinorrhea via the eustachian tube when the tympanic membrane remains intact. It may cause ossicular disruption and thereby severe impairment of hearing. Pluridirectional tomography has been successfully utilized in the evaluation of such fractures (Jongkees 1965; Davis 1971; Frey 1973). High-resolution CT scan in axial and coronal projection will delineate these structures well. A new high-resolution reconstruction program for the standard CT scan has shown very fine bone resolution for the evaluation of small bony structures and is presently available in new-generation scanners (Shaffer 1980). Opacification of mastoid air cells and soft-tissue injury are well seen by CT (Figs. 11-8, 11-9, 11-10). Fractures of the petrous apex and internal auditory canals are rare, and when they occur, may cause seventh- and eighth-nerve injury. Fractures of the cochlea and vestibule are uncommon. Fractures involving the clivus and the foramen magnum region are rarely seen, probably because they are usually fatal. A fracture of the jugular for-

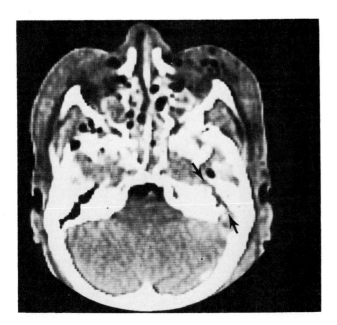

Figure 11-10 Fractures of the temporal bone and paranasal sinus. Axial CT scan through the face and temporal bones shows a fracture through the left petrous bone (arrow). There were also multiple fractures involving paranasal sinuses, with soft-tissue swelling of the face.

amen and hypoglossal canal should be suspected when ninth-, tenth-, eleventh-, or twelfth-cranial-nerve palsy occurs after head injury. Axial and coronal CT sections will delineate these fractures well.

Orbit

A fracture involving the superior rim of the orbit is not common; it normally occurs with a direct blow around the orbit. The most common trauma involving the orbit is a blowout fracture. When a blowout fracture is suspected by clinical examination or plain radiography, the patient should be reexamined by coronal CT of the orbit (Ghoshhajra 1980*b*). The coronal CT is ideal, as sections are taken at right angles to the floor of the orbit. Although the previous method of examination by pluridirectional tomography has been successful in demonstration of blowout fracture (Fuerger 1966; Dodick 1969), it fails to demonstrate entrapment of the orbital muscles and associated injury to the eyeball. Orbital or ocular hemorrhage can be easily diagnosed by CT. The

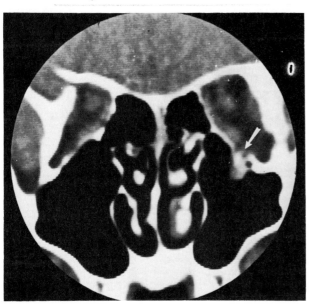

A

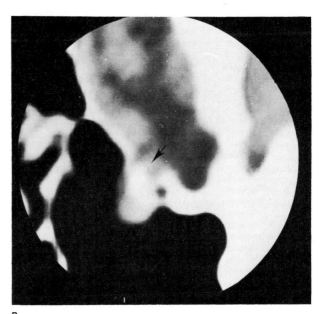

B

Figure 11-11 Blowout fracture of the orbit. **A.** Coronal CT scan of the orbit shows fracture involving the floor of the left orbit, with entrapment of the inferior rectus muscle (arrow). **B.** Magnified view of the left orbit shows a fractured bony fragment with muscle entrapment (arrow).

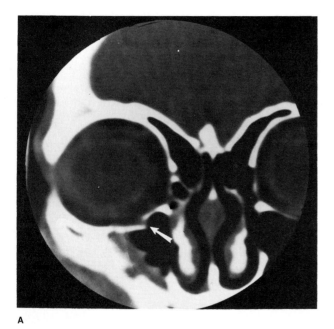

A

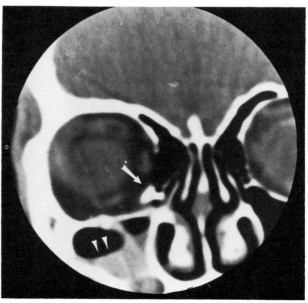

B

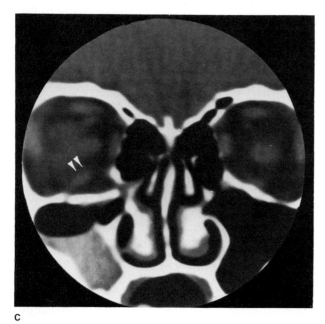

C

Figure 11-12 Blowout fracture of the orbit.   **A,B.** Serial coronal sections through the right orbit show a fracture through the floor of the right orbit extending to the medial wall (arrow). The right maxillary sinus shows an air-fluid level (arrowheads).   **C.** There is, in addition, superolateral displacement of the inferior rectus muscle (arrowheads) by a hematoma.

most common type of blowout injury involves the floor of the orbit, with frequent entrapment of the inferior rectus muscles causing diplopia (Fig. 11-11). Fracture of the medial orbital wall is not uncommon (Davidson 1965; Prasad 1975), occurring separately or as an extension of the inferior-wall fracture (Fig. 11-12). The limitation of movement is due either to entrapment of the orbital muscles or to intraorbital hematoma. A fracture may also involve the supraorbital region (Fig. 11-3). Fracture of the lateral wall is often associated with fracture of the zygoma. Posteriorly, injury to the orbit may fracture the greater or lesser wing of the sphenoid bone (Figs. 11-13, 11-14). These fractures may compromise the optic canal and superior orbital fissure. Injury to the optic nerve will cause loss of vision (Fig. 11-13). Compromise of the superior orbital fissure may cause superior orbital fissure syndrome.

Facial Bones

The most common facial injury involves the nasal bones. Nasal bone fractures are easily diagnosed by plain radiography. Other facial-bone injury commonly involves the orbital rim, floor of the orbit,

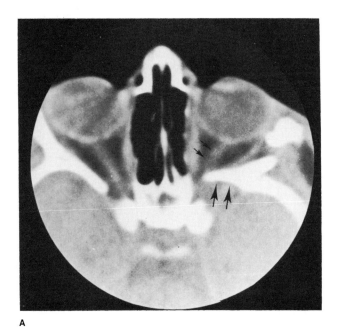

A

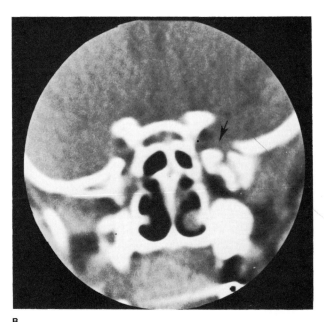

B

Figure 11-13 Fracture of the sphenoid wing with injury to the optic nerve. **A.** Axial CT scan through the orbit shows a fracture involving the lateral orbital wall (arrows), with anterior displacement of the sphenoid wing and impingement on the optic nerve (small arrows). **B.** Coronal section through the orbital cone shows comminuted fragments (arrow) at the optic foramen. *(Courtesy of Z.L. Deeb, M.D., University of Pittsburgh.)*

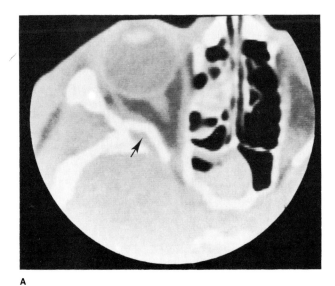

A

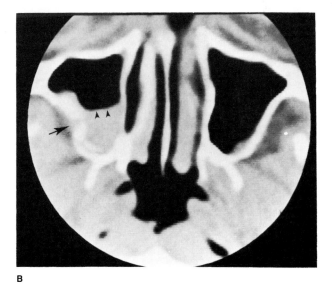

B

Figure 11-14 Fractures of the sphenoid wing and maxilla. **A.** Axial CT scan of the orbit shows a fracture of the greater wing of the sphenoid on the right (arrow). The optic canal is not compromised. There is also opacification of the right ethmoid sinuses. **B.** Section through the maxillary sinus shows depressed fracture (arrow) of the right lateral maxillary wall, with the air-fluid level within the maxillary sinus (arrowheads). *(Courtesy of Z.L. Deeb, M.D., University of Pittsburgh.)*

maxillary sinus, and zygoma. Fractures involving the nasal septum and pterygoid plates, though not uncommon, are often associated with fractures involving other bones. Fractures involving the zygomatic arch and mandible are best evaluated by plain radiography. CT provides a three-dimensional projection of the fracture involving the facial bones and helps in the planning of surgery.

Maxillary and Zygomatic Bones

Maxillary and zygomatic bones can be evaluated with axial and coronal projections (Figs. 11-14, 11-15). Fractures as well as soft-tissue abnormalities, especially the obstruction of nasal passages, are easily delineated by CT. Fractures involving the pterygoid plates and zygoma are best evaluted by coronal views (Fig. 11-15). Because of the anatomic configuration and location, fractures involving nasal bones, mandible, and zygomatic arch are best evaluated by standard plain radiography.

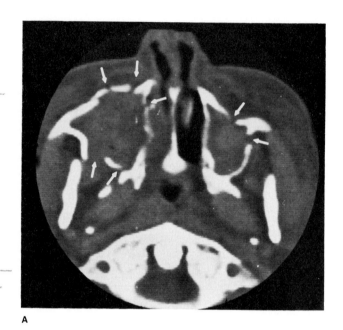

A

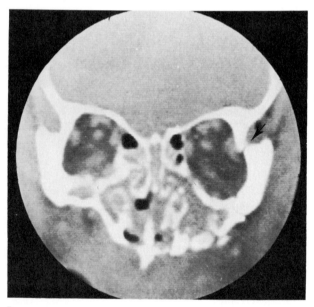

B

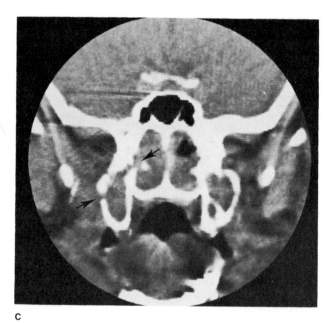

C

Figure 11-15 Fractures of maxilla and zygoma. **A.** Axial CT scan shows multiple fractures (arrows) involving the walls of both maxillary sinuses, with obliteration of the right nasal passage. **B.** Coronal section through the zygoma shows a fracture of the left zygoma (arrow). Again, multiple fractures involving both maxillae, with obliteration of air passage, are well demonstrated. **C.** Coronal section through the pterygoid processes shows extension of the fracture through the pterygoid plates (arrows).

CEREBROSPINAL FLUID FISTULA

When a fracture of the base of the skull accompanies an injury to the meninges, a communication of the intracranial subarachnoid space with the paranasal sinuses or middle ear occurs, resulting in cerebrospinal fluid (CSF) rhinorrhea or otorrhea. The clinical presentations of rhinorrhea or otorrhea are quite variable. There may be leakage of CSF or of blood mixed with CSF through the nose, postnasal space, or middle ear, depending on the location of the fistula. Severe cerebral injury in these patients may often be associated with fractures of the base of the skull. A CSF leakage may stop spontaneously. This is commonly seen when fracture of the petrous bone is involved. Occasionally CSF rhinorrhea, and rarely otorrhea, is precipitated by stress such as coughing or sneezing. Once the communication is established with the paranasal sinuses or middle ear, the incidence of recurrent meningitis or intracranial abscess formation from ascending infection is quite high. The diagnosis and accurate anatomic localization of these fistulas are thus imperative for proper medical and surgical management.

The accurate localization of the site of the fistula has always been a diagnostic challenge. Although isotope cisternography has been the procedure of choice for tracing CSF leakage, it lacks precise anatomic definition (DiChiro 1968). Other procedures, such as positive contrast (Pantopaque) and isotope ventriculography, have been utilized with some success in demonstrating the fistula tract (Allen 1972). Outlining of a CSF fistula with air during pneumoencephalography has also been reported (Marc 1973). Various tomographic changes of fracture sites in patients with CSF rhinorrhea have been described (Hurst 1974; Lantz 1980). The presence of intracranial air bubbles close to the fracture site and air within the fistulous tract during CT examination have been reported (Fox 1979; Levy 1978). Metrizamide CT cisternography has been used for successful localization of the site of CSF leakage (Drayer 1977; Manelfe 1977). Introduction of the new generation of CT scanners has further improved the precise localization of the site of CSF leakage utiliz-

ing metrizamide CT cisternography (Ghoshhajra 1979; Hilal 1980; Ghoshhajra 1980c; Naidich 1980; Manelfe 1982). Intermittent CSF rhinorrhea is a common manifestation of traumatic CSF leakage. Traumatic CSF otorrhea frequently stops spontaneously without intervention (Davis 1971; Frey 1973; Raaf 1967).

When symptoms of rhinorrhea or otorrhea persist, accurate anatomic demonstration of the fistula tract is imperative for surgical treatment. The conventional CT study may demonstrate the presence of intracranial air, and sections through the base of the skull will often demonstrate opacification or air-fluid level either in the paranasal sinuses or in the middle ear. Demonstration of fractures or disruption of the bony wall often requires high-resolution thin CT coronal sections. For precise anatomic demonstration of the fistula tract, further evaluation is necessary. Metrizamide cisternography using a newer-generation CT scanner appears to be the ideal modality at this time.

Technical Aspects

Metrizamide CT cisternography is a relatively simple procedure. Successful demonstration of the fistula tract depends on the presence and severity of the rhinorrhea or otorrhea during the examination. If the rhinorrhea or otorrhea is infrequent, the patient should be placed in a head-down position with frequent coughing, 24 h prior to the examination, so that active leakage can be reproduced at the time of the examination. The patient should be well hydrated prior to the examination by adequate oral fluid. A 10-mg dose of diazepam is given orally for premedication. Intrathecal administration of metrizamide at a dose of 5 to 6 cc in a concentration of 190 to 200 mg of iodine per milliliter is used by a lumbar route or C1-2 cisternal puncture. A slightly higher concentration and larger dose should be used when the leakage of CSF is profuse. The patient is then placed in a 60° Trendelenburg's position for 1 to 2 minutes. If no CSF leakage occurs in this position, the patient is asked to cough for induction of CSF leakage (Ghoshhajra 1980a). Actual leakage of CSF during the examination is a prerequisite for success in localizing a fistula tract. The metrizamide solution is injected under fluoroscopic control on a tilting table to direct the flow of the contrast agent into the head. If the patient has profuse CSF leakage, metrizamide can be introduced on the CT scanner.

Once the patient is taken to the CT room, a systematic approach to the scanning technique should be followed. Study in the axial plane is often complemented by further evaluation in the coronal or lateral decubitus position. The coronal or lateral decubitus views should be perpendicular to the axial plane. Often this may necessitate tilting the gantry or the table top and hyperextension of the patient's neck. Although this can be achieved in most cases, in patients with short necks or other physical problems these maneuvers may not be possible. In these patients, sagittal or coronal reformation, although less desirable, should be attempted. The tracing of a CSF leak is a tedious and time-consuming procedure. Four to six thin axial CT sections through the base of the skull will demonstrate distortions of the interhemispheric fissure or subfrontal sulci, suggesting the possible site of the fracture. The collection of CSF mixed with metrizamide can be seen in the paranasal sinus. Occasionally a Valsalva maneuver or sneezing may open the site of the leak and help demonstrate the fistula tract. If the leakage is profuse and yet metrizamide mixed with CSF is not seen in any of the sinuses during the examination, further evaluation should be done by lateral decubitus coronal sections or supine coronal sections. A high-resolution CT technique should be employed, using a 4- to 5-mm collimation of the x-ray beam with a 1-mm overlapping of the images or contiguous 1.5-mm thin sections.

A $2\times$ to $3\times$ magnification of the reconstructed image will adequately demonstrate the delicate anatomy of the subarachnoid space as well as the site of the fracture. Approximately four to six sections in coronal projection will be necessary, depending on the extent of the fracture and its location. All images are visualized in the standard as well as the reverse mode, if available simultaneously, using dual television monitors. In the standard mode it is sometimes difficult to differentiate an enhanced subarachnoid space from the adjacent bony structures. A reverse mode will differentiate the enhanced subarachnoid space (light-gray density) from the dark bony edges. The images are examined for deformity and distortion of subarachnoid spaces, cerebral herniation, bony defects, and the presence of metrizamide in the paranasal sinuses.

CSF rhinorrhea is most often secondary to fracture of the base of the skull constituting the anterior cranial fossa, although rarely it can be spontaneous or postsurgical. The most common site of leakage is the fractured cribriform plate. Such a fracture may extend anteriorly or posteriorly toward the planum sphenoidale. CSF leakage may also occur through the fractured frontal sinus. The other common site of CSF leakage is a fracture involving the floor of the sella turcica. CSF leak through a fractured posterior fossa is relatively uncommon. When it occurs, it commonly involves the petromastoid junction, causing otorrhea or rhinorrhea depending on the status of the tympanic membrane. When multiple fractures are present, with CSF rhinorrhea especially disrupting the sphenoid and ethmoid sinuses, accurate localization becomes difficult (Fig. 11-19). Opacification of the involved sinuses with metrizamide is seen, which may be due to multiple sites of leakage or to disruption of the wall of the sinuses.

Axial CT sections will often demonstrate distortion of the anterior interhemispheric fissure and subfrontal sulci indicating the possible site of the fracture and leakage (Figs. 11-16, 11-18). Anteroposterior extension of the fracture may often be demonstrated in these views (Fig. 11-18). Once the site of the fracture is identified or suspected on axial sections, further evaluation should be carried out by prone coronal projection (Figs. 11-16, 11-20). When profuse CSF leakage occurs during the examination, instead of prone coronal projection, supine coronal sections and occasionally lateral decubitus coronal sections may be helpful in demonstrating the accumulation of metrizamide mixed with CSF at the site of the fracture (Figs. 11-17, 11-18).

Herniation of the brain or leptomeninges is rarely seen immediately after trauma. Widening of

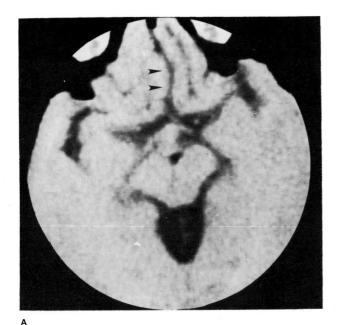
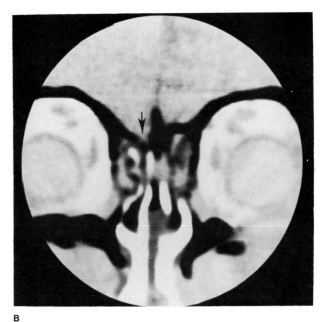

A   B

Figure 11-16 Depressed fracture of cribriform plate with CSF rhinorrhea. **A.** Axial section in metrizamide CT cisternography of a 56-year-old man with injury to the base of the skull and CSF rhinorrhea shows distortion of the anterior interhemispheric fissure (arrowheads). **B.** Coronal section in the prone position shows a fracture through the cribriform plate (arrow) with CSF leakage.

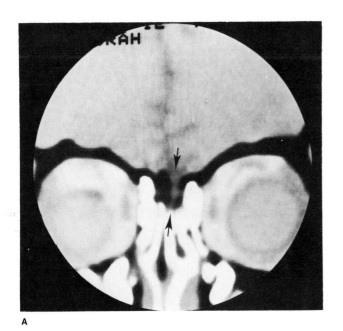
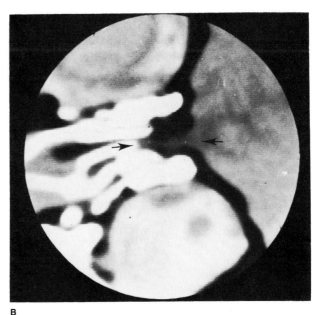

A   B

Figure 11-17 Diastatic fracture of cribriform plate with CSF rhinorrhea. **A.** Metrizamide CT cisternography in a coronal section (patient prone) of a 20-year-old woman with recurrent CSF rhinorrhea shows a diastatic fracture of the left cribriform plate with leakage of metrizamide (arrows). **B.** The metrizamide-mixed CSF leakage is best delineated in the left coronal decubitus view (arrows).

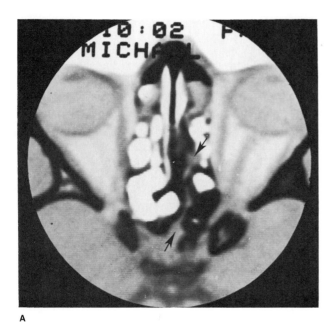

A

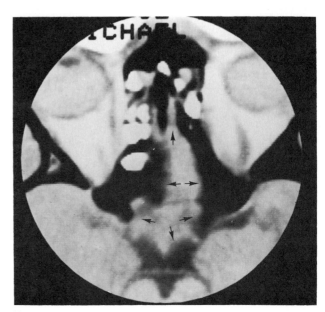

B

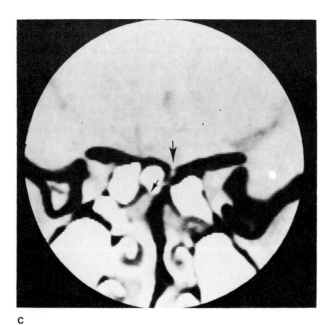

C

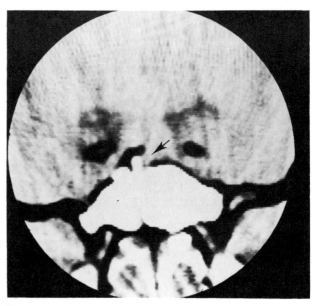

D

Figure 11-18   CSF rhinorrhea and cerebral herniation.   **A.** Axial section of a metrizamide CT cisternogram shows a fracture extending from the planum sphenoidale to the cribriform plate (arrows).   **B.** Axial section just above **A** shows cerebral herniation (arrows).   **C,D.** Prone coronal sections show the fracture of the planum sphenoidale and the floor of the sella turcica (arrow), with leakage of CSF (small arrow).   **E.** Supine coronal section through the anterior cranial fossa gives excellent demonstration of leakage through the fracture site (arrow).

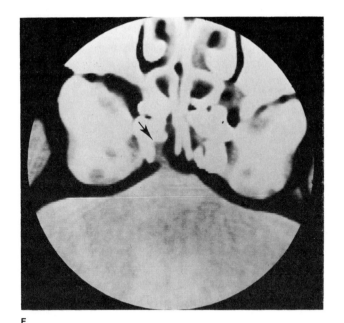

E

the fracture with herniation of leptomeninges may rarely occur as a delayed complication of trauma. Patients may present with intermittent or continuous CSF rhinorrhea. This cannot be differentiated from congenital encephalocele or meningocele purely on the basis of CT findings. The herniation of the brain or leptomeninges with extension of the subarachnoid space can easily be demonstrated in the axial as well as coronal CT (Figs. 11-18, 11-20).

Metrizamide CT cisternography is a relatively simple procedure with minimum morbidity, and it can be repeated when necessary. Incidence of headache, nausea, vomiting, and occasional seizures seen in metrizamide myelography is lower, probably because of the low dose and the faster clearance of the metrizamide from the subarachnoid space due to CSF leakage. High-resolution metrizamide CT cisternography is therefore the best examination for accurate localization of CSF leakage.

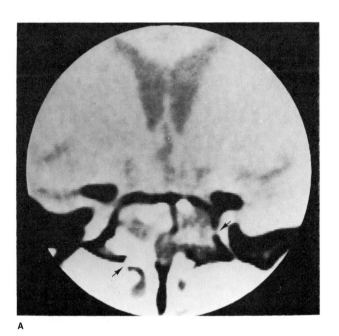

A

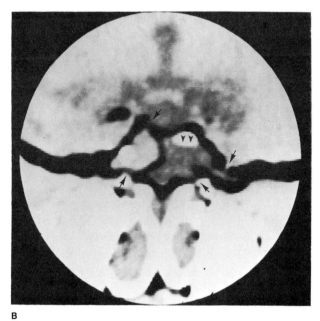

B

Figure 11-19 CSF rhinorrhea through multiple fractures. **A,B.** Metrizamide CT cisternography in coronal projections (patient prone) shows multiple fractures (arrows) involving the roof as well as the floor of the sphenoid sinuses. The concentration of metrizamide is higher in the left sphenoid sinus (arrowheads) than in the right because of profuse leakage through the fractured floor of the right sinus.

(Continued on p. 476.)

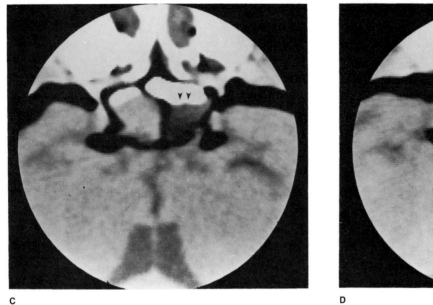

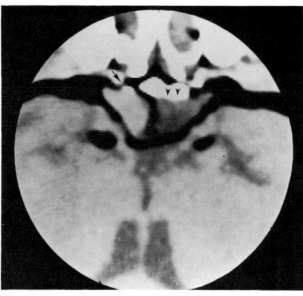

C

D

Figure 11-19 C,D. Supine coronal sections through the sphenoid sinus again demonstrate a higher concentration of metrizamide in the left sphenoid sinus (arrowheads).

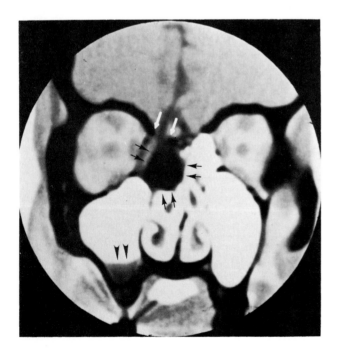

Figure 11-20 Leptomeningeal cyst with CSF rhinorrhea. Coronal section of metrizamide CT cisternography demonstrates a diastatic fracture (white arrows) of the roof of the right ethmoid sinus, with herniation of the subarachnoid space (black arrows) and leakage of metrizamide-mixed CSF into the right maxillary sinus (arrowheads). This patient had sustained a fracture of the base of the skull 12 years earlier. *(Courtesy of R.M. Desai, M.D. and V.S. Rishi, M.D., West Penn Hospital, Pittsburgh.)*

Bibliography

ALLEN BM et al: Fistula detection in cerebrospinal fluid leakage. *J Neurol Neurosurg Psychiatry* **35**:664–668, 1972.

AMBROSE J, GOODING M, UTTLEY D: EMI scan in the management of head injuries. *Lancet* **1**:847–848, 1976.

BECKER H, GRAU H, HACKER H, PLODER KW: The base of the skull: A comparison of computed and conventional tomography. *J Comput Assist Tomogr* **2** (1):113–118, January 1978.

BERGERON RT, RUMBAUGH CL: Skull trauma, in Newton TH, Pott DG (eds): *Radiology of the Skull and Brain*, vol. 1, *The Skull*. St. Louis, Mosby, 1971, pp 763–818.

CLAUSSEN CD, LOHKAMP FW, KRASTEL A: Computed tomography of trauma involving brain and facial skull (craniofacial injuries). *J Comput Assist Tomogr* **1** (4):472–481, October 1977.

DAVIDSON TM, OBSEN RM, NAHUM AM: Medial orbital wall fracture with rectus entrapment. *Arch Otolaryngol* **101**:33–35, January 1965.

DAVIS DO, RAUMBAUGH CL: Temporal bone, in Newton TH, Pott DG (eds): *Radiology of the Skull and Brain*, vol. 1, *The skull*. St. Louis, Mosby, 1971, pp 431–436.

DEVILLASANTE JM, TAVERAS JM: Computed tomography (CT) in acute head trauma. *Am J Roentgenol* **126**:765–778, 1976.

DICHIRO CG, et al: Isotope cisternography in the diagnosis and follow-up of cerebrospinal fluid rhinorrhea. *J Neurosurg* **28**:522–529, 1968.

DODICK JM, GALIN MA, BERRETT A: Radiographic evaluation of orbital blowout fracture. *Can J Opthalmol* **4**:370, 1969.

DRAYER BP, et al: Cerebrospinal fluid rhinorrhea demonstrated by metrizamide CT cisternography. *Am J Roentgenol* **129**:149–151, 1977.

DUBLIN AB: Fracture of the sella turcica, *Am J Roentgenol* **127**:969–972, 1976.

FISCHGOLD H, METZGER J: Tomography of the base of the skull, in Berrett A, Brunner S., Valvassori GE (eds): *Modern Thin Section Tomography*. Springfield, Ill, Charles C Thomas, 1973.

FOX JL, SCHIEBEL FG: Intracranial air bubbles localizing cerebrospinal fluid fistula. *J Comput Assist Tomogr* **3**:832–833, 1979.

FREY KW: Diagnosis of trauma of the temporal bone, in Berrett A, Brunner S, Valvassori GE (eds): *Modern Thin Section Tomography*. Springfield, Ill., Charles C Thomas, 1973, pp 78–79.

FUERGER GE, MILANSKAS AT, BRITTON W: The roentgenologic evaluation of blowout injuries. *Am J Roentgenol* **97**:614, 1966.

GHOSHHAJRA K: High resolution metrizamide CT cisternography for diagnosis and accurate localization of CSF rhinorrhea. Presented at the 65th Scientific Assembly and Annual Meeting of the Radiological Society of North America at Atlanta, Ga. November 1979.

GHOSHHAJRA K: Diagnosis and accurate localization of CSF rhinorrhea by high resolution CT cisternography. Presented at the International Symposium and Course on Computed Tomography, Las Vegas, 1980*a*.

GHOSHHAJRA K: Fracture of the base of the skull and its complications. CT: *J Comput Tomogr* **4** (4):271–276, December 1980*b*.

GHOSHHAJRA K: Metrizamide CT cisternography in CSF rhinorrhea. *J Comput Assist Tomogr* **4** (3):306–310, 1980*c*.

HAMMERSCHLAG SB, WOLPERT SM, CARTER BL: Computed tomography of the skull base. *J Comput Assist Tomogr* **1** (1):75–80, January 1977.

HILAL SK: CSF leaks. Presented at the International Symposium and Course on Computed Tomography, Las Vegas, 1980.

HURST NL: Communication between paranasal sinuses and meninges after trauma. *S Afr Med J* **48**:909, 1974.

JONGKEES LB: Facial paralysis complicating skull trauma, *Arch Otolaryngol* **81**:518–522, 1965.

LANTZ EJ, FORBES GS, BROWN ML, LAWS ER: Radiology of cerebrospinal fluid rhinorrhea. *Am J Neuroradiology* **1**:391–398, 1980.

LEVY JM, CHRISTENSEN FK, NYKAMP PW: Detection of a cerebrospinal fluid fistula by computed tomography. *Am J Roentgenol* **131**:344–345, August, 1978.

LOFSTROM JE: Injuries of the cranial vault and brain. *Radiol Clin North Am* **4**:323–340, 1966.

MANELFE C, GUERAUD B, TREMOULET M: Diagnosis of CSF rhinorrhea by computerized cisternography using metrizamide (letter). *Lancet* **2**:1073, 1977.

MANELFE C et al: Cerebrospinal fluid rhinorrhea *Am J Neuroradiology* **3**:25–30, 1982.

MARC JA, SCHECTER MM: The significance of fluid-gas displacement in the sphenoid sinus in post-traumatic cerebrospinal fluid rhinorrhea. *Radiology* **108**:603–606, September 1973.

MASTERS SG: Evaluation of head trauma: Efficacy of skull films. *Am J Neuroradiology Res* **1**:329–337, July/August 1980.

NAIDICH TP: Trauma, in Korbkin M, Newton TH (eds): *Computed Tomography 1977.* St. Louis, Mosby, 1977.

NAIDICH TP, MORAN CJ: Precise anatomic localization of atraumatic sphenoethmoidal cerebrospinal fluid rhinorrhea by metrizamide CT cisternography. *J Neurosurg* **53**:222–228, 1980.

NEW PFJ, SCOTT WR: *Computed Tomography of the Brain and Orbit (EMI Scanning).* Baltimore, Williams & Wilkins, 1975.

PRASAD SS: Blow-out fracture of the medial wall of the orbit. *Mod Probl Ophthalmol* **14**:493–505, 1975.

RAAF J: Post-traumatic CSF leaks. *Arch, Surg* **95**:648–615, 1967.

RAO KCVG: The role and limitation of CT in craniocerebral trauma. *CT: J Comput Tomogr* **4**:253–260, 1980.

RATZEN E: Paranasal sinuses, in Berrett A, Brunner S, Valvassori GE (eds): *Modern Thin Section Tomography.* Springfield, Ill, Charles C Thomas, 1973, pp 214–218.

SHAFFER KA et al: Manipulation of CT data for temporal bone imaging. *Radiology* **137**:825–829, 1980.

TAVERAS JM, WOOD EH: *Head Injuries and Their Complications,* vol 2, *Diagnostic Neuroradiology.* Baltimore, Williams & Wilkins, 1976, pp 1047–1090.

TSAI FY et al: Pituitary gland injury. Presented at the American Society of Neuroradiology, 18th Annual Meeting at Los Angeles, Calif., March 1980.

YOUNG HA, OLIN MS, SCHIDEK H: Fracture of the sella turcica. *Neurosurg* **7** (1):23–29, 1980.

ZATZKIN HR: Injuries to the Head, in *The Roentgen Diagnosis of Trauma.* Chicago, Year Book, 1965, pp 57–94.

ZIMMERMAN RA et al: Cranial computed tomography in diagnosis and management of acute head trauma. *Am J Roentgenol* **131**:27–34, July 1978.

12

CRANIOCEREBRAL TRAUMA

Pulla R. S. Kishore

Maurice H. Lipper

Perhaps the greatest impact of CT in the evaluation of patients with neurological disease has been in the diagnosis and management of head injury. The unique ability of CT to detect subtle differences in tissue density in a noninvasive manner in a short period of time has proved valuable in the detection of various traumatic intracranial lesions, especially hematomas. It has virtually replaced other radiologic investigations in suspected neurologic dysfunction secondary to head injury (Ambrose 1974; French 1977; Koo 1977; Merino-deVillasante 1976; Roberson 1979; Svendsen 1976; Zimmerman 1978a).

TECHNICAL AND CLINICAL FACTORS:

Before attempting to evaluate the role of CT in head trauma, the following factors must be considered.

Partial Volume Effect

A brief discussion of this phenomenon with respect to various traumatic lesions will facilitate understanding of the contents of this chapter (see also Chaps. 1 and 17). Partial volume effect results from scanning a structure or a lesion which occupies only part of the CT slice (Brooks 1976; McCullough 1976). Since the density at any point of the CT image is a result of the average attenuation of the entire slice thickness at that point, it does not contribute its full density to the image. As a result of this effect, an extracerebral subdural hematoma over the convexity measuring half or less of a slice thickness may merge with the bony calvarium and may not be detected on the CT image. This partial volume effect may also be the reason for the nonvisualization of small hematomas reported in some series (Levander 1975; Svendsen 1976). This phenomenon may also explain the experience of encountering a larger hematoma at surgery than expected from the CT image, as reported by French and Dublin (1977). A small intracerebral hematoma may be missed for the same reason.

Another area where partial volume effect may cause confusion is the region of the inferior frontal lobe, where the irregular floor of the anterior fossa projecting into the normal brain may simulate contusions (Fig. 12-1). To counteract this effect, one may scan with thinner overlapping slices or use a different angle.

Motion Artifact

Patient motion can produce artifacts which may obscure significant intracranial lesions (Fig. 12-2). Motion artifacts are accentuated by the presence of metallic fragments associated with missile injuries. Although this may be less of a problem with faster scanners, adequate immobilization is essential. This may be achieved by the use of restraining devices or sedation. The necessity of motion-artifact–free CT in trauma cannot be overemphasized, because a significant hematoma—especially an extracerebral one—can go undetected unless the patient is subjected to time-consuming angiography.

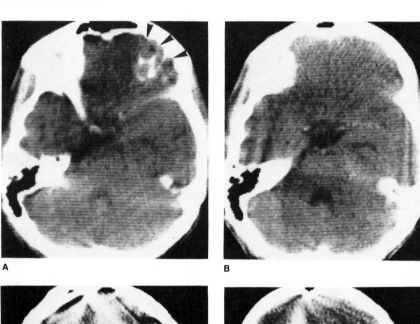

A   **B**

Figure 12-1 Artifact simulating contusion. **A.** A nonhomogeneous high-density zone is present in the frontal region (arrowheads), suggestive of an intracerebral contusion. **B.** An additional overlapping CT slice performed on the same patient reveals no abnormality. The "contusion" was thus an artifact caused by normally occurring bony irregularity on the floor of the anterior cranial fossa.

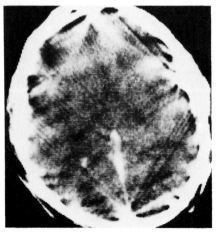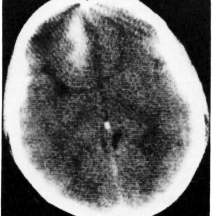

A   **B**

Figure 12-2 Artifact obscuring intracerebral hematoma. **A.** CT showing artifact caused by patient motion with no obvious lesion demonstrated. **B.** The same CT slice performed on the same patient after sedation reveals a frontal high-density zone compatible with an intracerebral hematoma.

Multiple Injuries

Associated multiple injuries, especially those involving the cervical spine, must be considered. Although the incidence of cervical spine injury associated with head injury varies in the literature, as many as 17 percent of fatal head trauma victims were known to have high spinal cord injury (Alcker 1978). Extreme care should be exercised in moving or manipulating the patient during the CT examination. A transtable lateral radiograph of the cervical spine should be obtained prior to CT to determine whether immobilization of the cervical spine is necessary if there is even a remote possibility of cervical spine trauma. In addition, when other severe life-threatening organ injuries are suspected, a limited CT examination may be performed to exclude the presence of a large intracranial lesion before the patient undergoes a major surgical procedure for injury of other organs.

Traumatic lesions demonstrable on CT include the following:

1. Edema: focal and diffuse
2. Contusion, laceration
3. Hematomas
   a. Intracerebral, acute and delayed
   b. Intraventricular
   c. Cortical and subcortical
   d. Extracerebral, subdural and epidural
4. Subarachnoid hemorrhage
5. Subdural hygroma
6. Fractures, displaced bone fragments, soft-tissue contusion, subgaleal hematoma, foreign bodies, and pneumocephalus
7. Posttraumatic
   a. Ischemic infarction
   b. Acute or delayed hydrocephalus
   c. Atrophy
   d. Abscess formation

CT FINDINGS IN HEAD INJURY

The incidence of traumatic cerebral lesions demonstrated on CT varies considerably, depending on patient selection, the severity of trauma, the interval between injury and CT, and the accessibility of a CT scanner. As few as 37 percent of the patients had CT abnormalities in one series (Baker 1974). In another series, 73 percent were reported to be abnormal (Paxton 1974). In one report on a series of 316 patients, 51 percent had an abnormal CT, with 38 percent having more than one detectable lesion (French 1977). Perhaps a more important observation is that only 13 percent of the neurologically intact patients demonstrated CT abnormalities, while 50 percent of the patients with a focal neurological deficit demonstrated lesions. Merino-de Villasante and Taveras in their retrospective study (1976) found that 75 percent of the patients with lateralized findings had discernible CT abnormalities. However, the above-mentioned reports were results of CT conducted at varying time intervals after different degrees of severity of trauma. An accurate assessment and understanding of traumatic CT lesions can be achieved only by studying patients with well-defined neurological deficit immediately following injury and sequentially thereafter, if necessary (Roberson 1979).

The authors' experience with 150 consecutive comatose patients who had suffered severe head trauma, with neurological impairment ranging from inability to follow simple commands to deep coma with posturing, loss of pupillary light reflexes, and loss of oculovestibular responses (Table 12-1), indicates that 40 percent of severe head injury patients can be expected not to have hemorrhagic lesions on CT and may be considered to have only diffuse

Table 12-1 Initial CT Findings in 150 Consecutive Patients with Severe Head Injury

Normal	47
Edema	13
Extracerebral hematoma	30
Intracerebral hematoma contusion	39
Combined intracerebral and extracerebral hematoma	21

brain injury and 60 percent can be expected to have hemorrhagic lesions. Nearly one-third of the patients (31 percent) had normal CT after severe head injury. Another 9 percent demonstrated low-density lesions only (Kishore, 1981). Thirty-nine (26 percent) had intracerebral hematomas and/or contusions, 30 (20 percent) had extraaxial hematomas, and 21 (14 percent) demonstrated combined intra- and extraaxial hematomas. The specific traumatic craniocerebral lesions demonstrable on CT are discussed in greater detail in the following sections.

Edema

The CT appearance of edema is that of low-density zones with attenuation value of 10 to 14 Hounsfield units (HU), less than that of white matter (22-36 HU). This may be focal, multifocal, or diffuse (Fig. 12-3). The last may be difficult to diagnosis because of the lack of normal brain density for comparison. Edema may be associated with mass effect leading to compression, distortion, and displacement of the adjacent ventricles. Generalized edema may manifest only as generalized compression and decrease in size of the ventricles. The compression may be so severe as to cause nonvisualization of the ventricular system and subarachnoid cisterns. (Auh 1980) (Fig. 12-4).

Adding confusion to the diagnosis of posttraumatic edema on CT is the fact that low-density areas may be due to causes other than edema. Low-attenuation substances such as lipids or cavitation and necrosis in subacute traumatic lesions may blend with small adjacent areas of hemorrhage, resulting in low-density zones. Conversely, edema may not be evident as low density if a simultaneous decrease in the lipid content counterbalances any decrease in attenuation caused by increased cerebral water content.

Finally, edema itself may not represent true posttraumatic edema and may be a result of ischemic infarction (Fig. 12-5), which does not have the same connotation as edema in terms of management and outcome (Miller 1980).

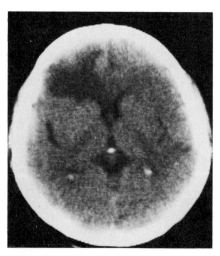 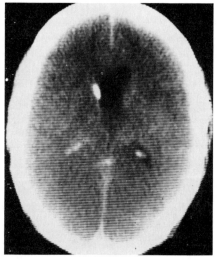 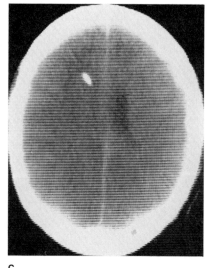

A   B   C

Figure 12-3 Edema.   **A.** CT performed on a 64-year-old male shows a frontal low-density zone with some compression of the frontal horn compatible with focal edema.   **B** and **C.** CT performed on a male aged 55 demonstrates bifrontal and right hemispheric low-density zones with compression of the lateral ventricle in keeping with multifocal edema.

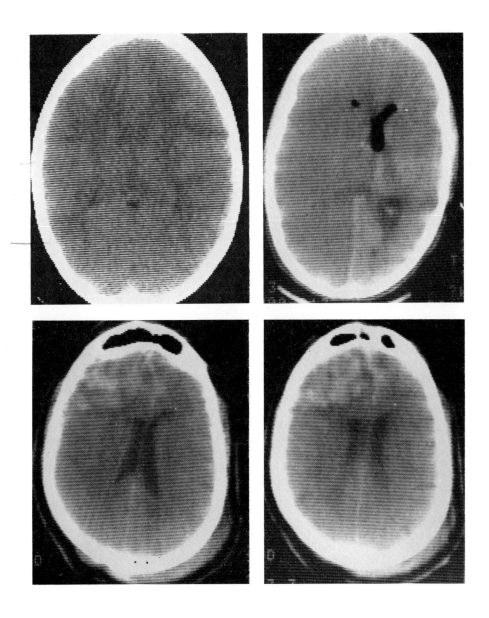

Figure 12-4 Excessively small ventricles. This nine-year-old female patient demonstrates nonvisualization of the ventricular system due to diffuse edema.

Figure 12-5 Hemispheric infarction from traumatic occlusion of internal carotid artery. CT of a female aged 16 reveals severe right hemispheric edema due to ischemic infarction as a result of internal carotid occlusion following trauma, as demonstrated by diffuse unilateral low density with ventricular compression and right-to-left shift. Intraventricular air is due to shunt procedure.

Figure 12-6 Multiple contusions with edema. Multiple bilateral frontal, temporal, and deep nonhomogeneous high-density zones with surrounding low density and ventricular compression. These features represent multiple contusions with surrounding edema.

Contusion

Contusions, which may be single or multiple, occur usually in the anterior frontal and temporal lobes (Fig. 12-6). They appear as areas of nonhomogeneous high-density zones with attenuation values of 50 to 67 HU. This appearance is due to the presence of multiple small areas of hemorrhage within the brain substance interspersed with areas of edema and tissue necrosis. Contusions may have varying proportions of high- and low-density areas, depending on the extent of hemorrhage, degree of edema, and time elapsed since injury. During the first 24 hours, increased density predominates; but with resolution of the hemorrhage, the amount of low density increases progressively until an appearance similar to that of edema is seen. On CT done several hours or days after injury, the contusions may be misinterpreted (Fig. 12-7) (French 1977).

A contusion usually has a poorly defined margin, often surrounded by a low-density zone representing edema. These areas are single or multiple and often demonstrate a mass effect with ventricular compression, distortion, and displacement. The initial high density and size of the contusion generally decreases, and CT resolution of the contusion is usually complete by 6 weeks, leaving no residual

changes or changes similar to porencephaly or focal atrophy, seen as CSF density; but occasionally the contusion may get larger as hemorrhage increases.

It may occasionally be difficult to differentiate between contusion and an extracerebral hematoma with intracerebral extension, especially in frontal and inferior temporal regions (Fig. 12-8). Approximately 15 percent of patients with severe head injury can be expected to have both extra- and intracerebral hemorrhages.

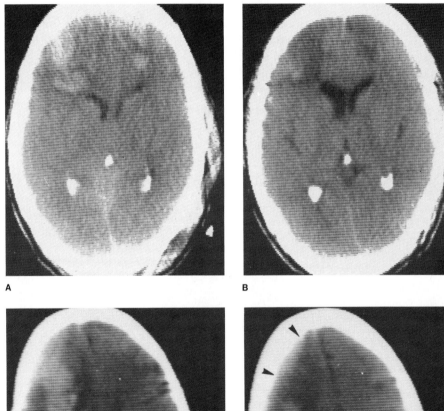

A   B

Figure 12-7 Contusion with resolution. **A.** Bilateral frontal nonhomogeneous high-density zones with surrounding edema and ventricular displacement compatible with contusions. **B.** CT performed 6 days later demonstrating almost complete resolution of the bifrontal contusions, with residual hypodense areas which may simulate edema.

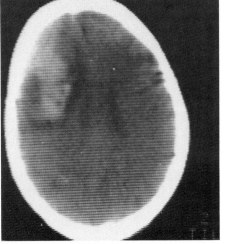
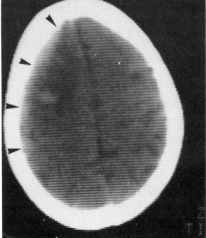

Figure 12-8 Contusion with intracerebral and subdural hematoma. A frontotemporal contusion and hematoma which merges imperceptibly with a thin subdural hematoma (arrowheads). This factor may render the recognition of the latter lesion difficult.

Intracerebral Hematoma

This is seen as a well-circumscribed, homogeneous, high-density zone with an attenuation of 70-90 HU, usually surrounded by areas of low density due to edema (Fig. 12-9). A recent lesion as small as 0.5 cm in diameter may be detected on CT because of the contrast between the high attenuation of the hematoma and the surrounding low-density brain tissue. The high attenuation value of a recent hematoma is attributed to clot retraction and the high absorption coefficient of the globin molecule of hemoglobin. This high density diminishes gradually because of disintegration of the blood components. During this resolution, a certain point in time is reached, usually 2 to 4 weeks after injury, when the attenuation is similar to that of the adjacent brain and the hematoma is termed *isodense,* being undetectable to the naked eye. At this stage the hematoma may be completely missed unless attention is paid to mass effect. It is important to be aware that a hematoma may be present intracerebrally, even in a patient with an apparently normal CT (Fig. 12-10) (Messina 1975). Contrast enhancement may assist in visualizing such isodense lesions (Zimmerman 1977). With further resolution an area of density similar to that of porencephaly may result.

Traumatic intracerebral hematomas may differ from those resulting from hypertension, aneurysms, or arteriovenous malformations in that the traumatic lesions are frequently of irregular contour. They tend to be poorly demarcated, with no uniformity of density. They may often be multiple and are usually located in the frontal or anterior temporal lobes, although they may occur in any intracranial location.

Although the majority of intracerebral hematomas develop immediately after head injury, they may show a delay in appearance (Fig. 12-11). Prior to the advent of CT, the time period for the development of delayed traumatic intracerebral hematomas was believed to be as late as several weeks after trauma (Baratham 1972). With increasing use of CT, however, it appears that most delayed hematomas occur during the first week after injury (Brown 1978; Diaz 1979). The authors, in their experience using serial CT, found that the majority (11 out of 12) developed during the first 48 hours following injury (Gudeman 1979). Delayed hematoma is usually associated with poor outcome (Gudeman 1979), with 50 percent of the patients dying subsequently. Although 50 percent of the delayed hemorrhages develop following decompression surgery, they may develop in patients with normal initial CT. A repeat CT at 48 hours or earlier should be obtained to detect the lesions in patients who undergo decompressive surgery or those who do not show improvement, even if they had a normal CT on admission.

Confusion may arise when an intracerebral he-

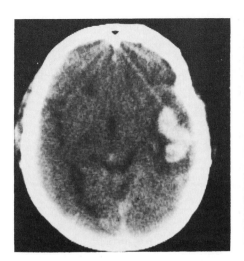 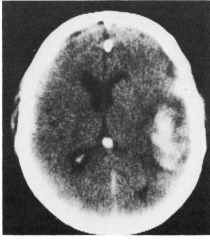

Figure 12-9 Traumatic intracerebral hematoma. A typical intracerebral hematoma in the temporal lobe is shown by a well-defined high-density zone surrounded by the low density of edema. Ventricular compression is present.

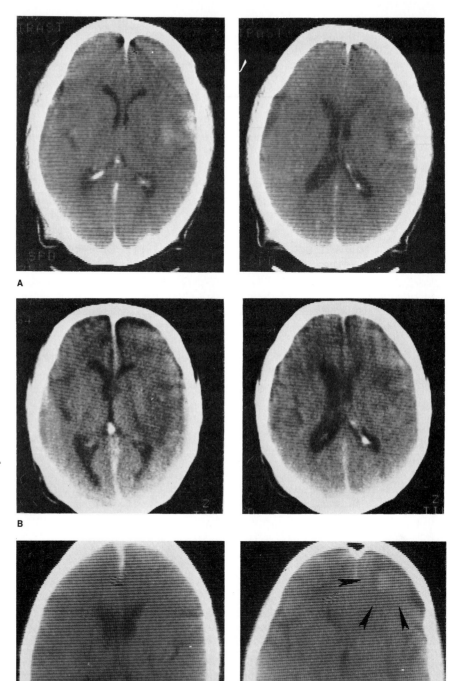

A

B

Figure 12-10 Contusion with resolution. **A.** Left insular/opercular contusion as seen on day 1 CT. **B.** The same lesion seen on day 14 when partial resolution of the contusion has occurred without surgical intervention, resulting in mass effect on the left lateral ventricle, with no definite high-density lesion visualized.

Figure 12-11 Delayed traumatic intracerebral hematoma. **A.** Day 1 CT demonstrating an extraaxial high-density zone in the right occipital region in keeping with an epidural hematoma (arrowheads). **B.** Study performed on day 4 after surgical removal of the epidural hematoma demonstrates a left frontal high-density zone which was not present on the original study, characteristic of a delayed traumatic intracerebral hematoma (arrowheads).

A   B

matoma located near the brain surface mimics an extracerebral hematoma. This may be distinguished by the relationship of the medial margin of the hematoma to the inner table. With an intracerebral hematoma, this margin usually forms an acute angle with the inner table, whereas with an extracerebral hematoma the angle is obtuse (Koo 1977).

Subdural Hematoma

Acute subdural hematomas usually appear as peripheral zones of increased density following the surface of the brain and having a concave inner margin and a convex outer margin adjacent to the inner table of the skull (Fig. 12-12). Although there is an occasional overlap in the appearance of the two types of extracerebral hematoma, the typical subdural lesion tends to be more diffuse than the epidural one. The extension of the latter is limited by the firm attachment of the dura mater to the calvarium. A subdural hematoma with a depth of as little as 5 mm is usually clearly demonstrable on CT. Thinner collections and occasionally even larger hematomas occurring along the high convexity may be missed because of the partial volume effect.

Sometimes the only clue to the presence of a large lesion may be the mass effect. A high convexity lesion may be more easily detected if the scanning is performed with the x-ray beam perpendicular to the affected region; this may be accomplished by tilting the patient's head or placing the patient in a lateral decubitus position (Svendsen 1976).

Although hematomas can sometimes be classified as acute, subacute, or chronic on the basis of the CT attenuation values, absolute reliance on such a classification may lead to an inaccurate diagnosis. Scotti et al. (1977) found a high degree of correlation between the CT density and the age of the hematoma: 100 percent of acute (within 7 days following injury) subdural hematomas showed as areas of increased density, 70 percent of the lesions classified as subacute (7 to 21 days) were isodense, and 76 percent of the chronic subdural hematomas (more than 22 days) were of decreased density. On the basis of this classification, a mistaken diagnosis of subacute or chronic subdural hematoma may be made if recent hemorrhage occurs into a chronic subdural collection, with resultant isodense appearance (Fig. 12-13). Similarly, in patients with a low hematocrit, an acute hematoma may have relatively low attentuation because of the low hemoglobin

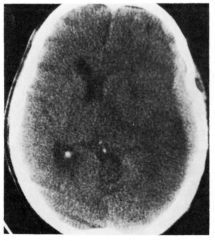 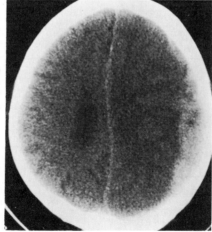 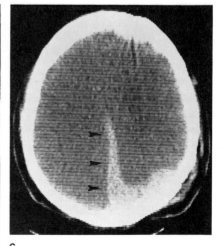

A **B** **C**

Figure 12-12 Acute subdural hematoma. **A** and **B.** Typical acute subdural hematoma as demonstrated by a peripheral zone of increased density following the surface of the brain, having a concave inner margin with ventricular shift to the contralateral side. **C.** Another case of acute interhemispheric subdural hematoma. Acute subdural hematoma in the parietal convexity extends into the posterior interhemispheric fissure (arrowheads).

Figure 12-13 Chronic subdural hematoma with rebleeding. **A.** A chronic subdural hematoma into which fresh bleeding has occurred from a recent head injury. This has resulted in a biconvex hemispheric extraaxial collection (arrowheads) which in part appears dense and in other parts isodense owing to the mixture of old and new clots. The chronicity of the lesion has given rise to the biconvex shape simulating an epidural collection. **B.** A bilateral subdural hematoma with blood-fluid levels (arrowheads) due to recent hemorrhage. A small meningioma in the right side is an incidental finding.

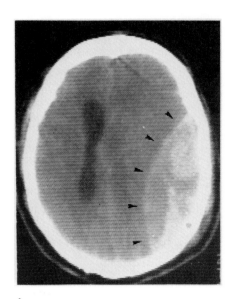

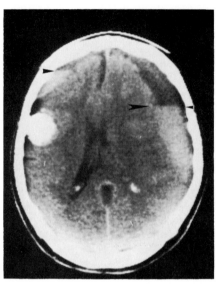

A   B

level and may mimic subacute or chronic lesions (New 1976; Smith 1981).

Because of the foregoing reasons, it is probably best to describe extracerebral lesions as hyper- or hypodense and to specify the size unless one is certain of all clinical factors. It is important to remember that the management of the patient with intracranial hematoma depends on the clinical condition, the size of the lesion, and the resultant brain compression rather than the "acute" or "chronic" nature of the lesion as determined by CT density. For therapeutic purposes, an acute lesion, especially if there is sufficient brain compression, requires decompressive surgery.

A subdural hematoma is usually associated with mass effect, which is seen as compression of the brain with obliteration of gyral markings over the affected hemisphere and midline displacement. If midline displacement away from the side of the lesion is not present or is less than expected, one must suspect lesions on the contralateral side. Approximately 40 percent of extracerebral hematomas are associated with other traumatic lesions such as cerebral contusions or hematomas in patients with severe head injury (Kishore, 1981).

As with intracerebral hematomas, the attenuation value of a subdural lesion decreases gradually over a period of weeks; this is dependent on the initial size and whether or not low-attenuation fluids such as CSF are mixed with the clot. When the hematoma reaches the isodense stage, it may not be visualized on CT unless a significant mass effect is present. Findings such as effacement of the sulci over the affected side and distortion of the ipsilateral ventricle should alert one to the presence of such a lesion (Fig. 12-14). Contrast-enhanced CT (CECT) may be of value in visualizing such lesions by causing enhancement of the membrane around the subdural hematoma or enhancement of the subdural collection itself as a result of seepage of the contrast material into the collection (Messina 1976) (Fig. 12-15). It has also been shown that as many as 40 percent of isodense subdural hematomas may be enhanced after 4 to 6 hours on a delayed CECT (Amendola 1977). The lesion may also be demonstrated by utilizing alteration in window and center settings, digital filtering techniques, and subtraction techniques (Larson 1977). Contrast infusion has been shown to demonstrate the isodense hematoma by visualizing the displacement of cortical veins and/or brain (Hayman 1979; Kim 1978). Also, CECT is extremely helpful in detection of bilateral isodense subdural hematomas. The absence of focal enhancement within the parenchyma on the CECT

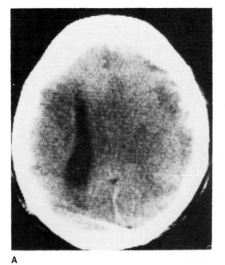

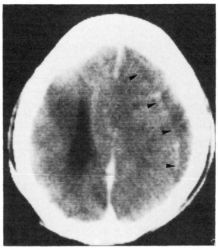

A   B

Figure 12-14 Isodense subdural hematoma. **A.** This illustrates the features of an isodense subdural hematoma with effacement of the sulci over the affected side and distortion of the ipsilateral ventricle. **B.** CECT shows enhancement of a peripheral membrane (arrowheads) at the interface between the brain and the subdural hematoma.

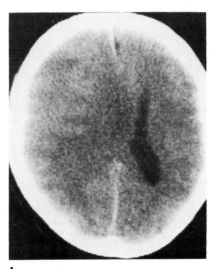

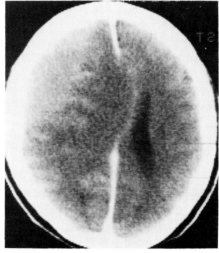

A   B

Figure 12-15 Isodense subdural hematoma. **A.** This demonstrates the presence of an isodense subdural hematoma seen as a mass effect with obliteration of sulci on the affected side, ipsilateral ventricular compression, and marked midline shift. **B.** The subdural hematoma has been made obvious by a delayed CT performed 4 hours after injection of contrast material. The previously isodense hematoma is now seen to enhance as a result of seepage of contrast into the collection.

in a patient with midline shift and a history of recent trauma should suggest the presence of an extracerebral lesion.

Further changes in the appearance of the subdural hematoma are probably due to absorption of fluid across the membrane, with a resultant decrease in attenuation value until it reaches that of CSF. The membrane's rich vascularity leads to its visualization on CECT. A chronic subdural hematoma is usually seen on CT as a biconvex low-density zone. A subdural hygroma developing acutely may also resemble a chronic subdural hematoma in appearance but does not have the biconvex configuration or enhancement of the membrane on CECT.

Occasionally a subdural hematoma may be seen in which sedimentation of corpuscular elements into the dependent portion of the hematoma has occurred, giving rise to the appearance of a low-attenuation zone in the supernatant area with increased density in the dependent portion. A subdural hematoma usually passes from an initial hyperdense value through the isodense stage into the

CSF density stage within a space of 3 to 6 weeks (Bergstrom 1977).

A diagnostic problem may arise in patients with focal atrophy, in which the dilated subarachnoid space may resemble a chronic subdural hematoma. On careful screening, one may see the CSF density extending into the enlarged sulci, thus differentiating it from a compressive lesion (Fig. 12-16). The CT image of a patient with hemiatrophy may be similar to that of an isodense hematoma. A relatively small lateral ventricle and absent or normal sulci over the convexity on the normal hemisphere, with midline shift to the atrophic side harboring a large ventricle in the case of hemiatrophy, can be mistaken for a hematoma on the normal side. However, wide windowing will permit the diagnosis of hemiatrophy by demonstrating a thicker bony calvarium on the side of the atrophy (Zilkha 1980). Additional findings such as enlarged sinuses and petrous bone associated with a small middle cranial fossa may be seen on the affected side.

Delayed Subdural Hematoma

Subdural hematomas, like intracerebral hematomas, may develop in a delayed manner either ipsilaterally or contralaterally following evacuation of a preexisting intracranial lesion (Fig. 12-17) (Lipper 1979). The delayed development of subdural hygromas

occurs in the frontal and temporal area. The hygromas are frequently bilateral. These are found to occur at varying time intervals following injury, usually between 6 and 46 days (French 1977). The authors' own experience with sequential CT of severe head injury patients indicates that 5 percent

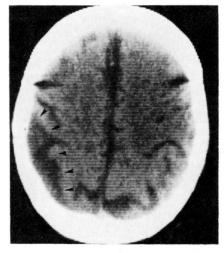

Figure 12-16 Cortical atrophy mimicking subdural hematoma. CT of an 89-year-old patient with cerebral atrophy which may suggest the presence of a posterior parietal chronic subdural collection (arrowheads). However, the extension of the peripheral low density into the sulci should confirm the presence of an enlarged subarachnoid space as seen in atrophy, rather than a collection.

Figure 12-17 Delayed subdural collection. **A.** Initial CT after trauma demonstrating a left temporal contusion and subdural hematoma (arrowheads). **B.** A CT performed 14 days later, after surgical evacuation of the hematoma, demonstrates a right frontoparietal peripheral low-density zone (arrowheads), consistent with a delayed contralateral extracerebral lesion.

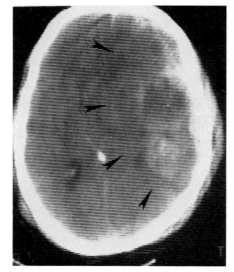

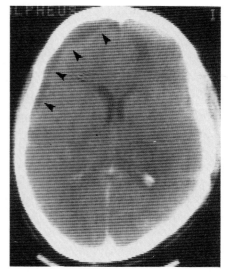

A

B

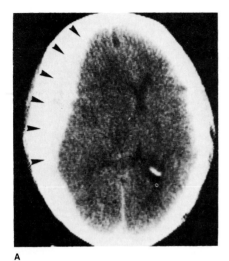 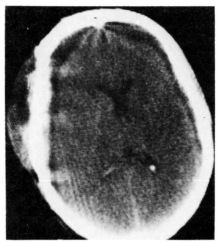

A   **B**

Figure 12-18 Subdural hygromas. **A.** A large right acute subdural hematoma (arrowheads). **B.** CT on day 14 following evacuation of the hematoma shows bifrontal peripheral low-density zones representing bilateral hygromas.

develop frontal hygromas. All the hygromas developed during the first 2 weeks after injury. These collections may disappear spontaneously by 3 months and probably do not require surgical evacuation (Fig. 12-18) (Lipper 1979).

Epidural Hematoma

On CT, an acute epidural hematoma is usually seen as a biconvex peripheral high-density lesion (Fig. 12-19). The biconvex appearance is caused by the firm dural adherence to the inner table. This lesion is usually denser on CT than a subdural hematoma because it is less likely to mix with CSF or brain. Occasionally, when associated with a large subdural hematoma on the contralateral side, a small epidural hematoma may not be seen in the initial scan, and may enlarge rapidly following surgical evacuation of the subdural hematoma (Fig. 12-20) (Nelson in press). This emphasizes the necessity of postoperative CT in these cases. Acute isodense epidural hematomas are rare compared to acute isodense subdural hematomas.

Although epidural and subdural hematomas can be differentiated by CT appearance, as described above, it may not always be possible to localize hematomas exactly to one or the other space. Approximately 20 percent of patients show blood in both spaces at surgery or autopsy (Jamieson 1968).

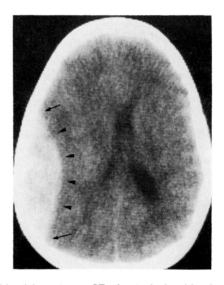

Figure 12-19 Epidural hematoma. CT of a typical epidural hematoma seen as a peripheral high-density zone with a biconvex appearance in the posterior parietal region (arrowheads). Note the obtuse angle at the junction with the inner table of the skull (arrows).

Intraventricular Hemorrhage

Intraventricular hemorrhage appears as high density within the ventricles (Fig. 12-21). The increased density disappears relatively quickly in comparison with intracerebral, subdural, and epidural hemato-

Figure 12-20 Delayed epidural hematoma. **A.** A moderately large left frontal subdural hematoma (arrowheads). **B.** CT performed one day later, after evacuation of the subdural hematoma reveals a biconvex high-density extraaxial collection in the right frontal region (arrowheads). An epidural hematoma was evacuated at surgery.

Figure 12-21 Intracerebral hematoma with intraventricular hematoma. **A.** A large traumatic hematoma in the right basal ganglion region with intraventricular hemorrhage seen as high density within the lateral ventricles on day 1 CT. **B.** NCCT performed after 4 days shows almost complete resolution of the intraventricular hematoma. (The basal ganglion hematoma has been surgically removed and a ventriculostomy tube is present in the lateral ventricle.)

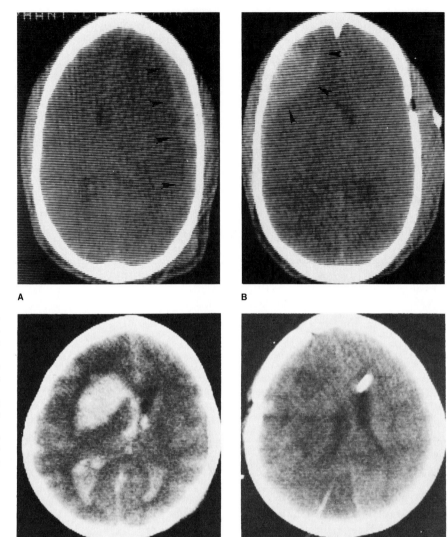

A   B

A   B

mas. The return to CSF density in the ventricles occurs within days, and clot density is rarely present after 1 week (Fig. 12-21). As with intracerebral hemorrhage, nonvisualization of hematoma in the ventricles may not imply total resolution of the clot. Occasionally sedimentation of the corpuscular elements occurs in the dependent portion of the ventricles, giving rise to some increased density in the dependent portion sharply demarcated from a CSF density in the uppermost portion (Fig. 12-22). This is frequently associated with intraparenchymal hemorrhage and appears to be more common than was realized before the advent of CT (French 1977; Roberson 1979; Zimmerman 1978a). Five percent of patients with severe head injury can be expected to have intraventricular hemorrhage (Roberson 1979). These reports indicate that intraventricular hemorrhage does not imply as grave a prognosis as was previously thought. Perhaps early CT recognition of ventricular enlargement, resulting in prompt therapeutic measures such as ventricular drainage, has improved the prognosis.

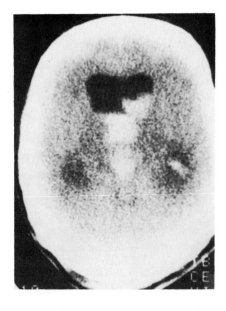
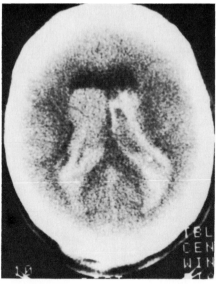

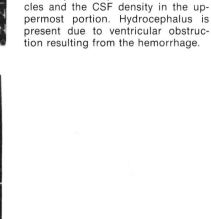

Figure 12-22 Traumatic intraventricular hemorrhage. Sedimentation of the corpuscular elements of the blood has occurred resulting in a sharp demarcation between the blood in the most dependent portion of the ventricles and the CSF density in the uppermost portion. Hydrocephalus is present due to ventricular obstruction resulting from the hemorrhage.

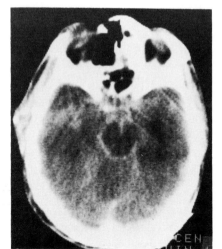
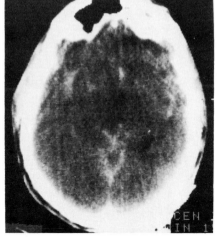

Figure 12-23 Traumatic subarachnoid hemorrhage. Increased density in the basal cisterns, sylvian fissures, interhemispheric fissure, and sulci denotes the presence of blood in these spaces as seen in a traumatic subarachnoid hemorrhage.

Other Acute Traumatic Lesions

Subarachnoid hemorrhage (SAH), frequently found in patients with head injury, is seen as zones of increased density in the basal cisterns, sylvian fissures, interhemispheric fissure, and sulci (Fig. 12-23). As may be expected, SAH is often present with other intracranial hematomas (Dolinskas 1978). The increased density on CT due to SAH rarely lasts more than a few days. The high density of the falx in older patients should not be mistaken for SAH,

and caution should be exercised in making the diagnosis of SAH on CT if there is high density only in the falcial region, not in any other subarachnoid space (Osborn 1980). (See chapter 17.)

Fractures with displaced bone fragments (Fig. 12-25), soft-tissue contusions, foreign bodies, and pneumocephalus are also easily recognizable on CT (Fig. 12-25). CT is also extremely valuable in the demonstration of lesions caused by gunshot wounds. Bone and bullet fragments are well demonstrated, as is the hemorrhagic track of the missile

Figure 12-24 Depressed skull fracture. **A.** A soft-tissue contusion is present in the frontal region. There is irregularity and inward projection of the portion of the inner table of the skull immediately adjacent to this area (arrowheads). **B.** The same CT slice with bone setting clearly demonstrates the frontal depressed skull fracture (arrowheads).

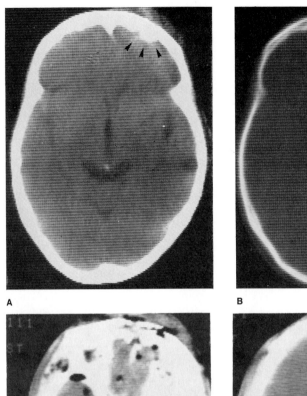

A

B

Figure 12-25 Multiple injury. CT images showing frontal soft tissue disruption, comminuted frontal fractures, multiple intracerebral hematomas and contusions, intraventricular hemorrhage, subarachnoid hemorrhage, and pneumocephalus. The latter is seen as multiple areas of low density equivalent to air density in the subarachnoid spaces and lateral ventricles.

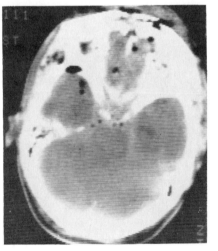

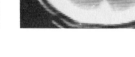

(Fig. 12-26). In patients with shearing injury, CT clearly demonstrates hemorrhage into the deep white matter, especially the corpus callosum (Fig. 12-31). These small hemorrhages are most often seen in the corpus callosum, internal capsule, upper brainstem, and corticomedullary junctures. The gross CT manifestations of shearing injury are often unimpressive and may be misleading relative to the much greater underlying gray and white matter damage (Zimmerman 1978*b*).

DELAYED SEQUELAE

Communicating *hydrocephalus* may develop following trauma as a result of blood in the subarachnoid space causing obstruction to the CSF pathways. Less commonly, non-communicating hydrocephalus may develop acutely secondary to hemorrhage within the ventricular system or around the aqueduct, obstructing the ventricular pathways. The lat-

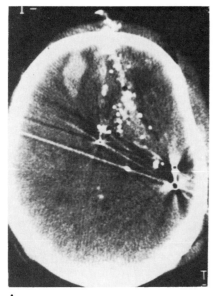

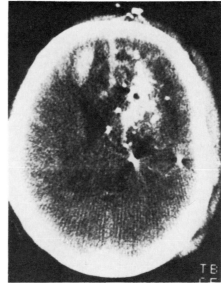

A   B

Figure 12-26 High-velocity missile injury. CT performed on a patient following a gunshot wound to the frontal region. **A.** Metallic fragments are noted extending from the midfrontal region to the left posterior parietal area. Note the streaking artifact caused by the metal. **B.** Hematoma is noted along the bullet path, as well as a right frontal intracerebral hematoma and blood in the anterior interhemispheric fissure.

ter type of hydrocephalus develops more rapidly compared to the one resulting from extraventricular obstruction.

The diagnosis of communicating hydrocephalus can be made on CT if there is a distended appearance of enlarged frontal horns, associated with dilatation of the temporal horns and the third and fourth ventricles. The absence of sulcal enlargement, and periventricular low density if present, are further evidence of hydrocephalus (Fig. 12-27) (Mori 1977). (See chapter 5.)

Serial CT evaluation of 200 consecutive severe head injuries revealed that hydrocephalus, if it is to develop, will do so by the end of the second posttrauma week in a majority (82 percent). Approximately 5.5 percent of all patients, or 8 percent of the survivors at 3 months after severe head injury, will have hydrocephalus (Gudeman, 1981).

Posttraumatic atrophy appears to be a more common cause of ventricular enlargement following severe head injury and can be distinguished from hydrocephalus by associated sulcal enlargement (Fig. 12-28). It may be seen in as many as 30 percent of severe head injury survivors (Gudeman, 1981). It is important not to confuse with ventricular enlargement the return of the ventricles to normal size following compression by brain swelling due to edema or hematomas in the immediate posttraumatic period.

Acute ischemic infarction, appearing as low-density areas, may be detectable within 24 hours of onset and by 7 days in over 60 percent of patients (Norton 1978). Ease of detection depends on the size of the lesion. The diagnostic yield is improved by nearly 15 percent by contrast infusion, with enhancement occurring most frequently between 1 and 4 weeks (Fig. 12-29) (Wing 1976; Yock 1975).

Posttraumatic abscess, occurring as the result of a penetrating injury or fracture or as a complication of surgery, takes the form of a low-density zone surrounded by a ring of enhancement following contrast infusion, usually associated with a large surrounding area of low density due to edema. Ventricular compression and displacement are also usually present. (See chapter 13.)

VALUE OF CT IN HEAD INJURY

Although the prognostic significance of CT in head injury needs further documentation, certain conclusions can be drawn from the various studies that

Figure 12-27 Communicating hydrocephalus. **A** and **B**. Initial CT performed on a 15-year-old male following head trauma reveals left frontal and temporal nonhomogeneous high-density zones (arrowheads) consistent with contusion associated with blood in the subarachnoid spaces. **C** and **D**. Study performed 1 month later reveals the features of communicating hydrocephalus as seen from the dilated ventricles, including enlargement of the frontal and temporal horns and third ventricle with periventricular low density (arrowheads) and the absence of sulcal enlargement.

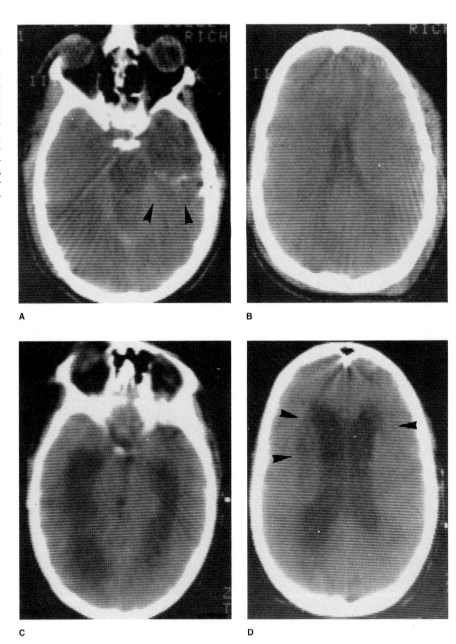

A

B

C

D

have been conducted so far. Needless to say, a patient with normal initial CT following head injury can be expected to have a good outcome unless secondary complications supervene, whether in the brain or other organs, especially pulmonary problems (Domingues de Silva, in press). Secondary complications in the brain, as mentioned earlier,

include the development of delayed extra- and intracerebral hemorrhage, transtentorial herniation, edema, and intracranial hypertension (Clifton 1980; Cooper 1979a; Gudeman 1979; Lipper 1979; Miller 1980; Tsai 1978).

Although attempts to correlate CT findings and intracranial pressure have led to conflicting reports

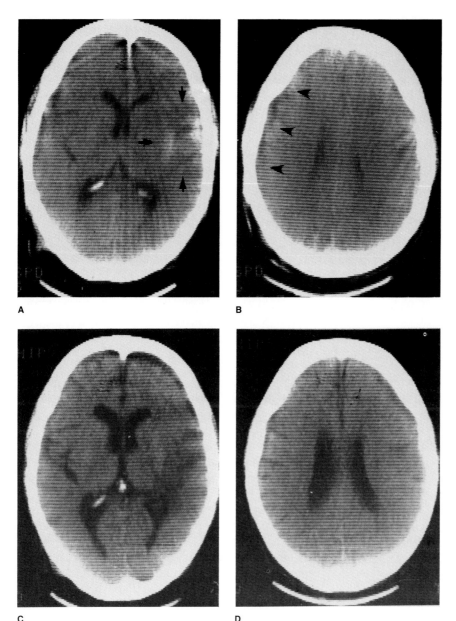

A

B

C

D

Figure 12-28 Posttraumatic atrophy. **A** and **B.** Admission CT on a male aged 55 showing a left temporal contusion (arrows) and low-density right fronto-temporal extraaxial collection (arrowheads). **C** and **D.** Repeat study performed after 3 months shows, in comparison with the above, enlargement of the lateral ventricles and cortical sulci, features consistent with posttraumatic atrophy.

(Auer 1980; Sadhu 1979), patients with normal initial CT can be expected to have normal intracranial pressure in 98 percent of cases during the first 24 hours (Kishore 1981). Furthermore, only 17 percent of patients may develop intracranial hypertension subsequently; and at least 91 percent of patients with normal initial CT have normal pressure during the first 48 hours following injury. On the other hand, 55 to 66 percent of patients with hemorrhagic lesions are likely to have intracranial hypertension. An increased incidence of poor outcome is noted in patients with contusions and increased intracranial pressure (Miller 1979).

Patients who develop delayed lesions on CT are more likely to have a poor outcome whether or not they had a normal initial CT (Cooper 1979a; Gude-

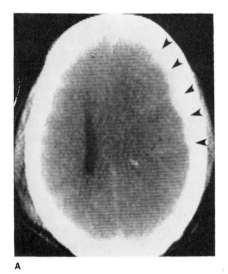
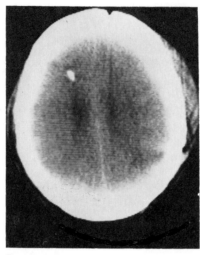
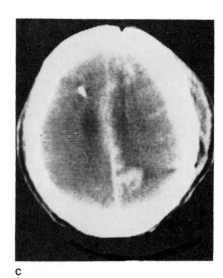

A   B   C

Figure 12-29   Traumatic cortical infarct.   **A.** Initial CT demonstrating a thin acute left subdural hematoma (arrowheads) with hemispheric edema, ventricular compression, and ventricular shift to the contralateral side.   **B.** Study performed 2 weeks later shows a left frontoparietal craniotomy with ill-defined low density over the left parietal region.   **C.** CECT shows extensive high parietal enhancement following the gyral pattern, typical of a parietal infarct.

man 1979; Lipper 1979). It is also well documented that a majority (75 percent) of patients with bilateral hemorrhagic lesions on CT during the first week end up in a persistent vegetative state or die (Sweet 1978); and 67 percent of patients with both intra- and extraaxial hemorrhagic lesions on initial CT can be expected to have a poor outcome, i.e., severe disability or worse (Kishore 1981). A case for repeat CT during the first week, preferably by the third day, is thus made in some reports (Clifton 1980; Cooper 1979a; Gudeman 1979; Kishore 1981). In one series (Clifton 1980), two thirds of patients who deteriorated after the first 48 hours had a new lesion on CT.

The location of the lesion in the brain as seen on CT is also important for prognosis. For example, it is well documented that patients with lesions involving the brainstem (Cooper 1979b, Tsai 1978) have poor outcome. Approximately 25 percent of those with primary brainstem injury survive in a permanent vegetative state (Tsai 1978). Unfortunately, a majority of brainstem lesions are not detectable on conventional CT because of artifacts in this region and because only 20 percent of brainstem

lesions are hemorrhagic, although partial or complete obliteration of the quadrigeminal cistern is frequently observed in patients with brainstem compression (Auh 1980). Cooper et al. (1979b) documented a similar poor outcome with brainstem injuries. Thus, if a brainstem hemorrhage is demonstrated on CT (Fig. 12-30), a poor outcome can be expected.

Shearing injuries involving the corpus callosum, if demonstrated on CT, indicate a poor outcome (Fig. 12-31). Seven of the eight patients with deep white-matter injuries involving the corpus callosum reported by Zimmerman et al. (1978b) ended up in a persistent vegetative state or died; they also noted a mortality rate of 40 percent in patients who had intraventricular in addition to intracerebral hemorrhage, as opposed to a 19 percent mortality for intracerebral hemorrhage alone.

Correlation has also been shown between atrophic changes seen on delayed CT (at the end of 3 months or 1 year) in surviving patients and the outcome (Gudeman 1981; Kishore 1978; Van Dongen 1980; Levin 1981). Although these correlations should be studied over an extended period of time,

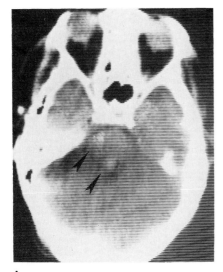

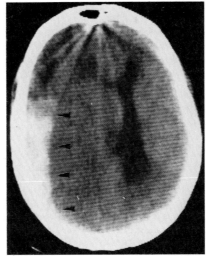

A   B

Figure 12-30 Brainstem hemorrhage. **A.** CT showing high-density zones in the pons and immediately anterior to the fourth ventricle (arrowheads). The presence of a brainstem hemorrhage was confirmed at autopsy. **B.** A large right subdural hematoma is also seen.

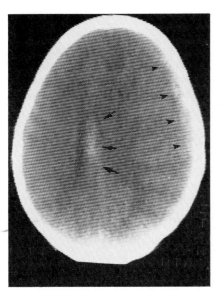

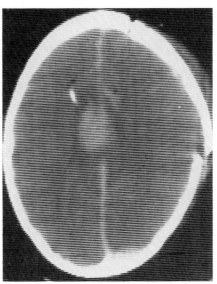

A   B

Figure 12-31 Hemorrhage in the corpus callosum. **A.** CT performed immediately following trauma reveals a high-density zone in the midline in the region of the corpus callosum (arrows). A thin left subdural hematoma (arrowheads) is present. **B.** CT performed 4 days later, following evacuation of the subdural hematoma, demonstrates marked increase in size of the corpus callosum hemorrhage.

it is fair to assume that patients with documented atrophic changes on a 3-month or 1-year CT scan can be expected to demonstrate corresponding neurological deficit.

In summary, (1) patients with normal CT can be expected to have a good outcome unless secondary complications supervene; (2) patients with lesions involving areas such as the brainstem, corpus callosum, and basal ganglia can be expected to have a poor outcome; (3) patients with bilateral hemorrhagic lesions or both intracerebral or intraventricular and extracerebral hemorrhages can be expected to have a worse outcome in a majority of instances; and finally, (4) patients who develop delayed lesions during the first week can be expected to have a poor outcome.

RADIOLOGIC WORKUP OF PATIENTS WITH HEAD INJURY

Contrast-Enhanced CT in Acute Head Injury

Although some authors have recommended the routine use of contrast enhancement in acute head injury (Tsai 1978), this is probably not necessary (French 1977). If NCCT reveals appropriate lesions (extra- or intracerebral hemorrhages) to account for a patient's neurological status, CECT may not provide additional pertinent information. However, if a patient presents with a history of recent trauma and no significant lesion is evident on CT, CECT should be performed if the patient's clinical status permits. Contrast enhancement may help in visualizing isodense lesions (Amendola 1977). CECT is essential if there is a mass effect as evidenced by ventricular compression or midline shift in the absence of mass lesions demonstrable on NCCT. Even if there is no evidence of mass effect on NCCT but the patient has a neurological deficit, CECT should be performed, because an isodense lesion, whether extra- or intracerebral, may be seen on CECT only, and this may obviate further invasive procedures such as angiography.

Not infrequently, a clear history is not available in patients with trauma (Figs. 12-14, 12-15). A patient may be harboring an isodense lesion from an apparently trivial trauma and present to the emergency room with recent injury and neurological deficit. CECT is helpful in bringing out the isodense lesion in such instances. It is important to remember that not all acute traumatic subdural hematomas present as hyperdense lesions on CT. A patient may rebleed into a low-density chronic subdural hematoma, and the admixture of recent clots and chronic low-density collection may appear isodense on CT. If two different densities are seen on CT, as shown in Figure 12-13, there is no need for CECT. However, even when a somewhat dense lesion is evident on CT following recent trauma, CECT is helpful in demonstrating the true nature of a lesion such as meningioma, as demonstrated by French (1978), thus differentiating an apparent hematoma from a tumor by enhancing additional areas beyond the high-density zones seen on NCCT (Fig. 12-32).

Value of Repeat CT During the First Week

As indicated earlier, a repeat CT during the first week, preferably on the third day if not earlier, should be obtained in all patients who do not show improvement in neurological status, whether they had a normal CT or had undergone surgery for an initial hemorrhagic lesion, because of the incidence

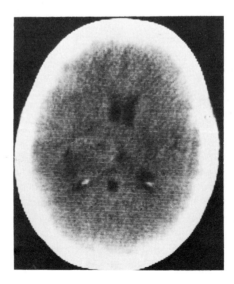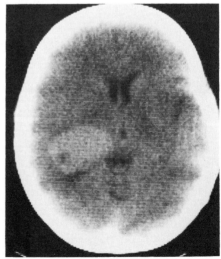

Figure 12-32 Differential diagnosis of resolving hematoma. An ill-defined mixed high- and low-density zone is present in the right posterior temporal region with resultant ventricular compression and displacement. CECT reveals enhancement of this region extending beyond the high-density zone previously noted. On NCCT this could easily be mistaken for a resolving hemorrhage, but CECT establishes the diagnosis of a neoplasm (astrocytoma).

of new lesions detected on CT in patients who show deterioration. Although the outcome for patients developing new lesions is poor, it should be kept in mind that these lesions may develop before detectable neurological deterioration or intracranial hypertension occurs. It has also been documented that decompressive surgery is beneficial in improving the outcome in some of these patients (Brown 1978; Diaz 1979).

Skull Radiography

The role of skull films in the evaluation of brain disorders has been debated since the advent of CT (Cumming 1980; DeSmet 1979; Masters 1980; Weinstein 1977), but we believe they are important in patients with head injury. Although it has been shown that even before the advent of CT, skull series did not affect the management of patients with head injury (Roberts 1972), it is known that 80 percent of fatal head injury patients have skull fracture at autopsy (Adams 1975), thus skull films may provide a clue as to the severity of initial injury. Basal skull fractures, not detectable on CT, may be demonstrated by skull radiography. However, CT provides accurate information regarding the exact location of intracranial fragments of a depressed fracture, in addition to the status of the intracranial contents. Perhaps CT should be the diagnostic examination of choice for initial evaluation of virtually every patient with significant head trauma, with plain skull films obtained after CT if critical to decision making in patient management.

Role of Angiography in Head Injury

As indicated in the beginning of the chapter, CT has virtually replaced angiography as the preferred method of investigation in head injury patients. Nevertheless, in spite of recent advances in CT technology facilitating "dynamic computed tomography," angiography remains the only means to detect vascular lesions resulting from head injury. Traumatic vascular lesions such as intimal tear of the internal carotid artery, occlusion, traumatic aneurysm, and arteriovenous fistula can be accurately evaluated only by angiography. Isodense hematomas that are not visible by other means can be detected only by angiography. Thus, when there is mass effect and an extracerebral hematoma is not detected on CT, angiography may be the only means to demonstrate such a hematoma. Angiography may also be necessary to detect an underlying aneurysm as a cause of intracerebral hematoma rather than trauma, when the clinical picture is confusing as to which event came first. Finally, arterial spasm following trauma can be evaluated only by angiography. Venous thrombosis also can be best evaluated by angiography, although CT signs consisting of increased density on CECT or high density due to thrombosis in the sinus area on NCCT have been reported (Buonanno 1978; Patronas 1981; Wendling 1978). In summary, angiography may be necessary when isodense or vascular lesions are suspected. The vascular lesion, whether it is the cause or the result of trauma, can be evaluated adequately only by angiography.

Bibliography

ADAMS JH: The neuropathology of head injuries, in Vinken PJ, Bruyn GW (eds): *Handbook of Clinical Neurology*, vol. 23, *Injuries of the Brain and Skull*. Amsterdam, Oxford, North-Holland Publishing Company, 1975, pp 35–65.

ALCKER GJ, et al: High cervical spine and craniocervical junction injuries in fatal traffic accidents. *Orthop Clin North Am* **9**:1103–1110, 1978.

AMBROSE J: Computerized x-ray scanning of the brain. *J Neurosurg* **40:**679–695, 1974.

AMENDOLA MA, OSTRUM BJ: Diagnosis of isodense subdural hematomas by computed tomography. *Am J Roentgenol* **129:**693–697, 1977.

AUER L, et al: Relevance of CAT-scan for the level of ICP in patients with severe head injury, in Shulman K et al (eds): *Intracranial Pressure IV.* Berlin, Springer-Verlag, 1980, pp 45–47.

AUH YH, LEE, SH, TOGLIA JU: The excessively small ventricle on cranial computed tomography: Clinical correlation in 75 patients. *J Comput Assist Tomogr* **4:**325–329, 1980.

BAKER HL, et al: Computer assisted tomography of the head: An early evaluation. *Mayo Clin Proc* **49:**17–27, 1974.

BARATHAM G, DENNYSON WG: Delayed traumatic intracerebral hemorrhage. *J Neurol Neurosurg Psychiatry* **35:**698–706, 1972.

BERGSTROM M, et al: Computed tomography of cranial subdural and epidural hematomas: Variation of attenuation related to time and clinical events such as rebleeding. *J Comput Assist Tomogr* **1:**449–455, 1977.

BROOKS RA, DICHIRO G: Principles of computer assisted tomography (CAT) in radiographic radioisotope imaging. *Phys Med Biol* **21:**689–732, 1976.

BROWN FD, MULLAN S, DUDA EE: Delayed traumatic intracerebral hematomas: Report of 3 cases. *J Neurosurg* **48:**1019–1022, 1978.

BUONANNO FS, MOODY DM, BALL MR, LASTER DW: Computed cranial tomographic findings in cerebral sinovenous occlusion. *J Comput Assist Tomogr* **2**(3):281–290, 1978.

CLIFTON GL, GROSSMAN RG, MAKELA ME, MINER ME, HANDEL S, SADHU V: Neurological course and correlated computerized tomography findings after severe closed head injury. *J Neurosurg* **52:**611–624, 1980.

COOPER PR, MARVILLA K, MOODY S, CLARK WK: Serial computerized tomographic scanning and the prognosis of severe head injury. *Neurosurgery* **5**(5):566–569, 1979a.

COOPER PR, MARAVILLA K, KIRKPATRICK J, MOODY SF, SKLAR FH, DIEHL J, CLARK WK: Traumatically induced brainstem hemorrhage and the computerized tomographic scan: Clinical pathological and experimental observations. *Neurosurgery* **4**(2):115–124, 1979b.

CUMMINS RO: Clinicians' reasons for overuse of skull radiographs. *Am J Neuroradiology* **1**(4):339–342, 1980.

DESMET AA, FRYBACK DG, THORNBURY JR: A second look at the utility of radiographic skull examination for trauma. *Am J Roentgenol* **132:**95–99, 1979.

DIAZ FG, YOCK DH JR, LARSON D, ROSKWOLD GL: Early diagnosis of delayed posttraumatic intracerebral hematomas. *J Neurosurg* **50:**217–223, 1979.

DOLINSKAS CA, ZIMMERMAN RA, BILANIUK LT: A sign of subarachnoid bleeding on cranial computed tomograms of pediatric head trauma patients. *Radiology* **126:**409–411, 1978.

DOMINGUES DA SILVA AA, KISHORE PRS, BECKER DP: Delayed CT changes and correlation with outcome in patients with normal initial CT (in press).

FORBES GS, et al: Computed tomography in the evaluation of subdural hematomas. *Radiology* **126:**143–148, 1978.

FRENCH BN, DUBLIN AB: The value of computerized tomography in the management of 1000 consecutive head injuries. *Surg Neurol* **7:**171–183, 1977.

FRENCH BN: Limitations and pitfalls of computed tomography in the evaluation of craniocerebral injury. *Surg Neurol* **10**(6):395–401, 1978.

GUDEMAN SK, KISHORE PRS, BECKER DP, LIPPER MH, GIREVENDULIS AK, JEFFRIES BF, BUTTERWORTH J: Computerized tomography in the evaluation of incidence and significance of post-traumatic hydrocephalus. *Radiology* **141:**597–402, 1981.

GUDEMAN SK, KISHORE PRS, MILLER JD, GIREVENDULIS AK, LIPPER MH, BECKER DP: The genesis and significance of delayed traumatic intracerebral hematoma. *Neurosurgery* **5:**309–313, 1979.

HAYMAN LA, EVANS RA, HINCK VC: Rapid-high-dose contrast computed tomography of isodense subdural hematoma and cerebral swelling. *Radiology* **131:**381–383, 1979.

HEINZ RE, WARD A, DRAYER BP, DUBOIS PJ: Distinction between obstructive and atrophic dilatation of ventricles in children. *J Comput Assist Tomogr* **4**(3):320–325, 1980.

JAMIESON KG, YELLAND JDN: Extradural hematoma: Report of 167 cases. *J Neurosurg* **29:**13–23, 1968.

KIM KS, HEMMATI M, WEINBERG PE: Computed tomography in isodense subdural hematoma. *Radiology* **128:**71–74, 1978.

KISHORE PRS, LIPPER MH, BECKER DP, DOMINGUES DE SILVA AA, NARAYAN RK: The significance of CT in the management of patients with severe head injury: Correlation with ICP. *Am J Neuroradiology* **2:**307–311, 1981.

KISHORE PRS, LIPPER MH, MILLER JD, GIREVENDULIS AK, BECKER DP, VINES FS: Post-traumatic hydrocephalus in patients with severe head injury. *Neuroradiology* **16:**261–265, 1978.

KOO AH, LAROQUE RL: Evaluation of head trauma by computed tomography. *Radiology* **123:**345–350, 1977.

LARSON GN, et al: Computer processing of CT images: Advances and prospects. *Neurosurgery* **1:**78–79, 1977.

LEVANDER B, STATTIN S, SVENDSEN P: Computer tomography of traumatic intra and extracerebral lesions. *Acta Radiol.* [Suppl. 346] *(Stockh)* pp 107–118, 1975.

LEVIN HS, MEYERS CA, GROSSMAN RG, SARWAR M: Ventricular enlargement after closed head injury. *Arch Neurol* **38:**623–629, 1981.

LIPPER MH, KISHORE PRS, GIREVENDULIS AK, MILLER JD, BECKER DP: Delayed intracranial hematoma in patients with severe head injury. *Radiology* **133:**645–649, 1979.

MASTERS SJ: Evaluation of head trauma: Efficacy of skull films. *Am J Neuroradiology* **1**(4):329–338, 1980.

MCCULLOUGH EC et al: Performance evaluation and quality assurance of computed tomography scanners, with illustrations from the EMI, ACTA, and Delta scanners. *Radiology* **120:**173, 1976.

MERINO-DE VILLASANTE J, TAVERAS JM: Computerized tomography (CT) in acute head trauma. *Am J Roentgenol* **126:**765–778, 1976.

MESSINA AV, CHERNICK NL: Computed tomography: The "resolving" intracerebral hemorrhage. *Radiology* **118:**609–613, 1975.

MESSINA A.V.: Computed tomography: Contrast media within subdural hematomas. *Radiology* **119:**725–726, 1976.

MILLER JD, GUDEMAN SK, KISHORE PRS, BECKER DP: CT, ICP and early neurological evaluation in the prognosis of severe head injury. *Acta Neurochir* [Suppl] *(Wien)* **28:**86–88, 1979.

MILLER JD, GUDEMAN SK, KISHORE PRS, BECKER DP: Post-traumatic brain edema on CT. *Adv Neurol* **28:**413–422, 1980.

MORI D, MARATA T, NAKANO Y, HANDA H: Periventricular lucency in hydrocephalus on computerized tomography. *Surg Neurol.* **8:**337–340, 1977.

NELSON AT, KISHORE PRS, LEE SH: Development of delayed epidural hematoma *Am J Neuroradiology* (in press).

NEW PF, ARONOW S: Attenuation measurements of whole blood and blood fractions in computed tomography. *Radiology* **121:**635–640, 1976.

NORTON GA, KISHORE PRS, LIN J: Contrast enhancement in cerebral infarctions on CT. *Am J Roentgenol* **131:**881–885, 1978.

OSBORN AG, ANDERSON RE, WING SD: The false falx sign. *Radiology* **134:**421–425, 1980.

PATRONAS NJ, DUDA EE, MIRFAKHRAEE M, WOLLMAN RL: Superior sagittal sinus thrombosis diagnosed by computed tomography. *Surg Neurol* **15**(1):11–14, 1981.

PAXTON R, AMBROSE J: The EMI scanner: A brief review of the first 650 patients. *Br J Radiol* **47**:530–565, 1974.

ROBERSON FC, KISHORE PRS, MILLER JD, LIPPER MH, BECKER DP: The value of serial computerized tomography in the management of severe head injury. *Surg Neurol* **12**:161–167, 1979.

ROBERTS F, SHOPFNER CE: Plain skull roentgenograms in children with head trauma. *Am J Roentgenol* **114**:230–240, 1972.

SADHU VK, SAMPSON J, HAAR FL, PINTO RS, HANDEL SF: Correlation between computed tomography and intracranial pressure monitoring in acute head trauma patients. *Radiology* **133**:507–509, 1979.

SCOTTI G et al: Evaluation of the age of subdural hematomas by computerized tomography. *J Neurosurg* **47**:311–315, 1977.

SMITH WP JR, BATNITZKY S, RENGACHARY SS: Acute isodense subdural hematomas: A problem in anemic patients. *Am J Neuroradiol* **2**(1):37–40, 1981.

SVENDSEN P: Computed tomography of traumatic extracerebral lesions. *Br J Radiol* **49**:1004–1012, 1976.

SWEET RC et al: Significance of bilateral abnormalities on the CT scan in patients with severe head injury. *Neurosurgery* **3**:16–21, 1978.

TSAI FY, HUPRICH JE, GRADNER FC, SEGALL HD, TEAL JS: Diagnostic and prognostic implications of computed tomography of head trauma. *J Comput Assist Tomogr* **2**:323–331, 1978.

VAN DONGEN KJ, BRAAKMAN R: Later computed tomography in survivors of severe head injury. *Neurosurgery* **7**:14–22, 1980.

WEINSTEIN MA, ALFIDI RJ, DUCHESNEAU PM: Computed tomography versus skull radiography. *Am J Roentgenol* **128**:873, 1977.

WENDLING LR: Intracranial venous sinus thrombosis: Diagnosis suggested by computed tomography. *Am J Roentgenol* **130**:978–980, 1978.

WING SD et al: Contrast enhancement of cerebral infarcts in computed tomography. *Radiology* **121**:89–92, 1976.

YOCK DH, MARSHALL WH: Recent ischemic brain infarcts at computed tomography: Appearances pre- and post-contrast infusion. *Radiology* **117**:599–608, 1975.

ZILKHA A: CT of cerebral hemiatrophy. *Am J Neuroradiology* **1**:255–258, 1980.

ZIMMERMAN RA, BILANIUK LT, GENNARELLI T, BRUCE D, DOLINSKAS C, UZZELL B: Cranial computed tomography in diagnosis and management of acute head trauma. *Am J Roentgenol* **131**:27–34, 1978a.

ZIMMERMAN RA, BILANIUK LT, GENNERALLI T: Computed tomography of shearing injuries of the cerebral white matter. *Radiology* **127**:393–396, 1978b.

ZIMMERMAN RD, LEEDS NE, NAIDICH TP: Ring blush associated with intracerebral hematoma. *Radiology* **122**:707–711, 1977.

13

INFECTIOUS DISEASES

Seungho Howard Lee

GENERAL CONSIDERATIONS

Central nervous system infections represent a group of life-threatening diseases that present a formidable challenge to physicians. Despite the development of effective antimicrobial agents and modern surgical techniques, significant mortality and morbidity with CNS infections persist. Since the introduction of computed tomography, there is evidence of a marked decrease in mortality among patients with brain abscesses, although the morbidity has not changed significantly (Rosenbaum 1978). CT correlation with pathology of the various CNS infections may aid in earlier diagnosis and bring about further decrease in morbidity and mortality.

The brain and spinal cord are well protected from direct spread of infectious disease processes by osseous and membranous coverings. However, once infection has involved the central nervous system, the brain is more sensitive to infection than other tissues. Microorganisms with weak pathogenic properties are capable of producing a fatal outcome when the central nervous system is involved. CNS infection may be a manifestation of a systemic disease (tuberculosis), or may be an independent process (meningococcal meningitis, encephalitis), or may be localized to a focal area (brain abscess). Possible reasons for the peculiar CNS response to microorganisms include certain structural peculiarities of the brain and its coverings, such as the absence of true lymphatics; differences in vascular supply in gray and white matter; the absence of capillaries in the subarachnoid space; intercommunication between intra- and extracranial venous systems via facial and emissary veins; and the presence of perivascular arachnoid space around the veins as well as around the large vessels (Virchow-Robin spaces) and the perivascular glial membrane. Cerebrospinal fluid also is an excellent culture medium for bacterial growth (Harriman 1976).

Infections reach the brain or meninges mainly by two routes: (1) hematogenous dissemination from a distant infective focus to the meninges, corticomedulllary junction, and choroid plexus; (2) direct extension by bony erosion from an adjacent focus of suppuration (otitis, mastoiditis, sinusitis), by transmission along anastomotic veins from the face, scalp, and orbits, and by transmission along cranial nerves following neurosurgery or traumatic craniocerebral wounds. Certain external factors serve to enhance the risk of intracranial infections, such as radiation; immunosuppressive or steroid therapy; cyanotic congenital heart disease; systemic illness such as diabetes mellitus, alcoholism, or cirrhosis; leukemia, lymphoma, or agammaglobulinemia; severe body stress; midline bony fusion defects; surgical or traumatic craniocerebral injury; and pulmonary or other systemic infections (Moore 1974).

BACTERIAL INFECTION

Epidural Empyema

Extension of infection from the paranasal sinuses or mastoid is the most frequent route of infection of the skull and epidural space. The infectious process is localized outside the dural membrane and beneath the inner table of the skull. The frontal region is most frequently affected, probably because of its close relationship to the frontal sinuses as well as the ease with which the dura can be stripped from the bone. Infection of the diploe (osteomyelitis) may spread through the inner table of the skull to produce an epidural abscess or may break through the

outer table to produce a subgaleal or subperiosteal abscess.

On NCCT, epidural infection appears as a poorly defined area of low density adjacent to the inner table of the skull. On CECT the low-density lentiform collection displaces the dura inward; if the collection lies in the midline, the attachment of the falx is displaced inward and separated from the adjacent skull, thus identifying its extradural location (Lott 1977; Kaufmann 1977). Thick, smooth-walled enhancement on the convex inner side represents inflamed dural membrane. The membrane enhancement is usually thicker in epidural than in subdural abscesses (Fig. 13-1). The underlying brain tissue appears normal (unless concomitant cerebritis is present), but there may be significant displacement of brain parenchyma if the epidural abscess is large. When the epidural abscess is situated on the convexity of one hemisphere, differentiation from a subdural empyema may be difficult on the basis of CT appearance alone; an associated and immediately adjacent area of bone destruction and subgaleal soft-tissue mass may provide a clue (Fig. 13-2). In addition, CT may demonstrate evidence of paranasal sinus or mastoid infection (fluid, soft-tissue thickening) and may complement skull radiography in demonstration of associated osteomyelitis. Occasionally angiography may be necessary to differentiate between epidural and subdural empyema (Handel 1974) (Fig. 13-1), and sometimes CECT in the coronal plane provides additional information by demonstrating inward displacement and/or thrombosis of the adjacent venous sinuses. Often epidural abscess is silent clinically, but focal seizures or neurologic deficits may result from compression or irritation of the underlying cerebral cortex. At surgery, the integrity of the dura is usually preserved because of its prophylactic role as a relatively impermeable barrier protecting the underlying brain.

Subdural Empyema

Subdural infection accounts for about 13 to 20 percent of all cases of intracranial bacterial infection and represents 5.1 percent of the space-occupying

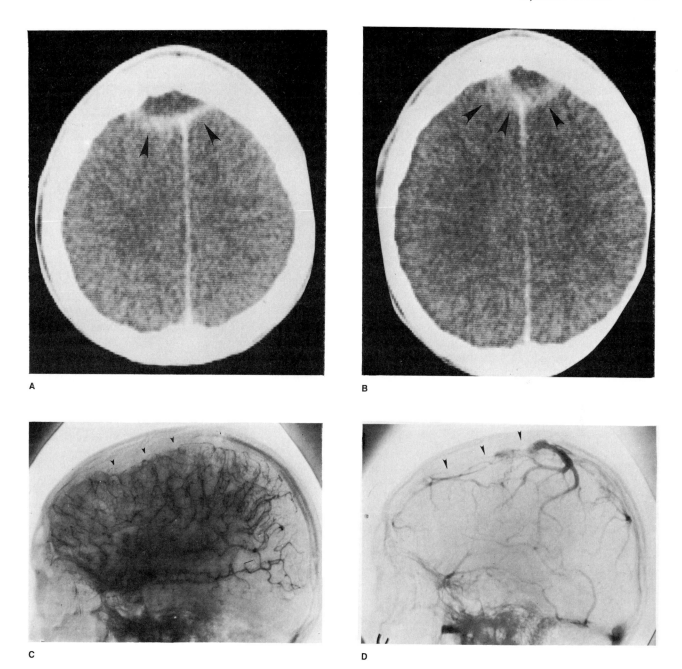

A

B

C

D

Figure 13-1 Epidural abscess. **A.** Biconvex hypodense lesion with contrast-enhanced dural margin (arrowheads) crosses the falx. **B.** Thick, irregular, nonhomogeneous membrane displaces the falx away from the inner table of the skull (arrowheads). **C.** Lateral cerebral angiogram, arterial phase, demonstrates avascular mass compressing the brain tissue (arrowheads). **D.** On venous phase, detachment of the superior sagittal sinus from the inner table of the skull (arrowheads) confirms its extradural location.

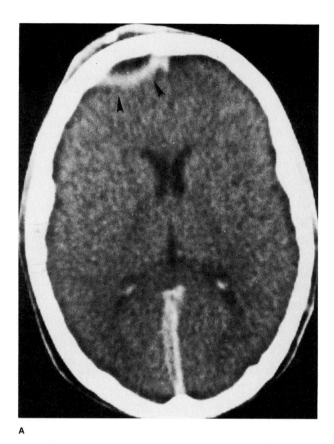

A

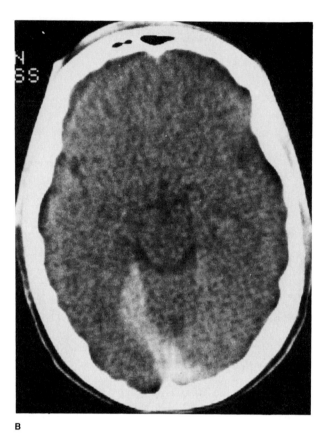

B

Figure 13-2 Frontal epidural abscess associated with subgaleal abscess and subdural empyema. Twenty-eight-year-old heroin addict sustained scalp infection following a minor head trauma. On NCCT (not shown), a hypodensity area in the frontal region was noted with no apparent mass effect or surrounding edema. **A.** On CECT, hypodense, lenticular epidural collection (arrowheads) is contiguous with the subgaleal abscess. Enhanced convex margin of the epidural abscess represents inflamed dural membrane. Enhancement of the posterior interhemispheric fissure represents subdural empyema. **B.** CECT at lower level shows enhancement along the tentorium cerebelli, which indicates extension of subdural empyema.

lesions in the subdural space (Weinman 1972; Galbraith 1974). It carried a mortality rate as high as 40 percent in the pre-CT era (Bhardari 1970; Weinman 1972; LaBeau 1973). Whenever progressive neurologic deterioration is associated with systemic manifestation of infection, this diagnosis should be strongly considered. The most common cause of subdural empyema is paranasal sinusitis (Kaufmann 1977). Less frequently, subdural empyema may be secondary to otitic infection, a penetrating wound of the skull, craniectomy, or osteomyelitis of the skull. The mechanism of subdural infection may be twofold: progressive retrograde thrombophlebi-

tis or (less likely) direct spread following penetration of the dura. The most common location of a subdural empyema is over the convexity of one or both hemispheres (80 percent), and bilateral involvement is frequent (Kaufmann 1977). Interhemispheric empyema is the next most frequent (12 percent), often occurring as an extension of the convexity collection. Rarely, the empyema may occur at the base of the brain or beneath the tentorium (Weinman 1972; Grinelli 1977) (Fig. 13-2).

NCCT demonstrates a crescentic or, more frequently, lentiform-shaped area of low density (0 to 16 HU) adjacent to the inner border of the skull.

This extracerebral hypodense collection represents pus. Adjacent cerebral and ventricular structures are compressed, and the subjacent brain surface is usually concave and smooth. On CECT, a narrow zone of enhancement of relatively uniform thickness separates the hypodense extracerebral collection from the brain surface (Fig. 13-3). This curvilinear enhancement is due to a combination of granulation tissue formation at the boundary of the empyema on its leptomeningeal surface and inflammation in the subjacent cerebral cortex (Grinelli

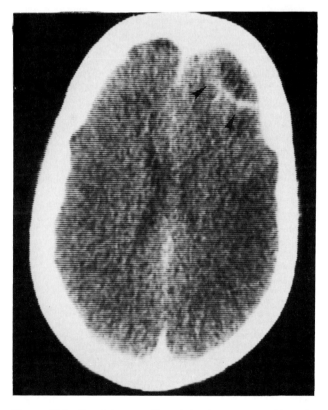

Figure 13-3 Frontal convexity subdural empyema with early cerebritis. CECT shows a thin, convex marginal enhancement outlining a lentiform hypodense collection in the frontal region (arrowheads). The marginal enhancement on the brain surface is usually uniformly thinner than that of the epidural abscess membrane but may be irregular (arrows), depending on the degree of inflammatory reaction in the leptomeninges and subjacent cerebral cortex. Regional hypodense area in the parietal lobe with compression of ipsilateral ventricle represents mass effect due to early cerebritis.

1977) (Fig. 13-4). The margins of the enhanced zone may show varying degrees of irregularity and thickness (Stephanov 1979; Sadhu 1980) which, in association with the underlying gyral enhancement due to venous thrombosis or cerebritis, may be of great help in differentiating the empyema from chronic subdural hematoma. Frequently, septic venous thrombosis leads to edema, hemorrhage, infarction, cerebritis, or brain abscess. The concomitant CT findings may be demonstrated in addition to the presence of the subdural empyema (Chap. 15).

The spindle shape of an interhemispheric subdural empyema is determined by the rigid falx cerebri medially and a combination of neovascularization in the abscess membrane and a disruption of the blood-brain barrier laterally (Figs. 13-4, 13-5). Hyperemia in the adjacent normal brain also plays a role in outlining an interhemispheric collection. Occasionally an interhemispheric subdural empyema may appear crescentic in shape (Joubert 1977; Sadhu 1980). When definite enhancement of the borders of an extracerebral fluid collection cannot be identified on CT as encountered early in the course of the disease despite substantial clinical evidence (Dunker 1981), angiography should be performed. Angiographic findings are enlarged inflammatory meningeal arteries, vasospasm of the large arteries at the base of the brain, and multiple cortical arterial occlusions, spasm, or prolonged flow (Rao 1978; Kim 1976; Sadhu 1980; Luken 1980).

Meningitis

Haemophilus influenzae and *Escherichia coli* in neonates and young children and meningococci and pneumococci in adolescents and adults account for the majority of instances of suppurative meningitis. The leptomeninges offer comparatively little resistance to infection, and the common initial response to these invading organisms is meningeal vascular congestion, edema, and minute hemorrhages. The underlying brain and its ependymal surfaces remain intact. CT may be normal at this stage (Claveria 1976; Zimmerman 1976) and may continue to be normal if treatment is instituted promptly and ad-

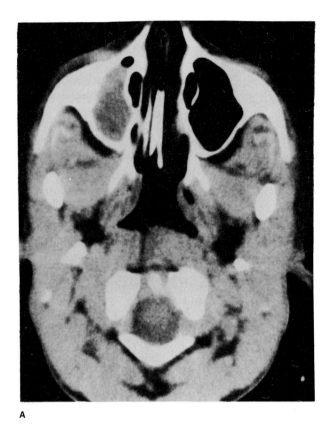

A

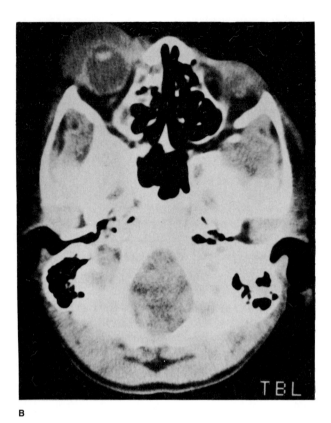

B

Figure 13-4 Subdural empyema associated with leptomeningitis and cerebritis. Right maxillary sinusitis **(A)** extends into the right orbit **(B)**. CECT at the base **(C)** shows marked contrast enhancement at the basal cistern representing extensive leptomeningitis. **D.** A thin, crescentic, left hemispheric subdural empyema (arrowheads) with marked contrast enhancement of the underlying gyri (cerebritis, venous thrombosis) and of the interhemispheric fissure (leptomeningitis). **E.** CECT following surgical evacuation of the left subdural em-

pyema demonstrates occurrence of the right subdural empyema with underlying cerebritis (arrowheads). Frontal interhemispheric subdural empyema can be seen on both sides of the falx cerebri (arrow). **F.** On CECT, convexity level shows a large interhemispheric subdural empyema delineated by a thick falx cerebri on medial side (arrowheads) and an early membrane formation on the lateral side. Note also gyral contrast enhancement on both hemispheres.

equately. Once infection progresses, however, the subpial cortex of the brain and the ependymal lining of the ventricles show evidence of inflammatory reaction. On NCCT, increased density in the basal cistern, interhemispheric fissure, and choroid plexuses frequently simulates contrast enhancement, probably because of a combination of hypervascularity in the acutely inflamed leptomeninges and choroid plexuses and fibrinous or hemorrhagic exudate in the subarachnoid space in the interhemispheric fissure and/or the basal cistern. The lateral and third ventricles are symmetrically compressed and extremely small (Auh 1980), perhaps because

of diffuse brain swelling representing both cortical congestion and edematous white matter. The cortical congestion is often less severe than in encephalitis. Focal areas of low density representing focal edema may be seen on CT. Abnormal contrast enhancement of bandlike or gyral configuration in the leptomeningeal and cortical zones may be observed, resulting from the vascular congestion of the meninges and also from disruption of the blood-brain barrier (Figs. 13-4, 13-6).

CT is useful in the early detection of complications of meningitis following subsidence of the acute inflammatory phase. Arterial or venous vas-

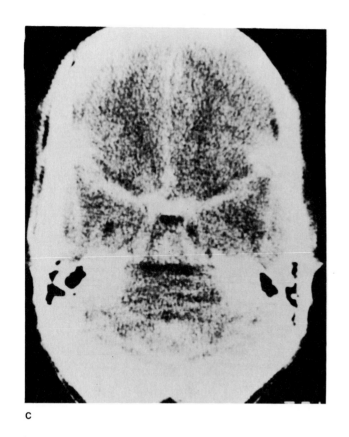

C

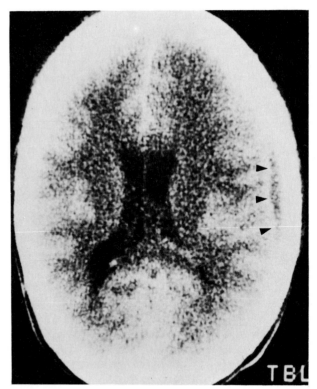

D

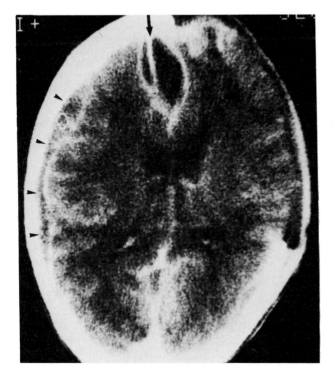

E

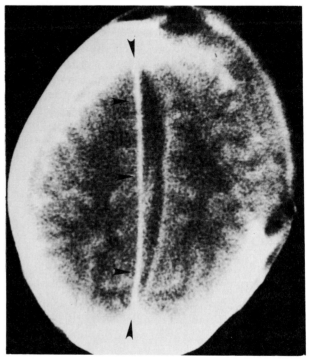

F

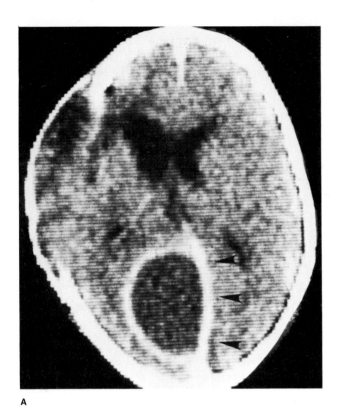

A

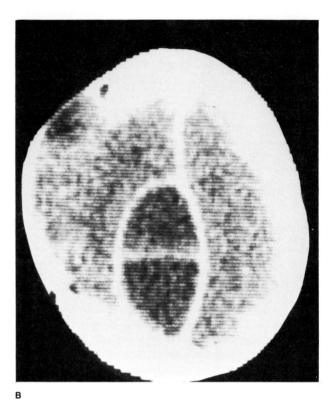

B

Figure 13-5. Interhemispheric subdural empyema in 8-year-old boy following surgery for otitis media. **A.** On CECT, the biconvex pus collection is clearly delineated by enhanced falx cerebri medially (arrowheads) and enhanced membrane laterally. The central low density (10 to 20 HU) represents pus collection, and the shift of the falx cerebri is due to the ex-pansible force of the abscess under increased pressure. Operative defect is noted in the temporal region. **B.** CECT at the high convexity level in the same patient demonstrates further extension of the subdural empyema. In addition, septation due to membrane formation within the empyema is shown by midline horizontal linear enhancement.

culitis or thrombosis may lead to areas of cerebral infarction. In such cases CT demonstrates diffuse or localized areas of low density within the brain parenchyma, usually conforming to the distribution of the involved vessels (Fig. 13-7). Focal dilatation of the ventricles may be noted adjacent to an area of encephalomalacia as a late sequel of this chain of events. The low-density areas of encephalomalacia and/or atrophy show a predilection for the frontal regions and are most frequently observed with *H. influenzae* meningitis (Cockrill 1978). Purulent exudate may collect at the base of the brain, particularly in the basal cisterns and convexities, causing communicating hydrocephalus as a result of impaired absorption of CSF from the subarachnoid space

(Figs. 13-6, 13-8). Ependymal inflammation in the ventricles may result in hydrocephalus from obstruction of the fourth ventricle or secondary to intraventricular septation and compartmentalization (Schultz 1973). Consequently, a portion of the ventricles—temporal horn or fourth ventricle—can be trapped and may present as an expanding mass lesion (Zimmerman 1978) (Fig. 13-9). Focal areas of periventricular calcification may evolve in neonates during the initial weeks following onset of severe bacterial meningitis complicated by ventriculitis (Kotagal 1981).

Development of subdural effusion is a common and well-recognized complication of leptomeningitis. Loculations of fluid between the thickened men-

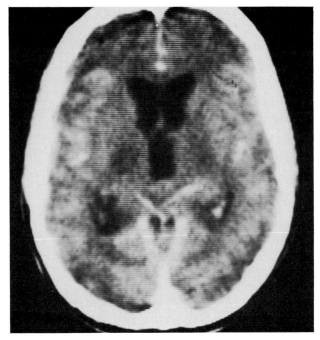

A

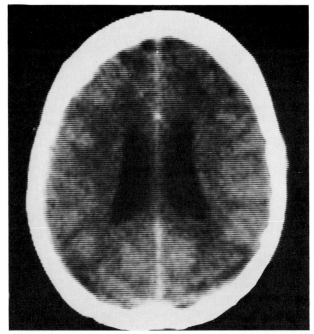

B

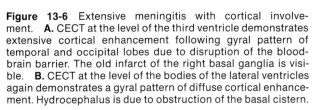

Figure 13-6 Extensive meningitis with cortical involvement.   **A.** CECT at the level of the third ventricle demonstrates extensive cortical enhancement following gyral pattern of temporal and occipital lobes due to disruption of the blood-brain barrier. The old infarct of the right basal ganglia is visible.   **B.** CECT at the level of the bodies of the lateral ventricles again demonstrates a gyral pattern of diffuse cortical enhancement. Hydrocephalus is due to obstruction of the basal cistern.

Figure 13-7 Hemispheric infarct following meningitis. Eight-year-old girl with congenital hypothyroidism presented with seizure and hemiparesis. At 2 years of age she suffered severe *Shigella* meningoencephalitis resulting in carotid artery occlusion at the basal cistern. CT discloses an infarct. *(Courtesy of Dr. Raymond Truex, St. Christopher's Hospital, Philadelphia, Pa.)*

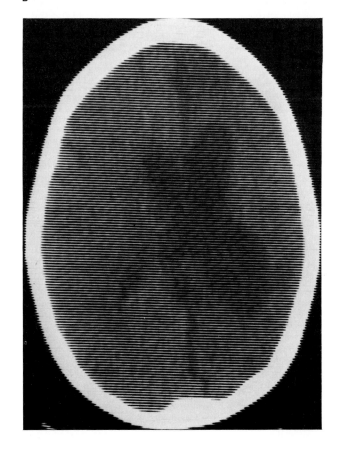

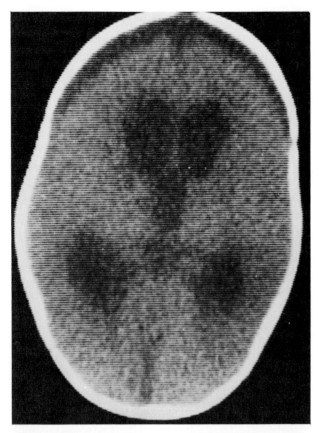

inges occur over the base of the brain and on the surfaces of the cerebral hemispheres (Fig. 13-8). Subdural empyema may develop from a preexisting postmeningitis subdural effusion. Another late result of postmeningitic subdural effusion is calcification in the walls of the effusion (Nelson 1969; Claveria 1976).

◀ **Figure 13-8** Subdural effusion following meningitis. Three-month-old infarct with pneumococcal meningitis developed into hydrocephalus and frontal subdural effusion bilaterally.

Figure 13-9 (Below) Trapped ventricles. Four-year-old child with history of tuberculosis meningitis. A shunt was placed for hydrocephalus. **A.** The trapped fourth ventricle shows a rounded appearance and may present as an expanding mass. Dilated temporal horn is noted. **B.** In this CT, taken at a higher level, the trapped trigone of the lateral ventricle is also seen.

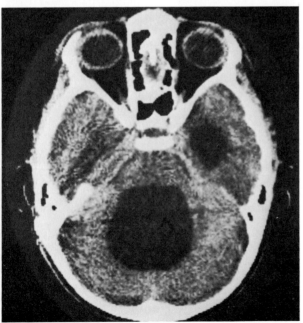

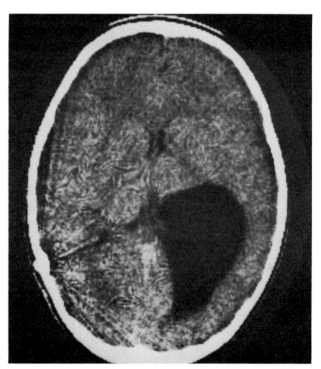

A

B

Cerebritis

Cerebritis is initially manifested by an area of low density in the white matter with poorly defined borders and regional (Fig. 13-3) or widespread (Fig. 13-10) mass effect reflecting vascular congestion and edema. There may be little or no contrast enhancement at this early stage. Further progression of the inflammatory process leads to cerebral softening and petechial hemorrhage, reflecting progressive damage to the blood-brain barrier. At this stage, CECT reveals mottled irregular areas of enhancement, mostly in the regional gray matter (New 1980) (Figs. 13-4, 13-6). The appearance of contrast enhancement often simulates the gyral patterns of cerebral infarction. Patchy, irregular enhancement of the white matter may also be noted (Fig. 13-11). Experimental studies of the evolution of brain abscess following direct inoculation of organisms have

demonstrated ring enhancement in the cerebritis stage (Enzmann 1979). The degree and extent of the mass effect is evidently out of proportion to that of the gyral enhancement. This finding may be of aid in the differential diagnosis from cerebral infarction when clinical findings are equivocal.

Aneurysms of inflammatory origin may be bacterial, syphilitic, or mycotic. Although all are termed mycotic, a bacterial etiology is the most common. These aneurysms originate mainly as an embolic complication of bacterial endocarditis, but less commonly aneurysms form as a complication of cardiac surgery, meningitis, cavernous sinus thrombophlebitis, or osteomyelitis. The most frequent location is at peripheral branches of the middle cerebral artery, followed by the anterior cerebral artery, the internal carotid artery, and the basilar artery. Progressive weakening of the elastica and the media of the aneurysm wall may result in rupture, with hem-

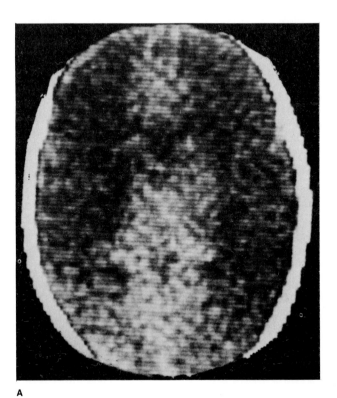 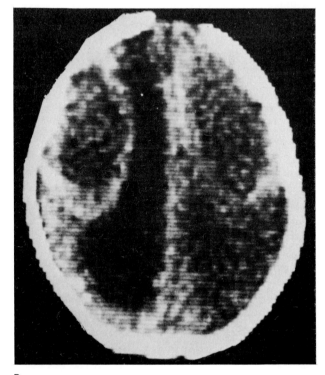

A   **B**

Figure 13-10 Diffuse cerebritis involving both hemispheres. **A.** NCCT shows diffuse extensive hypodensity of both hemispheres involving both white and gray matter. **B.** Follow-up CT demonstrates multiple abscess formation.

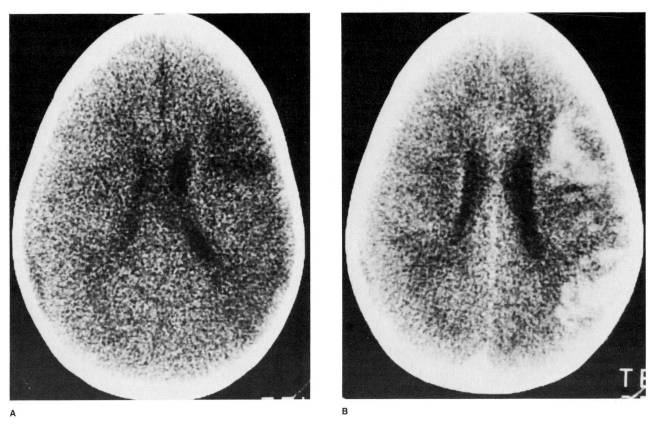

A   B

Figure 13-11   Cerebritis involving both gray and white matter.   **A.** NCCT shows poorly defined regional hypodense areas in the left frontal and parietal lobes.   **B.** CECT exhibits intense patchy enhancement in the white matter of the frontal lobe and gyral enhancement in the parietal lobe.

orrhage into the adjacent cortex or into the subarachnoid or subdural spaces. CT clearly demonstrates the results of aneurysm rupture, but the aneurysm itself is demonstrated only occasionally. Meningitis, cerebral abscess, or cerebral infarction may be associated with mycotic aneurysms.

Abscesses

Development of a brain abscess as a complication of leptomeningitis is unusual, but development of leptomeningitis secondary to an underlying brain abscess is common (Butler 1974). Brain abscesses typically occur as a result of preceding extracerebral infection. The extracerebral sources of infection can be divided into local (otitis media, mastoiditis, par-

anasal sinusitis, facial cutaneous infection, dental abscess, penetrating skull injury) and systemic (pulmonary infection, bacterial endocarditis, osteomyelitis, and congenital cyanotic heart disease with right-to-left shunt). Most venous-blood–borne abscesses are situated in subcortical white matter and appear on gross inspection as ill-defined areas of infected encephalomalacia (suppurative cerebritis). Arterial-blood–borne abscesses often commence in gray matter rather than in white matter and are located in the distribution of the middle cerebral artery, with a strong tendency toward multiplicity (disseminated microabscesses). In about one-quarter of cases of brain abscess, the source of the infection is uncertain (Kerr 1958) and sterile abscesses on smear and culture are not uncommon. Anaerobic organisms are isolated in the majority of abscesses, but multiple organisms are frequently found. Overall, the most commonly cultured organism currently is *Streptococcus*.

The center of cerebral softening in cerebritis may undergo necrosis and liquefaction, resulting in an abscess. On CT, mass effect on the ventricular system or the midline structures is noted in more than 80 percent of brain abscesses (Nielsen 1977). On NCCT, an ill-defined, low-density area is almost always seen (Claveria 1976; Nielsen 1977; Stevens 1978). Frequently a ring of slightly high density surrounding a central area of low density is noted (Paxton 1974; Joubert 1977; Stevens 1978; Whelan 1980).

Attenuation values within the central low-density area may vary between 4 and 28 HU. According to Mauersberger (1981), the average density value for the contents of an abscess was 11 HU, while the necrotic center of a glioblastoma revealed an average value of 23 HU. The high-density ring represents the abscess capsule and enhances densely following intravenous contrast injection (Figs. 13-12, -14, -18). Whelan (1980) reported several examples of dense nodules with further enhancement on CECT and suggested that this pattern was due to hemorrhagic infarction associated with vascular thrombosis and embolism in patients with sepsis. Visuali-

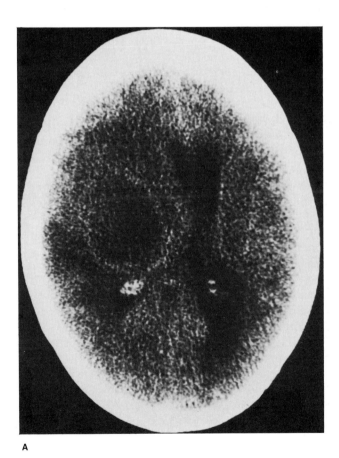

A

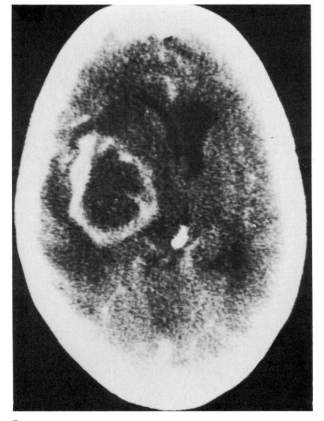

B

Figure 13-12 Temporal lobe abscess with thick, irregular capsule. **A.** NCCT shows a round, ringlike, hyperdense capsule differentiated from central low density (pus) and marked surrounding edema in the white matter. The compressed ipsilateral ventricle has shifted. **B.** On CECT, densely enhanced abscess capsule is evident. The irregular, thick wall of the capsule is not usual in pyogenic abscess. Central low density represents pus collection and does not change after IV contrast injection. The differentiation from glioblastoma may be extremely difficult in this case.

zation of gas within the abscess cavity indicates that the abscess was caused by gas-forming organisms (New 1976; Nielsen 1977). The presence of gas collections within the brain with no antecedent history of penetrating craniocerebral trauma or surgical intervention (Fig. 13-13) may permit a specific diagnosis of abscess.

On CECT, the central low-density area in the cavity does not change in appearance or CT number. Oval or circular peripheral ringlike contrast enhancement is an almost constant finding, delineating the formation of an abscess capsule. The degree of contrast enhancement of the capsule is reported to vary from 11.6 to 74 HU (Nielsen 1977; New 1976). The wall is usually thin (3 to 6 mm) and of uniform thickness (Figs. 13-14, 13-18). Not infrequently, however, an irregularly thick wall of an

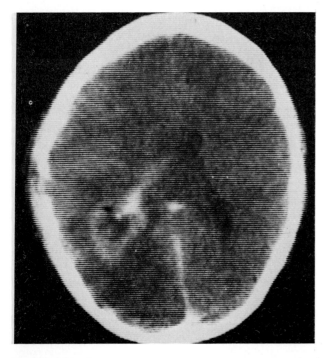

Figure 13-13 Postsurgical abscess cavity with air and ventriculitis. A small amount of gas present within the abscess cavity is the result of surgical intervention. Contrast enhancement within the ventricle represents ependymitis due to extension of infection from the abscess. Although presence of gas within the abscess produced by gas-forming organisms is diagnostic of a pyogenic abscess, its CT detection is extremely rare.

abscess cavity measuring up to 12 to 15 mm may mimic the wall of a glioblastoma (Figs. 13-12, 13-15).

Pathologically the abscess capsule consists of three layers: an inner layer of granulation tissue, a relatively thick middle layer of collagen, and an outer layer of reactive glial tissue. The collagen layer plays a major role in encapsulation of the infected brain tissue and is derived from fibroblasts which can be found in the meninges and in the walls of neophyte vessels (Waggener 1974; Moore 1974). Thinning of the medial margin of the capsule is frequently observed and is thought to be due to the relatively poor vascular supply of the white matter. This may account for the tendency of abscesses to rupture into the ventricular system and to form daughter abscesses in the white matter. Delay in capsule formation on the deep medial side of the abscess makes the wall less firm than on the side adjacent to the gray matter. Although medial thinning of the abscess wall on CT has been reported in 48 percent of cerebral abscesses (Stevens 1978), increased thickness of the medial wall of the capsule has also been frequently found (Fig. 13-15). The smoothness of the innermost layer of the cavity wall on CT is thought to be strongly suggestive of abscess diagnosis (Stevens 1978). The innermost layer of the wall, on the other hand, is irregular on pathological specimens because it contains uneven layers of necrotic debris and inflammatory granulation tissue (Harriman 1976).

Inasmuch as the simmering infection serves as an ongoing stimulation to vascular proliferation, leakage of protein-containing fluid from neophyte capillaries in an abscess wall is a constant feature and represents a major source of the accompanying edema (Waggener 1974). Edema in the white matter around the lesion is almost a constant finding (80 to 90 percent) on CT (Paxton 1974; Nielsen 1977). The volume of the surrounding edematous white matter is often greater than that of the abscess and is therefore responsible for much of the mass effect (Fig. 13-12).

The varying CT features of cerebral abscess described above are probably a reflection of different stages in the evolution of the abscess (Nahser 1981) and also a function of the host's reaction to infec-

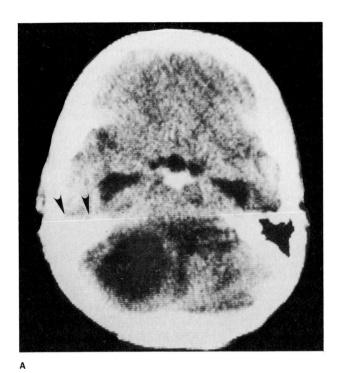

A

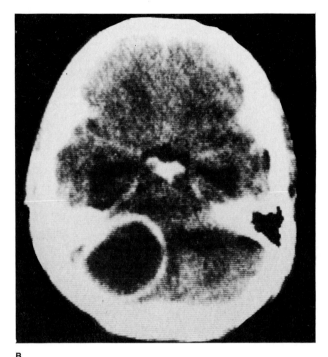

B

Figure 13-14 Cerebellar abscess. Eighteen-year-old with mastoiditis developed cerebellar abscess. **A.** NCCT shows the right mastoid is dense and without air cells (arrow) in comparison with the opposite side. A large, round, low density in the right cerebellar hemisphere displaces the fourth ventricle to the contralateral side. **B.** CECT shows a ringlike abscess cavity, well demarcated by a thin wall of uniform thickness contiguous to the petrous bone.

tion. If all the parameters of the abscess ring, such as thickness variability, patient's age, outside diameter, average value of CT numbers in the center, maximum wall thickness, and edema-to-ring ratio are considered, the correct diagnosis of abscess can be made with 84 percent accuracy (Coulan 1980).

Cerebellar abscesses constitute 2 to 18 percent of all brain abscesses (Fig. 13-14). They are less likely to be encapsulated but have a better prognosis than supratentorial abscesses if recognized early and treated surgically, prior to the onset of irreversible brainstem damage (Morgan 1975).

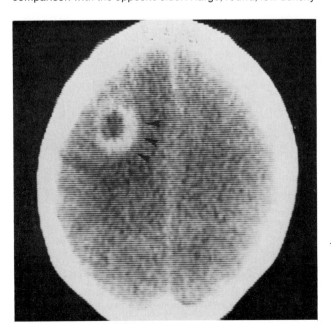

◀ **Figure 13-15** Frontal abscess. Twenty-four-year-old woman with pneumococcal abscess of the lung developed posterior frontal abscess. On CECT, thick and irregular capsule, especially on the medial side adjacent to the white matter (arrowheads), is noted; this is contrary to the usual pathological finding of thinner, less-firm capsule toward the white matter because of its poor vascularity.

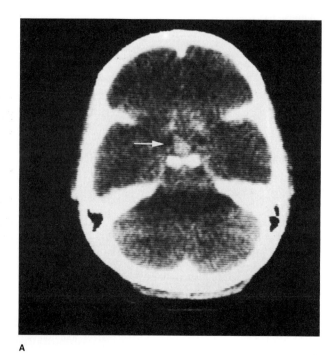

A

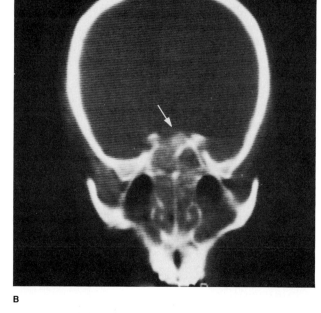

B

Figure 13-16 Intrasellar abscess. **A.** CECT demonstrates a triangular enhancement in the sella (arrow). **B.** Coronal view discloses pansinusitis with opacification and fluid levels. Opacified sphenoid sinus with infected mucocele communicates with the intrasellar abscess (arrow) by way of the destroyed floor of the sella. Complete resolution of intrasellar abscess occurred following surgery and vigorous antibiotic therapy.

Pituitary or intrasellar abscess should be suspected if the radiological and clinical features of a rapidly expanding mass in the sella are combined with a history of recurrent episodes of meningitis and rhinorrhea. Preoperative radiologic diagnosis of intrasellar abscess was considered impossible prior to the CT era (Lindholm 1973; Rudwan 1977). CECT demonstrates a focal area of intense contrast enhancement within the sella (Fig. 13-16). Abscess may also develop in an intrasellar tumor, in which circumstance the prognosis is grave (Zorub 1979).

Detection of septation within an abscess cavity (Fig. 13-17) or of development of daughter abscesses, either contiguous or noncontiguous, or of multiple abscesses (Fig. 13-18) is of utmost importance in surgical or medical management. Of particular interest to surgeons is the fact that a ring pattern on CECT does not necessarily imply a firm

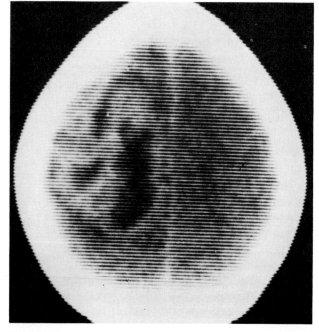

Figure 13-17 Multiseptation within the abscess cavity. A large abscess cavity with irregular nonuniform wall contains multiple thick septations. Satisfactory surgical results can be expected after total excision of all the compartments within the cavity.

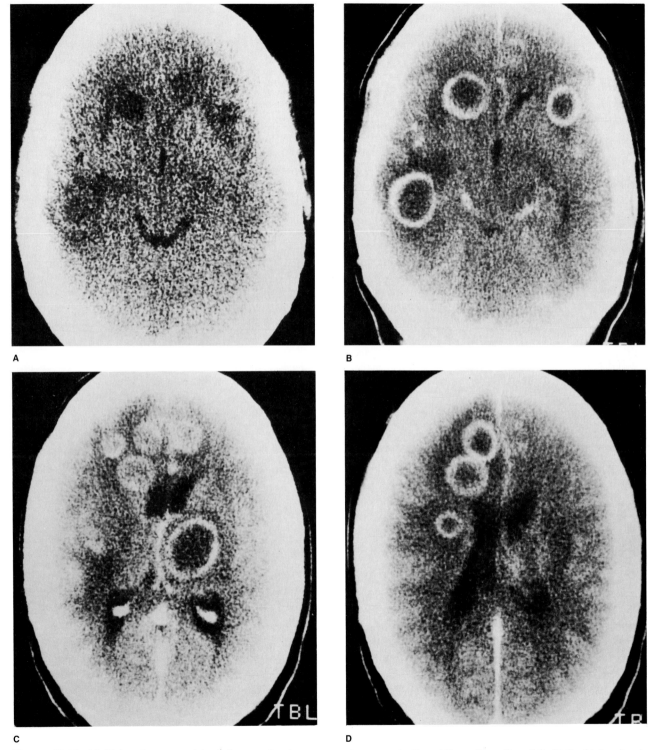

A

B

C

D

Figure 13-18 Multiple abscesses (staphylococcal) of unknown origin in 25-year-old man. **A.** NCCT shows multiple round, hypodense areas in both hemispheres. Faint ringlike hyperdense capsules are visible. **B.** CECT reveals multiple abscesses in the white matter. **C** and **D.** At the higher level, numerous cavities in the white matter, corticomedullary junction of both frontal lobes, and deep gray matter are present.

capsule at surgery or in pathological specimens; firmness of the capsule wall appears to be a time-dependent phenomenon seen in patients with clinical symptoms lasting more than 2 weeks (Whelan 1980). The duration of symptoms is thus helpful in predicting the firmness of the capsule in association with ring enhancement on CT. CT is also helpful in the follow-up of multiple abscesses during medical and surgical treatment and in the selection of patients who would benefit from surgical intervention (Kobrine 1981).

Clinical improvement with medical therapy has been correlated with a decrease in both the degree of contrast enhancement of the ring and the amount of surrounding edema (Robertheram 1979; Kamin 1981). Persistence of ring enhancement following surgical drainage may signify a poor result with recurrence of the abscess (Claveria 1976), but prolonged enhancement in the postoperative period without clinical deterioration has been reported to resolve spontaneously within 3 to 4 months (Robertheram 1979). Delayed postsurgical contrast enhancement may be due to vascular granulation tissue present about the circumference of the previous abscess and may not represent persistence of the abscess capsule. Steroids may help reduce the inflammatory edema associated with brain abscesses (Wallenfang 1981) but can also suppress the contrast enhancement completely. The CT diagnosis may then be quite difficult in spite of strong clinical evidence suggesting an abscess. Also, withdrawal of steroids may result in a rebound increase in degree of enhancement (Robertheram 1979).

The greatest dangers for the patient with an abscess are raised intracranial pressure (with the risk of cerebral herniation due to mass effect) and rupture of the abscess into the ventricle. It is thus extremely important to determine the severity of the associated edema as well as the accurate size of an abscess, and CT is certainly the least invasive and perhaps the best diagnostic modality in distinguishing surrounding edema from abscess cavity. Demonstration of coexisting contrast-enhanced ring and contrast enhancement of the adjacent ventricular wall indicates rupture of an abscess into the ventricle with ependymitis (Figs. 13-13, 13-19). The prognosis in this situation is poor.

Ependymitis

Spread of infection to the ventricles may follow leptomeningitis (usually resulting from retrograde extension of the infection via the lateral recesses of the fourth ventricle) or may follow spontaneous or iatrogenic rupture of an abscess cavity directly into the ventricles. Acute bacterial ependymitis shows distinct thin contrast enhancement along the ventricular wall regionally or more diffusely (Zimmerman 1976; Nielsen 1977) (Figs. 13-19, 13-20). Intraventricular septations and compartmentalization due to organization of intraventricular exudate and debris (Schultz 1973) and blockage of intraventricular foramina by purulent exudate lead to noncommunicating hydrocephalus. The loculated infection in the ventricles acts as a reservoir of infected material. CT not only precisely depicts the size and

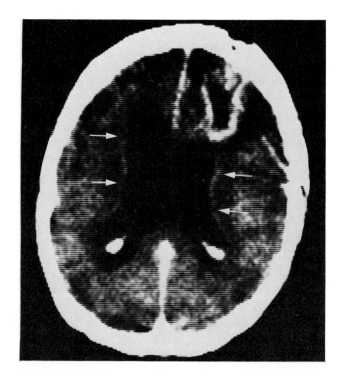

Figure 13-19 Abscess with ependymitis. CECT shows a slightly deformed abscess cavity due to surgical drainage in the left frontal lobe with direct extension of infection into the ipsilateral frontal horn. Thin curvilinear enhancement of the inflamed wall (arrows) of dilated lateral ventricles is seen. *(Courtesy of Dr. Dean Rich, Bryn Mawr Hospital, Philadelphia.)*

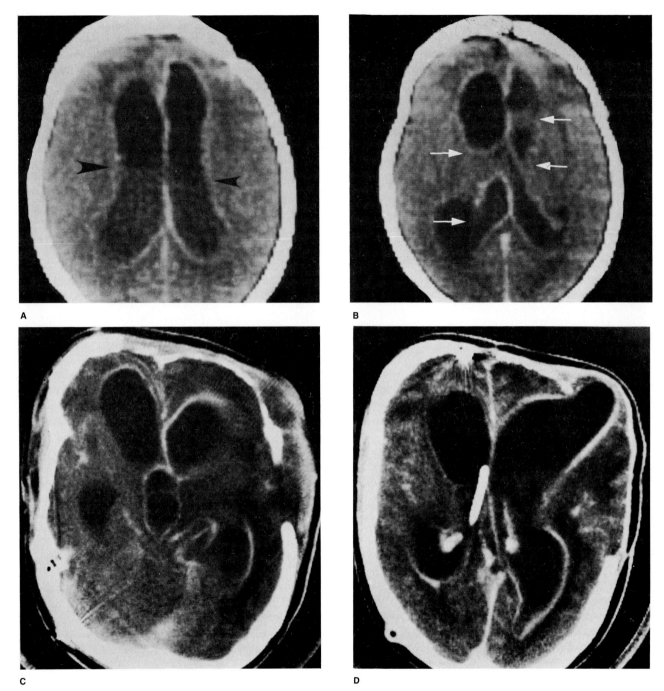

A

B

C

D

Figure 13-20 Ependymitis with septations following surgery for frontal sinusitis and abscess. **A.** On CECT extensive ependymitis shows as a thin contrast enhancement along the ventricular wall. CSF levels in the ventricles (arrowheads) are due to layering of pus in the dependent posterior halves of the bodies of dilated lateral ventricles. Frontal craniotomy defect is the result of surgery for frontal abscess secondary to frontal sinusitis. **B.** CECT at lower level demonstrates intraventricular septations (arrows) resulting in multiple compartmental-ization. Note again extensive enhancement of the inflamed ventricular wall. **C** and **D.** A young man sustained multiple craniofacial fractures following a gas-tank explosion. Post-surgical evacuation of the extracerebral collection was complicated by the wound infection and drainage of pus in the shunt tube. CECT demonstrates intense linear contrast en-hancement along the walls of the ventricular system. Pus-CSF fluid levels are also noted in the lateral ventricles. Noncom-municating hydrocephalus is evident.

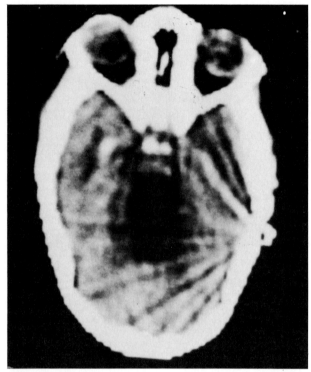

A

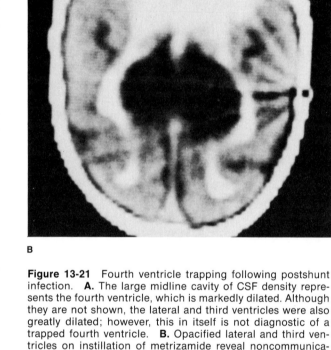

B

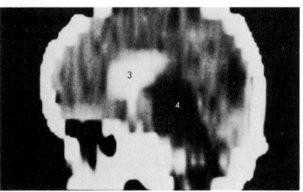

C

Figure 13-21 Fourth ventricle trapping following postshunt infection. **A.** The large midline cavity of CSF density represents the fourth ventricle, which is markedly dilated. Although they are not shown, the lateral and third ventricles were also greatly dilated; however, this in itself is not diagnostic of a trapped fourth ventricle. **B.** Opacified lateral and third ventricles on instillation of metrizamide reveal noncommunication with the fourth ventricle. **C.** Sagittal reformation in the midline clearly demonstrates marked dilatation of the fourth ventricle (4) extending supratentorially with no communication with the opacified third ventricle (3).

shape of the ventricles but also may suggest the presence of intraventricular septations and compartmentalization (Fig. 13-20). Trapping of the fourth ventricle because of obstruction of outlets and the aqueduct may ensue as a result of ependymitis following diffuse meningitis or shunt infection. This may act as an expanding mass in the posterior fossa which may require direct shunting

procedure (Zimmerman 1978) (Figs. 13-9, 13-21). Occasionally, ventricular instillation of low-dose, low-concentration metrizamide is necessary to demonstrate intraventricular compartmentalization or ventricular trapping (Fig. 13-21). Subependymal gliosis in chronic fungal or tuberculous ependymitis may show marked irregularity of ventricular margins with contrast enhancement (Fig. 13-34).

GRANULOMATOUS INFECTION

Tuberculous Infection

Tuberculous meningitis results from the hematogenous dissemination of bacilli from a primary lesion in the thorax, abdomen, or genitourinary tract. Small granulomas located in the cerebral cortex or in the meninges may rupture into the subarachnoid space, initiating a widespread meningeal infectious process. The very young and the very old are mainly affected, with the highest incidence in the first 3 years of life (Pfuetze 1966). The fibrinous pachymeningitis is associated with a purulent exudate accompanied by a vascular inflammatory response and formation of granulation tissue, which can result in communicating hydrocephalus with obstruction at the level of the basal cistern. Constriction of the major vessels at the base of the brain and in the sylvian fissures is seen in response to direct insult by the infecting organism (vasculitis) and as a result of the surrounding meningeal inflammation. Cerebritis, caseous granuloma formation (tuberculoma), and arterial or venous infarctions are further complications seen in association with tuberculous meningitis. True tuberculous abscess of the brain, as opposed to tuberculoma is very rare.

On NCCT, the basal cisterns may be partially obscured by the presence of inflammatory tissue and exudate. Obliterated and asymmetrical suprasellar and basal cisterns may be identified (Fig. 13-22). On CECT, the involved cisterns are uniformly and intensely enhanced, with an appearance that may resemble that of subarachnoid hemorrhage on NCCT or the images obtained with subarachnoid metrizamide (Enzmann 1976) (Fig. 13-22). The basal cisterns are most frequently affected, although frequently the sylvian cisterns and other subarachnoid

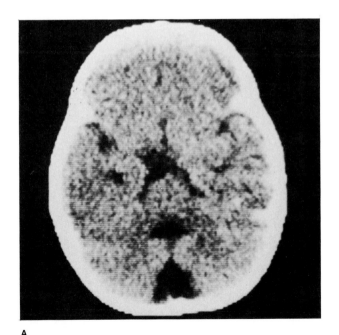

A

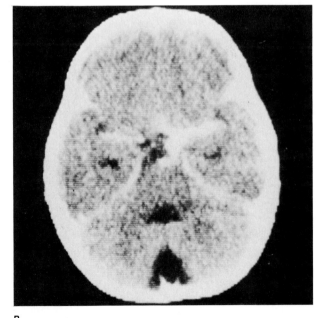

B

Figure 13-22 Tuberculous meningitis. Two-year-old child with choreoathetoid movement of face and arms. Cerebral angiogram demonstrated narrowing of the supraclinoid internal carotid arteries (not shown). **A.** NCCT demonstrates partial obliteration of suprasellar cistern. **B.** CECT demonstrates marked enhancement at the basal cisterns extending into both sylvian fissures and tentorial margins and mimicking subarachnoid hemorrhage or metrizamide.

spaces are involved (Armitsu 1979; Casselman 1980). Hydrocephalus secondary to blockage of the basal cisterns is a common sequela of tuberculous meningitis and is usually persistent, without progression or improvement in spite of antituberculous therapy (Price 1978; Stevens 1978). Calcification of the meninges at the base of the brain has been demonstrable 18 months to 3 years after the onset of the disease in 48 percent (Lorber 1958). Calcification within tuberculoma is not so common and ranges from 1 to 13 percent (Lorber 1958).

Cerebral *tuberculoma* is a rare manifestation of tuberculosis in the United States. The infrequency of the disease often results in diagnostic oversight. Definitive diagnosis may be particularly difficult since 42 percent of patients with intracranial tuberculomas have no evidence of extracranial disease (Mayers 1978). The clinical features of intracerebral tuberculoma are rarely distinguishable from other space-occupying intracranial lesions (Anderson 1975). A tuberculoma is composed of a caseous center surrounded by a ring of granulomatous tissue and may be spherical or multiloculated and single or multiple. Tuberculomas are found in any part of

the cerebral or cerebellar tissue and in the epidural, subdural, and subarachnoid spaces (Harriman 1976). On NCCT, varying image patterns have been reported: a tuberculoma may be isodense (Welchman 1979) or hyperdense or occasionally of mixed density (Lee 1979). After contrast injection, ringlike enhancement (Fig. 13-23) is commonly seen (Welchman 1979); but homogeneous enhancement (Claveria 1976; Peatfield 1979), irregular heterogeneous enhancement (Price 1978; Lee 1979) (Fig. 13-24), or absence of enhancement have also been described. The ring, when it is present, tends to be unbroken and is usually of uniform thickness (Hirsh 1978). It may be smooth or irregular in outline. This ringlike enhancement is attributed to enhancement of the capsule as well as the surrounding gliotic tissue. The density of the tissue within the ring is similar to that of the surrounding brain (Welchman 1979) (Fig. 13-23), in contradistinction to the central low density of pyogenic bacterial abscess cavities. Tuberculomas may spontaneously become cystic, fibrous, or calcified, but their chief risk lies in their liability to spill into the meninges. The "target sign" described by Welchman (1979) represents a central

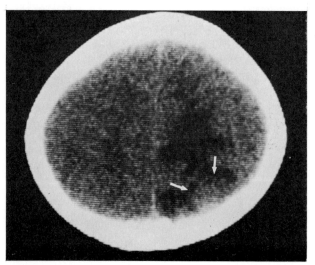

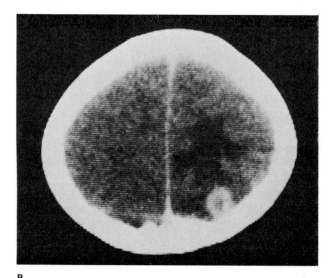

A   B

Figure 13-23 Tuberculoma. **A.** NCCT shows edema in the white matter and an isodense round cortical lesion (arrows). **B.** CECT shows a thick, ringlike lesion in the cortex. The center of the lesion remains isodense, with no change on contrast injection. *(Courtesy of J. H. Suh, M.D., Severance Hospital, Yonsei University, Seoul, Korea.)*

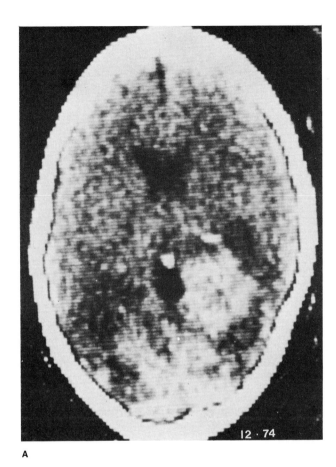

A

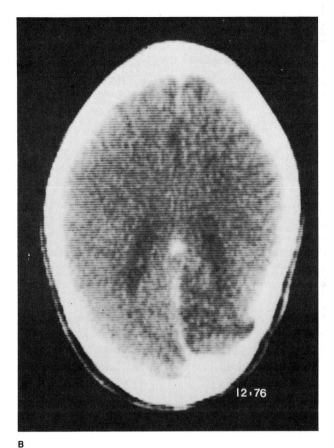

B

Figure 13-24 Tuberculoma. On NCCT, mixed, irregular density in the occipital lobes (not shown) was noted. **A.** CECT shows nonhomogeneous enhancement mimicking malignant glioma. Cerebral angiogram (not shown) demonstrated avascular mass. Culture and smear of the surgical specimen disclosed the correct diagnosis. **B.** Two years later, following surgery and antituberculous medical therapy, repeat CECT shows almost complete resolution. *(Reproduced by permission from Lee et al., Pa. Med., 82:36–38, 1979.)*

nidus of calcification or central enhancement surrounded by a ring of enhancement and is strongly suggestive of tuberculoma. Disproportionate surrounding edema and mass effect are usual but not prominent findings.

Tuberculomas may be predominantly extracerebral in location and attached to the dura (Welchman 1979) (Fig. 13-25). These en plaque tuberculomas closely resemble meningiomas, both clinically and operatively. Multiple tubercules may be found within the brain at the corticomedullary junction and in the paraventricular regions, because of extensive hematogenous spread, usually from miliary

tuberculosis of the lungs. On NCCT, the nodules may not be identified because of their isodensity, but on CECT, numerous small, round, discrete nodules are readily detected (Witham 1979) (Fig. 13-26). Occasionally, centrally decreased density within the nodule may be visualized, but edema adjacent to the tubercle is not a common finding (Whelan 1981). Midline shift or ventricular compression are not usual or prominent findings, most probably because of the relative paucity of edema and diffuse involvement of both hemispheres. These tuberculous nodules may undergo complete resolution after antituberculosis therapy. CT is essential both in es-

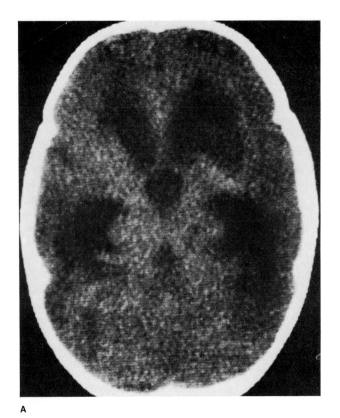

A

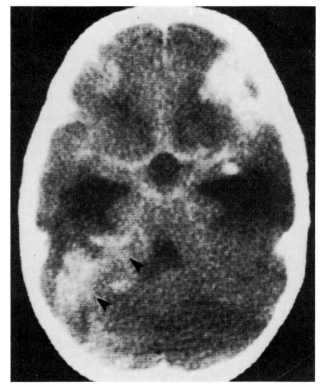

B

Figure 13-25 Tuberculomas, intracerebral and extracerebral. **A.** NCCT shows obliteration of the basal cistern and slightly increased density along the tentorial margins. Noncommunicating hydrocephalus (third and lateral ventricles) is due to obstruction at the level of the basal cistern. **B.** CECT demonstrates extradural granulomas (en plaque tuberculomas) along the right tentorial margin (arrowheads) and in the basal subarachnoid cistern. Irregular, mixed contrast-enhancing lesion in the left frontal lobe represents intracerebral tuberculoma.

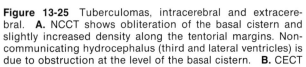

A

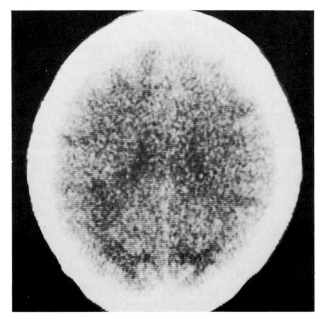

B

tablishing the diagnosis of tuberculous meningitis and tuberculomas and in monitoring the response of the tuberculous lesions and the associated hydrocephalus to therapy.

Intracranial Sarcoidosis

Involvement of the central nervous system is a rare occurrence in systemic sarcoidosis. Although 4 to 7 percent of patients with sarcoidosis present with neurological manifestations, the incidence of intracranial involvement in patients with known sarcoidosis is about 15 percent (Silverstein 1965; Weiderholt 1965). Rarely, CNS involvement may be the only manifestation of this disease (Cahill, 1981; Griggs 1973). Sarcoid may present at any age (Robert 1948) but is most common in the third and fourth decades, usually in females. Two patterns of intracranial involvement have been identified: (1) as a granulomatous leptomeningitis, and (2) as an intra-

cerebral mass. Granulomatous leptomeningitis may occur diffusely or as a circumscribed process at the skull base, involving the optic chiasma, pituitary gland, floor of the third ventricle, and hypothalamus. Communicating hydrocephalus is a common result. The second pattern of CNS sarcoid, less commonly seen, consists in noncaseating granulomas either scattered diffusely in the brain parenchyma or as a single large mass which mimics a brain neoplasm (Saltzman 1958; Silverstein 1965; Robert 1948; Griggs 1973).

On CT, sarcoidosis may thus present as hydrocephalus secondary to leptomeningitis (Fig. 13-27) or an obstructing mass lesion (Bahr 1978; Kendall 1978; Kumpe 1979) (Fig. 13-28). Patients with sarcoid granulomatous leptomeningitis and resulting communicating hydrocephalus may occasionally show contrast enhancement of the basal cisterns (Morehouse 1981). Differentiation from other causes of communicating hydrocephalus may be difficult unless the patient has proved pulmonary sarcoid-

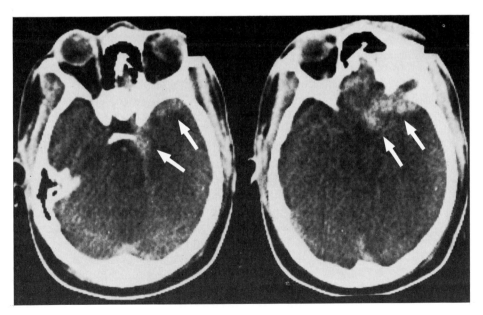

Figure 13-27 Leptomeningeal sarcoid granulomas. On CECT, extensive granulomas present as nonhomogeneous densities in the temporal fossa along the sphenoid bone (arrows) and in the parasellar region (arrows).

◄ **Figure 13-26** Multiple tuberculomas. Hematogenous dissemination in 24-year-old with miliary tuberculosis and tuberculous peritonitis. **A.** NCCT shows mild ventricular compression bilaterally, but no apparent density changes are noted. **B.** CECT shows numerous discrete nodules in the cortex and corticomedullary junction. No apparent edema is present. Complete resolution was noted following vigorous antituberculosis therapy.

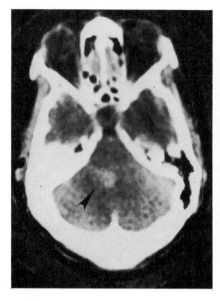
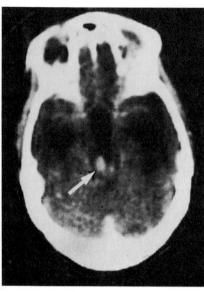

Figure 13-28 Parenchymal sarcoid granulomas. CECT demonstrates sarcoid granulomas in the brainstem (arrowhead) and midbrain (arrow).

osis. Granulomatous masses usually appear as a hyperdense area on NCCT, with further homogeneous enhancement on CECT. In a patient with known sarcoidosis, the intracranial mass may be suspected to represent sarcoid granulomas. When there is no evidence of peripheral sarcoidosis, differentiation from a meningioma or other hyperdense contrast-enhancing intracranial neoplasm may be difficult unless CSF analysis or biopsy is performed. Differentiation from other pathological entities, such as carcinomatous metastases or multiple intracerebral granulomas following other chronic infectious processes, is not possible when multiple hyperdense nodular lesions are seen involving the brain parenchyma, with further increase in density on CECT. Unlike most metastases, sarcoid granulomatous masses within the parenchyma rarely demonstrate surrounding edema. Sarcoid granulomas shrink in size following treatment with steroids.

VIRAL INFECTION

Manifestations of viral diseases of the CNS on CT differ from those of bacterial or fungal etiology by their tendency to diffuse parenchymal involvement and the frequent absence of distinctive gross alterations in the involved parenchyma. An exception to this statement is herpes encephalitis.

Herpes simplex virus, type 1, is the most common cause of sporadic viral encephalitis in the United States. Herpetic encephalitis is characterized by a fulminant necrotizing encephalitis with petechial hemorrhages, with early involvement of the subfrontal and medial temporal regions. Mortality is high (in the vicinity of 70 percent). The success of treatment, particularly with adenine arabinoside, depends on early diagnosis and institution of therapy before the development of coma (Whitley 1977). Even in the presence of characteristic CT findings strongly suggestive of herpes infection, definitive diagnosis must be based on positive fluorescein antibody staining or culture of virus from brain biopsy.

The most commonly noted CT findings in herpes infection are a poorly marginated hypodense area (63 to 64 percent), mass effect (50 to 52 percent) and nonhomogeneous contrast enhancement (50 to 57 percent) (Davis 1978; Leo 1978). The earliest and predominant CT finding is the low-density abnormality in the temporal and frontal lobes, which are also characteristics sites of involvement in gross pathologic specimens (Davis 1978; Leo 1978) (Fig.

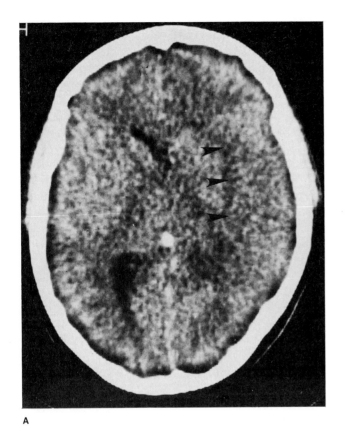

A

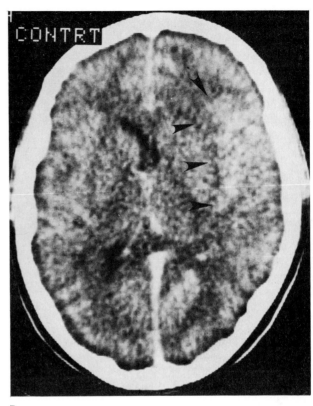

B

Figure 13-29 Herpes simplex (type 1) encephalitis. **A.** NCCT exhibits poorly defined mixed-density area in the temporal lobe (arrowheads), with effacement of the ipsilateral ventricle. **B.** On CECT, patchy areas of enhancement involve the temporal and frontal lobes (arrowheads).

13-29). The low-density area may later extend to involve the deep frontal or occipital lobes, but isolated frontal or occipital lobe involvement is uncommon (Ketonen 1980). The low density in the early period probably represents a combination of tissue necrosis and focal brain edema. Abrupt transition to normal density at the lateral margin of the lenticular nucleus has been considered characteristic (Zimmerman 1980) (Figs. 13-29, 13-30).

The mass effect is manifested either as a midline shift or as a focal mass causing compression of the ventricles or sylvian cisterns. This is usually concomitant with a low-density area and persists for more than a month (Davis 1978). Occasionally there may not be a midline shift owing to bilateral balanced involvement (Fig. 13-30).

The pattern of contrast enhancement may be gyral (Davis 1978), linear streaks at the periphery of the low-density lesion (Enzmann 1978) (Fig. 13-30), patchy (Fig. 13-29), or multiple ringlike (Ketonen 1980) (Fig. 13-30). Occasionally, the location of the enhancement does not correspond to the areas of low density (Davis 1978). The wide variation in appearance of the enhancement pattern may be due to the nonspecificity of the compromised blood-brain barrier in the area of rapid progressive hemorrhagic necrosis. Subarachnoid enhancement suggestive of meningeal involvement on CECT and intracerebral hemorrhage depicted on NCCT as a well-defined mass (Zegers de Beyl 1980) or as ill-defined linear streaks of increased density (Enzmann 1978) are uncommon findings. These CT ab-

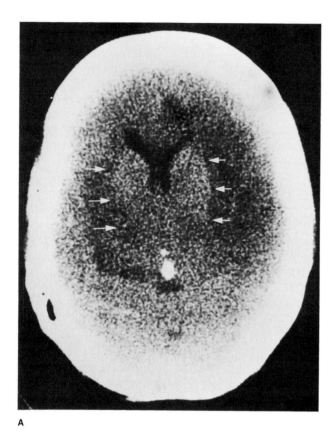

A

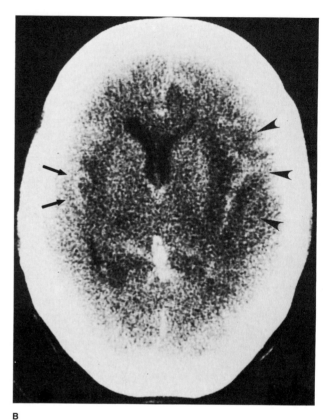

B

Figure 13-30 Herpes simplex (type 1) encephalitis. **A.** On NCCT, extensive low-density lesions in both temporal lobes, more on the left than the right, are clearly demarcated by the lateral margin of the basal ganglia (arrowheads). **B.** CECT shows different patterns of contrast enhancement: linear streaks (arrowheads) on the left and ringlike figures (arrows) on the right. Absence of midline shift is due to bilateral, balanced involvement.

normalities are usually not seen in the initial 5 to 7 days after onset of illness (Zimmerman 1980; Greenberg 1981) although the earliest recorded occurrence of contrast enhancement was at 3 days after the onset of signs and symptoms (Davis 1978). Contrast enhancement may be detectable until 2½ months after disease onset (Ketonen 1980). Thus, a normal CT in the initial symptomatic period does not exclude the diagnosis of herpes simplex encephalitis. Radionuclide brain imaging, with dynamic and static delayed scintiscans, may be of value in detecting early changes in the initial period.

Late follow-up CT typically demonstrates widespread low density (encephalomalacia) involving the temporal and frontal lobes, indicating extensive involvement of the brain, which is often not appreciated early in the course of the disease.

The primary role of CT in the evaluation of herpes simplex encephalitis is to confirm the clinical diagnosis and to indicate the best site for biopsy as well as to exclude the presence of an abscess or tumor. Early definitive diagnosis is essential prior to treatment with adenine arabinoside, since this chemotherapeutic agent may be neurotoxic, mutagenic, and carcinogenic.

Infection with *herpes simplex virus, type 2* in the newborn infant may be acquired transplacentally or during delivery, presumably secondary to genital and perineal infection in the mother. Early intra-uterine infection with type 2 virus is known to have marked neurotrophic teratogenic potential and has been associated with microcephaly, micrencephaly, intracranial calcification, microphthalmia, and retinal dysplasia (South 1969). Disseminated encephalitis in infants produces widespread calcifications conforming to an atrophic cerebral hemisphere. On NCCT, microcephaly with grossly dilated ventricles and thin cortical mantle are noted. Masses of calcifications are scattered throughout white and gray matter and may have a periventricular distribution (Dublin 1977).

Other causes of congenital calcification of the brain include toxoplasmosis, rubella, and cytomegalovirus. Toxoplasmosis and rubella calcifications are evenly distributed in necrotic brain substance but may be compressed by hydrocephalus and thus mimic the periventricular subependymal calcifications of cytomegalovirus. Occasionally, cortical and subcortical white-matter calcification is found in cytomegalovirus infection (Harwood-Nash 1970; Malloy 1963).

FUNGAL INFECTION

Fungal infections represent nontuberculous granulomatous diseases which may be acute and fulminant. Infection may be meningeal, parenchymal (fungal "abscess"), or both. In most instances, the primary portal of entry is the lungs, but fungal osteomyelitis or lymphadenitis may precede brain involvement. The frequency of CNS fungus infection has increased significantly in recent years, because of opportunistic organisms in patients receiving steroids or immunosuppressive drugs (Britt 1981).

Although a variety of opportunistic organisms may involve the central nervous system, not all of the entities have a characteristic pattern that suggests the diagnosis purely on the basis of CT findings. Most often CT is useful in demonstrating and localizing the parenchymal or meningeal involvement, and confirmation as to the specific fungus involved is based on a variety of CSF studies, most often the CSF culture.

CT features of fungus infection are varied and nonspecific (Enzmann 1980). In general, ringlike contrast enhancement in fungal infection, frequently observed in patients free of additional systemic derangements, probably reflects the host's ability to wall off the organisms, with a better prognosis.

Cryptococcal (torular) meningitis is perhaps the most common fungal infection of the brain. A thick, immobile exudate is noted at the base of the brain, topographically similar to a tuberculous exudate. Large parenchymal granulomatous "abscesses" (toruломas) also simulate tuberculomas. CT may show poorly marginated hypodense lesions in the white matter with minimal or no contrast enhancement (Fig. 13-31). Intraparenchymal torulomas may exhibit ringlike (Long 1980) or focal homogeneous contrast-enhanced areas with or without circumferential edema (Fujita 1981). Nine of 12 patients reported by Long (1980) had a variety of nonspecific

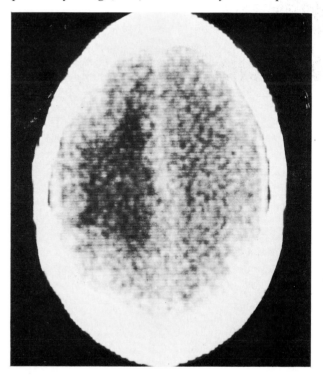

Figure 13-31 Cryptococcal granuloma. CT shows poorly marginated, extensive, hypodense lesion in the white matter with no contrast enhancement.

CT changes such as ventricular dilatation, cortical atrophy, and focal ischemic changes. Calcification may be present on follow-up studies. In immunosuppressed organ-transplant recipients (Britt 1981), cryptococcal and *Listeria* infections are more frequently seen as meningitis than intraparenchymal granulomas. Basal cisterna contrast enhancement or latent development of subdural hygroma may be seen.

Coccidioides imitis is a dust-borne fungus endemic to the southwestern part of the United States, especially the San Joaquin Valley of California, as well as portions of Mexico and central South America (Fraser 1978). It is spread by inhalation of the spore, which is present in soil. Only 0.02 to 0.2 percent of cases progress to the disseminated form involving the brain, meninges, and other systemic organs (Einstein 1974). Pathologically, CNS coccidioidomycosis is characterized by thickened, congested leptomeninges with multiple granulomas, which are especially prominent in the basal cisterns and result in communicating hydrocephalus. Vasculitis also occurs, but occlusions are rare. Ependymitis and periventricular diffuse focal white-matter and deep gray-matter lesions (focal granulomas without calcification) are also seen (McGahan 1981). The most common CT findings are hydrocephalus (86 percent) and abnormal basal or convexity cisternal contrast enhancement (71 percent) (Dublin 1980; Enzmann 1976).

Candida albicans is increasingly associated with nervous system infection, particularly in patients with diabetes mellitus or those with altered immune status caused by immunosuppressive or cytotoxic drugs or broad-spectrum antibiotics or steroids. Candidiasis of the CNS is characterized by scattered granulomatous microabscesses, leptomeningitis, and numerous thrombosed vessels. CT demonstrates areas of poorly circumscribed low density without contrast enhancement in immunosuppressed patients (Enzmann 1980). Cavity formation of various thicknesses with an isodense or slightly hypodense center may be encountered in patients with no predisposing systemic illness (Fig. 13-32). Noteworthy is the central density, which is higher than that of bacterial abscesses except for tuberculosis.

Aspergillus fumigatus usually appears as an opportunistic infection and reaches the brain in most cases by hematogenous dissemination from a primary focus in the lung or by direct extension from the ear, nose, or paranasal sinuses. Solitary brain abscess, thrombosis with hemorrhagic necrosis, and massive subarachnoid and intracranial hemorrhage are known to occur (Visudhiphan 1973). Enzmann (1980) and Grossman (1981) reported nonspecific, poorly circumscribed areas of subtle low density with little or no contrast enhancement and mass effect. However, a ring configuration representing a well-formed, thick, and regular abscess capsule has been noted on CECT (Claveria 1976). Compared to neuropathologic findings, the CT findings generally underestimated the extent of involvement.

Nocardia asteroides infection may demonstrate multiple extensive hypodense lesions on NCCT, with ringlike appearance on CECT (Fig. 13-33). A rare case of *Cladosporium trichoides* following a penetrating craniocerebral injury has recently been reported (Kim 1981). CT showed a round lesion in the edematous frontal white matter above the original site of injury. The center of the lesion showed near-isodensity with no contrast enhancement. Intense contrast enhancement was present in the walls of the cavity and the ventricles. The ependymitis along the ventricular wall was thick, irregular, and not contiguous (Fig. 13-34). At surgery, a firm subcortical mass, with extensive granulomatous inflammation, was found. No fluid was present within the cavity. *Toxoplasma gondii* infection may exhibit either nonspecific low density or ringlike enhancement on CT (Enzmann 1980).

PARASITIC INFECTIONS

Cysticercosis

Cysticercosis is one of the most common parasitic diseases to affect the brain. Humans serve as the intermediate hosts of *Taenia solium*, the pork tape-

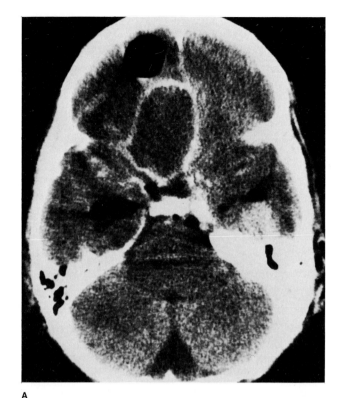

A

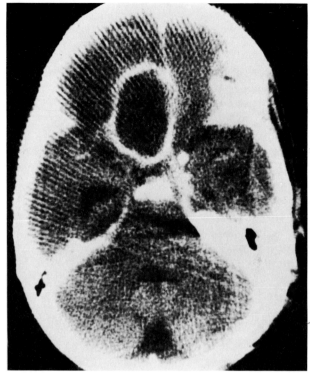

B

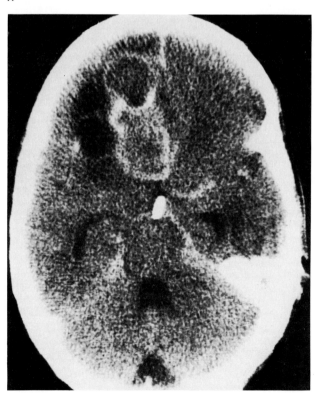

C

Figure 13-32 *Candida* granuloma. Eighteen-year-old involved in severe motor vehicle accident who sustained multiple basal skull fractures. **A.** Basal skull CECT shows multiple pneumocephalus and left temporal lobe hemorrhage. A large cavity in the right frontal lobe contains an isodense center and irregular wall. Aspiration and culture grew *Candida albicans.* **B** and **C.** Follow-up CT, after treatment with amphotericin B, demonstrates thicker cavity wall and development of a daughter cavity. Resorption of temporal lobe hematoma and pneumocephalus is noted.

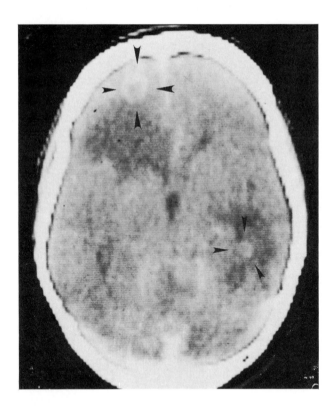

Figure 13-33 Nocardial "abscess." CECT shows two discrete round lesions in the right frontal and left temporal lobes. Peripheral contrast enhancement (arrowheads) and extensive surrounding edema are present.

Figure 13-34 *Cladosporium* granuloma. **A.** CECT shows a large, thin, ringlike cavity in the frontal lobe with surrounding white matter edema. Thick, irregular enhancement in the ventricular wall represents ependymitis. **B.** CECT, following surgical and medical treatment, demonstrates marked decrease in the size of the cavity and the extent of edema. Dilatation of the left lateral ventricle is due to obstruction of the foramen of Monro by ependymal granulomas (arrowheads).

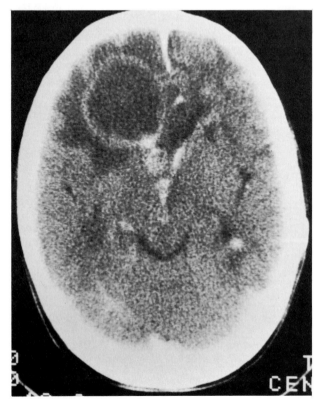

A

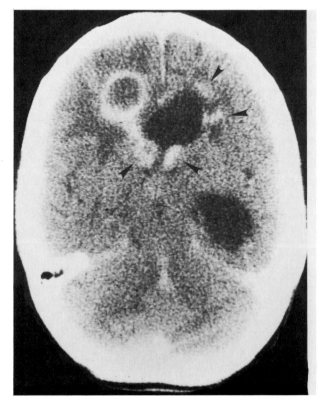

B

worm, in this disease, which is prevalent in parts of Asia, India, Africa, Europe, and Latin America. There appears to be a recent increase in the incidence of cysticercosis in the United States, perhaps due to an increase in travel to and from endemic areas. The central nervous system is the most frequently infected organ system, with reported incidence of CNS involvement as high as 92 percent of cases (Dixon 1961). Classification by anatomic localization include meningeal (39 percent), intraventricular (17 percent), parenchymal (20 percent), mixed (23 percent), and intraspinal (1 percent) (Carbajal 1977).

Meningeal involvement is manifested by extracerebral cysts, arachnoiditis, vasculitis, or a combination of these. Since the walls of subarachnoid cysts are not visible on CT before or after contrast injection and the density of the fluid contents of

these cysts is identical to that of CSF, the detection of these cysts is based on focal areas of apparent enlargement of the subarachnoid spaces. Breakdown of these cysts provokes an arachnoiditis which may exhibit focal contrast enhancement, and occurrence of one or more cysts in the basal cisterns may obstruct cerebrospinal fluid pathways, with resultant communicating hydrocephalus. Vasculitis associated with the meningeal cysticercal infestation may cause arterial narrowing, with thrombosis and resultant cerebral infarction.

Solitary or multiple intraventricular cysts may be attached to the ventricular walls or may be free-floating. Larger cysts may cause focal expansive deformities of the affected ventricle. A large cyst or cluster of cysts within the fourth ventricle and its expansion may simulate entrapment of the fourth ventricle (Fig. 13-35). Noncommunicating hydro-

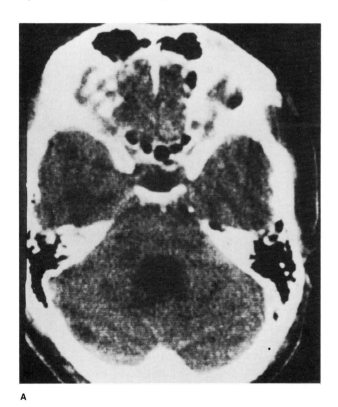

A

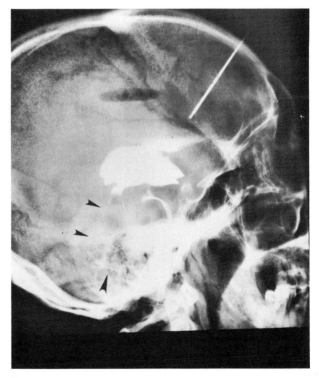

B

Figure 13-35 Cysticercosis in the fourth ventricle. **A.** Apparent dilatation of the fourth ventricle and obstructive hydrocephalus. On close inspection, the density within the fourth ventricle is slightly lower than that of cerebrospinal fluid. **B.**

On positive-contrast ventriculogram, the fourth ventricle is faintly outlined (arrows). At surgery, multiple cysts were delivered from the fourth ventricle. *(Courtesy of Man Chung Han, M.D., Seoul National University Hospital, Seoul, Korea.)*

cephalus due to obstruction of the foramen of Monro, unilateral or bilateral, or of the fourth ventricle is a common finding. Uniform enhancement in an isodense cyst in the anterior third ventricle (Jankowski 1979) and ringlike enhancement in the fourth-ventricle cyst (Zee 1980) are rare findings and may not represent enhancement of the cyst wall. Usually, cysts are not identified on CT because of their thin walls, approximately CSF-equivalent cyst contents, and lack of contrast enhancement (Carbajal 1977; Benson 1977). Measurements of the density of the cyst fluid range from 0 to 10 HU. Large cysts often appear slightly lower in density than the CSF.

Living larvae create parenchymal masses up to 2 or 3 cm in diameter within the substance of the brain. On CT, these appear as rounded cystic structures of CSF-equivalent density (Fig. 13-36). Rarely,

isodense or hyperdense masses are noted (Sim 1980). Since there is little reaction of the surrounding brain prior to the death of the larva, contrast enhancement or focal edema around the cyst is rarely observed in association with living cysticerci. This lack of inflammatory reaction about cysticercus cysts is a striking feature of the disease and is probably related to poor antigenicity of the wall of the parasite and inaccessibility of cysticercal antigens within the CNS because of an intact blood-brain barrier (Biagi 1974).

However, at the termination of cohabitant status with the brain parenchyma, ringlike or nodular contrast enhancement occurs, often accompanied by surrounding focal edema (Fig. 13-37). The exact mechanism of the acute inflammatory reaction in the presence of dying cysticerci but not with living larvae is not known. Perhaps when antigenic stim-

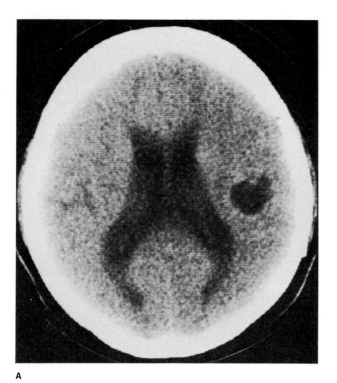

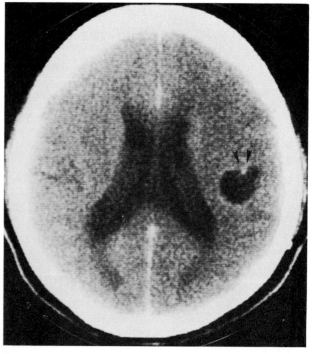

A   B

Figure 13-36 Living intraparenchymal cysticercus. **A.** NCCT demonstrates a rounded cystic structure of CSF-equivalent density in the white matter of the parietal lobe. No surrounding edema is present. **B.** CECT shows no contrast enhancement around the cyst, but the scolex (arrowheads) is slightly enhanced, indicating the living cysticercus. *(Courtesy of Dr. S. Y. Kim, Kyung Hee University Medical School, Seoul, Korea.)*

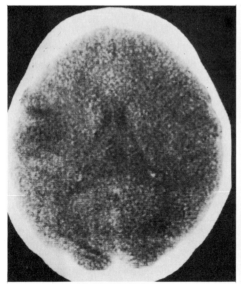
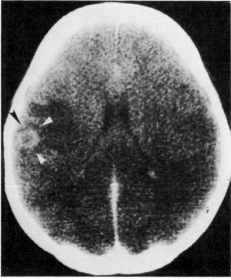

A B

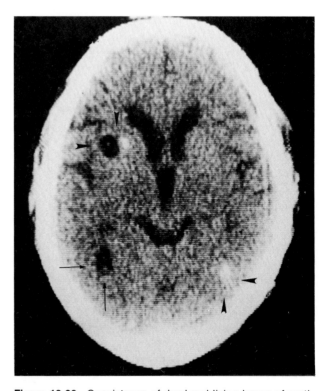

Figure 13-37 Dead intraparenchymal cysticercus. **A.** NCCT shows ill-defined low-density lesion in the parietal lobe. **B.** CECT demonstrates ringlike enhancement around the cyst and surrounding edema.

ulation from cysticerci ceases the immunological balance is disrupted, and the brain may then react to dead foreign bodies, resulting in acute inflammation.

Calcifications are a manifestation of dead larvae and may require 10 years or more to develop (Dixon 1961). Calcifications are seen only with the parenchymal form, not with ventricular or cisternal cysts. Usually they are located in the gray matter or near its junction with the white matter, but they are sometimes seen in the basal ganglia and occasionally in the midst of the white matter (Santin 1966) (Fig. 13-38). Calcification may involve both the wall and contents of the cyst. It typically appears round or slightly oval and is from 7 to 16 mm in size (Carbajal 1977). These wholly or partially calcified spheres frequently contain an eccentric small nodular calcification measuring 1 to 2 mm in diameter which represents the scolex of the erupted larva (Jankowski 1979). Both dead larvae with calcifications and living larvae may coexist in cases of reinfestation (Fig. 13-38). Vasculitis may develop in the vicinity of these lesions and lead to cortical arterial occlusion and infarction.

The differentiation of meningeal cysticercosis from arachnoid cyst and intradural epidermoid cyst, as well as the differentiation of intraventricular cysticercosis from colloid cyst, ependymal cyst,

Figure 13-38 Coexistence of dead and living larvae of cysticercosis. NCCT exhibits a rounded, low-density living larva (arrows) in the right occipital lobe and calcified cysts (arrowheads) in the right basal ganglia and the left occipital lobe. Calcification is a manifestation of dead larvae, occurring usually after 10 years and seen only with parenchymal forms.

or intraventricular epidermoid depends heavily on appropriate clinical information. Parenchymal cysticercosis can simulate primary or metastatic neoplasm, pyogenic abscess, and fungal infection. Cerebral infarctions must be considered in the differential diagnosis when enhancement around the cyst wall exists on CECT.

Hydatid Disease

Hydatid disease due to *Echinococcus granulosus* is usually manifested by cysts in the liver and lungs. Only 2 percent of hydatid infestations involve the CNS (Dew 1934).

Hydatid cysts of the brain are usually large and solitary, lying just a few millimeters below the cortex. Extradural cysts have been reported (Ozgen 1979). Multiple cysts are rare, but daughter cysts are not infrequent after inadvertent rupture or intentional puncture of a solitary cyst (Adams 1976).

On CT, a hydatid cyst appears as a large intraparenchymal cystic lesion, spherical in shape, with sharply defined borders. The density of the cyst contents is similar to that of water or CSF (Ozgen 1979) (Fig. 13-39). Severe distortion and shift of the ventricular system and hydrocephalus due to partial obstruction of cerebrospinal fluid pathways are usual findings. The lack of contrast enhancement at the periphery and of edema surrounding the cyst (Abbassioun 1978) serves to differentiate this lesion from cerebral abscess. Differentiation of an extracerebral hydatid cyst from arachnoid cyst may not be possible by CT alone.

Paragonimiasis

Paragonimus westermani is endemic in the Far East but recently has been decreasing in incidence. The freshwater crawfish is the intermediary. Owing to its common infestation of the lung, the ova of this fluke are commonly disseminated hematogenously and deposited in the brain parenchyma, meninges, and ventricles (Kim 1955).

Three forms of reaction of CNS tissue to paragonimiasis, namely, chronic arachnoiditis, granuloma, and encapsulated abscess, have been described (Kim 1961). On CT, isodense or mixed-density masses with ringlike or nodular contrast enhancement and perilesional edema are noted in early infestation of brain parenchyma (Figs. 13-40,

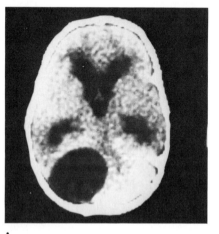
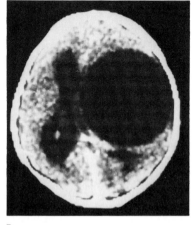
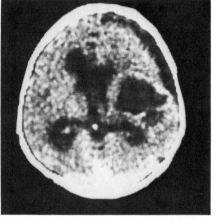

A   B   C

Figure 13-39 Hydatid cysts. **A.** A large cyst in the occipital lobe with no contrast enhancement of the capsule or perifocal edema. **B.** A large supratentorial hydatid cyst compressing the ipsilateral ventricle. **C.** Postsurgery view of *B* demonstrates reexpansion of the lateral ventricle. Marked decrease in size of the cyst with minimal rim enhancement. *(Reprinted with permission from Abbasioun et al., J Neurosurg 49:408–411, 1978.)*

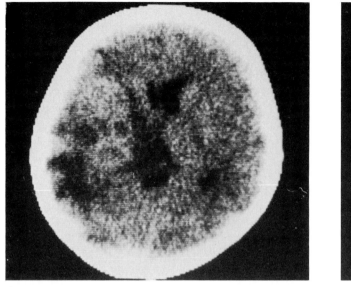

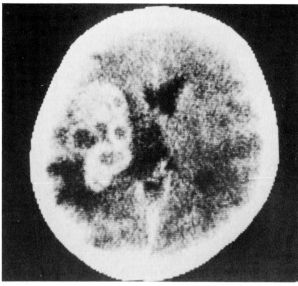

A

B

Figure 13-40 Paragonimiasis: intraparenchymal. **A.** On NCCT, irregular mixed-density lesion in the temporoparietal lobe is associated with focal edema. **B.** On CECT, multiple ova are clearly demonstrated as ringlike enhancement.

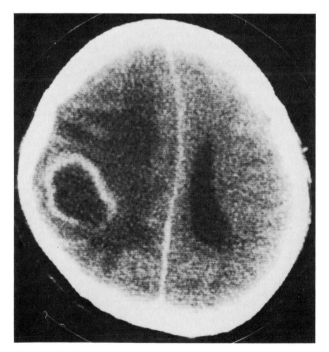

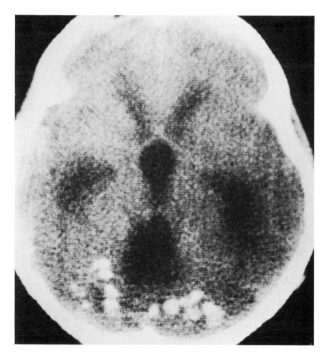

Figure 13-41 Paragonimiasis: intraparenchymal abscess. CECT shows a rounded lesion with peripheral enhancement and extensive edema, which represents encapsulated abscess.

Figure 13-42 Paragonimiasis: intraventricular and intraparenchymal. Fourth and third ventricles are dilated and filled with multiple cysts. Shell-like calcifications in the cerebellum are late manifestations of dead ova.

13-41). Differential diagnosis from other infectious diseases or even primary or metastatic tumors on the basis of CT findings alone at this stage is extremely difficult without appropriate clinical information. Intraventricular cysts show approximately CSF-equivalent density with no contrast enhancement (Fig. 13-42). Shell-like conglomerate calcification in the later stages is characteristic (Sim 1980), although spotty calcifications have also frequently been observed (Fig. 13-42).

Bibliography

ABBASSIOUN K et al: CT in hydatid cyst of the brain. *J Neurosurg* **49**:408–411, 1978.

ADAMS H: *Greenfield's Neuropathy.* Chicago, Year Book, 1976, pp. 227–278.

ANDERSON JM, MACMILLAN JJ: Intracranial tuberculoma: An increasing problem in Britain. *J Neurol Neurosurg Psychiatry* **38**:194–201, 1975.

ARMITSU T et al: CT in verified cases of tuberculous meningitis. *Neurology* **29**:384–386, 1979.

AUH YH, LEE SH, TOGLIA JU: Excessively small ventricles on cranial CT: Clinical correlation in 75 patients. *CT: J Comput Tomogr* **4**:325–329, 1980.

BAHR AL, KRUMBHOLZ A, KRISTT D, HODGES FJ: Neuroradiological manifestations of intracranial sarcoidosis. *Radiology* **127**:713–717, 1978.

BENSON JR et al: CT in intracranial cysticercosis. *J Comput Assist Tomogr* **1**(4):464–471, 1977.

BHARDARI T, SARKAN N: Subdural empyema: A review of 37 cases. *J Neurosurg* **32**:35–39, 1970.

BIAGI F, WILLIAMS K: Immunologic problems in the diagnosis of human cysticercosis. *Ann Parasitol Hum Comp* **49**:509–513, 1974.

BRITT RH, ENZMANN DR, REMINGTON JS: Intracranial infection in cardiac transplant recipients. *Ann Neurol* **9**:107–119, 1981.

BUTLER IJ, JOHNSON RT: Central nervous system infection. *Pediatr Clin North Am* **21**(3):649–668, 1974.

CAHILL DW, SALCUMAN M: Neurosarcoidosis—A review of the rare manifestation. *Surg Neurol* **15**(3):204–211, 1981.

CARBAJAL JR et al: Radiology of cysticercosis of the CNS, including CT. *Radiology* **125**:127–131, 1977.

CASSELMAN ES et al: CT of tuberculous meningitis in infants and children. *J Comput Assist Tomogr* **4**(2):211–216, 1980.

CLAVERIA LE, DU BOULAY GH, MOSELEY IF: Intracranial infections: Investigations by C.A.T. *Neuroradiology* **12**:59–71, 1976.

COCKRILL HH et al: CT in leptomeningeal infections. *Am J Roentgenol Radium Ther Nucl Med* **130**:511–515, 1978.

COULAN CN, SESHUL M, DONALDSON J: Intracranial ring lesions: Can we differentiate by CT? *Invest Radiol* **15**(2):103–112, 1980.

DAVIS JM et al: CT of herpes simplex encephalitis with clinicopathological correlation. *Radiology* **129**:409–417, 1978.

DEW HR: Hydatid disease of the brain. *Surg Gynecol Obstet* **59**:312–319, 1934.

DIXON HBF, LIPSCOMB FM: *Cysticercosis: An Analysis and Followup of 450 Cases.* Privy Council, Medical Research Council Report, no. 229, London, Her Majesty's Stationery Office, 1961, pp. 1–57.

DUBLIN AB, MERTEN DF: CT in the evaluation of herpes simplex encephalitis. *Radiology* **125**:133–134, 1977.

DUBLIN AB, PHILLIPS HE: CT of disseminated cerebral coccidioidomycosis. *Radiology* **135**:361–368, 1980.

DUNKER RO, KHAKOO RA: Failure of computed tomographic scanning to demonstrate subdural empyema. *JAMA* **246**(10):1116–1118, 1981.

EINSTEIN HE: Coccidioidomycosis of the CNS. *Adv Neurol* **6**:101–105, 1974.

ENZMANN DR, BRANT-ZAWADZKI M, BRITT RH: Computed tomography of central nervous system infections in immunosuppressed patients. *Am J Neuroradiol* **1**:239–243, 1980.

ENZMANN DR, BRITT RH, YEAGER AS: Experimental brain abscess evolution: Computed tomographic and neuropathologic correlation. *Radiology* **133**:113–122, 1979.

ENZMANN DR et al: CT of herpes simplex encephalitis. *Radiology* **129**:419–425, 1978.

ENZMANN DR, NORMAN D, MAIN J, NEWTON TH: CT of granulomatous basal arachnoiditis. *Radiology* **120**:341–344, 1976.

FEELY MP, DEMSEY PJ: Assessment of the post-operative course of excised brain abscess by computed tomography. *Neurosurgery* **5**(1):49–52, 1979.

FRASER RG, PARE JAP: *Diagnosis of Diseases of the Chest*, 2d ed. Philadelphia, Saunders, 1978, vol. 2, pp. 778–787.

FUJITA NK et al: Cryptococcal intracerebral mass lesions: The role of CT and non-surgical management. *Ann Intern Med* **94**:382–388, 1981.

GALBRAITH JG, BARR VW: Epidural abscess and subdural empyema. *Adv Neurol* **6**:257–267, 1974.

GREENBERG SB et al: CT in brain biopsy–proven herpes simplex encephalitis: Early normal results. *Arch Neurol* **38**:58–59, 1981.

GRIGGS RC, MANESBERRY WR, CONDEMI JJ: Cerebral mass due to sarcoidosis: Regression during corticosteroid therapy. *Neurology* **23**:981–989, 1973.

GRINELLI VS, BENTSON JR, HELMER E, WINTER J: Diagnosis of interhemispheric subdural empyema by CT. *J Comput Assist Tomogr* **1**(2):99–105, 1977.

GROSSMAN RI et al: CT of intracranial aspergillosis. *J Comput Assist Tomogr* **5**(5):646–650, 1981.

HANDEL SF, KLEIN WC, KIM YU: Intracranial epidural abscess. *Radiology* **111**:117–120, 1974.

HARRIMAN DGE: *Greenfield's Neuropathology*. Chicago, Year Book, 1976, pp. 238–247.

HARWOOD-NASH DC et al: Massive calcification of the brain in a newborn infant. *Am J Roentgenol* **108**:528–532, 1970.

HIRSH LF, LEE SH, SILBERSTEIN SD: Intracranial tuberculomas and the CAT scan. *Acta Neurochir (Wien)* **45**:155–161, 1978.

JANKOWSKI R, ZIMMERMAN RD, LEEDS NE: Cysticercosis presenting as a mass lesion at the foramen of Monro. *J Comput Assist Tomogr* **3**(5):694–696, 1979.

JOUBERT MD, STEPHANOV S: CT and surgical treatment in intracranial suppuration. *J Neurosurg* **47**:73–78, 1977.

KAMIN M, BIDDLE D: Conservative management of focal intracerebral infection. *Neurology* **31**:103–106, 1981.

KAUFMANN DM, LEEDS NE: CT in the diagnosis of intracranial abscesses. *Neurology* **27**:1069–1073, 1977.

KENDALL BE, TATELER GLV: Radiological findings in neurosarcoidosis. *Br J Radiol* **51**:81–92, 1978.

KERR FWL, KING RB, MEAGHER JN: Brain abscess: A study of 47 consecutive cases. *JAMA* **168**:868–872, 1958.

KETONEN L, KOSKINIEMI ML: CT appearance of herpes simplex encephalitis. *Clin Radiol* **31**:161–165, 1980.

KIM KS, WEINBERG PE, MAGIDSON M: Angiographic features of subdural empyema. *Radiology* **118:**621–625, 1976.

KIM RC et al: Traumatic intracerebral implantation of *Cladosporium trichoides. Neurology* **31:**1145–1148, 1981.

KIM SK: Cerebral paragonimiasis. *J Neurosurg* **12:**89–94, 1955.

KIM SK, WALKER AE: Cerebral paragonimiasis. *Acta Psychiatr Neurol Scand* **36:**153, 1961.

KOBRINE A, DAVIS DO, RIZZOLI HV: Multiple abscesses of the brain: Case report. *J Neurosurg* **54:**93–97, 1981.

KOTAGAL S, TANTANASIRIVONGSE S, ARCHER C: Periventricular calcification following neonatal ventriculitis. *J Comput Assist Tomogr* **5**(5):651–653, 1981.

KUMPE DA, RAO KCVG, GARCIA JH, HECK AF: Intracranial neurosarcoidosis. *J Comput Assist Tomogr* **3**(3):324–330, 1979.

LABEAU J et al: Surgical treatment of brain abscess and subdural empyema. *J Neurosurg* **38:**198, 1973.

LEE SH, KUMAR ARV, LORBER B: Tuberculosis of the CNS presenting as mass lesions: Diagnostic dilemma. *Pa Med* **82:**36–38, 1979.

LEO JS et al: CT in herpes simplex encephalitis. *Surg Neurol* **10:**313–317, 1978.

LINDHOLM J, RAMUSSEN P, KORSGAARD O: Intracellar or pituitary abscess. *J Neurosurg* **38:**616–626, 1973.

LONG JA et al: Cerebral mass lesion in torculosis demonstrated by CT. *J Comput Assist Tomogr* **4**(6):766–769, 1980.

LORBER J: Intracranial calcification following tuberculous meningitis in children. *Acta Radiol* **50:**204–210, 1958.

LOTT T et al: Evaluation of brain and epidural abscess by CT. *Radiology* **122:**371, 1977.

LUKEN MG, WHELAN MA: Recent diagnostic experience with subdural empyema. *J Neurosurg* **52:**764–771, 1980.

MALLOY PM, LEYMAN RM: The lack of specificity of neonatal paraventricular calcification. *Radiology* **80:**98–102, 1963.

MAUERSBERGER W: The determination of absorption values as an aid in CT differentiation between cerebral abscess and glioblastoma. *Adv Neurosurg* **9:**36–40, 1981.

MAYERS MM, KAUFMANN DF, MILLER MM: Recent cases of intracranial tuberculomas. *Neurology* **28:**256–260, 1978.

MCGAHAN JP: Classic and temporary imaging of coccidioidomycosis. *Am J Roentgenol* **136:**393–404, 1981.

MOORE GA, THOMAS LM: Infections including abscesses of the brain, spinal cord, intraspinal and intracranial lesions. *Surg Ann* **6:**413–417, 1974.

MOREHOUSE H, DANZIGER A: CT findings in intracranial neurosarcoid. *Comput Tomogr* **4:**267–270, 1981.

MORGAN H, WOOD MW: Cerebellar abscesses: A review of 7 cases. *Surg Neurol* **3:**93–96, 1975.

NAHSER HC et al: Development of brain abscesses—CT compared with morphological studies. *Adv Neurosurg* **9:**32–35, 1981.

NELSON JD, WATTS CC: Calcified subdural effusion following bacterial meningitis. *Am J Dis Child* **117:**730–733, 1969.

NEW PFJ, DAVIS KR: The role of CT scanning diagnosis of infections of the central nervous system, in Remington J, Swartz M (eds): *Current Clinical Topics in Infectious Diseases.* New York, McGraw-Hill, 1980, pp. 1–33.

NEW PFJ, DAVIS KR, BALLANTINE HT: Computed tomography in cerebral abscess. *Radiology* **121**:641–646, 1976.

NIELSEN H, GYLDENSTADT C: CT in the diagnosis of cerebral abscess. *Neuroradiology* **12**:207–217, 1977.

ÖZGEN T et al: The use of CT in the diagnosis of cerebral hydatid cysts. *J Neurosurg* **50**:339–342, 1979.

PAXTON R, AMBROSE J: The EMI scanner: A brief review of the first 600 patients. *Br J Radiol* **47**:530–565, 1974.

PEATFIELD RC, SHAWDON HH: Five cases of intracranial tuberculoma followed by serial CT. *J Neurol Neurosurg Psychiatry* **42**:373–379, 1979.

PFUETZE KH, RADNER DB (eds): *Clinical Tuberculosis: Essentials of Diagnosis and Treatment.* Springfield, Charles C Thomas, 1966.

PRICE HI, DANZIEGER A: CT in cranial tuberculosis. *Am J Roentgenol* **130**:769–771, 1978.

RAO KCVG, WILLIAMS JP, BRENNAN TG, KOSNIK E: Interhemispheric subdural empyema. *Child Brain* **4**:106–113, 1978.

ROBERT F: Sarcoidosis of the central nervous system. *Brain* **71**:451–475, 1948.

ROBERTHERAM EB, KESSLER LA: Use of computerized tomography in nonsurgical management of brain abscess. *Arch Neurol* **36**:25–26, 1979.

ROSENBAUM ML et al: Decreased mortality from brain abscesses since advent of CT. *J Neurosurg* **49**:659–668, 1978.

ROVIRA M, ROMERO F, TORRENT O, IBARRA B: Study of tuberculosis by CT. *Neuroradiology* **19**:137–141, 1980.

RUDWAN MA: Pituitary abscess. *Neuroradiology* **12**:243–248, 1977.

SADHU VK, HANDEL SF, PINTO RS, GLASS, TF: Neuroradiologic diagnosis of subdural empyema and CT limitation. *Am J Neuroradiol* **1**:39–44, 1980.

SALMON JH: Ventriculitis complicating meningitis. *Am J Dis Child* **124**:35–40, 1972.

SALTZMAN GF: Roentgenologic changes in cerebral sarcoidosis. *Acta Radiol [Diagn] (Stockh)* **50**:235–241, 1958.

SAMSON DS, CLARK K: A current review of brain abscess. *Am J Med* **54**:201–210, 1973.

SANTIN G, VARGAS J: Roentgen study of cysticercosis of CNS. *Radiology* **86**:520–528, 1966.

SCHULTZ P, LEEDS NE: Intraventricular septations complicating neonatal meningitis. *J Neurosurg* **38**:620–626, 1973.

SILVERSTEIN A, FEUER, MM, SILTZBACH LE: Neurologic sarcoidosis: Study of 18 cases. *Arch Neurol* **12**:1–11, 1965.

SIM BS: CT findings of parasitic infestations of the brain in Korea. *J Korean Neurosurg Soc* **9**(1):7–18, 1980.

SOUTH MA et al: Congenital malformation of the CNS associated with genital type (type 2) herpes virus. *J Pediatr* **75**:13–18, 1969.

STEPHANOV S et al: Combined convexity and parafalx subdural empyema. *Surg Neurol* **11**:147–151, 1979.

STEVENS EA et al: CT brain scanning in intraparenchymal pyogenic abscesses. *Am J Roentgenol* **130**:111–114, 1978.

VISUDHIPHAN P et al: Cerebral aspergillosis: Report of 3 cases. *J Neurosurg* **38**:472–476, 1973.

WAGGENER JD: The pathophysiology of bacterial meningitis and cerebral abscesses: An anatomical interpretation. *Adv Neurol* vol. 6, 1974.

WALLENFANG TH, REULEN JG, SCHURMANN K: Therapy of brain abscess. *Adv Neurosurg* **9**:41–47, 1981.

WEIDERHOLT WC, SIEKERT RG: Neurological manifestations of sarcoidosis. *Neurology* **15**:1147–1154, 1965.

WEINMAN D, SAMARASHINGHE HHR: Subdural empyema. *Aust N Z J Surg* **41**:324, 1972.

WELCHMAN JM: CT of intracranial tuberculomata. *Clin Radiol* **30**:567–573, 1979.

WHELAN MA, HILAL SK: Computed tomography as a guide in the diagnosis and followup of brain abscesses. *Radiology* **135**:663–671, 1980.

WHELAN MA, STERN J: Intracranial tuberculoma. *Radiology* **138**:75–81, 1981.

WHITLEY J et al: Adenine arabinoside therapy of biopsy-proven herpes simplex encephalitis. *N Engl J Med* **287**:289–294, 1977.

WITHAM RR, JOHNSON RH, ROBERTS DL: Diagnosis of miliary tuberculosis by cerebral CT. *Arch Intern Med* **139**:479–480, 1979.

ZEE CS, et al: Unusual neuroradiological features of intracranial cysticercosis. *Radiology* **137**:397–497, 1980.

ZEGERS DE BEYL D, NOTERMAN J, MARTELART A, FLAMENT-DURAND J, BALERIAUX D: Multiple cerebral hematoma and viral encephalitis. *Neuroradiology* **20**:47–48, 1980.

ZIMMERMAN RA, PATEL S, BILANIUK LT: Demonstration of purulent bacterial intracranial infections by computed tomography. *Am J Roentgenol* **127**:155–165, 1976.

ZIMMERMAN RA, BILANIUK LT, GALLO E: CT of the trapped fourth ventricle. *Am J Roentgenol* **130**:503–506, 1978.

ZIMMERMAN RD, et al: CT in the early diagnosis of herpes simplex encephalitis. *Am J Roentgenol* **134**:61–66, 1980.

ZORUB DS et al: Invasive pituitary adenoma with abscess formation: Case report. *Neurosurgery* **5**(6):718–722, 1979.

CEREBRAL VASCULAR ANOMALIES

Karel TerBrugge

Krishna C.V.G. Rao

Seungho Howard Lee

Cerebral vascular anomalies, which comprise aneurysms and vascular malformations, commonly present with a history of subarachnoid hemorrhage. Frequently with aneurysm there are a variety of clinical findings, such as transient ischemic attacks or signs of cranial nerve involvement. On the other hand, with vascular malformations seizures may be the presenting clinical symptom. CT is the first modality of examination providing an approach to selecting the patients as well as the time when the definitive study, cerebral angiography, should be performed.

INTRACRANIAL ANEURYSMS AND SUBARACHNOID HEMORRHAGE

An aneurysm is an abnormal focal enlargement of an artery. Aneurysms can be classified according to their appearance as saccular or fusiform. The etiological classification of aneurysms includes congenital, arteriosclerotic, mycotic, and dissecting. By far the most common type is the congenital, or so-called berry, aneurysm which is thought to be due to a defect in the tunica media (Crawford 1959; Crompton 1966). With advancing age, arteriosclerotic changes are thought to cause further weakening of the already defective tunica media, and this may result in enlargement or rupture of the aneurysm (Crompton 1966; Richardson 1941; Nystrom 1963; DuBoulay 1965; Sarwar 1976a).

The incidence of intracranial aneurysms in the general population is approximately 3 percent (Chason 1958; Housepian 1958). The aneurysm involves the carotid system in 95 percent and the vertebral basilar system in 5 percent of the cases (Locksley 1966). The anterior communicating artery is the single most common site (30 percent), followed by the posterior communicating artery (25 percent) and the middle cerebral artery (20 percent), according to Locksley (1966). Approximately 20 percent of patients with an intracranial aneurysm have more than

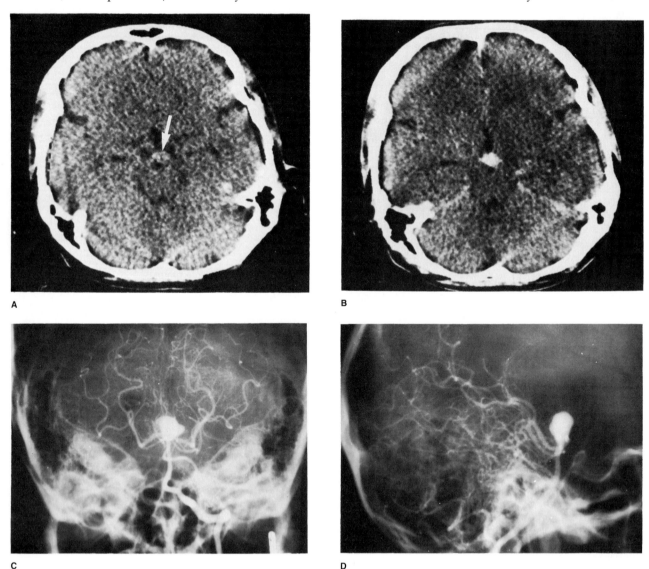

A

B

C

D

Figure 14-1 Basilar artery aneurysm. **A.** The NCCT shows a rounded area of slightly increased density at the level of the interpeduncular cistern (arrow). **B.** Enhancement occurs on CECT. **C, D.** Angiograms disclose a large aneurysm arising from the tip of the basilar artery.

one aneurysm demonstrated at angiography (McKissock 1964; Locksley 1966; Kendall 1976*b*). The great majority of the aneurysms are small in size (diameter less than 1 cm) and present with subarachnoid hemorrhage (DuBoulay 1965; Locksley 1966). The large-size (diameter between 1 and 2.5 cm) and giant-size (diameter greater then 2.5 cm) aneurysms usually do not present with subarachnoid hemorrhage but with clinical symptoms related to their localized mass effect and pressure upon the adjacent brain and cranial nerves (Bull 1969; Morley 1969; Sarwar 1976*a,b,*; Scotti 1977; Nadjmi 1978; Deeb 1979; Pinto 1979; Thron 1979).

The *CT appearance* of intracranial aneurysms depends on whether the entire lumen of the aneurysm is patent or whether there is a partial or complete thrombosis of the aneurysm. If the entire lumen of the aneurysm is patent, the lesion can be seen on CT as a rounded or elongated area of slightly increased density (Fig. 14-1) (Scotti 1977; Handa 1978;

Pinto 1979). After intravenous injection of contrast material the lumen of the aneurysm will show homogeneous enhancement and the margin of the lesion will be well defined (Scotti 1977; Handa 1978; Pinto 1979; Yock 1980). This appearance is easily explained on the basis of a hyperdense blood pool which is subsequently opacified by circulating iodine contrast material (Pressman 1975*b*; Pinto 1979; Yock 1980).

Partially thrombotic aneurysms have a different appearance, which is related to the presence of the thrombus and the degree of patency of the lumen within the aneurysm. On NCCT they show as a central or eccentric hyperdense region within an isodense or calcific area. The lesions are rounded or lobulated in appearance, and the margins are well defined. The central and peripheral zones are enhanced by contrast material, while the isodense zone is not (Fig. 14-2) (Lukin 1975; Sarwar 1976*a*; Scotti 1977; Perrett 1977; Handa 1978; Nadjmi 1978;

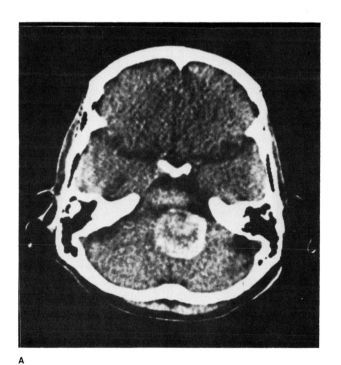

A

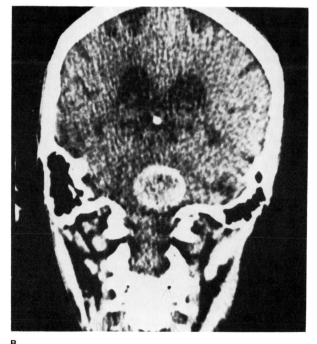

B

Figure 14-2 Posterior inferior cerebellar artery (PICA) aneurysm. **A.** The NCCT shows a rounded lesion adjacent to the left cerebellopontine angle cistern with a peripheral rim of calcification. **B.** The coronal CT shows the lesion to the left of the midline, superior to the foramen magnum. A central hypodense area is present with a rim of calcification. (*Continued on p. 550.*)

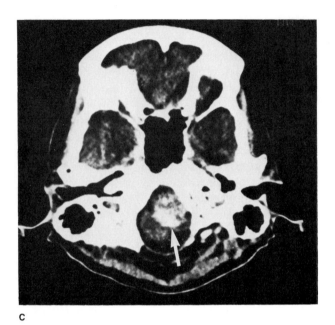

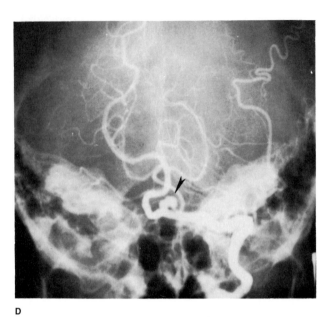

C   D

Figure 14-2 (Cont.)   **C.** The CECT at the level of the foramen magnum shows the lesion to be extraaxial in location, and there is eccentric enhancement in part of the lesion (arrow).   **D.** Angiogram shows the PICA aneurysm on the left side, consisting of a large thrombosed part and a small patent lumen.

Babu 1979; Pinto 1979; Thron 1979; Schubiger 1980). The CT appearance of a partially thrombotic aneurysm is due to a central or eccentric patent lumen of the aneurysm which enhances following contrast infusion. This lumen is surrounded by thrombotic material which is isodense on CT. The peripheral wall of the aneurysm consists of fibrous tissue, which is hyperdense on CT and often calcified. This rim of tissue contains increased vascularity, which is thought to be a meningeal response to the enlarging aneurysm, and enhancement of this tissue may be a phenomenon similar to the dural enhancement in other locations (Pinto 1979).

The *completely thrombosed aneurysm* exhibits a central area of isodensity or slightly decreased density and a peripheral rim of increased density and often calcific density (Fig. 14-3). The peripheral rim of increased density may show enhancement after contrast infusion (Nadjmi 1978; Pinto 1979). The central area of isodensity represents thrombus within the aneurysm, while the peripheral ring enhancement is thought to be due to increased microvascularity within the tissue along the wall of the aneurysm similar to dural enhancement (Pinto

1979). Meningioma or malignant glioma may mimic giant aneurysms (larger than 1 cm), but the lack of edema in aneurysms should rule out the tumors (Pinto 1979).

Ectasia of the intracranial arteries, and in particular the basilar artery, can be diagnosed on CT (Peterson 1977; Scotti 1978; Deeb 1979). The ectatic basilar artery may be seen crossing the prepontine cistern toward a cerebellopontine angle cistern as an elongated band-like structure of increased density on the NCCT. Homogeneous enhancement occurs after contrast infusion (Fig. 14-4). Tortuous vertebral-basilar arteries may be associated with cranial nerve syndromes and may result in hydrocephalus resulting from transmitted pulsation of the ectatic fusiform dilated vertebral basilar artery. CT has proved excellent for screening such cases, possibly obviating angiography (Deeb 1979) (Fig. 14-4).

The *differential diagnosis* of lesions which may mimic a small aneurysm consists mainly of variations from the normal vascular anatomy, such as looping of vessels or prominent veins. Depending on the clinical situation, angiography is often necessary to sort out these diagnostic problems. The

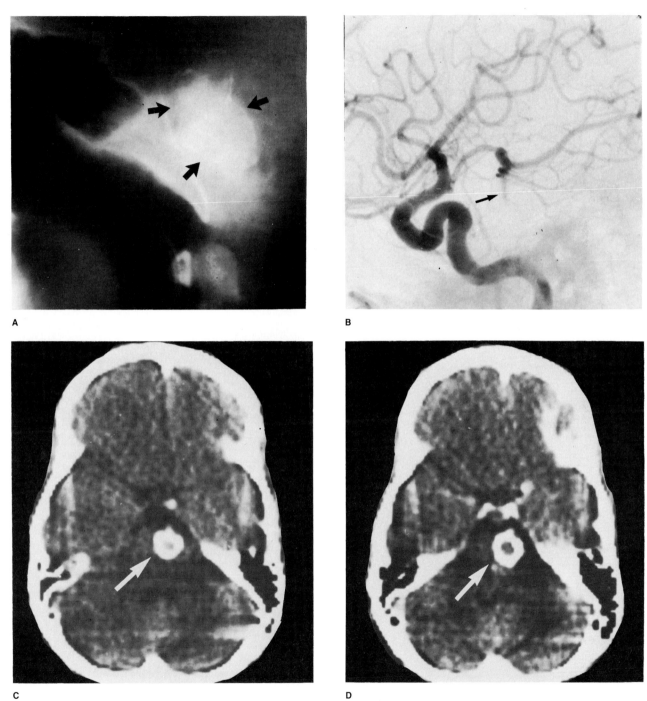

Figure 14-3 Completely thrombosed aneurysmal dilatation of basilar artery. **A.** Tomography in the lateral projection shows a partially calcified mass with curvilinear calcification posterior to the clivus (arrows). **B.** Carotid angiogram shows opacification of the distal basilar artery (arrow). Vertebral an-giogram (not shown) revealed no opacification of the basilar artery. **C, D.** The NCCT and CECT show a rounded lesion with a hypodense center and a peripheral rim of calcification located along the anterior aspect of the pons (arrow). *(Courtesy of Dr. G. Wortzman, Toronto General Hospital.)*

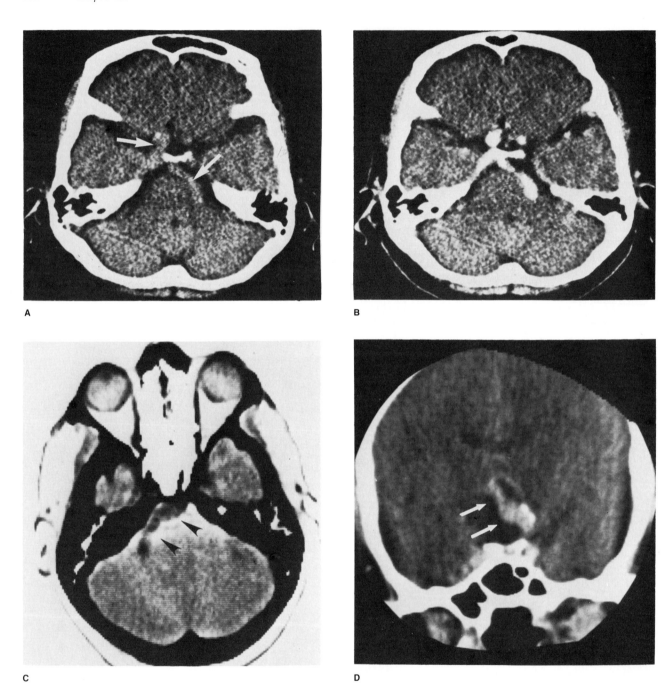

Figure 14-4 Ectasia of the basilar and carotid arteries. **A.** The NCCT shows an elongated band of hyperdensity which courses from the left cerebellopontine angle cistern toward the prepontine cistern (arrow). An elongated hyperdense area is noted along the right side of the suprasellar cistern (arrow). **B.** Enhancement of the lesions is present on CECT. Angiography confirmed ectasia of the basilar and right internal carotid artery system. **C, D.** Ectasia of the basilar artery. Axial and coronal CECT show ectasia of the vertebral basilar artery along its entire course in another patient.

CT appearance of large and giant aneurysms may be mimicked by a number of disease processes and depends to a certain degree on the location of the lesion. In the posterior fossa, large aneurysms may simulate intra- and extraaxial lesions (Handa 1978; Thron 1979). The extraaxial lesions which most often mimic an aneurysm are acoustic neuromas and meningiomas. Epidermoid tumors and chordomas may occasionally exhibit a CT pattern similar to large aneurysms. Intraaxial tumors which sometimes have a CT appearance mimicking large aneurysms are gliomas, medulloblastomas, ependymomas, choroid plexus papillomas, and metastatic disease (Byrd 1978). Para- and suprasellar lesions which may have a CT appearance similar to large aneurysms include pituitary adenomas, meningiomas, craniopharyngiomas, third ventricular tumors, and metastatic disease (Fig. 14-5) (Perrett 1977; Handa 1978; Babu 1979). Important features of large aneurysms on CT are the absence of surrounding edema and the presence of curvilinear peripheral calcifications. These characteristics are extremely

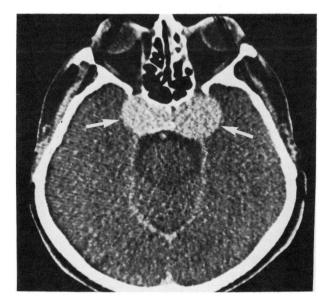

Figure 14-5 Bilateral internal carotid artery aneurysms. Homogeneous enhancement reveals two rounded lesions (arrows), each of which is located in the parasellar cistern, with extension toward the sella turcica simulating a pituitary adenoma or possible meningioma. Angiography confirmed presence of giant internal carotid aneurysms.

uncommon in neoplastic disease, with the exception of craniopharyngiomas. In such cases, rapid sequence (dynamic) CT scanning following intravenous bolus injection may be of help in distinguishing an aneurysm from a tumor (Fig. 14-6).

The advent of CT has led to postponement of invasive neuroradiological methods such as angiography. Past experience has indicated that many large and giant-size aneurysms were diagnosed on CT as neoplastic disease, and the possibility of a vascular abnormality was often not considered (Lukin 1975; Perrett 1977; Handa 1978; Nadjmi 1978; Babu 1979; Pinto 1979; Thron 1979). Therefore, awareness of the CT appearance of the large aneurysms is important, and angiography is indicated if the possibility of such an aneurysm cannot be excluded on CT. *Angiography* will generally establish the diagnosis but demonstrates only the part of the aneurysm with circulating blood. The mass effect related to the thrombus in the partially thrombotic aneurysm is often much better appreciated with CT. Angiography may be frankly misleading in the totally thrombosed aneurysm, which may show only as a nonvascular mass lesion (Fig. 14-7) (Nadjmi 1978; Pinto 1979; Thron 1979). Aneurysms may increase in size, and further growth of the aneurysm can be correctly diagnosed by means of CT, while a change in the patent lumen part of the aneurysm is better demonstrated by means of angiography (Fig. 14-8). CT can also be used to assess the postoperative status of an aneurysm, and it is the method of choice to investigate the remaining lumen of an inoperable giant aneurysm in patients who have undergone proximal ligation of the parent artery (Fig. 14-9) (Handa 1978).

The *CT detection* of intracranial aneurysms is greatly dependent on the size and location of the aneurysm. Since most aneurysms are small and located along the base of the skull, their detection has so far been limited by the spatial resolution of the CT system. A good-quality scan with thin slices and overlapping cuts along the base of the skull will detect an aneurysm larger than 5 mm in diameter, but at present angiography remains the method of choice to detect the small aneurysm with a diameter less than 5 mm.

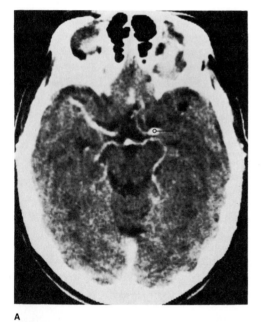

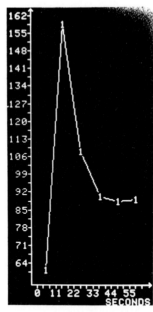

Figure 14-6 Dynamic CT scanning. **A.** CECT reveals a round area of hyperdensity (small circle) in the left side of the circle of Willis. **B.** Rapid-sequence CT scanning of the same region with a cursor was performed following intravenous bolus injection of contrast material. A time-density curve shows a rapid initial rise and fall, indicating the vascular structure. Angiography confirmed the presence of an aneurysm arising from the distal end of the internal carotid artery. This curve may be compared with the slow rise-and-decline curve, characteristic of a tumor, seen in a case of tuberculum sellae meningioma (**C, D**).

A

B

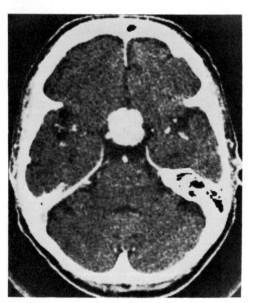

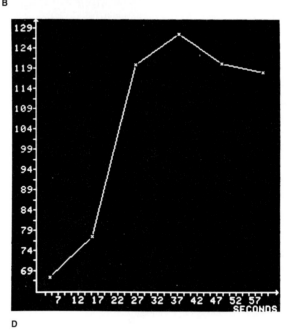

C

D

The advent of CT has significantly changed the method of investigation and management of patients with *subarachnoid hemorrhage* (Kendall 1976b; Liliequist 1977; Scotti 1977; Weir 1977; Modesti 1978). The mortality of patients with subarachnoid hemorrhage is high in the first few days after the ictus and is related to the mass effect of an intracranial hematoma (Weir 1977; Weisberg 1978). CT has proved to be the method of choice in the demonstration of subdural, subarachnoid, and intracerebral or intraventricular hemorrhage (Hayward 1977) (Fig. 14-10). Approximately 75 percent of pa-

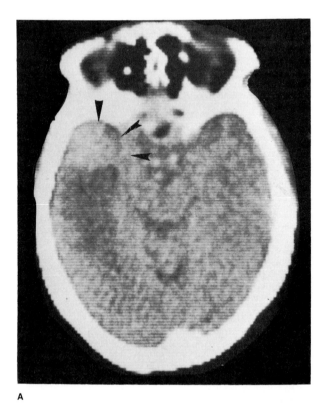

A

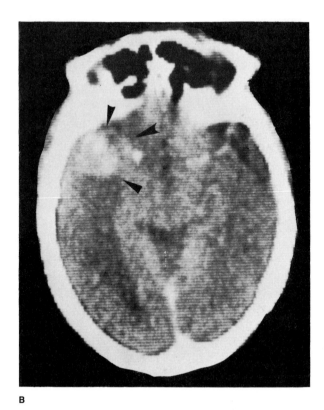

B

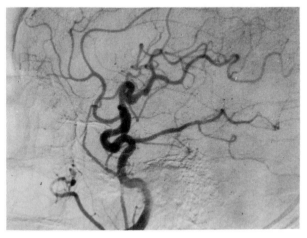

C

Figure 14-7 Thrombosed giant middle cerebral artery aneurysm. **A.** NCCT shows a moderately hyperdense area with surrounding low density. **B.** CECT shows homogeneous enhancement of the center with further peripheral enhancement, findings suggestive of a meningioma. **C.** Angiogram in lateral projection shows an avascular mass. The fusiform middle cerebral artery aneurysm was confirmed at surgery.

tients with subarachnoid hemorrhage have a ruptured aneurysm and 5 percent an arteriovenous malformation; in 15 percent no cause for bleeding is identified, based on angiography (Bjorkesten 1965).

In the first few days after the ictus, CT identifies blood in the subarachnoid space in approximately 80 percent of cases. The accuracy of detection of recently extravasated blood in the subarachnoid space declines with time, and generally no blood can be demonstrated 1 week after the ictus (Scotti 1977; Weir 1977; Modesti 1978). A false negative CT scan is not uncommon in patients with good neurological grades and therefore probably indicates a relatively small amount of blood in the subarachnoid space. This phenomenon is, however, not necessarily associated with a better clinical outcome (Weir 1977).

Various patterns can be recognized on CT in patients with subarachnoid hemorrhage, depending

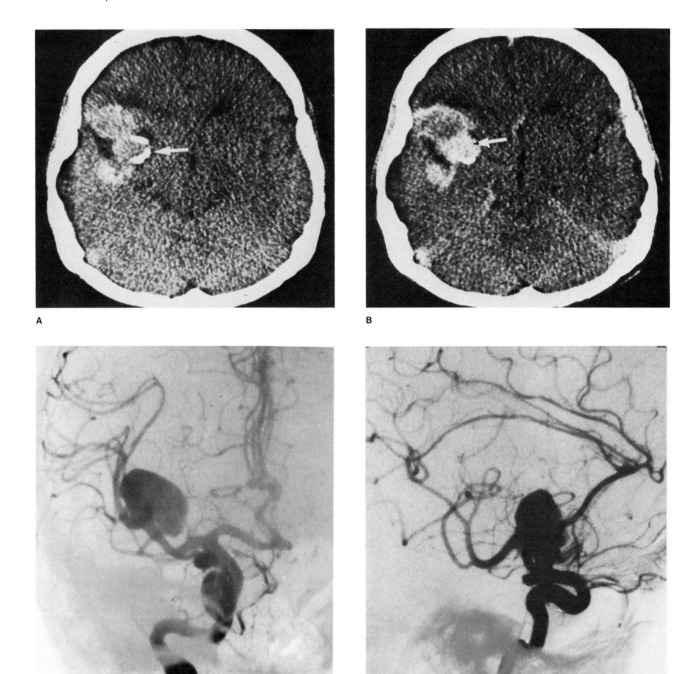

A

B

C

D

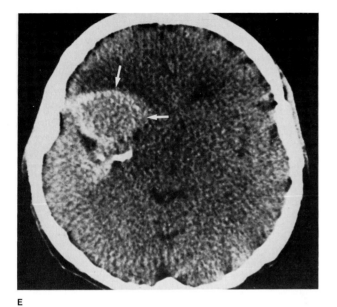

E

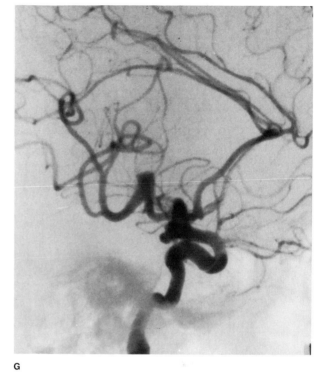

G

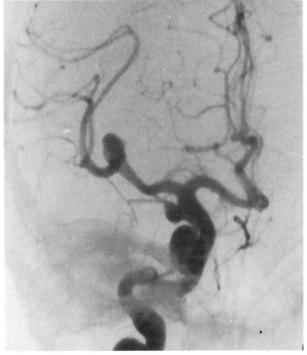

F

Figure 14-8 Giant middle cerebral artery aneurysms. **A.** The nonenhanced scan shows a lobulated lesion within the right sylvian fissure with rimlike calcification (arrow). **B.** After contrast infusion, eccentric enhancement is present (arrow). **C, D.** Angiogram in frontal and lateral projection shows a giant middle cerebral artery aneurysm. **E.** One-year follow-up without specific treatment shows increase in size of the thrombosed aneurysm (arrows). **F, G.** Angiogram shows that the patent lumen of the aneurysm has diminished dramatically since the initial examination.

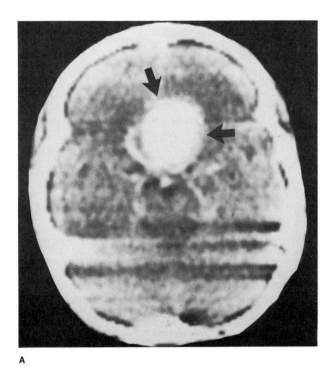

A

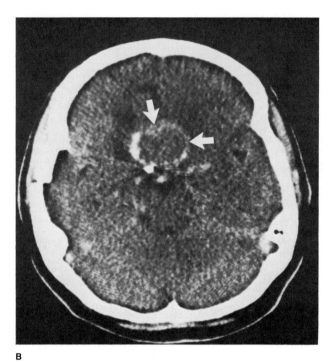

B

Figure 14-9 Giant anterior communicating artery aneurysm. **A.** Homogeneous enhancement of a rounded lesion at the level of the suprasellar cistern (arrows). Angiography revealed a giant anterior communicating artery aneurysm, and proximal ligation of the parent anterior cerebral artery was done. **B.** Six-month follow-up CECT shows no evidence of abnormal enhancement, and the aneurysm is completely thrombosed (arrow).

on the location of the ruptured aneurysm (Scotti 1977; Modesti 1978; Yock 1980). The anterior communicating artery aneurysm tends to bleed into the interhemispheric fissure and suprasellar cistern. The cingulate and callosal gyri are often outlined by blood. Frequently blood is also present around the brainstem and in the sylvian fissure (Fig. 14-11). Asymmetrical presence of blood in the sylvian fissure has been shown to occur with ruptured anterior communicating artery aneurysms and does not exclude that possibility (Yock 1980). The internal carotid and posterior communicating artery aneurysm tend to bleed into the suprasellar cistern and adjacent sylvian fissure. Blood is less frequently present within the interhemispheric fissure. Middle cerebral artery aneurysms invariably bleed into the sylvian fissure and adjacent suprasellar cistern. Aneurysms arising from the tip of the basilar artery bleed into the interpeduncular cistern around the brainstem and the suprasellar cistern, while bleeding into the sylvian and interhemispheric fissure is uncommon. Ruptured aneurysms arising from the posterior inferior cerebellar artery are often associated with false negative findings on the CT unless the bleeding is massive. In most cases, blood can be seen outlining the brainstem.

Care should be taken to distinguish the *normal falx* from recently extravasated blood into the interhemispheric fissure (Lim 1977). The posterior or retrocallosal aspect of the falx can be visualized in 88 percent of normal patients, while the anterior aspect is visualized on CT in 38 percent of patients without subarachnoid hemorrhage (Zimmerman 1982). When the increased density in the interhemispheric fissure does not extend into the paramedian sulci or does not show any change from previous CT, the diagnosis of normal falx is established (Osborn 1980).

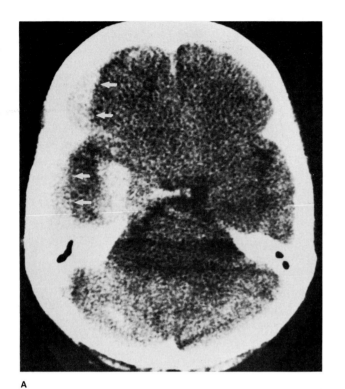

A

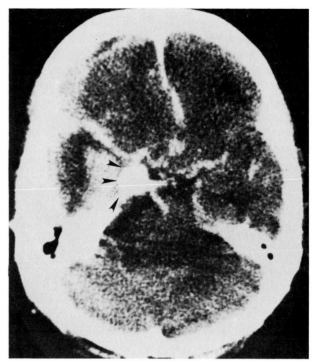

B

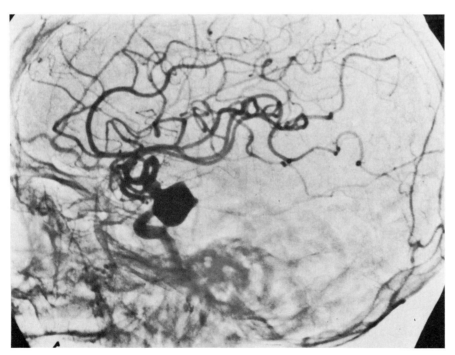

C

Figure 14-10 Internal carotid aneurysm: rupture into intracerebral, subarachnoid, and subdural spaces in a 70-year-old woman with no history of trauma. **A.** NCCT shows a medial temporal lobe hematoma and subdural hematoma (arrows) in the frontal and temporal regions. **B.** CECT shows a large aneurysm (arrowheads) originating from the internal carotid artery. **C.** Lateral cerebral angiogram confirms the location and origin of the bleeding aneurysm.

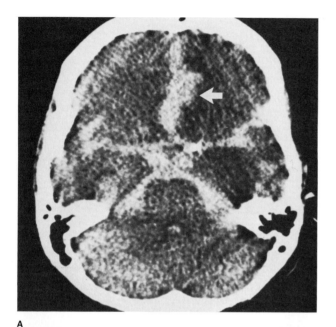

A

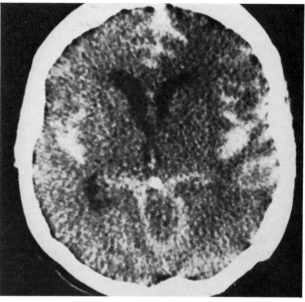

B

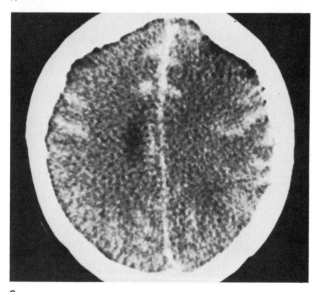

C

Figure 14-11 Subarachnoid hemorrhage following ruptured anterior communicating artery aneurysm.   **A.** The hyperdense recently extravasated blood outlines the suprasellar, interpeduncular, ambient, and sylvian cisterns. A localized hematoma is present along the anterior inferior aspect of the interhemispheric fissure (arrow).   **B.** The sylvian fissure and anterior interhemispheric fissure with the callosal and cingulate sulci are outlined with blood.   **C.** The interhemispheric fissure and sulci over the convexity are outlined with blood.

The ability to localize the ruptured aneurysm by means of CT is greatly improved if localized *hematoma* is present. Aneurysms arising from the anterior cerebral arterial complex tend to bleed into the adjacent frontal lobes and the septum pellucidum. A septal hematoma is present in 30 percent of ruptured anterior communicating artery aneurysms and invariably indicates the particular location of the aneurysm (Fig. 14-12) (Hayward 1976; Scotti 1977; Yock 1980), although the authors have seen such a hematoma from a ruptured pericallosal artery aneurysm and a posterior communicating artery aneurysm. Temporal lobe and basal ganglia hematomas occur with middle cerebral, posterior communicating, and internal carotid artery aneurysms (Fig. 14-10). The comma-shaped sylvian fissure hematomas are characteristic of ruptured middle cerebral artery aneurysm and are easily distinguishable from the external-capsule hematomas which occur in primary intracerebral hemorrhage in patients with hypertension (Fig. 14-13). Hayward (1976) reported 90 percent accuracy in the ability of CT to distinguish primary intracerebral hemorrhage from intracerebral hematoma caused by a ruptured intracranial aneurysm.

CT is of limited value in identifying, in cases of

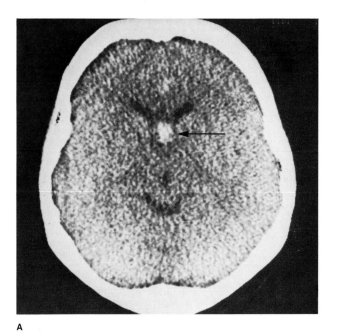

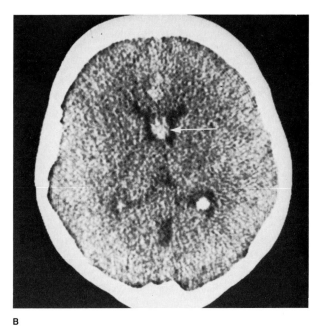

A

B

Figure 14-12 Septal hematoma due to anterior communicating artery aneurysm. **A, B.** A rounded area of increased density is present at the level of septum pellucidum (arrow), indicating a septal hematoma. An anterior communicating aneurysm was demonstrated at angiography.

multiple intracranial aneurysms, which one has bled if a nonspecific CT pattern is encountered. However, when localized hematoma is present in addition to the subarachnoid hemorrhage, the accuracy of CT may approach 100 percent (Aalmaani 1978).

Depending on the location of the aneurysm, contrast enhancement will allow for direct visualization of the aneurysm in 30 to 76 percent of the cases of subarachnoid hemorrhage and is therefore recommended (Ghoshhajra 1979; Yock 1980). When subarachnoid hemorrhage is associated with intracerebral or *subdural hematomas,* without a history of trauma, subdural hematoma of arterial origin (aneurysm or arteriovenous malformation) should be considered (Rengachary 1981). In such cases, CECT is indicated to elicit the source of bleeding (Fig. 14-10).

The advent of CT has greatly changed the role of angiography in the investigation and follow-up of patients with subarachnoid hemorrhage. The need for emergency angiography is diminished, and angiography can be delayed until the patient's condition stabilizes and surgery is contemplated. An-

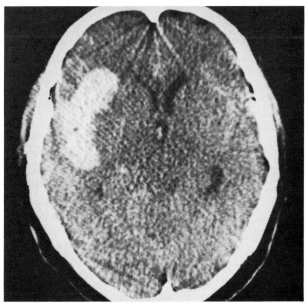

Figure 14-13 Sylvian fissure hematoma following middle cerebral artery ruptures: A large, comma-shaped, well-defined area of increased density at the level of the sylvian fissure indicates a sylvian fissure hematoma. Angiography demonstrated a right middle cerebral artery aneurysm.

giography should be directed primarily toward detailed demonstration of the vessels adjacent to the abnormality shown on CT.

The frequency of neurological deterioration of patients with subarachnoid hemorrhage is well known. CT has a definite role in the follow-up of these patients. Rebleeding of the aneurysm and ventricular enlargement are readily shown on CT. The development of *ventricular enlargement* appears to be a much more common phenomenon than previously realized and occurs in the first few days after the ictus in up to 60 percent of cases of subarachnoid hemorrhage (Modesti 1978). However, in contrast to the preliminary study by Davis et al (1980), the CT findings in patients with *vasospasm* are not as impressive in the author's opinion, and although CT may show cerebral edema and infarction, it often fails to show any change in a patient with angiographic evidence of severe vasospasm (Liliequist 1977; Ghoshhajra 1979). A negative CT, however, might be useful in such cases, since it would exclude rebleeding and ventricular enlargement and therefore might indirectly indicate vasospasm in a patient who is clinically deteriorating, although consistent correlation between vasospasm and clinical deterioration has not been proved.

CT should be the first investigative procedure in patients with possible subarachnoid hemorrhage. The study should be done as early as possible after the ictus and, if clinically indicated, should be done as an emergency procedure. CT accurately diagnoses, in addition to the subarachnoid hemorrhage, a significant intracranial hemorrhage or ventricular enlargement which may require immediate neurosurgical intervention. In cases where, in addition to the subarachnoid hemorrhage, a small localized hematoma is present, cerebral angiography and surgery may be postponed until the condition of the patient stabilizes. A negative CT scan does not exclude the possibility of recent subarachnoid hemorrhage, and in these circumstances a lumbar puncture is warranted. If the lumbar puncture reveals evidence of subarachnoid hemorrhage, digital intravenous angiography and/or arteriography is indicated when the condition of the patient stabilizes.

INTRACRANIAL VASCULAR MALFORMATION

Vascular malformations are developmental malformations of the vascular bed. They are classified into four groups: capillary telangiectasis, cavernous angioma, arteriovenous malformation, and venous malformation. An increase in the size of the malformation may occasionally be demonstrated, and progressive destruction of the adjacent brain tissue may occur, but there is no evidence of neural tissue proliferation and therefore no evidence of neoplastic disease (Russell 1977).

Capillary Telangiectasis

These lesions are composed of dilated capillary blood vessels which vary greatly in caliber; the vessels are separated by normal neural tissue. The lesions are a relatively common incidental finding at autopsy but are rarely symptomatic. They are uncommonly associated with hemorrhage. In the hereditary form, called Rendu-Osler-Weber disease, multiple cutaneous and mucosal lesions are present. This form is often symptomatic. The lesions of telangiectasis are most often located in the pons, but other sites include the cerebral cortex and subcortical white matter. Angiographically a blush may be demonstrated in the capillary phase within the malformation, but most often the angiogram is negative (Poser 1957; Roberson 1974). Patients frequently present with focal areas of hemorrhage. The CT may demonstrate cerebellar atrophy in capillary telangiectasis (Assencio-Ferreira 1981), although actual CT demonstration of the lesion itself has, to our knowledge, not been reported. We have seen one case of telangiectasia pathologically confirmed. NCCT demonstrated two hyperdense lesions with slight enhancement on CECT (Fig. 14-14). These findings are nonspecific.

Cavernous Hemangioma

Cavernous hemangiomas are composed of large sinusoidal vascular spaces which are closely clustered

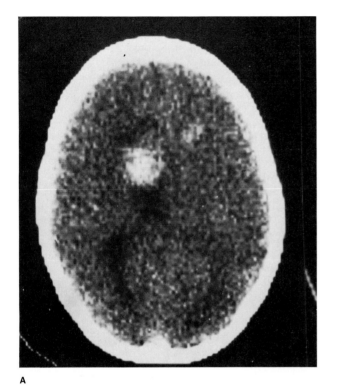

A

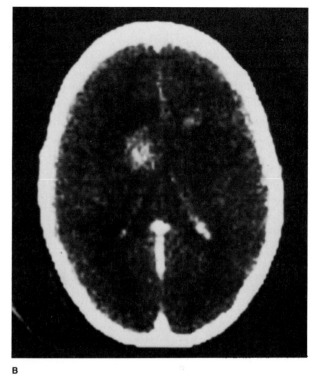

B

C

Figure 14-14 Telangectasia. **A.** Two small hemorrhagic areas are seen on NCCT. **B.** No change in density on CECT. **C.** A capillary blush is noted on angiography (arrows). Subsequently proved following surgery. *(Courtesy of Dr. A. J. Kumar, Johns Hopkins Hospital.)*

together; the vessels are not separated by normal neural tissue. Hemangiomas represent the rarest form of vascular malformation but are clinically important because they are often symptomatic, causing seizures. They are commonly within the intracerebral hemispheres, particularly in the subcortical region. Calcification is present in 30 percent of cases. Angiography is frequently normal, although prolonged injection angiography may demonstrate feeding arteries, a capillary blush, and abnormal draining veins (Numaguchi 1979). CT findings consist of a hyperdense and often partially calcified lesion which shows fairly homogeneous enhancement of minimum degree (Fig. 14-15A) or no enhancement (Fig. 14-15B) depending on whether they are partially or completely thrombosed. The

lesion is not associated with mass effect or surrounding edema except when recent hemorrhage is present (Bartlett 1977; Ito 1978; Numaguchi 1979; Ramina 1980). Occasionally the CT appearance may be indistinguishable from a meningioma (Ishikawa 1980), but the location of the lesion is often intracerebral.

Arteriovenous Malformation

This is a vascular malformation in which there is an intimate topographic admixture of arteries and veins. It represents the most common form of vascular malformation. It is clinically important because it is often symptomatic. According to LeBlanc (1979), 55 percent of arteriovenous malformations present with intracranial hemorrhage, 36 percent

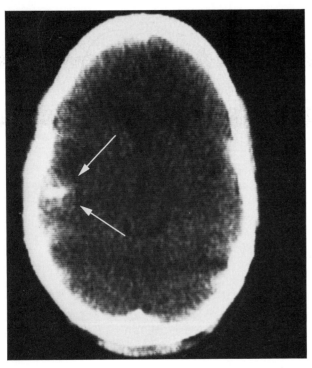

A

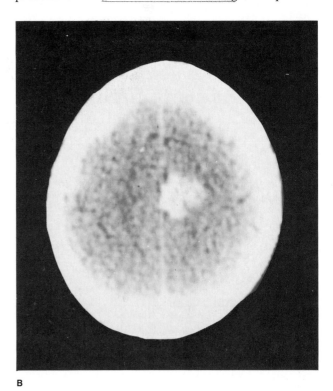

B

Figure 14-15 Cavernous hemangioma. **A.** NCCT shows calcified lesion in the temporal lobe in a 33-year-old woman with seizures. CT number measures 90 HU. CECT (not shown) failed to demonstrate obvious enhancement, but, on measurement, increase of 60 to 150 HU in the same area was noted. At surgery, partially thrombosed cavernous hemangioma with dystrophic calcification and an old and a recent hemorrhage were found. **B.** Another cavernous hemangioma. CECT shows a calcified parasagittal lesion without evidence of contrast enhancement or surrounding edema. Angiography failed to show any vascular abnormality, but a cavernous hemangioma was proved at surgery. *(Courtesy Dr. G. Wortzman, Toronto General Hospital.)*

with a seizure disorder, and 9 percent with headaches and progressive neurological deficit. Approximately 12 percent of patients with subarachnoid hemorrhage were found to have an underlying arteriovenous malformation (Hayward 1976). The lesions may occur in all parts of the central nervous system but are commonly located in the distribution of the middle cerebral artery along the cortex of the brain. The brain parenchyma adjacent to an arteriovenous malformation shows destructive and atrophic changes (TerBrugge 1977; Russell 1977). Calcifications are often present within the vascular channels as well as in the adjacent brain parenchyma (Figs. 14-16, 14-17).

The angiographic appearance of an arteriovenous malformation is that of abnormally dilated and tortuous feeding arteries and a racemose tangle of increased vascularity, which drains early into tortuous and elongated veins. Occasionally the malformation may become partially or completely thrombosed, and angiography may fail to show any evidence of it.

The CT appearance of intracranial arteriovenous malformation, when not associated with recent hemorrhage, is fairly characteristic (TerBrugge 1977; Pressman 1975; Kendall 1976a). The lesion most commonly presents on NCCT as an area of mixed density. Focal areas of hyperdensity are interspersed with areas of decreased density. The margins of the lesions are poorly defined and irregular in outline. After contrast infusion, the lesion will show nonhomogeneous enhancement (Fig. 14-16).

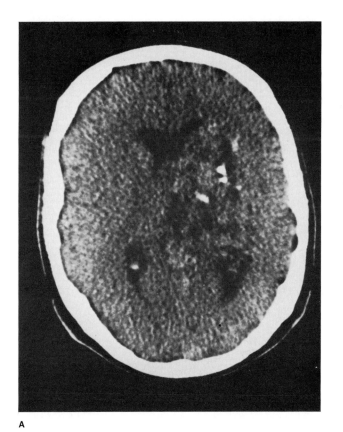
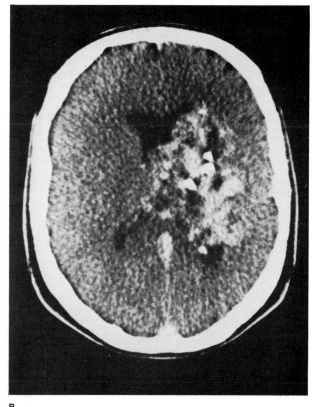

A

B

Figure 14-16 Arteriovenous malformation (AVM). **A.** A large, poorly defined area of mixed density interspersed with calcifications is present within the basal ganglia and thalamus on the left side. **B.** On CECT, nonhomogeneous enhancement occurs. Note persistence of focal areas of decreased density and absence of edema surrounding the angiographically proved AVM.

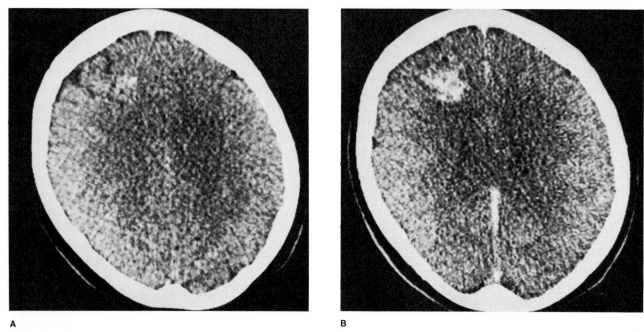

A   B

Figure 14-17   Arteriovenous malformation (AVM).   **A.** A focal area of cortical atrophy is noted on NCCT, with minute calcifications.   **B.** Nonhomogeneous enhancement is present on CECT. The margins are poorly defined, without evidence of edema, in this angiographically proved AVM.

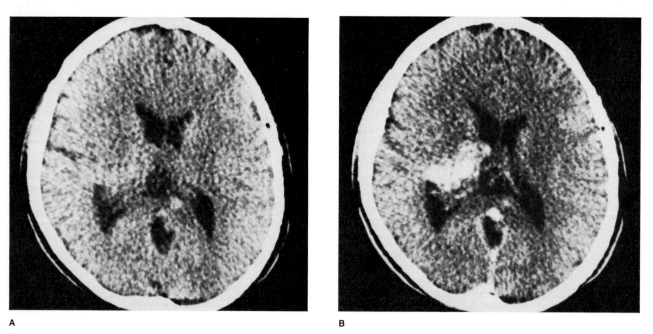

A   B

Figure 14-18   Arteriovenous malformation (AVM).   **A.** Ventricular asymmetry with focal compression of the body of the lateral ventricle is present on NCCT.   **B.** On CECT, nonhomogeneous enhancement of lesion with poorly defined margins adjacent to the body of the lateral ventricle is noted without evidence of surrounding edema. AVM proved at angiography.

Feeding arteries and draining veins may be recognized on CT. The lesion may be associated with focal atrophy (Fig. 14-17) and localized mass effect (Fig. 14-18), but surrounding edema is extremely uncommon (LeBlanc 1979; TerBrugge 1977).

A significant number of arteriovenous malformations will not show an abnormality on NCCT and become apparent only after contrast infusion, which is therefore a mandatory part of the examination (TerBrugge 1977). CECT will show nonhomogeneous enhancement and poorly defined margins of the lesion (Fig. 14-19).

One may observe areas of increased density, usually in the range of 40 to 50 HU, on NCCT (Michels 1977). Postulated explanations for this baseline increased density implicate the presence of local gliosis and hemosiderosis (New 1975), mural thrombus or calcification, or an increased blood pool (Pressman 1975). CECT demonstrates enhancement of the central angiomatous mass and visualization of adjacent vessels (Fig. 14-19).

A small number of arteriovenous malformations exhibit a predominantly hyperdense appearance and are heavily calcified (Fig. 14-20). Enhancement may be difficult to detect in such angiographically occult arteriovenous malformations with CT number measurements (Kramer 1977; Golden 1978; Sartor 1978; Bell 1978; Teraco 1979; LeBlanc 1981). Delayed high-dose CT scanning is of little value in the evaluation of patients with angiographically occult, thrombosed arteriovenous malformations (Hayman 1981). Contrast enhancement of these calcified, thrombosed arteriovenous malformations, as mentioned earlier under cavernous hemangiomas, probably depends on the degree and extent of thrombosis.

Unusual patterns of arteriovenous malformation on CT have been described in which a well-defined area of decreased density was a prominent feature (Fig. 14-21). These cases presumably reflect patients who have had previous episodes of hemorrhage associated with the arteriovenous malformation

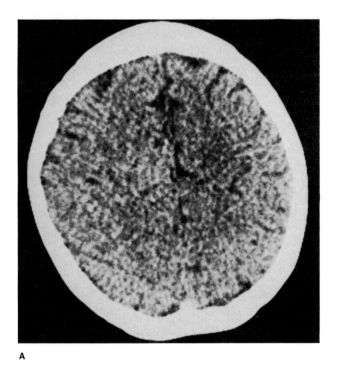

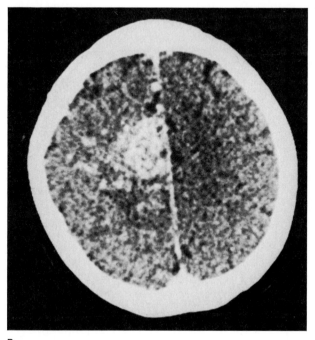

A   **B**

Figure 14-19 Arteriovenous malformation. **A.** NCCT shows slightly increased density. **B.** On CECT there is nonhomogeneous enhancement of the lesion with poorly defined margins representing central angiomatous mass. Multiple peripheral dotlike enhancement sites represent adjacent enlarged vessels.

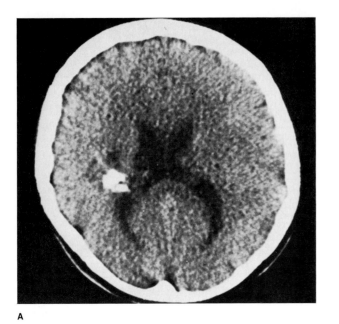

A

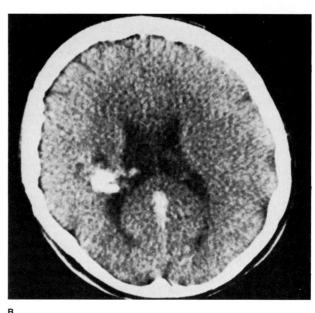

B

Figure 14-20 Thrombosed arteriovenous malformation (AVM). **A.** NCCT shows a small, predominantly calcified lesion adjacent to the trigone of the right lateral ventricle. **B.** CECT shows subtle enhancement detectable only by CT number measurements. Angiogram proved to be normal. A thrombosed AVM was proved at surgery.

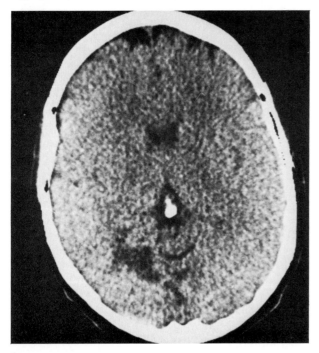

A

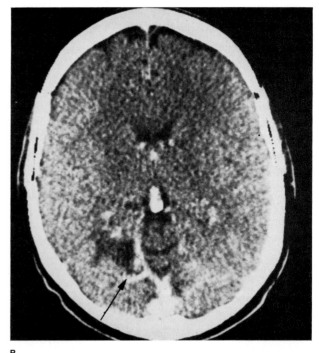

B

Figure 14-21 Arteriovenous malformation (AVM) associated with resolving hematoma. **A.** NCCT shows a triangular, well-defined area of decreased density along the medial aspect of the right occipital lobe. **B.** CECT shows abnormal enhancement present along the margin of the lesion. An enlarged draining vein is noted along the edge of the tentorium (arrow). Angiography demonstrated a small occipital AVM which, by clinical history, probably had bled 2 years prior to this examination.

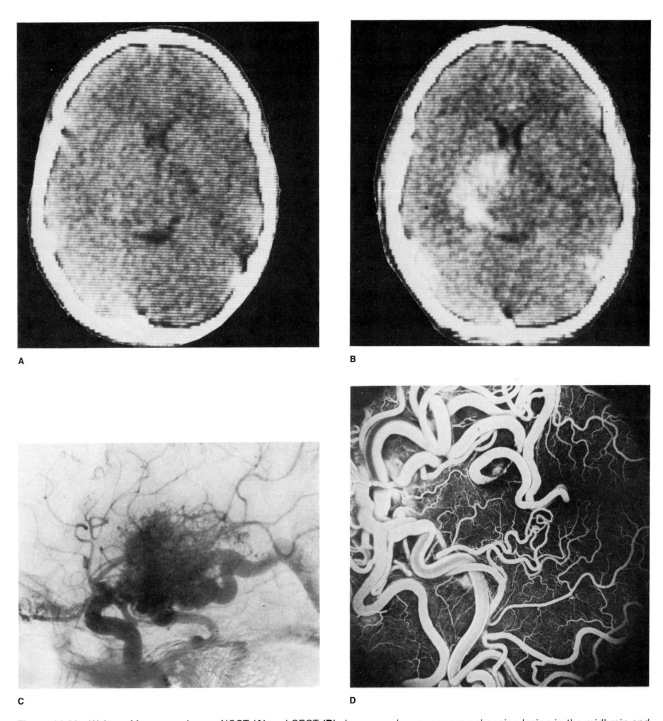

Figure 14-22   Wyburn-Mason syndrome. NCCT **(A)** and CECT **(B)** show a nonhomogeneous enhancing lesion in the midbrain and thalamus.   **C.** Angiogram demonstrates the vascular malformation, with extension of vascular anomaly along the optic nerve into the orbit.   **D.** Racemose retinal angiomatosis shown by fluorescein angiography.

with subsequent resolving hematoma and "cyst" formation (Daniels 1979; Britt 1980). On careful inspection, a partial curvilinear enhancement at the margin of the cystlike lesion, without surrounding edema or mass effect, may give a clue as to the presence of underlying arteriovenous malformation. Occasionally, in rupture of arteriovenous malformations, extravasation of blood into the preexisting cystic cavities presents as intraparenchymal blood-fluid levels (Richmond 1981). Spontaneous closure of the arteriovenous malformation of the basal ganglia is demonstrated on CT as nonenhancing, well-demarcated hypodensity with focal dilatation of adjacent lateral ventricle (Sartor 1978).

A characteristic but rare form of arteriovenous malformation has been described in the midbrain associated with ipsilateral angiomatosis of the retina and presence of a cutaneous nevus in the distribution of the trigeminal nerve, called *Wyburn-Mason syndrome* (Wyburn-Mason 1943). CECT usually demonstrates a nonhomogeneous density of varying size, most commonly in the midbrain (Fig. 14-22). The orbital component of the vascular malformation around the optic nerve, which is always on the same side as the retinal angiomas and the intracranial AVM, may not be detected by CT unless high-resolution thin sections are obtained or the orbital vascular component is very large. The extent of the orbital as well as intracranial vascular anomaly can be confirmed by angiography.

Another variant of the arteriovenous malformation is the *aneurysm of the vein of Galen,* which consists largely of an impressive aneurysmal dilatation of the varix of the great vein of Galen which may cause compression of the midbrain and aqueduct. The CT findings in patients with aneurysm of the vein of Galen are fairly characteristic (MacPherson 1979; Spallone 1979). A well-defined, hyperdense, rounded or triangular mass lesion in the region of the vein of Galen is noted on NCCT. Homogeneous enhancement occurs after contrast infusion (Fig. 14-23). Hydrocephalus is invariably present. CT is of great value in the postoperative assessment of these patients in demonstrating the development of thrombosis within the cavity of the varix, as well as in the recognition of hydrocephalus and possible subdural effusions (Diebler 1981).

The accuracy of CT in the detection of pial and

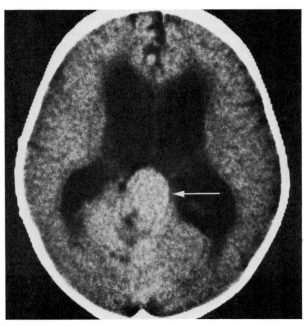

A

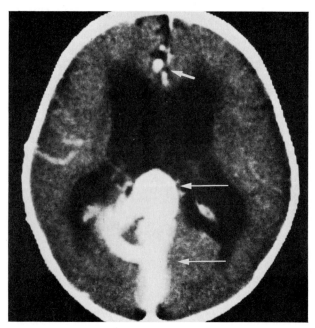

B

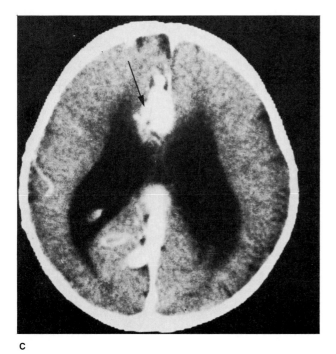

C

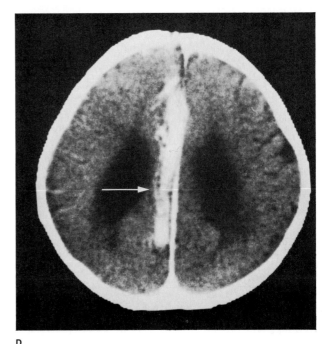

D

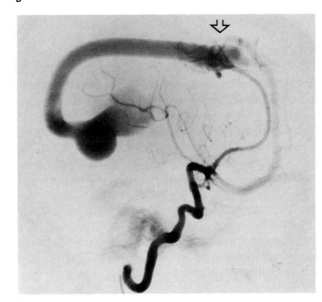

E

F

Figure 14-23 Midline arteriovenous malformation (AVM) with aneurysmal dilatation of inferior longitudinal sinus and vein of Galen. **A.** An elongated area of slightly increased density is present at the level of the vein of Galen (arrow). **B.** CECT. Enhancement outlines the enlarged anterior cerebral arteries (small arrow) and the engorged vein of Galen and straight sinus (large arrows.) **C, D.** Enhancement of the vascular mal-

formation along the anterior-superior aspect of the corpus callosum (black arrow) and the ectatic inferior longitudinal sinus (white arrow). **E, F.** Angiogram in the frontal and lateral projection shows a midline AVM (arrow) with secondary enlargement of the inferior longitudinal sinus and vein of Galen. *(Courtesy of Dr. D. Harwood-Nash, Toronto Hospital for Sick Children.)*

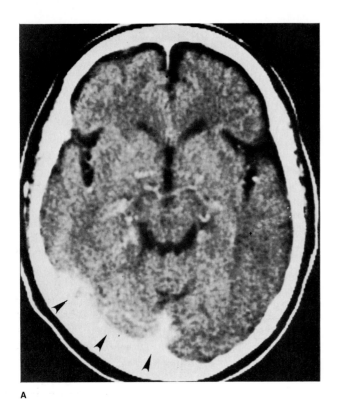

A

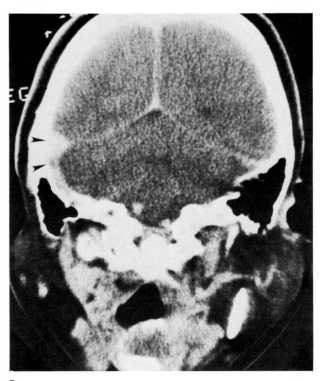

B

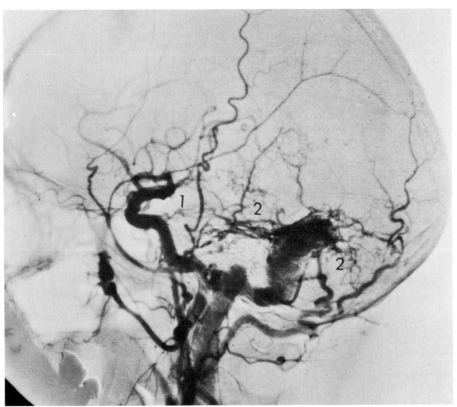

C

Figure 14-24 Dural arteriovenous malformation. Axial **(A)** and coronal **(B)** CECT images demonstrate contrast enhancement along the right transverse sinus (arrowheads). This CT finding could represent a normal transverse sinus and is nonspecific. **C.** Lateral cerebral angiogram shows multiple dural branches from internal (1) and external (2) carotid arteries, supplying the dural arteriovenous malformation with rapid shunting into the transverse sinus and jugular vein.

mixed pial and dural type of arteriovenous malformation is reported to be as high as 100 percent when good-quality scans are done with and without contrast enhancement (TerBrugge 1977). False negative results, however, are common in the pure dural type of arteriovenous malformation (Fig. 14-24).

Approximately 50 percent of patients with an arteriovenous malformation present with intracranial hemorrhage (LeBlanc 1979). Bleeding often occurs into the subarachnoid space or into the ventricular system, less often into the brain parenchyma (Fig. 14-25), and rarely into the subdural space (Rengachary 1981). Intracranial hemorrhage may occasionally obscure arteriovenous malformation on initial CT. Therefore, follow-up CT, subsequent to resorption of hemorrhage, may be necessary to demonstrate the underlying AVM. Furthermore, whenever a cortical hematoma is identified in a young patient who is normotensive, an underlying vascular malformation should be strongly suspected and angiography should be done (Solis 1977; Cone 1979).

Angiography remains the definitive method of diagnosis of arteriovenous malformation and will certainly be required to demonstrate the anatomy of the malformation before treatment is planned.

Venous Angioma

This vascular malformation is composed solely of veins. The abnormality consists either of an enlarged single vein with many tributaries or a compact group of such veins. They represent the rarest type of vascular malformation. They occur in both the cerebrum and cerebellum, but the most frequent site is the spinal cord and its meninges. They are clinically often asymptomatic, but they may be associated with subarachnoid or intracerebral hemorrhage or with seizures.

The angiogram shows a normal arterial and capillary phase with multiple venules draining in an umbrella-type pattern toward an engorged draining vein, which is often positioned perpendicular to the cortex. NCCT is normal in the majority of cases, although sometimes a rounded hyperdense area is noted. CECT shows a rounded or linear area of enhancement which is not associated with mass effect or surrounding edema (Michels 1977; Fierstein 1979) (Fig. 14-26).

A variant of venous malformation is the encephalofacial angiomatosis of *Sturge-Weber disease.* This rare condition consists in the association of an extensive capillary-venous malformation affecting one cerebral hemisphere with a homolateral cutaneous nevus or port-wine stain in the trigeminal nerve distribution, together with contralateral hemiparesis and Jacksonian epilepsy. Plain skull films may show characteristic "tram line" type calcification along the cortical gyri. The affected brain is atrophied, and the overlying leptomeninges are thickened. The angiogram shows a decrease in number or a complete absence of cortical superficial veins and enlargement of the deep cerebral venous system (Bentson 1971). On NCCT there is cortical atrophy with superficial cortical calcification (Welch 1980). Enhancement of the involved cortex occurs after contrast infusion (Fig. 14-27). The ipsilateral cranial vault is thickened and the hemicranium is most often smaller in size as compared with the normal opposite side. Ipsilateral enlargement of the hemicranium is uncommon (Enzmann 1977).

The value of CT in embolization of cerebral AVM rests on detection of complications, mainly infarction and hemorrhage, following interventional procedure. On CT, tantalum powders mixed with embolizing materials give rise to metal artifacts, but silicone spheres do not (Fig. 14-28). Dynamic scanning with fast scanning time may be of assistance in evaluation of the dynamic changes of blood flow associated with embolization of AVM.

CT should be the first investigation in patients with possible vascular malformations. Both NCCT and CECT are mandatory in the investigation of patients with intracranial vascular malformations. The degree of accuracy in the detection of an abnormality in such patients is high, although frequently angiography may be necessary to establish the definitive diagnosis. CT is not able to exclude the possibility of a pure dural vascular malformation, and angiography is mandatory in such cases. CT is superior to angiography in the demonstration of completely thrombosed vascular malformations and in the diagnosis of intracranial hemorrhage, which is frequently a complication associated with intracranial vascular malformation.

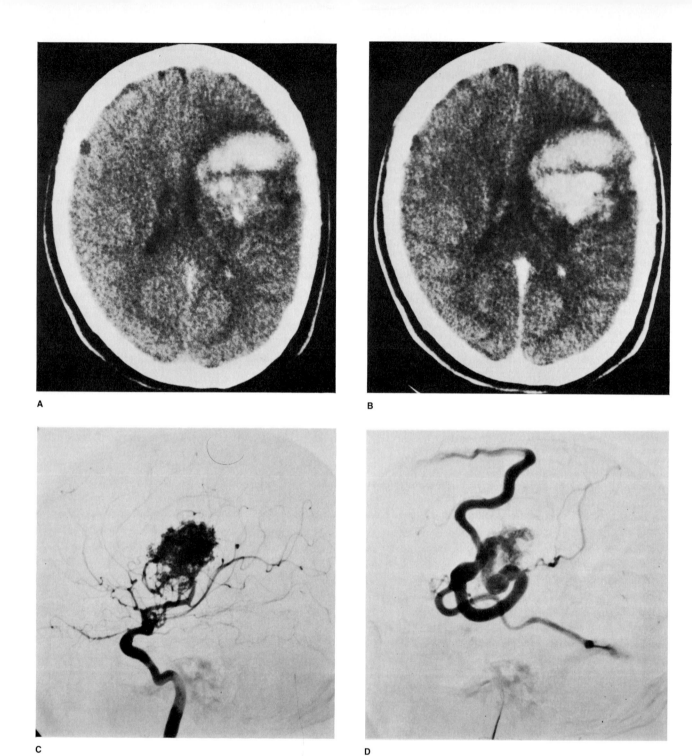

Figure 14-25 Calcified arteriovenous malformation presenting with hematoma. **A.** NCCT shows a large intracerebral hematoma anteriorly and a hyperdense mass with punctate calcifications posteriorly. **B.** CECT exhibits intense enhancement of the calcified posterior lesion. **C, D.** Lateral angiograms demonstrate a frontoparietal arteriovenous malformation supplied by middle cerebral artery branches and drained by cortical veins.

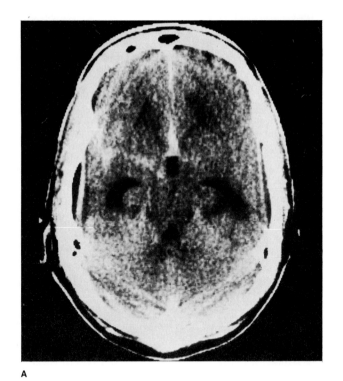

A

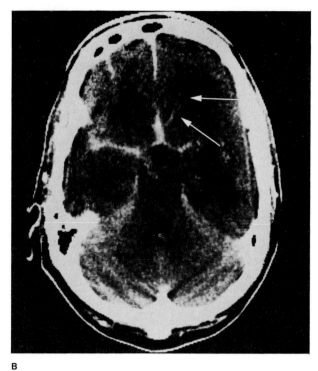

B

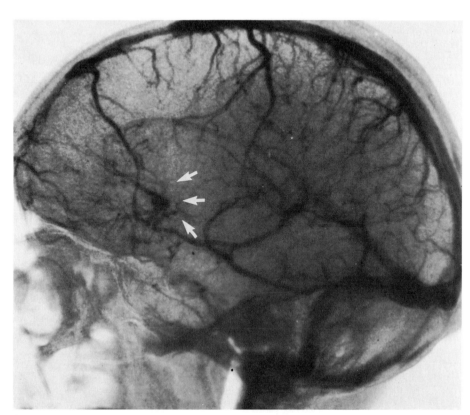

C

Figure 14-26 Venous angioma.
A. NCCT shows no abnormality.
B. CECT shows linear enhancement along the medial border of the frontal horn (arrows), representing draining veins. No surrounding edema or mass effect is noted. **C.** Angiogram reveals irregular vessels in medusa-like pattern, converging into the draining vein (arrows). No arterial or capillary abnormality is noted.

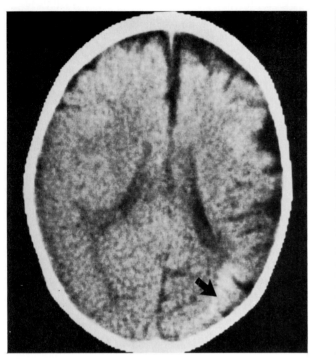

A

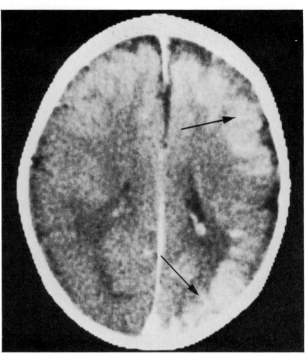

B

Figure 14-27 Sturge-Weber syndrome. **A.** NCCT shows cortical atrophy with calcification along the cortex (arrow) in 1-year-old child. **B.** Enhancement after contrast infusion along the cortex of the left frontal and parietal lobe (arrow). *(Courtesy Dr. D. Harwood-Nash, Toronto Hospital for Sick Children.)*

Figure 14-28 Arteriovenous malformation. **A.** NCCT and CECT demonstrate dense serpiginous enhancement due to the vascular malformation. **B.** The angiogram before embolization demonstrates the vascular malformation. **C.** NCCT and CECT demonstrate the silicone spheres and polyvinyl alcohol foam (Ivalon) within the region of the vascular malformation. *(Continued on p. 578.)*

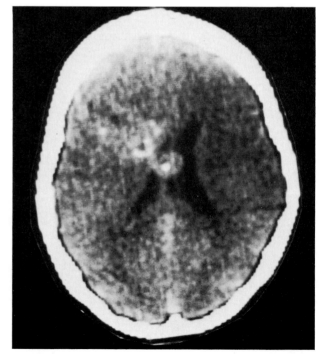

A (NCCT)

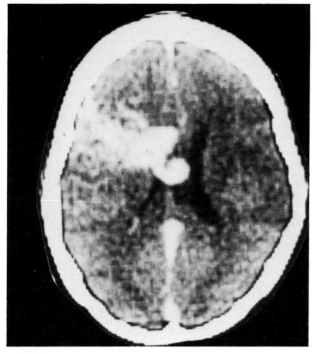

A (CECT)

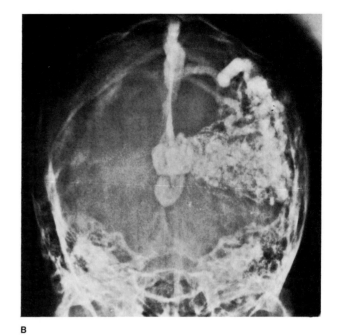

B

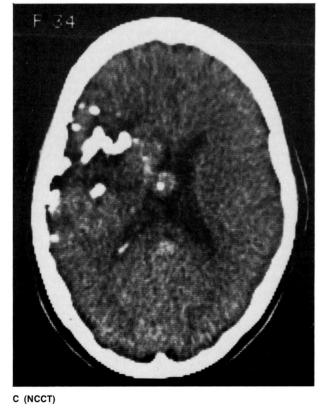

C (NCCT)

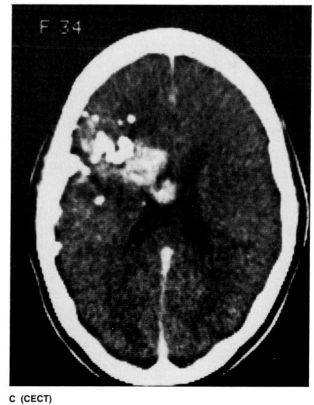

C (CECT)

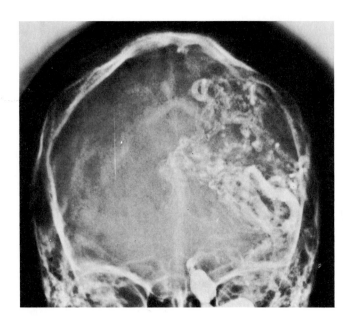

Figure 14-28 (Cont.) **D.** Angiogram following embolization demonstrates reduction in the flow.

Bibliography

AALMAANI WS, RICHARDSON AE: Multiple intracranial aneurysms: Identifying the ruptured lesion. *Surg Neurol* **9**:303–305, 1978.

ASSENCIO-FERREIRA VJ et al.: Computed tomography in ataxia-telangiectasia. *J Comput Assist Tomogr* **5**(5):660–661, 1981.

BABU VS, EISEN H: Giant aneurysm of anterior communicating artery simulating third ventricular tumor. *Comput Tomogr* **3**:159–163, 1979.

BARTLETT JE, KISHORE PRS: Intracranial cavernous angioma. *Am J Roentgenol Radium Ther Nucl Med* **128**:653–656, 1977.

BELL BA, KENDALL BE, SYMON L: Angiographically occult A-V malformations of the brain: *J Neurol Neurosurg Psychiatr* **41**:1057–1064, 1978.

BENTSON JR, WILSON GH, NEWTON TH: Cerebral venous drainage pattern of Sturge-Weber syndrome. *Radiology* **101**:111–118, 1971.

BJORKESTEN G, HALONEN V: Incidence of intracranial vascular lesions in patients with subarachnoid hemorrhage investigated by four-vessel angiography. *J Neurosurg* **23**:29–32, 1965.

BRITT RH, SILVERBERG GD, ENZMANN DR, HANBERRY JW: Third ventricular choroid plexus arteriovenous malformation simulating a colloid cyst. *J Neurosurg* **52**:246–250, 1980.

BULL JWD: Massive aneurysms at the base of the brain. *Brain* **92**:535–570, 1969.

BYRD SE, BENTSON JR, WINTER J, WILSON GH, JOYCE PW, O'CONNOR L: Giant intracranial aneurysms simulating brian neoplasms on computed tomography. *J Comput Assist Tomogr* **2**:303–307, 1978.

CHASON JL, HINDMAN WM: Berry aneurysms of the circle of Willis: Results of a planned autopsy study. *Neurology* **8**:41–44, 1958.

CONE JD, MARAVILLA KR, COOPER PR, DIEHL JT, CLARK WK: Computed tomography findings in ruptured arteriovenous malformation of corpus callosum. *J Comput Assist Tomogr* **3**:478–482, 1979.

CRAWFORD T: Some observations on the pathogenesis and natural history of intracranial aneurysm. *J Neurol Neurosurg Psychiatry* **22**:259–266, 1959.

CROMPTON MR: Mechanism of growth and rupture in cerebral berry aneurysm. *Br Med J* **1**:1138–1142, 1966.

DANIELS DL, HAUGHTON WM, WILLIAMS AL, STROTHER CM: Arteriovenous malformation simulating a cyst on computed tomography. *Radiology* **133**:393–394, 1979.

DAVIS JM, DAVIS KR, CROWELL RM: Subarachnoid hemorrhage secondary to ruptured intracranial aneurysm: prognostic significance of cranial CT. *Am J Neuroradiol* **1**:17–21, 1980.

DEEB ZL, JANETTA PJ, ROSENBAUM AE, KERBER CW, DRAYER BP: Tortuous vertebro-basilar arteries causing cranial nerve syndromes: Screening by computed tomography. *J Comput Assist Tomogr* **3**:774–778, 1979.

DIEBLER C, et al.: Aneurysms of the vein of Galen in infants aged 2 to 15 months. Diagnosis and natural evolution. *Neuroradiology* **21**:185–197, 1981.

DUBOULAY GH: Some observations on the natural history of intracranial aneurysms. *Br J Radiol* **38**:721–757, 1965.

ENZMANN DR, HAYWARD RW, NORMAN D, DUNN RP: Cranial computed tomographic scan appearance of Sturge-Weber disease: Unusual presentation. *Radiology* **122**:721–724, 1977.

FIERSTEIN SB, PRIBRAM HW, HIESHIMA G: Angiography and computed tomography in the evaluation of cerebral venous malformations. *Neuroradiology* **52**:246–250, 1979.

GHOSHHAJRA K, SCOTTI L, MARASCO J, BAGHAINAIINI P: C.T. detection of intracranial aneurysms in subarachnoid hemorrhage. *Am J Roentgenol Radium Ther Nucl Med* **132**:613–616, 1979.

GOLDEN JB, KRAMER RA: The angiographically occult cerebrovascular malformation. *J Neurosurg* **48**:292–296, 1978.

HANDA J, NAKANO Y, AII J, HANDA H: Computed tomography with giant intracranial aneurysms. *Surg Neurol* **9**:257–263, 1978.

HAYMAN LA, FOX AJ, EVANS RA: Effectiveness of contrast regimens in CT detection of vascular malformations of the brain. *AJNR* **2**:421–425, 1981.

HAYWARD RD: Intracranial arteriovenous malformations. *J Neurol Neurosurg Psychiatry* **39**:1027–1033, 1976.

HAYWARD RD, O'REILLY GVA: Intracerebral hemorrhage. *Lancet* **1**:1–4, 1977.

HOUSEPIAN EM, POOL JL: A systematic analysis of intracranial aneurysms from the autopsy file of the Presbyterian Hospital, 1914-1956. *J Neuropathol Exp Neurol* **17**:409–423, 1958.

ISHIKAWA M et al.: Computed tomography of cerebral cavernous hemangiomas. *J Comput Assist Tomogr* **4**(5):587–591, 1980.

ITO J, SATO I, TANIMURA K: Angiographic and computed tomography findings of a convexity cavernous hemangioma. *Jpn J Clin Radiol* **23**:204–205, 1978.

KENDALL BE, CLAVERIA LE: The use of computed axial tomography for the diagnosis and management of intracranial angiomas. *Neuroradiology* **12**:141–160, 1976a.

KENDALL BE, LEE BCP, CLAVERIA E: Computerized tomography and angiography in subarachnoid hemorrhage. *Br J Radiol* **49**:483–501, 1976b.

KRAMER RA, WING SD: Computed tomography of angiographically occult cerebral vascular malformations. *Radiology* **123**:649–652, 1977.

LEBLANC R, ETHIER R: The CT appearance of angiographically occult arterio-venous malformation of the brain. *Canad J Neuroscience* **8**:7–13, 1981.

LEBLANC R, ETHIER R, LITTLE JR: Computerized tomography findings in arteriovenous malformations of the brain. *J Neurosurg* **51**:765–772, 1979.

LILIEQUIST B, LINDQUIST M, VALDIMARSSON E: Computed tomography and subarachnoid hemorrhage. *Neuroradiology* **14**:21–26, 1977.

LIM ST, SAGE DJ: Detection of subarachnoid blood clot and other thin flat structures by computed tomography. *Radiology* **123**:79–84, 1977.

LOCKSLEY HB: Report on the cooperative study of intracranial aneurysms and subarachnoid hemorrhage. *J Neurosurg* **25**:219–239, 1966.

LUKIN RR, CHABERS AA, MCLAURIN R, TEW J: Thrombosed giant middle cerebral aneurysms. *Neuroradiology* **10**:125–129, 1975.

MCKISSOCK W, RICHARDSON A, WALSH L, OWE E: Multiple intracranial aneurysms. *Lancet* **1**:623–626, 1964.

MACPHERSON P, TEASDALE GM, LINDSAY KW: Computed tomography in diagnosis and management of aneurysm of the vein of Galen. 1979.

MICHELS LG, BEAVSON JR, WINTER J: Computed tomography of cerebral venous angiomas. *J Comput Assist Tomogr* **1**:149–154, 1977.

MODESTI LM, BINET EF: Value of computed tomography in the diagnosis and management of subarachnoid hemorrhage. *Neurosurgery* **3**:151–156, 1978.

MORLEY TP, BARR HWK: Giant intracranial aneurysms: Diagnosis, course and management. *Clin Neurosurg* **16**:73–94, 1969.

NADJMI M, RATZKA M, WODARZ M: Giant aneurysms in C.T. and angiography. *Neuroradiology* **16**:284–286, 1978.

NEW PFJ, SCOTT WR: *Computed Tomography of the Brain and Orbit (EMI Scanning).* Baltimore, Williams & Wilkins, 1975, pp 317–331.

NUMAGUCHI Y, KISHIKAWA T, FUKUI M, SAWADA K, KITAMUZA K, MATSUURA K, RUSSELL WJ: Prolonged injection angiography for diagnosis of intracranial cavernous hemangiomas. *Radiology* **131**:137–138, 1979.

NYSTROM SHM: Development of intracranial aneurysms as revealed by electron microscopy. *J Neurosurg* **20**:329–337, 1963.

OSBORN AG, ANDERSON RE, WING SD: The false falx sign. *Radiology* **134**:421–425, 1980.

PEACH B: Arnold-Chiari malformation. *Arch Neurol* **12**:613–621, 1965.

PERRETT LV, SAGE MR: Computerized tomography and giant intracranial aneurysms. *Aust Radiol* **21**:308–312, 1977.

PETERSON NT, DUCHESNEAU PM, WESTBROOK EL, WEINSTEIN MA: Basilar artery ectasia demonstrated by computed tomography. *Radiology* **122**:713–715, 1977.

PINTO RS, KRICHELL II, BUTLER AR, MURALI R: Correlation of computed tomographic angiographic and neuropathological changes in giant cerebral aneurysms. *Radiology* **132**:85–92, 1979.

POSER CM, TAVERAS JM: Cerebral angiography in encephalotrigeminal angiomatosis. *Radiology* **68**:327–336, 1957.

PRESSMAN BD, KIRKWOOD JR, DAVIS DO: Computerized transverse tomography of vascular lesions of the brain: I. Arteriovenous malformations. *Am J Roentgenol Radium Ther Nucl Med* **124**:208–215, 1975.

PRESSMAN BD, GILBERT GE, DAVIS DO: Computerized transverse tomography of vascular lesions of the brain: II. Aneurysms *Am J Roentgenol Radium Ther Nucl Med* **124**:215–219, 1976b.

RAMINA R, INGUNZA W, VONOFAKOS D: Cystic cerebral cavernous angioma with dense calcification. *J Neurosurg* **52**:259–262, 1980.

RENGACHARY SS, SZYMANSKI DC: Subdural hematomas of arterial origin. *Neurosurgery* **8**(2):166–172, 1981.

RICHARDSON JC, HYLAND HH: Intracranial aneurysms: Clinical and pathological study of subarachnoid and intracerebral hemorrhage caused by berry aneurysms. *Medicine* **20**:1–83, 1941.

RICHMOND T et al.: Intraparenchymal blood fluid levels: new CT sign of arteriovenous malformation: rupture *Am J Neuroradiol* **2**:577–579, 1981.

ROBERSON GH, KASE CS, WOLPOW ER: Telangiectases and cavernous angiomas of the brain stem: "Cryptic" vascular malformations. *Neuroradiology* **8**:83–89, 1974.

RUSSELL DS, RUBINSTEIN LJ: Pathology of tumors of the nervous system, 4th ed. E. Arnold, Edinburgh, 1977, pp. 126–145.

SAITO I, SHIGENU T, ARITAKE K, TANISHIMA T, SANO K: Vasospasm assessed by angiography and computerized tomography. *J Neurosurg* **51**:466–475, 1979.

SARTOR K: Spontaneous closure of cerebral arteriovenous: malformation demonstrated by angiography and computed tomography. *Neuroradiology* **15**:95–98, 1978.

SARWAR M, BATNITZKY S, SCHECHTER MM: Tumorous aneurysms. *Neuroradiology* **12**:79–97, 1976a.

SARWAR M, BATNITZKY S, SCHECHTER MM, LIEBESKIND A, ZIMMER AE: Growing intracranial aneurysms. *Radiology* **120**:603–607, 1976b.

SCHUBIGER O, VALAVANIA A, HAYEK J: Computed tomography in cerebral aneurysms with special emphasis on giant intracranial aneurysms. *J Comput Assist Tomogr* **4**:24–32, 1980.

SCOTTI G, ETHIER R, MELANCON D, TERBRUGGE KG, TCHANG S: Computed tomography in the evaluation of intracranial aneurysms and subarachnoid hemorrhage. *Radiology* **123**:85–90, 1977.

SCOTTI G, DEGRAND C, COLOMBO A: Ectasia of the intracranial arteries diagnosed by computed tomography. *Neuroradiology* **15**:183–184, 1978.

SOLIS OJ, DAVIS KR, ELLIS GT: Dural arteriovenous malformation associated with subdural and intracerebral hematoma: A C.T. scan and angiographic correlation. *Comput Tomogr* **1**:145–150, 1977.

SPALLINE A: Computed tomography in aneurysms of the vein of Galen. *J Comput Assist Tomogr* **3**;779–782, 1979.

TERACO H, HOZI T, MATSUTANI M, OKEDA R: Detection of cryptic vascular malformation by computerized tomography. *J Neurosurg* **51**:546–551, 1979.

TERBRUGGE KG, SCOTTI G, ETHIER R, MELANCON D, TCHANG S, MILNER C: Computed tomography in intracranial arteriovenous malformations. *Radiology* **122**:703–705, 1977.

THRON A, BOCKENHEIMER S: Giant aneurysms of the posterior fossa suspected as neoplasms on computed tomography. *Neuroradiology* **18**:93–97, 1979.

WEIR B, MILLER J, RUSSELL D: Intracranial aneurysms: A clinical, angiographic and computerized tomographic study. *Can J Neurol Sci* **4**:99–105, 1977.

WEISBERG LA, NICE C, KATZ M: *Cerebral Computed Tomography: A Text-Like Atlas.* Philadelphia, Saunders, 1978, pp. 87–105.

WELCH K, NAHEEDY MH, ABROMS IF, STRAND RD: Computed tomography of Sturge-Weber syndrome in infants. *J Comput Assist Tomogr* **4**:33–36, 1980.

WYBURN-MASON R: The Vascular Abnormalities and Tumors of the Spinal Cord and Its Membranes, Kingston, London, 1943.

YOCK DH, LARSON DA: Computed tomography of hemorrhage from anterior communicating artery aneurysms, with angiographic correlation. *Radiology* **134**:399–407, 1980.

ZIMMERMAN RD, YURBERG E, LEEDS NE: The falx and interhemispheric fissure on axial computed tomography: I. Normal anatomy. *Am J Neuroradiol* **3**:175–180, 1982.

15

STROKE

Herbert I. Goldberg

Stroke is the third of the leading causes of death in the United States, exceeded only by heart disease and cancer (*Report to the President* 1964–65). It kills over 200,000 people each year in this country (Kurtzke 1980) and affects close to 400,000 (Whisnant 1971). The incidence rate and death rate from stroke increase dramatically with age (Eisenberg 1964). About 15 to 35 percent of patients will die with each episode of cerebral infarction (Eisenberg 1964; Matsumoto 1973); a much higher mortality—60 to 80 percent—occurs with cerebral hemorrhage (Whisnant 1971). Those who survive are usually left with permanent disability. With the increasing mean population age in this country, stroke will become an even greater medical and social problem. Accurate and early diagnosis may improve the mor-

bidity and mortality rates in the future as newer and more effective therapies currently being tested are instituted.

The advent of computed tomography (CT) in the early 1970s greatly facilitated the diagnosis and management of stroke and added significantly to our understanding of the pathophysiologic brain alterations it causes in humans. With CT it is now possible for the first time to noninvasively and reliably diagnose and distinguish between stroke resulting from cerebral infarction and that resulting from cerebral hemorrhage. In addition, other brain lesions that at times may clinically present as stroke-like syndromes, such as primary or metastatic brain tumor, brain abscess, or subdural hematoma, can usually be clearly differentiated by the CT examination. In most instances it is no longer necessary to perform cerebral angiography to exclude a possible surgical lesion in patients in whom the clinical diagnosis of stroke may have been in doubt. In some strokes the initial CT findings are of uncertain etiologic significance; however, follow-up scans after 2 to 3 weeks will usually demonstrate a characteristic evolution of the CT alterations, establishing the correct diagnosis.

The high spatial- and density-resolution capabilities of CT result in one of the most accurate methods available for identifying and localizing an infarction within the brain. Ischemic infarction, hemorrhagic infarction, and intracerebral hematoma are usually readily differentiated. CT also permits identification of the acute and chronic sequelae that may develop after an ischemic event. These include, in the acute phase, brain swelling and conversion of a bland into a hemorrhagic infarct and in the chronic phase, cystic parenchymal change, cortical atrophy, and focal ventricular dilatation.

In CT evaluation of stroke, additional and frequently valuable information may be gained when CT scans are performed both before and after the intravenous administration of contrast material. Contrast-enhanced CT greatly aids recognition of other types of brain lesions that may present clinically as stroke and permits detection of up to 13 percent of infarcts which are invisible on noncontrast CT scans (Masdeu 1977; Wing 1976). Athough the underlying nature of the vascular pathology causing an infarction is not directly revealed by CT, frequently distinguishing pathophysiologic alterations will be evident on CECT which, in combination with the alterations seen on NCCT, will suggest the correct diagnosis between two major causes of infarction—embolism and primary cerebral vasoocclusive disease. In this differentiation, follow-up NCCT and CECT scans are frequently valuable during the first 2 to 3 weeks, as distinctive differences in the temporal evolution of these two conditions may be revealed. The differentiation of these two varieties of infarction has important therapeutic implications.

Besides diagnosing large-artery, atherosclerotic, or embolic occlusive disease, the CT may reveal alterations which suggest involvement of smaller arteries and other etiologies for the stroke. Hypertensive vascular disease which primarily affects small penetrating arteries (arteriolosclerosis) usually shows ischemic change in the deep gray masses and in the periventricular white matter. In some cases of primary and secondary arteritis the CT patterns of ischemia, in conjunction with other CT alterations and the patient's age, sex, and clinical history, will suggest the correct diagnosis. Cerebral sinovenous thrombosis will frequently demonstrate unique CT changes.

Although intracerebral hematomas all appear relatively similar on CT regardless of their etiology, presenting as circumscribed homogeneous regions of increased density, their various causes may be suggested by the location of the hemorrhage and associated changes which may be revealed on pre- or postcontrast scans. This frequently permits differentiation of hematomas caused by hypertension, trauma, tumor, venous thrombosis, arteriovenous malformation, and aneurysm.

Stroke may be classified as being caused by decreased circulation to the brain (infarction) or by intracerebral hemorrhage. The former produces brain injury from ischemic necrosis, while the latter causes brain damage by compression necrosis and vascular disruption. The incidence of the major causes of stroke, based on a communitywide survey of diagnoses in Rochester, Minn., during the years 1955 through 1969, before the introduction of CT, was as follows: for cerebral infarction, 79 percent, with embolism at 8 percent included in this group; for intracerebral hemorrhage, 10 percent; for subarachnoid hemorrhage, 6 percent; and ill-defined causes, 5 percent (Matsumoto 1973). Kinkel (1976), utilizing CT, found a much higher incidence of intracerebral hemorrhage as a cause for supratentorial stroke (26 percent). In this series a high percentage of cases were clinically misdiagnosed as to the type of stroke: 43 percent with cerebral hemorrhage were clinically thought to have cerebral infarction, and 14 percent with cerebral infarction were diagnosed as having cerebral hemorrhage. A recent clinical survey by Mohr (1980), from the records of the Harvard Cooperative Stroke Registry, in which all appropriate laboratory aids were employed, including CT, four-vessel cerebral angiography, and CSF examination, found cerebral embolism to account for 31 percent of all strokes, atherosclerotic thrombosis 33 percent, and lacunar infarcts 18 percent. Hypertensive intracerebral hemorrhage caused 11 percent of the strokes, and hemorrhage from ruptured aneurysm and vascular malformation 7 percent. The high incidence of cerebral embolism (31 percent) in this clinical series is in agreement with an autopsy study of Fisher and Adams (Mohr 1980), in which cerebral embolism caused 32 percent of the strokes.

Transient ischemic attacks (TIA) are acute neurological deficits which clear completely within 24 hours. These attacks are caused by a short period of reduced blood flow to the eye or brain which does not result in permanent tissue damage. The reduced circulation may result from either small emboli or severe cerebrovascular occlusive disease, the latter usually in association with a transient reduction in arterial pressure (Ruff 1981).

Recovery from a TIA occurs because of the rapid return of normal arterial perfusion pressure to the affected brain tissue. When the TIA is related to a severe vascular stenosis, either a rise in blood pressure or return to a normal cardiac rate and rhythm, depending on the inciting cause, could reestablish the normal perfusion pressure; when caused by emboli, either rapid clot lysis or the rapid establishment of adequate collateral blood flow could account for complete clearing of the ischemic symptom. A TIA is an important warning sign of a possible subsequent major stroke. The CT scan is

Table 15-1   Causes of Cerebral Infarction

Arterial occlusive disease
  Atherosclerotic occlusion
  Embolism
  Hemodynamic ischemia
  Arteriolosclerosis (lacunar disease)
  Vasculitis
  Moyamoya disease
Anoxic ischemia
Venous thrombosis

Table 15-2   Causes of Intracerebral Hemorrhage

Hypertensive vascular disease (arteriolosclerosis)
Aneurysm
Vascular malformation
Hemorrhagic arterial and venous infarction
Mycotic aneurysm
Amyloid angiopathy
Premature neonatal germinal matrix
Hemorrhagic hematologic disorders

usually normal after a TIA (Kinkel 1976; Bradac 1980). There have, however, been reports of CT abnormalities with TIAs such as focal low densities in up to 20 percent of the cases (Buell 1979; Ladurner 1979; Perrone 1979). These abnormalities may be related to previous small silent infarcts and not to the current TIA episodes (Bradac 1980).

Tables 15-1 and 15-2 list the major causes of cerebral infarction and non-traumatic intracerebral hemorrhage.

Although cerebral angiography is the only technique short of pathologic examination that may specifically localize and indicate the nature of the vascular disease in some of the categories in Tables 1 and 2, not infrequently CT alterations are apparent which may be strongly suggestive of many of them. The use of intravenous contrast material after NCCT and the obtaining of follow-up studies in many instances significantly aids in determination of the correct vascular etiology of the stroke, as does correlation of the CT changes with the patient's age, sex, history, and neurological findings.

CEREBRAL INFARCTION

Ischemic stroke has been reported to result in a positive CT scan in from 66 to 98 percent of cases (Bradac 1980; Buell 1979; Campbell 1978; Kinkel 1976). The percentage that become positive increases if follow-up CT scans are performed (Campbell 1978; Inoue 1980) and if CT is performed both before and after intravenous contrast administration (Norton 1978; Weisberg 1980; Wing 1976). The CT may become faintly positive as early as 3 hours after the onset of symptoms, but usually a low-density abnormality will become evident between 24 and 72 hours (Inoue 1980). The size and location of the infarct, along with the degree of patient motion, significantly influences the time at which the lesion will first be detected. Small lesions that are usually not associated with significant edema may not become evident until very late, when necrotic tissue absorption has produced a well-demarcated, hypodense cystic lesion. Infratentorial infarcts (cerebellum and brainstem) have a lower incidence of detection, with focal abnormality apparent in from 31 to 44 percent of cases (Campbell 1978; Kingsley 1980). Brainstem infarcts are usually not identified, because they are frequently very small and because of the inherent large spatial artifacts in this region produced by the dense petrous ridges.

Newer-generation fast CT scanners should result in increased early stroke detection, since image-degrading patient motion will present less of a problem. Detection rates of only 40 to 50 percent were found for ischemic strokes within 48 hours utilizing the slower early-model scanners (Davis 1975). Recently Inoue et al. (1980) reported that approximately 90 percent of supratentorial infarcts that eventually became positive on sequential CT scanning were evident by 24 hours. All scans obtained between 25 and 35 days after the ictus revealed a focal abnormality in this series.

Whereas CT will frequently reveal abnormality during the first week after an infarction, the radionuclide scan usually does not become positive until the second week (Blahd 1971; Di Chiro 1974). The detection rates for both types of studies are approximately equal during the second week for both supra- and infratentorial infarctions, but CT provides a much greater specificity (Campbell 1978; Masdeu 1977; Lewis 1978; Chiu 1977).

The CT alterations that develop and evolve over time with ischemic infarction reflect the pathologic changes that are occurring in the brain tissue. In the first few hours after a large cerebral artery occlusion, widespread tissue damage can be recognized microscopically, involving the gray and white matter. In the central regions of the infarct, coagulation necrosis may develop in all tissue elements. At the periphery of the infarction, where damage is less severe, there is disintegration of nerve cells, myelin sheaths, and oligodendroglia, along with varying lesser degrees of damage to the astrocytes; the microglia and blood vessels are preserved. The small blood vessels and tissues are infiltrated with polymorphocytic leukocytes, which reach their maximum concentration at 3 days and then begin to decline. They are replaced by phagocytic mononuclear cells, which become evident by the fifth day. These cells continue to increase through the fourth week, removing the products of enzymatic digestion of neuronal and myelin disintegration. Beginning around Day 5, proliferation of capillary endothelial cells becomes evident at the margins of the infarct. During the next several weeks these new capillaries greatly increase in number. They first grow into cortex and deep gray areas of infarction and later into the white-matter regions. As the process of tissue breakdown continues, the phagocytes become fat-laden and then degenerate, leaving cystic spaces filled with yellowish fluid. Astrocytes also undergo hypertrophy and hyperplasia, laying down collagen fibers which contribute to tissue repair at the infarct margins. After several months the necrotic tissue has been replaced by cystic spaces containing fluid and a variable number of fat-filled phagocytes. The margin between the infarct and the adjacent normal brain tissue is sharply defined during all stages of the infarct evolution.

Arterial Occlusive Diseases

Large-Artery Thrombotic Infarction (Atherosclerotic Occlusion)

Between 8 and 24 hours after the onset of ischemic symptoms, the NCCT may reveal a poorly marginated, mottled region of slight hypodensity involving

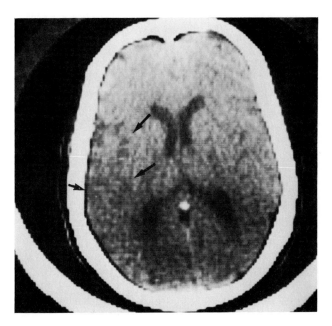

Figure 15-1 Early infarct, middle cerebral artery territory: poorly defined nonhomogeneous hypodensity involving right temporal region with patchy involvement of the cortex and underlying white matter (arrows). Bilateral occipital low density secondary to machine artifact. (See follow-up CT, Fig. 15-2A.)

both the cortex and the underlying white matter down to the ventricular surface (Figs. 15-1, 15-4A) (Baker 1975; Davis 1975; Yock 1975). The hypodensity becomes more distinct after a few days and assumes a triangular or wedge-shaped configuration with its base on the brain surface. The low density is confined within the vascular territory of the occluded artery (Figs. 15-2, 15-3). When the internal carotid artery or the proximal segment of the middle cerebral artery is occluded, the low density may extend into the basal ganglia and the internal capsule region (Figs. 15-3, 15-4, 15-20). This initial low-density pattern represents tissue necrosis with intracellular edema (cytotoxic edema) (Alcala 1978). Little or no mass effect is evident during the initial 24 hours of the infarct. Detection of infarct changes during the first 24 hours is dependent on the size of the infarct, the degree of the ischemic insult, and the availability of scans of high contrast resolution with minimal artifacts from patient motion.

Between the third and the fifth day the region of infarction becomes a more homogeneous low-density area with sharper margins. Its hypodensity increases over that of earlier scans (Figs. 15-2A, 15-4B) (Davis 1975; Inoue 1980). Pathologically, tissue necrosis and intracellular edema reaches its maximum at this time. This results in a variable degree of mass effect which depends on the size and degree of infarction. Swelling may be mild to severe, with the CT revealing either focal or diffuse compression of the ventricular system and midline shift (Figs. 15-2B, 15-3, 15-4B). With large infarcts, early signs of tissue swelling may become evident before 24 hours. At this time there may be obliteration or effacement of sulci and the sylvian fissure on the side of the infarct, and the ipsilateral ventricle may be slightly smaller (Fig. 15-4). Mass effect of some degree is reported in from 21 to 70 percent of infarcts (Masdeu 1977; Wing 1976; Yock 1975) and is most marked between the third and fifth days. With large hemispheric infarctions brain swelling may be considerable, with the development of a marked midline shift. This may result in posterior cerebral artery occlusion with occipital lobe infarction from transtentorial herniation (Fig. 15-5). With small infarcts there may be no mass effect or only slight focal ventricular distortion. Brain swelling begins to decrease after the first week and usually completely resolves in 12 to 21 days.

With embolic infarcts, considerable further brain swelling may develop, predominantly vasogenic in nature, when antegrade circulation is reestablished following clot lysis. This frequently occurs, usually between the second and fourteenth day after the infarction, and results in the leakage of increased amounts of fluid from the ischemically damaged capillary bed when exposed to the high reperfusion pressure.

The low density of infarction remains strictly confined to the distribution of the arterial system involved or to the watershed or border zone between major arterial distributions (Fig. 15-2). This sharp localization is due to the hypodensity representing cellular necrosis and edema, which is mainly intracellular (cytotoxic), in contrast to the vasogenic form of edema, which is extracellular and

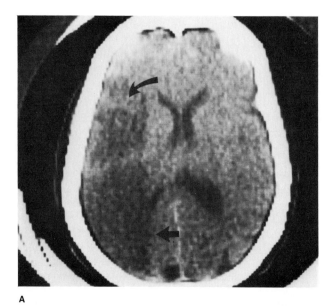

A

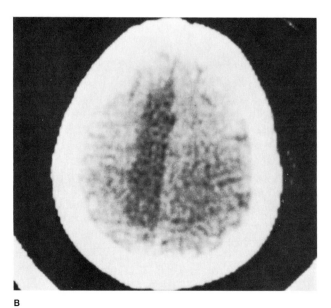

B

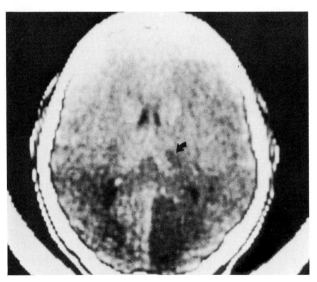

C

Figure 15-2 Major cerebral infarct territories in 3- to 5-day-old infarcts. **A.** Peripheral middle cerebral artery territory infarct (same patient as in Fig. 15-1): well-defined homogeneous hypodensity involving cortex and underlying white matter in right posterior temporal and lateral occipital region. The basal ganglia region is normal, indicating that the proximal middle cerebral artery segment from which the lenticulostriate supply arises is not occluded. Linear demarcation at watershed between infarct hypodensity in middle cerebral artery territory and normal tissue density of posterior cerebral artery territory (straight arrow). Hypodensity of cortex and white matter in anterior temporal region is nonhomogeneous, suggesting incomplete infarction in this region (curved arrow). Right lateral

spreads along white matter tracts and is commonly associated with brain tumor and inflammatory disease.

The low-density pattern associated with infarction can usually be differentiated from that seen with tumor and inflammatory disease. With infarction the region of decreased density usually involves both the gray and the white matter, while with tumor and inflammation it is mainly situated within the white matter, although it may extend to the cortex. With infarction the margins of the hypodensity are sharply demarcated, with a square or wedge-shaped configuration, and are located within or between arterial distributions, whereas with tumor and abscess the low density tends to spread diffusely within the white matter in a pseudopod-

ventricle is compressed and shifted slightly to left of midline. **B.** Anterior cerebral artery territory infarct: rectangular, well-defined, homogeneous hypodensity involving the cortex and underlying white matter in the superior medial aspect of the right hemisphere. There is sharp margination of the hypodensity at the watershed region with the middle cerebral artery territory laterally and the posterior cerebral artery territory posteriorly. The hypodensity extends inferiorly on lower sections to the level of the roof of the lateral ventricle. **C.** Posterior cerebral artery territory infarct. Hypodensity involving posterior thalamus on the left (arrow) along with sharply defined cortical white-matter region in the medial posterior occipital area.

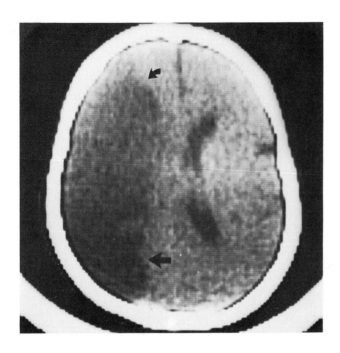

Figure 15-3   Four-day-old complete right middle cerebral artery territory infarction. Obliteration of right lateral ventricle and marked midline shift to the left. Homogeneous hypodensity involving lateral basal ganglia and all cortical white-matter regions of peripheral middle cerebral artery distribution. Sharp linear margination anteriorly at junction with anterior cerebral artery territory (curved arrow) and posteriorly with posterior cerebral artery territory (straight arrow).

Figure 15-4.   A. Early signs of mass effect with large middle cerebral artery territory infarct: CT obtained at about 12 hours after stroke. Poorly defined region of slight hypodensity involving basal ganglia (curved arrow) and frontotemporal region (straight arrows) on left side. The cortical sulci and sylvian fissure are obliterated on the left side and there is slight compression of the left frontal horn.   **B.** Marked mass effect and increased left middle cerebral artery territory hypodensity approximately 2 days after **A.** (*Courtesy of Robert G. Peyster, M.D., Hahnemann Medical College.*)

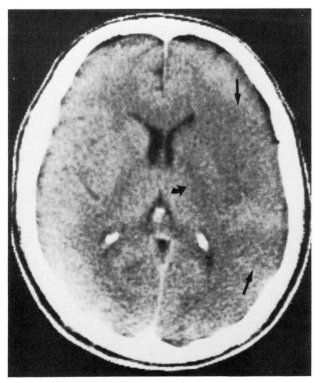
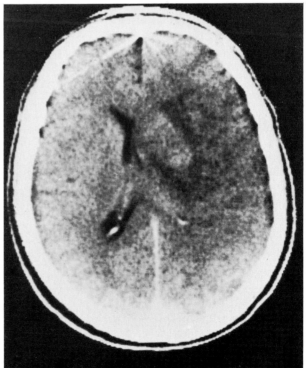

A   **B**

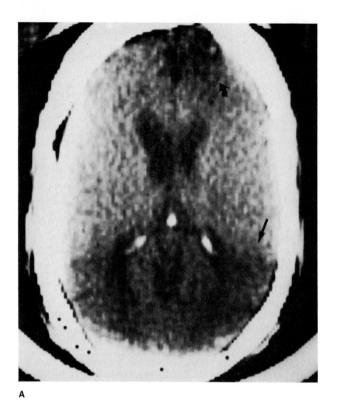

A

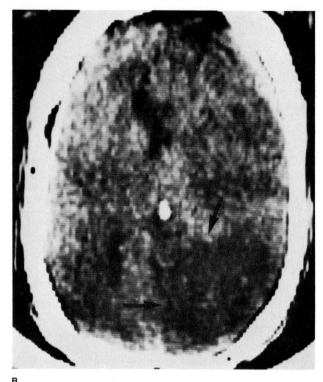

B

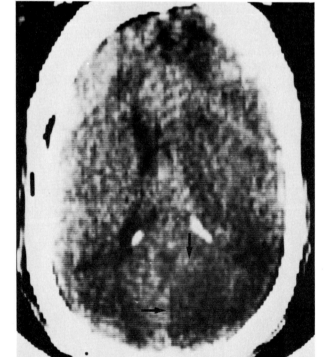

C

Figure 15-5 Infarct swelling, causing tentorial herniation and secondary posterior cerebral artery territory infarct. **A.** Infarct hypodensity without mass effect in 1-day-old infarct involving left middle cerebral artery temporal parietal region (straight arrow) and left anterior cerebral territory (curved arrow). **B.** Four days after **A** (similar brain level) CT reveals a marked increase in left middle cerebral artery territory hypodensity, mass effect, and midline shift. There were clinical signs of left tentorial herniation. Hypodensity now also involves distal left posterior cerebral artery territory (arrows). **C.** CT section 1 cm above **B** revealing hypodensity from occipital infarct (arrows) in the territory of the posterior cerebral artery.

like manner, has ill-defined rounded margins, and is usually not limited to an arterial division or to adjacent arterial branches.

During the second and third weeks, isodense to slightly hyperdense curvilinear bands and nodular regions frequently develop within hypodense areas of the infarct (Inoue 1980). They are located mainly in gray matter and result from hyperemia related to new capillary ingrowth and improved collateral circulation in thrombotic infarcts while some of the hyperdensity may be caused by petechial hemorrhage in embolic infarct. The hyperdensity appears most commonly as slightly hyperdense bands in the expected location of the cortical ribbon and are most prominent at the margins of the infarct (Fig. 15-6). They may also occur in cortical regions, more centrally in the infarct, and in the deep gray masses. They tend to produce a mottled appearance at the margins of the infarct, which then become less

sharply defined than on earlier poststroke scans. The infarcted white matter usually does not show any density increase and remains hypodense. As the edema resolves in the white matter between the second and the fourth weeks, its low density becomes even more marked than previously, owing to the accumulation of abundant fat-laden phagocytes in the infarct tissues at this time.

Starting at about 4 to 5 weeks and continuing for the next 2 to 3 months, the infarct region becomes more sharply outlined on CT, with its hypodensity becoming more homogeneous and approaching that of cerebral spinal fluid (Davis 1975; Inoue 1980). The isodense cortical bands usually convert to low-attenuation zones. Pathologically there is cystic cavitation of the necrotic infarcted brain tissue, prominent lipid content, and gliosis (Yates 1976). The cystic change predominantly affects the white matter and the region of the basal ganglia, where tissue

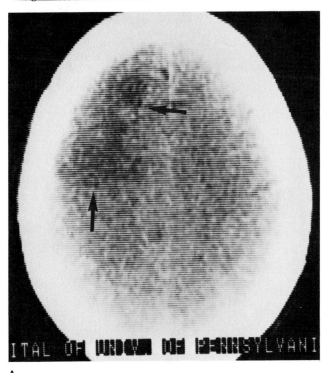

A

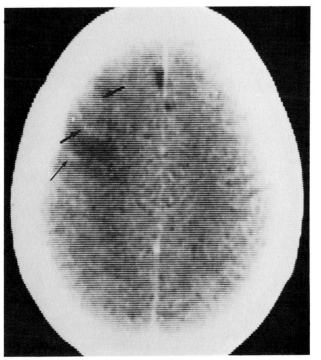

B

Figure 15-6 Development of isodense cortical bands on NCCT in right middle cerebral territory infarct. **A.** Relatively homogeneous hypodensity involving the cortical gray and underlying white matter at day 3 (arrows). **B.** At day 12 isodense bands representing the infolded cortical ribbon (arrows) extend down into white matter hypodensity. Infarct appears smaller with indistinct margins because cortex at periphery of infarct has become isodense (see Figure 15-13 CECT).

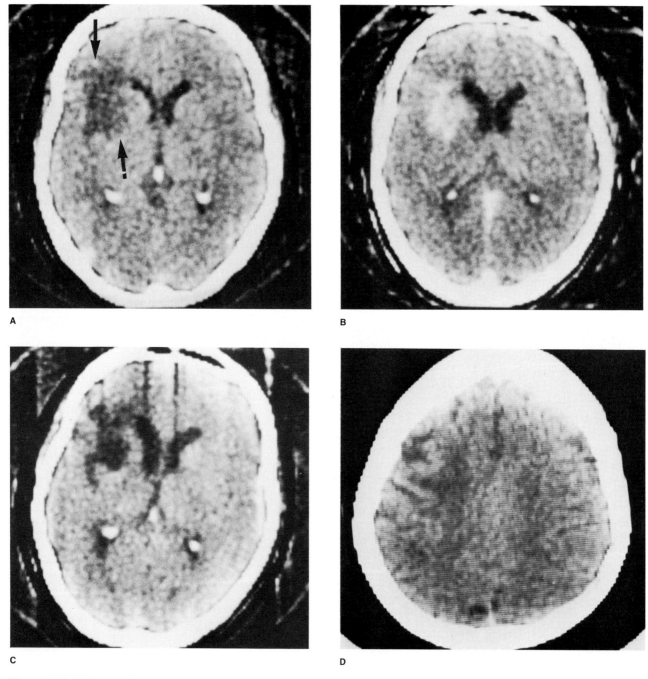

A

B

C

D

Figure 15-7 Infarct evolution to chronic phase. **A.** NCCT at 3 days: hypodensity in anterior basal ganglia and frontal middle cerebral territory (arrows); compression of frontal horn. **B.** CECT at 10 days: enhancement throughout infarct region; lack of frontal horn compression. **C.** NCCT at 4 months: more marked and well defined infarct hypodensity; enlargement of right frontal horn and sylvian fissure with midline shift to right. **D.** CT at higher level: enlargement of cortical sulci on right with white-matter hypodensity.

necrosis is generally most severe. The infarct appears smaller because of absorption of necrotic tissue and contraction from gliosis (McCall 1975). The adjacent portion of the lateral ventricle dilates and extends toward the region of infarction. A shift of the brain midline to the side of the infarct may also develop with large lesions. The overlying cortex frequently reveals atrophic change, with enlargement of adjacent sulci and cisterns (Fig. 15-7). With some cortical infarcts, sulcal enlargement may be the only long-term abnormality (Fig. 15-8). The chronic brain changes usually become stable by the end of the third month.

CONTRAST ENHANCEMENT   CECT has been of great value in the diagnosis and characterization of infarcts. A significant percentage of infarcts reveal contrast enhancement, which usually first appears during the second week after the onset of symptoms (Fig. 15-9). Early studies reported contrast enhancement in only about 60 percent of cerebral infarcts (Wing 1976; Masdeu 1977); recent studies have observed enhancement in upward of 82 to 88 percent of infarcts evaluated between the second and fourth weeks (Pullicino 1980; Lee 1978). In a study of supratentorial infarcts with serial CT examinations, 93

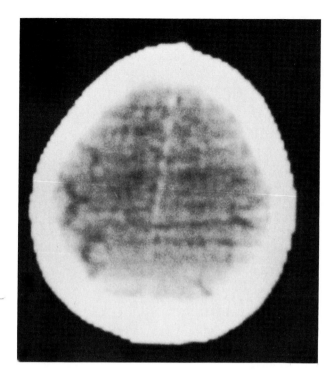

Figure 15-8 Sulcal enlargement from an old cortical infarct: asymmetric enlargement of right parietal sulci with normal white-matter density. On lower sections right sylvian fissure is enlarged.

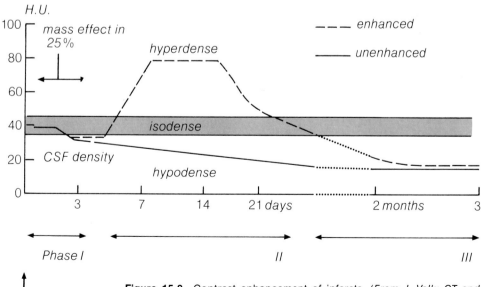

Figure 15-9 Contrast enhancement of infarcts. (*From J. Valk: CT and Cerebral Infarctions, New York, Raven Press, 1980.*)

percent of those which developed an abnormality showed contrast enhancement between the second and third week (Inoue 1980). There has been a wide range in the reported incidence of enhancement occurring during the first week of the infarct, from zero to 62 percent (Weisberg 1980; Lee 1978). This large variation probably reflects differences in infarct etiology in these series. Those series which have a high percentage of embolic and hemodynamic infarcts (see next section) reveal a high incidence of early enhancement because these infarcts are reperfused early at systemic arterial pressure levels which will reveal blood-brain barrier abnormalities not evident in persistently anemic infarcts. Hayman et al. (1981), employing high-dose contrast infusion (80 g iodine) along with immediate and delayed (3 hours) CT scans, had a 72 percent incidence of enhancement (13 of 18) within the first 28 hours. Most of the patients with early enhancement had embolic infarcts. In addition, these authors found that enhancement which occurred predominantly on the 3-hour-delayed scans had a grave prognostic implication; four of seven patients with this type of enhancement subsequently developed hemorrhagic infarcts and died. None of the patients with only immediate enhancement on high-dose scans had this sequela.

Contrast administration either at high dose (Hayman 1981) or by rapid injection (Heinz 1979; Norman 1981) during the first 24 hours of an infarct or later may reveal characteristic nonenhancing abnormalities in an otherwise normal CT. With both these techniques the cortical gyri and deep gray matter in the infarct region may demonstrate a deficiency in contrast blush of the capillary bed which will be evident in the surrounding uninvolved gray matter and in homologous regions of the opposite hemisphere. With the high-dose technique advocated by Hayman et al. (1981), routine scanning methods which may utilize slow scanning times will demonstrate this change. With the rapid-injection technique (dynamic CT), however, 40–50 ml of contrast must be injected in about 5 seconds and four to six fast scans (5 seconds or less) obtained in rapid sequence, that is, 2 to 3 seconds apart (Fig. 15-10) (Norman 1981). This latter technique requires CT equipment with these special capabilities.

The intensity of enhancement begins to decline after the third week. It will usually persist for 6 to 7 weeks and with large infarcts up to 12 weeks (Weisberg 1980; Pullicino 1980). It may rarely last for as long as 9 months (Norton 1978).

The amount of radiographic contrast injected greatly influences the intensity of enhancement. Weisberg (1980) observed that only 5 percent of 100 patients with infarction demonstrated contrast enhancement after injection of a 50-ml bolus of a 60 percent iodinated contrast agent (14 g of iodine), whereas enhancement occurred in 65 percent of 100 patients after a drip infusion of 300 ml of a 30 percent contrast agent (42 g of iodine).

The mechanism of CT contrast enhancement appears to be identical to that producing delayed uptake in a radionuclide brain scan and is related to abnormality in the blood-brain barrier. Anderson et al. (1980), in a cat stroke model, found a strong positive correlation between tissue concentrations of ^{99m}Tc, sodium pertechnetate, and methylglucamine iothalamate in the area of infarct and the surrounding brain tissues at all time intervals, indicating a similarity in the temporal profile in these two studies. The radionuclide, however, revealed a consistently higher brain-blood ratio than the iodinated contrast material. This probably accounts for the slightly higher incidence of positive nuclide scans than of standard-dose CECT scans. Depending on the dose of contrast given, at some time periods its brain-blood ratio may be below the level of tissue concentration that can be resolved on CT. Masdeu et al. (1977), in a study in humans, found a slightly higher incidence of positive radionuclide brain scans with infarction when compared with CECT at 2 weeks (72 percent versus 63 percent), using a standard contrast dose. Gado et al. (1975) have shown in human studies that CT contrast enhancement is primarily a result of contrast material in the extracellular space. Only a small degree of contrast enhancement can be explained by tissue hypervascularity, except perhaps when large blood pools are present, as with arteriovenous malformation.

The pathophysiologic abnormality that permits passage of contrast material into the extravascular space is a breakdown in the blood-brain barrier mechanisms of the capillary endothelium (Fishman

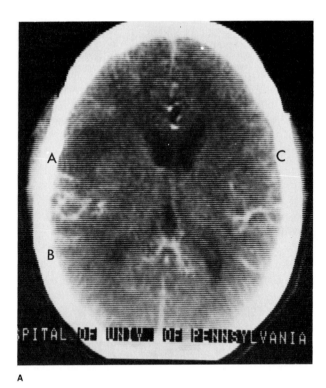

A

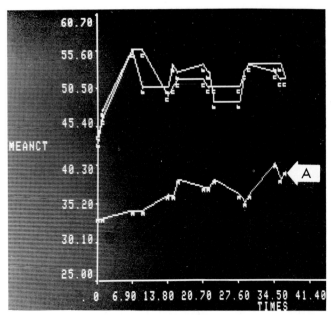

B

Figure 15-10 Ischemic changes on rapid-sequence CT: 2-day-old right middle cerebral territory infarct. **A.** High-speed CT scan (2.4-second scan time) 12 seconds after rapid intravenous injection of 40 ml contrast. Absence of surface vessels and cortical gyral blush in right posterior frontal region (A; normal cortical blush in regions B and C). **B.** Time-density curves following bolus contrast injection in region A (area of infarct) and regions B and C (normal cortical regions) in **A.** Time in seconds displayed on horizontal axis and CT density (H units) on vertical axis. Curves B and C (upper) display a rapid rise and decline of contrast density, reflecting normal initial circulation of the contrast bolus through the brain. The subsequent fluctuations in the curves reflect to a large extent recirculation of the bolus. Curve A over the infarct indicates a slow circulation probably in association with a defective blood-brain barrier. It seems likely that some of the slow density increase of the infarct results from leakage of contrast from poorly filled, damaged capillaries.

1975; Anderson 1980). Brain capillaries, unlike those in other parts of the body, restrict the passage of most large molecules through their walls because of tight endothelial cell junctions. Ischemic insult to the brain damages the blood-brain barrier, permitting large molecules to leak into the extravascular space. Although animal studies have shown that after infarction produced by a permanent arterial occlusion, capillary leakage may become evident at about 4 hours (O'Brien 1974), the CECT or the isotope brain scan will usually not become positive until after the first week (Blahd 1971; Inoue 1980). This appears to be related to persistent severe ischemia of the infarct region during the first week due to limited collateral or antegrade circulation. As a result of this low flow, insufficient contrast is delivered to the infarct for enhancement to be demonstrated even in the presence of a severely disturbed blood-brain barrier. By 7 to 10 days brain swelling is less, and this improves collateral circulation and results in sufficient leakage of contrast from infarct capillaries to be visualized. Concomitantly, considerable neovascular capillary proliferation is occurring around areas of necrosis, and these vessels have an incompetent blood-brain barrier (Dudley 1970; Yamaguchi 1971; Hayman 1980; Anderson 1980). This neovascularity is responsible for persistence of contrast enhancement during the next 4 to 8 weeks as the reparative process is completed.

Contrast enhancement may develop before the usual 7 to 10 days if perfusion at the infarct increases significantly (Hayman 1980). Large-molecule leakage at a disturbed blood-brain barrier varies directly with the systemic blood pressure level (Klatzo 1972).

Contrast enhancement tends to occur early with embolic infarcts (after clot lysis) and with hemodynamic infarcts.

Contrast enhancement develops primarily in the cortex and deep gray masses (Inoue 1980). The gray matter is considerably more vascular than white matter. The cortex at the margins of the infarct tends to show enhancement earliest, since collateral circulation is initially more adequate to this region (Fig. 15-11). Delayed scans may demonstrate enhancement extending into the underlying white matter. This may be caused either by diffusion of contrast material leaked from the more numerous cortical capillaries or by its slower buildup in white matter related to lower blood flow in this tissue. Vasogenic edema fluid accumulates primarily in white matter, which may further decrease its circulation (Klatzo 1972).

The pattern of infarct enhancement usually has a heterogeneous appearance, which may be related to avascular regions of coagulation necrosis or to variability in the degree of collateral recirculation to different portions of the infarct (Fig. 15-12). At times the enhancing pattern is homogeneous, suggesting incomplete tissue necrosis and more uniform reperfusion of the infarct (Fig. 15-7). With both these patterns the cortical ribbon and basal ganglia are the regions that predominantly enhance when immediate scans are obtained; with delayed scans after contrast (30 minutes to 3 hours), both homogeneous and heterogeneous enhancement may also develop in the white matter (Fig. 15-13). Norton (1978) reported that the patterns of enhancement were homogeneous in 22 percent and heterogeneous in 59 percent of infarcts.

Infarct enhancement may also show a multifocal linear, bandlike configuration or central, peripheral, or ring patterns (Norton 1978; Pullicino 1980). The linear bandlike and the central patterns usually represent different regions of enhancement in the cor-

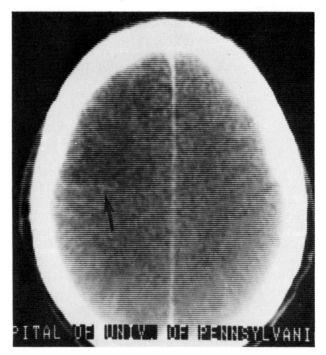

A

B

Figure 15-11 Marginal enhancement in 3-day-old infarct. **A.** NCCT demonstrating wedge-shaped hypodensity involving the cortex and white matter within the right middle cerebral artery territory (arrows). **B.** CECT reveals slight linear enhancement at posterior margin of the infarct (arrow), most probably in the cortex of the infolded convolution. (See Figure 15-13 for progression of enhancement at day 12.)

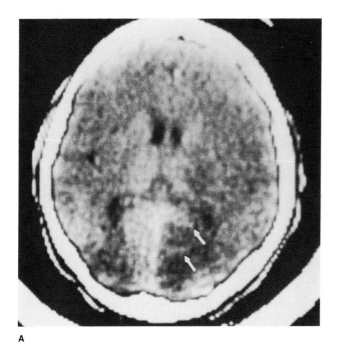

A

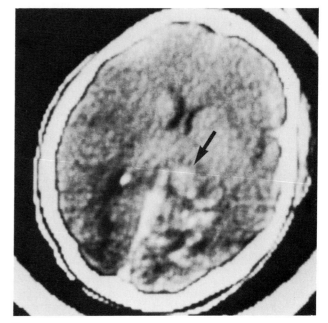

B

Figure 15-12 Heterogeneous enhancement of posterior cerebral artery territory infarct at day 10 (same patient as Figure 15-2C at day 3). **A.** NCCT reveals poorly defined hypodensity in left occipital and posterior thalamic region which contains bands and nodules of isodensity (arrows). **B.** CECT reveals linear and nodular regions of enhancement roughly corresponding in location to the isodense areas within the infarct in **A.** Homogeneous region of enhancement in posterior thalamus (arrows).

tical ribbon within and surrounding the area of infarction (Fig. 15-13). Since the cortical ribbon extends into the depth of the brain a variable distance around the sulci, a region of cortical enhancement may appear at times to be situated within white matter. The central pattern may also represent enhancement in the deep gray masses (Fig. 15-7). Differences in these enhancement patterns probably occur because of variations in collateral reperfusion and in the degree of necrosis in different regions of the infarct.

The peripheral enhancing pattern appears as a rim of enhancement which assumes a roughly hemispheric configuration about the lateral gray matter and deep white-matter margins of the infarct. This pattern would tend to develop about areas of hemispheric infarction when there is necrosis in both

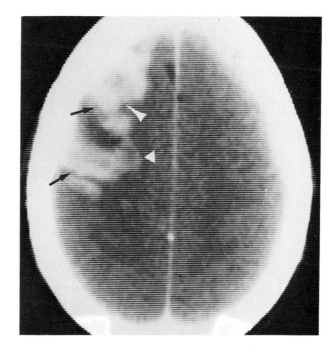

Figure 15-13 CECT: cortical ribbon (gyriform) enhancement (arrows) right middle cerebral artery territory at day 12. Some enhancement of white matter (arrowheads) on delayed CECT at 45 min. See NCCT, Figure 15-6, for isodense bands corresponding to the regions of cortical ribbon enhancement.

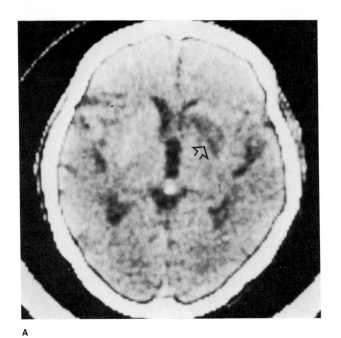

A

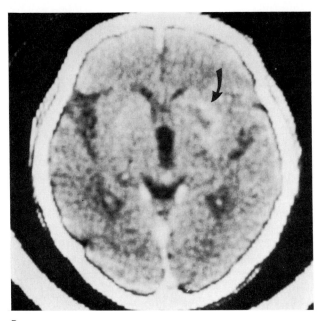

B

Figure 15-14 Ring enhancement in 9-day-old infarct in basal ganglia–anterior capsule region. **A.** NCCT reveals hypodensity involving left anterior capsule–basal ganglia region (arrow) with compression of adjacent frontal horn. CT was normal 7 days before. **B.** CECT demonstrates ring enhancement within outer margin of hypodensity (arrow).

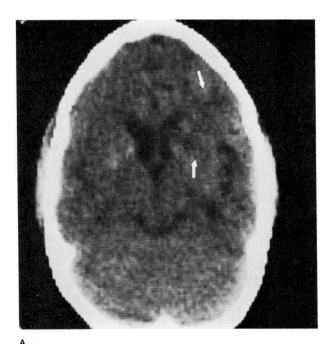

A

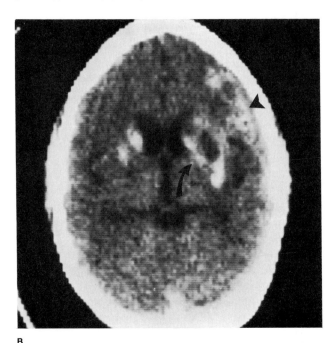

B

Figure 15-15 Left basal ganglionic, middle cerebral artery, and right anterior ganglionic infarct at day 16, secondary to bilateral middle cerebral artery emboli from cardiomyopathy (subsequent autopsy confirmation). **A.** NCCT: hypodensity of left basal ganglionic and presylvian region (arrows) with com-pression of frontal horn. **B.** CECT demonstrates irregular ring enhancement of left basal ganglia (arrow) along with patchy enhancement in the left cortex (arrowhead) and in the right anterior basal ganglia.

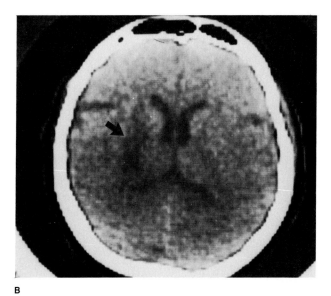

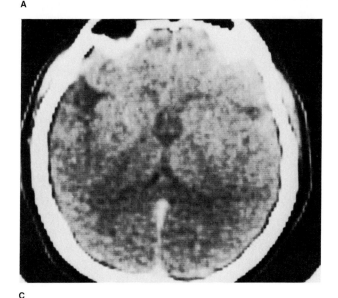

Figure 15-16 Masking of recent infarct with enhancement. **A** and **B.** NCCT, contiguous sections: large right basal ganglia–capsular hypodensity (arrows). **C.** CECT: region of infarct hypodensity in **A** and **B** isodense after enhancement. Similar change was noted on adjacent sections.

gray and white matter as indicated by homogeneous hypodensity in both these regions on NCCT.

The ringlike enhancing pattern is most commonly seen around necrotic infarcts in the basal ganglia (Fig. 15-14) but may also develop around those in the white-matter portion of a hemispheric infarct when there is incomplete non-necrotic involvement of the overlying cortex. Basal ganglia infarcts may be small, resulting from a single lenticulostriate artery occlusion (Fig. 15-14), or large,

when multiple lenticulostriate arteries are blocked secondary to proximal middle cerebral artery occlusion. With the latter, associated infarction may be present in the peripheral middle cerebral artery territory (Fig. 15-15). Central coagulation necrosis commonly develops with basal ganglia infarcts because of inadequate collateral channels to this territory. Ring enhancement develops from the rich neovascular ingrowth in surrounding unaffected portions of the basal ganglia. When the ring pattern surrounds a necrotic white-matter infarct, the ring results from a combination of overlying cortical and peripheral deep white-matter neovascular ingrowth.

In most cases contrast enhancement will elevate a low-density region to one of higher-than-normal tissue density. Occasionally a zone of hypodensity becomes isodense with the surrounding brain on CECT (Fig. 15-16), and the infarction may not be recognized if only CECT is obtained. Wing et al. (1976) noted this postcontrast normalization phenomenon occurring in about 5 percent of recent infarcts. Conversely, they also observed that in 11 percent of the infarcts that enhanced, the NCCT was normal (Fig. 15-17).

The central, peripheral, and ring enhancement patterns present an appearance which may strongly resemble that of tumor or abscess. With infarction, however, most of the mass effect has usually resolved when enhancement appears, and the entire lesion (low density and area of enhancement) is confined to the territory of one vascular distribution in a wedge-shaped or rectangular pattern. There is usually also involvement of cortex. The combination of these changes, which are generally not present with tumor or inflammatory disease, should in most cases reliably differentiate these conditions. If the diagnosis is still uncertain, follow-up CT study should clearly differentiate infarction from the other conditions. With infarction the enhancement usually disappears or markedly decreases in 3 to 4 weeks and atrophic changes develop over the next 1 to 3 months, as evidenced by focal ventricular dilatation and enlargement of overlying cortical sulci.

Weisberg (1980) observed that patients in whom the infarct showed enhancement had a better prognosis than those without enhancement: there were no deaths in a group of 50 patients who had enhancement, whereas 5 of 35 patients without enhancement died after their cerebral infarction. Functional recovery from motor, sensory, visual, and language disturbances was better for patients who showed enhancement and whose follow-up scans showed no residual low-density area, indicating absence of brain necrosis. These findings are in contrast to those of Pullicino and Kendall (1980), who recently reported that enhancing infarcts in their series had a significantly *poorer* prognosis than those without enhancement. They also found that enhancement was more common with larger infarcts and in those that had mass effect. These two factors would probably account for the more adverse prognosis associated with enhancement in their series.

Embolic Infarction

Embolic infarction is probably much more frequent than concluded on clinical grounds. Adams and

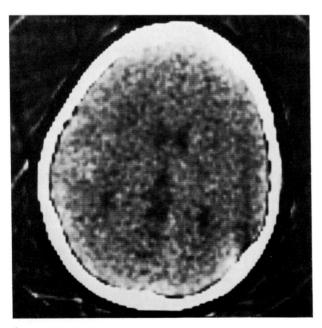

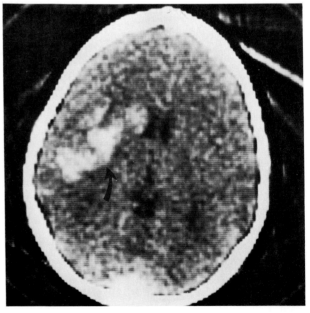

A

B

Figure 15-17 Enhancement of isodense middle cerebral artery territory infarct. **A.** NCCT: no definite abnormality evident. **B.** CECT: extensive enhancement in basal ganglia and parasylvian region.

Vander Eecken (1953) indicate that it is responsible for 50 percent of infarcts. Lhermitte et al. (1970) found in an autopsy study that 68 percent of middle cerebral artery occlusions were embolic in origin. Cerebral emboli frequently originate from heart disease and from atheromatous disease in the aorta or the carotid or vertebral arteries.

Yock (1981) recently identified emboli on NCCT in the middle and anterior cerebral arteries. They appeared as a focal hyperdensity at the usual location near major bifurcations in these vessels. The emboli had peak attenuation values of 84 to 214 HU, which indicated that most consisted of calcific material with or without thrombus. Those with a density of less than 95 HU may represent only dense clot.

With embolic infarction the temporal evolution of early CT changes is different from those seen with atherosclerotic thrombotic infarcts. Whereas atherosclerotic occlusion usually results in a relatively permanent arterial obstruction, the embolic occlusion frequently fragments and undergoes lysis between the first and fifth day, resulting in reestablishment of normal antegrade circulation. This exposes the infarcted brain tissue to a much higher perfusion pressure than was present before clot lysis, when circulation depended on the adequacy of collateral channels. The hemodynamic consequences of clot lysis are responsible for the differences in the CT alterations with embolic infarction. The CT scan performed prior to lysis of an embolus will be similar to that present with an atherosclerotic occlusion, except that there may be infarcts in more than one vascular distribution of approximately the same age (Fig. 15-18). After fragmentation and dissolution of the embolus, the rise in perfusion pressure results in a marked increase in blood flow in and around the infarcted tissue, which frequently becomes higher than normal, and increased breakdown of the blood-brain barrier. This hyperemia develops because there is a loss of normal autoregulatory control of blood flow in the infarct region.

Autoregulation is a unique intrinsic property of normal cerebral vasculature which maintains blood flow at a constant level over a wide range of arterial pressures. This control is located mainly in the ar-

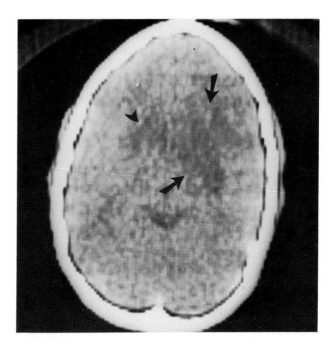

Figure 15-18 Bilateral embolic middle cerebral artery territory infarctions at 36 hours (same patient as in Figure 15-15). Large, poorly defined hypodensity involving basal ganglia and posterior frontal region on left (arrows). Similar but smaller area of hypodensity on right (arrowhead).

terioles, which constrict with rising pressure and dilate with falling pressure. In the normal person the limits of autoregulation extend over a mean arterial pressure ranging from about 50 mmHg to 140 mmHg. The control of this mechanism appears to be mediated through an intrinsic myotonic stretch reflex in the arteriolar wall. In addition, changes in blood and tissue chemical factors such as carbon dioxide, lactic acid, and molecular oxygen concentrations may alter arteriolar diameter and affect autoregulation. Increased carbon dioxide and lactic acid concentrations and decreased oxygen tension cause vasodilation. Vessels with loss of autoregulation may lose their response to these chemical regulators. Infarction, as well as other conditions which cause brain injury such as trauma, infection, subarachnoid hemorrhage, and tumor, results in loss of normal autoregulation and varying degrees of vasoparalysis in the vascular bed of the affected region.

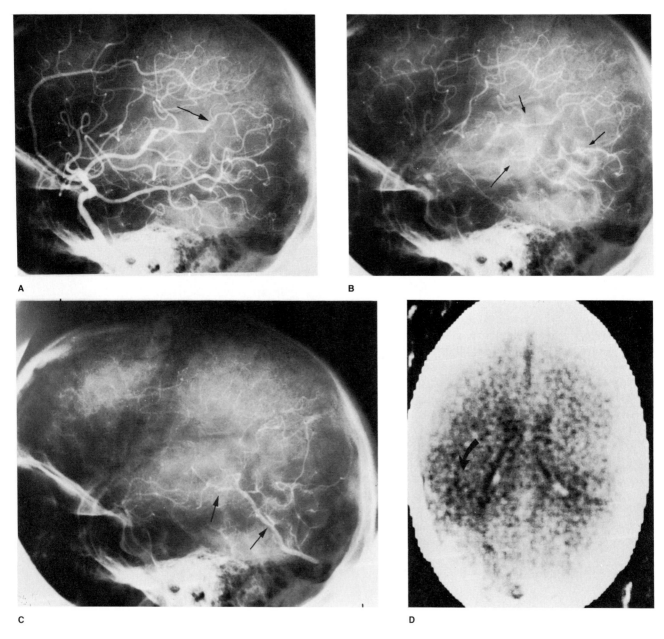

A

B

C

D

Figure 15-19   Embolic infarction reactive hyperemia (luxury perfusion) at day 5 following major clot lysis and reestablishment of antegrade circulation.   **A.** Lateral right carotid angiogram, mid-arterial phase, revealing small embolic fragment partially occluding the angular gyrus artery distally (arrow).   **B.** Lateral right carotid angiogram, late arterial phase, revealing early appearance of a prominent gyriform capillary blush (reactive hyperemia) in the posterior temporal–inferior parietal region (arrows).   **C.** Lateral right carotid angiogram, capillary phase, revealing early venous filling (luxury perfusion) in the posterior temporal–inferior parietal region (arrows).   **D.** NCCT at time of angiogram. Suggestion of ill-defined slight hypodensity in right posterior temporal–parietal region (arrow).   **E.** CECT: gyriform enhancement in right posterior temporal–parietal region (arrows).   **F.** NCCT 4 months after stroke. Well-defined region of marked hypodensity involving cortex and underlying white matter (arrow) in the right posterior temporal–parietal region, associated with ventricular dilatation.

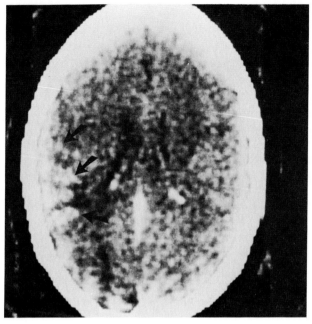

E

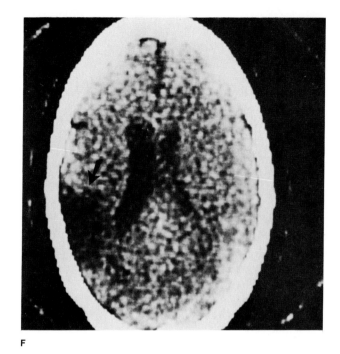

F

Loss of autoregulation may persist for several weeks following infarction; its duration is dependent on the severity of the ischemic injury. During this time circulation in these regions passively follows changes in perfusion pressure, as the arterioles no longer have the capacity to dilate or constrict in response to blood pressure change. The local tissue acidosis which develops within the area of infarction due to build-up of acid metabolites causes vasoparalysis (Myer 1957; Lassen 1966; Kassik 1968). This results in arteriolar dilatation, with blood flow becoming markedly increased with the reestablishment of normal perfusion pressure. Lassen (1966) has characterized this hyperemia as "luxury perfusion," because blood flow to the tissues is above its normal metabolic requirements. The *hyperemic (luxury perfusion) reaction* associated with loss of autoregulation becomes evident only after the return of normal perfusion pressure to the region of infarction, as will occur after lysis of an embolic occlusion. With persistent arterial occlusion this reaction is not seen, except possibly at the margins of the infarct, which could be supplied by antegrade flow through

nonoccluded vessels. Not infrequently some degree of hypertension develops after infarction, which produces further arteriolar dilatation, resulting in a higher rate of blood flow. Cerebral angiography in the first few weeks after dissolution of an embolus usually reveals dilated cortical arterioles and gyral hyperemia associated with early filling of regional draining veins (Fig. 15-19) (Cronqvist 1967, 1968; Ferris 1966; Irino 1977a, 1977b; Leeds 1973; Pitts 1964). Concomitantly the radionuclide brain scan will demonstrate a region of high activity in the dynamic flow sequence (Yarnell 1975; Soin 1976). Focal elevation of cerebral blood flow may also be revealed with the Xe 133 technique (Cronqvist 1967, 1968; Hoedt-Rasmussen 1967; Paulson 1970).

Infarct hyperemia (luxury perfusion) generally causes some regions which were hypodense on CT obtained before revascularization to become isodense or slightly hyperdense on NCCT (Fig. 15-20). This change develops mainly in the cortex and deep gray matter because these regions have a large capillary bed which passively dilates after reperfusion. Rapid-sequence CT scanning after bolus contrast

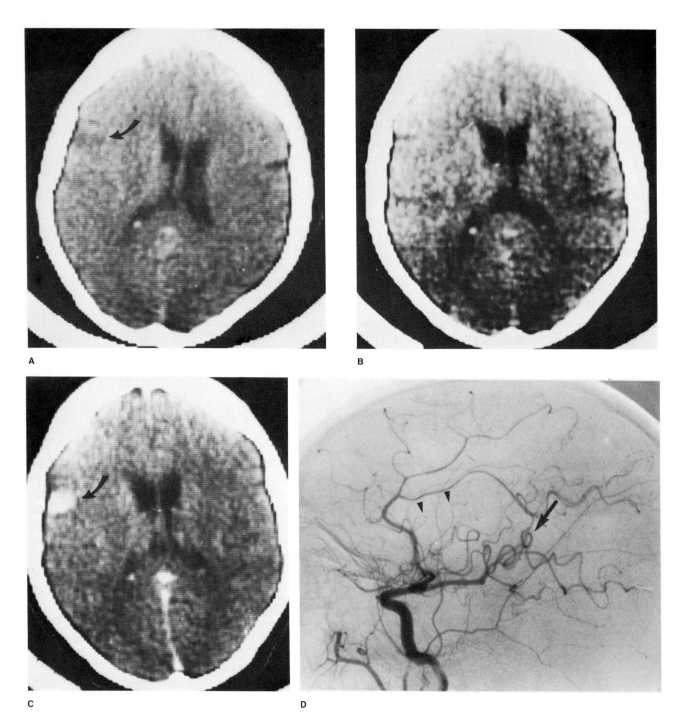

Figure 15-20 Embolic infarction, conversion on NCCT of hypodense tissue to isodensity after reestablishment of antegrade circulation. **A.** NCCT on day 3 reveals cortical hypodensity in the posterior frontal region (arrow). **B.** NCCT on day 8 fails to demonstrate hypodensity. **C.** CECT on day 8 reveals cortical enhancement (arrow) in region of hypodensity in **A.** **D.** Lateral carotid angiogram on day 9 demonstrates embolic occlusion of posterior inferior (arrow) and parietal branches (arrowheads) of middle cerebral artery tributary. Avascular parietal region fills well on subsequent films from distal anterior cerebral artery branches. There is relatively normal antegrade circulation into region of CT abnormality in posterior frontal area (arrowheads) suggesting previous lysis of embolic fragment. Large ulcerated plaque at origin of internal carotid artery is probable source of emboli (not shown).

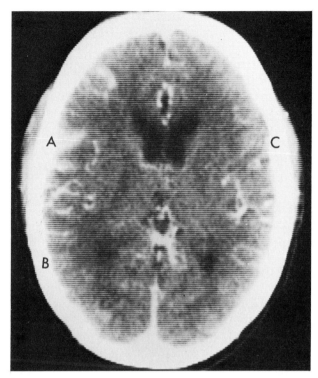

A

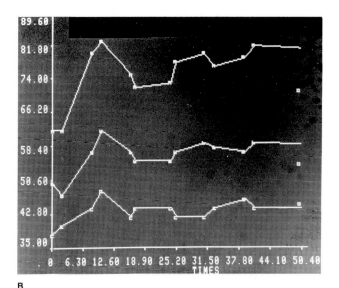

B

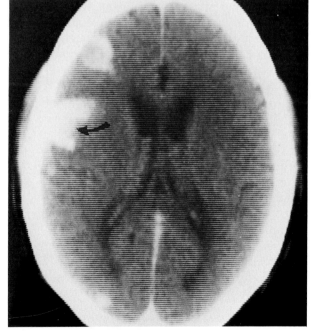

C

Figure 15-21 Hyperemic changes on rapid-sequence bolus injection CT. Probable embolic infarction at day 10. **A.** Rapid-sequence CT approximately 6 seconds after contrast bolus arrival at brain. Maximum vascular phase contrast density at this time. Highest cortical contrast density at location *A*, site of ischemic circulatory changes at day 2 (Fig. 15-10). Locations *B* and *C* over uninvolved cortical regions on previous CT. **B.** Time-density curves of locations *A*, *B*, and *C* in **A**. Graph parameters are the same as in Figure 15-10B. Curve *A* (upper) demonstrates a more rapid and greater rise and a fall of contrast density than curves *B* (middle) and *C* (lower) during their first passage through the brain. Secondary density increase of curve *A* reflects tissue enhancement due to a defective blood-brain barrier and high tissue perfusion pressure. **C.** CT 30 minutes after **A**. Increased cortical enhancement (arrow) with spread of enhancement into adjacent white matter as evidenced by thickening of the cortical ribbon (compare with **A**) and obliteration of the intergyral white-matter hypodensity.

injection may demonstrate the luxury perfusion reaction (Fig. 15-21). Besides the elevation in blood volume, some of the cortical density increase may be the result of the petechial hemorrhages (Inoue 1980). Because of its much lower capillary volume, the white matter does not appreciably contribute to the hyperemic reaction. The density increase in the cortex is usually diffuse but may be spotty, depending on the degree of fragmentation and lysis of the embolus. The NCCT may have a normal appearance, but usually the underlying white matter remains hypodense (Fig. 15-19).

Prominent enhancement develops following lysis of the embolus, usually appearing as a cortical gyral pattern (Fig. 15-19) with frequent involvement of the basal ganglia. The high reperfusion pressure potentiates spread of enhancement into the adjacent white matter (Fig. 15-21). Enhancement appears in most cases by the fifth day and frequently develops earlier, depending on the time it takes for clot lysis to occur. Enhancement is related to disturbance in the blood-brain barrier and, to a lesser extent, hyperemia. Kohlmeyer (1978), evaluating the relationships between CT and cerebral blood flow, found that enhancement was usually not associated with luxury perfusion unless the enhancement develops during the first 3 to 5 days after the stroke. These observations suggest that early enhancement, since it is associated with increased cerebral blood flow, may indicate embolic infarction after clot lysis. Enhancement and luxury perfusion are potentiated by high reperfusion pressure. Hayman et al. (1981) recently described an ominous enhancement pattern in infarcts 9 to 28 hours old that were mainly embolic in origin. The enhancement appeared 1 to 3 hours after intravenous infusion of 80 g of iodine. The enhancement pattern consisted of a large, frequently wedge-shaped, inhomogeneous zone of increased density which involved the cortex and extended down through the white matter to the ventricle (Fig 15-22). Over half the patients with this pattern (four of seven) subsequently developed hemorrhagic infarcts and died. No other "double dose" CECT pattern could be associated with development of hemorrhagic infarction.

Brain swelling is frequently present when enhancement develops with embolic infarcts. This is because enhancement usually becomes evident between the second and fifth day, a time period when infarct brain swelling is maximal. This is in contrast to the general lack of mass effect at the time enhancement appears with atherosclerotic thrombotic infarcts at 10 to 14 days. Brain swelling with embolic infarcts may further increase after the appearance of enhancement, because the increased perfusion pressure resulting from clot lysis potentiates the formation of vasogenic edema (Olsson 1971). In the extreme case, hemorrhagic infarction may develop which further increases the degree of mass effect.

HEMORRHAGIC INFARCTION   This is in most instances an adverse sequela of embolic infarction related to the effects of high-pressure reperfusion of severe ischemic brain. Fisher and Adams (1951) found that in 66 hemorrhagic infarcts, only three were not clearly caused by embolism. Jorgensen and Torbik (1964) observed that 80 percent of embolic infarcts were found at autopsy to be hemorrhagic. Angiography in combination with CT has confirmed the relationship between fragmentation and lysis of the embolus and hemorrhagic infarction (Irino 1977b; Davis 1975, 1977). In the report of Davis et al. (1977), three patients with hemorrhagic infarction all had clinical evidence of an embolic stroke, and in two, cerebral angiography documented the embolic occlusion before there was clinical or CT evidence of the hemorrhagic infarct. In one patient, a repeat cerebral angiogram at the time of neurologic deterioration and appearance of the hemorrhagic infarct on CT revealed lysis of a previously demonstrated embolic occlusion. Hemorrhagic infarction may also occur with atherosclerotic thrombotic infarcts in patients with coagulation disorders and in those on antithrombotic therapy

Figure 15-22 Enhancement on delayed high-contrast dose CT during the first day after the infarct. **A.** NCCT 20 hours after infarct reveals obliteration of the right sylvian fissure and ill-defined slight hypodensity in right posterior frontal region (arrow). **B.** Immediate high-contrast dose CT demonstrates absence of enhancement. **C.** Delayed high-dose CT 3 hours after **B.** Marked enhancement of the cortex in the right frontal region (short arrow) extending in a wedge-shaped fashion deep into the white matter in the middle and posterior frontal region (large arrow). There is in addition enhancement in the region of the right basal ganglia. **D.** Autopsy section of brain 8 days later at same level as CT scans. There is hemorrhagic infarction in region of enhancement on delayed CT in **C** (arrows) and anemic infarction with small cortical petechial hemorrhage in nonenhanced region of adjacent middle cerebral artery territory. (*From Hayman LA et al. 1981.*)

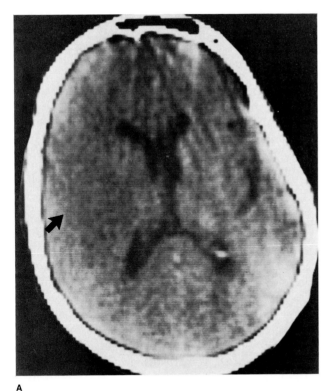

A

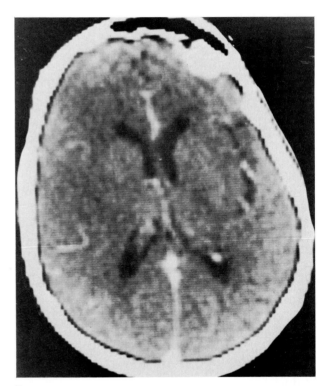

B

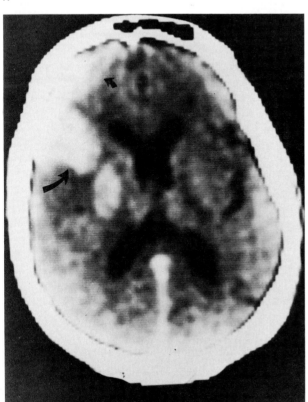

C

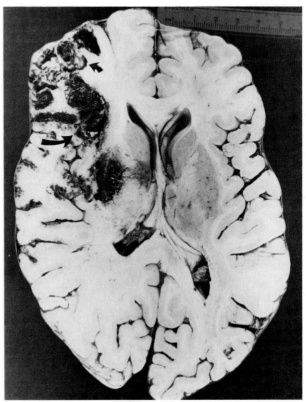

D

(Wood 1958). The incidence of hemorrhagic infarction has been reported to range between 18 and 23 percent (Fisher 1951; Davis 1977; Hayman 1981).

Small areas of petechial hemorrhage are identified pathologically on the periphery of many otherwise bland infarcts, but in hemorrhagic infarcts the petechial hemorrhage is more marked and spread diffusely throughout, though predominantly in the cortex and deep gray matter (Adams 1968). It may involve only areas of cortex located in the depth of sulci. On occasion an area of frank hemorrhage develops from leakage of blood out of small arteries and capillaries into the perivascular spaces. Microscopically these vessels may not show evidence of ischemic damage, which is usually very severe in the surrounding brain parenchyma.

Hemorrhagic infarct is more likely to develop when tissue necrosis is marked. In animal studies, prolonging the initial period of ischemia from 6 to 24 hours before reperfusion increases the incidence of hemorrhagic infarction from 40 to 60 percent (Kamijyo 1977). Increasing blood pressure (Laurent 1976) and the use of heparin (Wood 1958) have also been shown to result in hemorrhagic transformation of some infarcts produced by permanent arterial occlusions. Clinical experience with carotid endarterectomy has similarly shown that reestablishing increased perfusion pressure by surgical removal of the obstructing atheromatous plaque during the first several weeks after a recent infarct may cause conversion of an anemic into a hemorrhagic infarct.

In a serial CT study by Cronqvist (1976), the initial CT scan obtained during the first 5 days revealed only a low-density lesion within the brain in six out of seven patients who developed hemorrhagic infarcts. In one patient the initial scan at 2 days demonstrated hemorrhagic infarction. In the six with initial low-density lesions, hemorrhagic infarction became evident between 5 and 21 days after the onset of the stroke. In another study, Davis et al. (1977) reported that 10 of 12 stroke patients who developed secondary abrupt neurologic deterioration revealed hemorrhagic infarct on CT within 5 days of the initial stroke. Two of the patients had had earlier scans which showed no evidence of hemorrhage. Four developed the hemorrhagic in-

farct after 1 day, three after 2 days, one after 4 days, and two at 5 days.

The hemorrhagic infarct will in most instances reveal a very characteristic CT appearance, which can usually be readily differentiated from that of an intracerebral hematoma (Davis 1975). The hemorrhage primarily involves the cortex (Fig. 15-23), either alone, as confluent petechiae, or with occasional secondary extension into the underlying white matter (Davis 1977). It may also involve the deep gray matter if the embolus initially arrests in the middle cerebral artery proximal to or at the origins of the lenticulostriate arteries (Fig. 15-24). Cortical hemorrhage generally appears as a ribbon or bandlike region of slightly to moderately increased density. It has unsharp margins and assumes the wavy configuration of the cortical gyri. The surrounding white matter is hypodense, and its involvement is limited to the same vascular distribution as the region of hemorrhage. This pattern may be diffuse over a large region of the cortex or may be more localized to the depth of one or more sulci. The hemorrhage may be nonhomogeneous or speckled in appearance (Figs. 15-24, 15-26). At times the petechial hemorrhage is mild and, because of volume averaging, may elevate the low density only up to the isodense range (Alcala 1978). If the hemorrhage extends into the white matter, it may resemble an intracerebral hematoma, from which differentiation may be difficult (Fig. 15-25). An intracerebral hematoma is usually homogeneously dense, with a rounded to oval configuration and sharp, distinct borders. White-matter extension of hemorrhagic infarct, in contrast, may be wedge-shaped to rectangular and is not usually homogeneously dense; its border may be somewhat indistinct.

On CECT, hemorrhagic infarction will usually develop contrast enhancement in the already dense cortical and basal ganglia and, to a variable degree, in the surrounding isodense cortex (Fig. 15-26). The intracerebral hematoma does not show enhancement in the area of hemorrhage.

Clinical deterioration and increased mass effect usually occurs when hemorrhagic infarction develops; they are related to the extravasated blood in

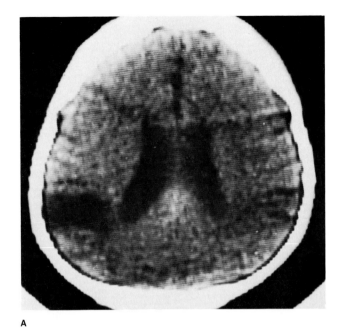

A

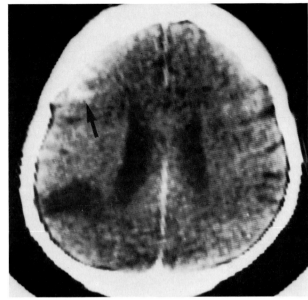

B

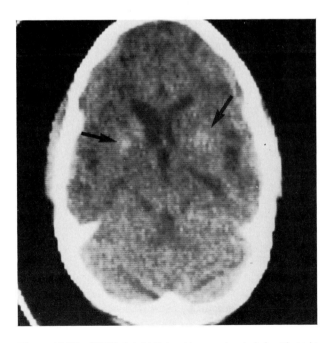

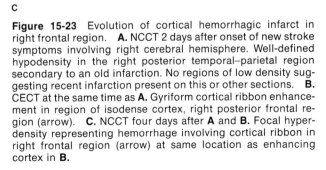

C

Figure 15-23 Evolution of cortical hemorrhagic infarct in right frontal region. **A.** NCCT 2 days after onset of new stroke symptoms involving right cerebral hemisphere. Well-defined hypodensity in the right posterior temporal–parietal region secondary to an old infarction. No regions of low density suggesting recent infarction present on this or other sections. **B.** CECT at the same time as **A.** Gyriform cortical ribbon enhancement in region of isodense cortex, right posterior frontal region (arrow). **C.** NCCT four days after **A** and **B.** Focal hyperdensity representing hemorrhage involving cortical ribbon in right frontal region (arrow) at same location as enhancing cortex in **B.**

Figure 15-24 NCCT: faint bilateral hemorrhagic infarctions in the region of the basal ganglia (arrows), 2 weeks after bilateral middle cerebral artery embolic occlusion.

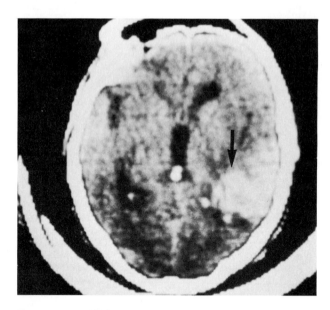

the brain and the increase in vasogenic edema resulting from the higher perfusion pressure at the infarct after clot lysis.

Hemodynamic Infarction

Cerebral ischemic episodes may develop in patients with vasoocclusive disease when there are temporary alterations in circulatory dynamics (Denny-Brown 1960; Brierley 1976). This mainly occurs in older patients with hypertension or cardiac arrhythmias who have a fixed vascular lesion in an extra or intracranial artery (Ruff 1981). The vascular lesion could be either a severe stenosis or an occlusion of long standing (Fig. 15-27).

Cerebral blood-flow studies have demonstrated disturbed autoregulation in this group of patients (Kindt 1967); any decrease in perfusion pressure, therefore, may cause a proportional decrease in cerebral blood flow either focally or diffusely. Depending on the length of time the perfusion pressure is reduced and its severity, the patient may incur a transient ischemic attack, a reversible isch-

Figure 15-25 White matter extension of hemorrhagic infarction caused by middle cerebral artery embolus from heart (autopsy confirmation). NCCT: well-defined high density cortical hemorrhagic involvement in middle and posterior left temporal region with deep white matter extension posteriorly down to the level of the lateral wall of the ventricle (arrow).

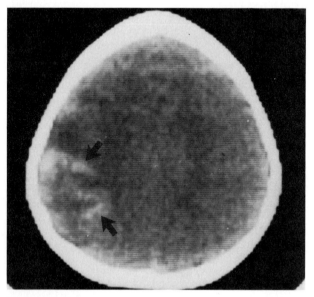

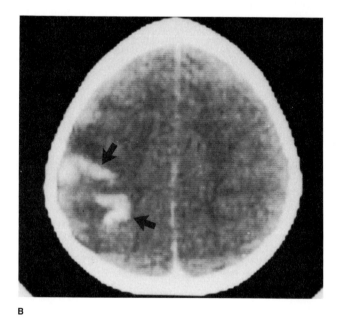

A   B

Figure 15-26 Contrast enhancement of cortical hemorrhagic infarct. **A.** NCCT: patchy gyriform cortical hemorrhagic involvement in the right superior posterior parietal region (arrows). Ischemic infarct hypodensity involving adjacent cortex and underlying white matter. **B.** CECT: enhancement in region of hemorrhagic cortical ribbon (arrows).

emic neurologic deficit, or an infarction. In many of these patients, the stroke occurs while they are asleep at night, probably brought about by a nocturnal reduction of blood pressure. In some hypertensive persons, a reduction in blood pressure, even to only a normotensive level, can result in severe focal cerebral ischemia in the brain already perfused through a stenosed artery or collateral circulation. Cardiac arrhythmias, which can reduce both cardiac output and blood pressure, may cause hemodynamic infarction. Not infrequently, when a patient is first examined after a stroke, blood pressure has returned to its usual level and the cardiac arrhythmia has cleared. Correction of the hemodynamic alteration reestablishes brain-perfusion pressure at its normal level and accounts for the early appearance on angiography of luxury perfusion (Fig. 15-27 A–D) and abnormalities in the blood-brain barrier on CT (Fig. 15-27E, F) (Ito 1976).

The regions of the brain most severely affected by hemodynamic infarction are the border zones, or watershed area (Romanul 1964; Brierley 1976), located at the junctions of the anterior, middle, and posterior cerebral artery circulations. Border zones

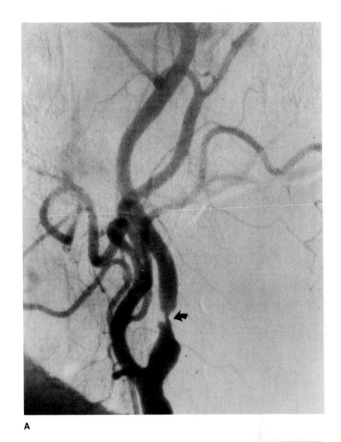

A

Figure 15-27 Watershed infarct at day 3. **A.** Cervical carotid angiogram: severe stenosis with ulceration near origin of internal carotid artery (arrow). **B.** Lateral carotid angiogram, mid-arterial phase. Slowed intercranial circulation as evidenced by distal middle cerebral artery branch filling (arrowhead) lagging behind filling of high scalp tributaries of the external carotid artery (arrow). Normally the distal middle cerebral branches fill before those of the external carotid artery.

(Continued on p. 612.) B

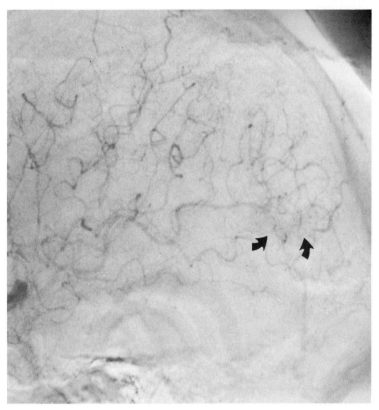

C

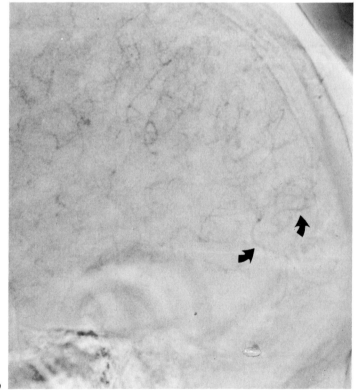

D

Figure 15-27 (Cont.) **C.** Lateral carotid angiogram, late arterial phase. Faint cortical blush at temporal occipital watershed junction (arrows). **D.** Lateral carotid angiogram, early capillary phase. Early venous filling (arrows) from region of capillary blush in **C.** **E.** NCCT: no abnormality on this section or at other levels. **F.** CECT: cortical enhancement at same region as angiographic hyperemia in temporal occipital watershed (arrows).

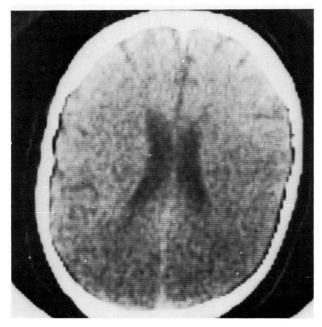

E

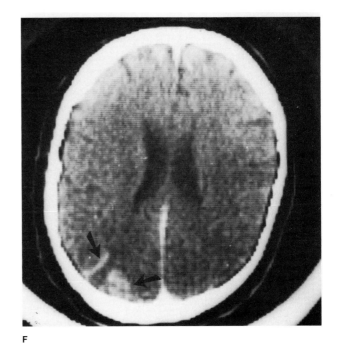

F

are most vulnerable to ischemic injury from a generalized reduction in perfusion pressure, because they are the terminal areas of supply of each major artery and therefore have the lowest perfusion pressure in these vascular distributions. If significant occlusive disease develops in the large arteries at the base of the brain or extracranially, ischemic damage in the watershed region may develop from even a mild reduction in blood pressure, because the occlusive disease reduces distal perfusion pressure to a level at which autoregulation produces maximum vasodilatation. At this point no further compensation for additional pressure reduction is possible, particularly in the watershed zone, and ischemic injury occurs. The watershed region tends to shift into the territory of the involved vascular system. The parietal occipital border zone is the region most susceptible to hemodynamic ischemic injury, as it is the most peripheral region of the anterior, middle, and posterior cerebral arterial circulations to the cerebral hemispheres.

On CT, the cortical luxury-perfusion pattern in hemodynamic infarction is similar to that seen with embolic infarction after clot lysis but occurs earlier and in a different distribution. It is usually present when the patient is first seen during the initial 24 hours. NCCT will in most instances appear normal (Fig. 15-27E) but may show slight density reduction in the white matter. This may only become evident in later scans or may not develop at all. The ischemic injury frequently remains localized to the cortex, which histologically reveals incomplete infarction, with the damage limited to neurons in the third or the fifth and sixth cortical layers, or both. This variety of infarction is frequently referred to as *laminar necrosis*. If the ischemic insult is severe, all layers of the cortex will be involved, along with the underlying white matter (Brierley 1976). On CECT, a cortical gyral blush develops, predominantly in the parietal-occipital watershed region (Fig. 15-27F). Enhancement may persist for only a few days or may last for several weeks, depending on the severity of the initial ischemic damage.

Hemodynamic watershed infarction may on occasion be hemorrhagic in nature (Brierley 1976). This may occur if the initial ischemia is very severe or the reperfusion pressure is high, as may develop with hypertensive disease.

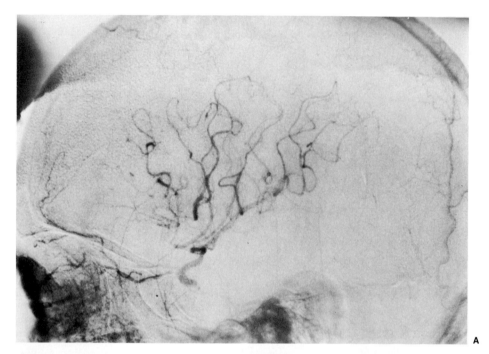

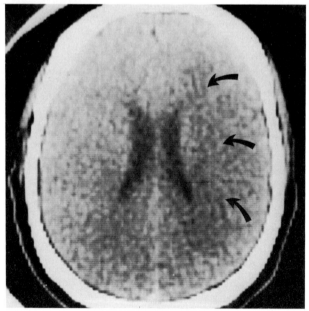

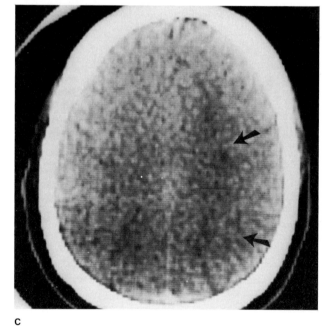

Figure 15-28 Deep watershed infarct. **A.** Lateral carotid angiogram, mid-arterial phase. Internal carotid artery completely occluded in neck at origin (not shown). Retrograde ophthalmic artery flow to intracranial carotid and middle cerebral arteries. Very slow filling and washout of middle cerebral artery branches. **B.** NCCT 3 days after stroke: poorly defined diffuse slight hypodensity in left periventricular white matter (arrows). **C.** NCCT, day 3, at supraventricular level: slight white-matter hypodensity on the left extends more superficially in parietal-occipital watershed region (arrows). **D.** NCCT at 4 months: well-defined more hypodense region in left central white matter extending superficially in parietal-occipital watershed region (arrows). **E.** High-convexity-level CT at 4 months. Increased prominence of cortical sulci on left at distal middle cerebral–anterior cerebral artery watershed territory.

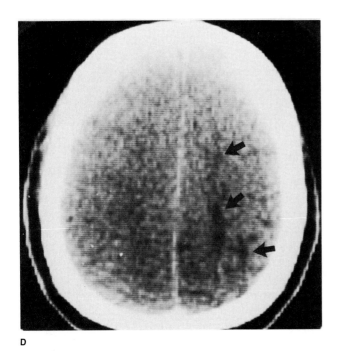

D

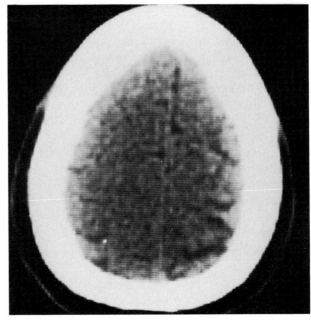

E

The chronic change of incomplete (laminary) cortical infarction on CT is sulcal dilatation (Fig. 15-8). It generally becomes evident after 2 to 3 months in the region where the gyral enhancement pattern was demonstrated. In cases with more profound ischemia resulting in complete cortical infarction and white-matter involvement, the affected cortex, initially isodense, becomes hypodense during the next 4 to 6 weeks; the underlying white matter, which may originally have been slightly hypodense, becomes a more sharply demarcated region of hypodensity. The adjacent portion of the lateral ventricle usually dilates. Some surrounding sulci may also enlarge because of incomplete infarction in the bordering cortex.

Another CT pattern associated with hemodynamic infarction is hypodensity involving mainly the deep periventricular white matter. This alteration tends to occur when there is a long-standing carotid occlusion and chronic ischemia in the hemisphere from poor collateral circulation (Fig. 15-28A). It is not entirely clear why the white matter is preferentially involved in these circumstances. It is possible that with chronic ischemia there is a

change in the blood-flow relationship between the cortex and white matter, with greater flow going to cortical areas. This might occur because of a more pronounced effect of autoregulatory vasodilatation in the cortical vascular bed, which is about four times greater than that in the white matter, and the potentially higher perfusion pressure in the cortical arterioles, which are closer to the supplying vessels on the brain surface. The combination of these two factors would tend to result in shunting of circulation away from the white matter. A reduction in arterial perfusion pressure might then cause a significant ischemia only in the white matter and not in the cortex.

This white-matter involvement is primarily located adjacent to the superior lateral border of the lateral ventricle, in the region of the body and trigone (Fig. 15-28B). This area is not only a terminal field of supply for the penetrating (ventriculopetal) transmedullary white-matter arteries originating on the brain surface but is also a deep watershed zone between these arteries and the short arterial branches radiating outward from the lateral ventricle (ventriculofugal tributaries) (De Reuck 1971).

The ventriculofugal arteries originate from two sources. They are the terminal tributaries of the lenticulostriate artery branches which supply the lateral aspect of the caudate nucleus as well as tributaries of branches from the anterior choroidal and posterior lateral choroidal arteries which supply the ventricular wall.

A severe episode of hypotension or reduction in cardiac output, such as may occur following myocardial infarction or during surgery, can result in extensive bilateral cortical infarction with accentuation in the watershed distribution even in patients without preexisting vascular disease (Brierley 1976). White-matter involvement is not usual but may occur in cases with severe circulatory deficiency or, more commonly, if there is associated hypoxia (DeReuck 1978). In addition, the terminal territories of the lenticulostriate supply to the basal ganglia may also be affected. The main areas of basal ganglia involvement are the inferomedial portion of the head of the caudate nucleus, the upper and outer border of the head and body of the caudate nucleus, and the upper part of the anterior third of the putamen (Brierley 1976). The thalamus is usually not significantly affected. Watershed infarction may also occur in the cerebellum, in the boundary between the areas supplied by the superior cerebellar and posterior inferior cerebellar arteries. In the acute phase the gray-matter regions may be isodense on NCCT and show enhancement on CECT. In the chronic stage, depending on the severity of the initial oligemia, the gray matter may demonstrate hypodense necrotic areas or diffuse atrophic change. White matter may become hypodense, particularly in the periventricular regions.

Intracerebral Arteriolar Disease

Occlusive disease of the intraparenchymal arterioles may be the sole or major vascular involvement in several disease entities. *Arteriolosclerosis* is the pathologic process mainly encountered in patients with long-standing hypertension. The long, penetrating lenticulostriate arteries and arterioles supplying the internal capsule and basal ganglia region are the ones most commonly involved with this disease process (Prineas 1966; Fisher 1979). To a lesser extent the penetrating arteries to the brainstem and cerebral white matter are affected. Pathologically, arteriolosclerosis resembles atherosclerosis of the larger arteries in that there may be fibroblastic intimal proliferation with increased collagen fibers, but in addition wall thickening and stenosis from hyalin deposition in the subintimal, medial, and outer layers of the arteries also occur. Microaneurysms develop from wall weakening due to the hyalin degeneration (Russell 1963; Cole 1967) and may lead to thrombosis of the vessel or intracerebral hemorrhage, both of which are prevalent in hypertensive persons.

Amyloid or congophilic angiopathy is another type of small-vessel disease which occurs with increasing incidence in the elderly. It is reported to be present in 46 percent of those over 70 years of age (Vinters 1981). The disease, unlike arteriolosclerosis, affects only the intracortical arterioles and does not involve the penetrating arteries to the white matter, basal ganglia nuclei, brainstem, or cerebellum. The occipital and parietal cortex is most commonly involved. The disease is associated with Alzheimer's plaques in patients without a familial history of Alzheimer's disease. Dementia is commonly associated with amyloid angiopathy. Occasionally, intracerebral hemorrhage situated mainly in the cortex and superficial white matter and frequently associated with subarachnoid hemorrhage occurs, in contrast to hypertensive intracerebral hemorrhages, which are usually centered more deeply in the white matter and rarely involve the cortex or extend into the subarachnoid space.

Several varieties of collagen arteritis may affect the small intracerebral arteries, including polyarteritis nodosa, lupus erythematosus, and Wegener's granulomatosis. Granulomatous arteritis, infectious or allergic, primarily involves the intracerebral arterioles but may affect the larger surface arteries. Some forms of central nervous system infection, including viral meningoencephalitis, purulent meningitis, mucormycosis meningitis, and syphilitic angiitis, may have prominent intraparenchymal arterial involvement.

LACUNAR INFARCTS The arteriolosclerotic vascular disease process associated with the chronically hypertensive patient frequently produces small lacunar infarcts, most commonly located in the basal ganglia–internal capsule territory. These are in the distribution of the six to twelve lenticulostriate penetrating arteries which arise from the proximal anterior and middle cerebral arteries. Other arteries to this territory arise from the anterior choroidal artery. Severe neurologic deficit may develop from occlusion or significant stenosis of even one of these small penetrating vessels (Fisher 1965), which range in size at their origin from about 0.2 to 0.8 mm in diameter. The lacunar infarcts may be as small as 0.5 cm in maximum diameter or less or as large as 2.5 cm in maximum diameter. The variation in infarct size is determined by the site of lenticulostriate artery occlusion (origin or peripheral branch) and the caliber of the individual artery at its origin (Fisher 1979).

Lacunar infarcts assume a cylindrical to conical configuration and extend through a portion of the basal ganglia and internal capsule, often terminating in the periventricular white matter. The location of the infarct in the basal ganglia depends on which striate artery is occluded (Manelfe 1981). When a middle cerebral artery lenticulostriate branch is occluded, the infarct may involve a greater or lesser portion of either the putamen along with the superior and periventricular part of the knee and posterior limb of the internal capsule and body of the caudate nucleus (Fig. 15-16), or the lateral aspects of the head of the caudate nucleus and anterior limb of the internal capsule (Fig. 15-29). When the anterior cerebral striate artery (recurrent artery of Heubner) is involved, the medial inferior portion of both the head of the caudate nucleus and anterior limb of the internal capsule are affected. When anterior choroidal striate arteries are occluded (Fig. 15-30), the infarct involves the globus pallidus, the inferior part of the knee and posterior limb of the internal

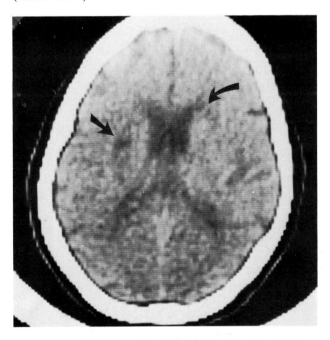

Figure 15-29 Middle cerebral–lenticulostriate artery territory lacunar infarct, with anterior limb of internal capsule superiorly and adjacent anterior portion of putamen on right (straight arrow). Suggestion of very small lacunar infarct in head of anterior lateral caudate nucleus (curved arrow).

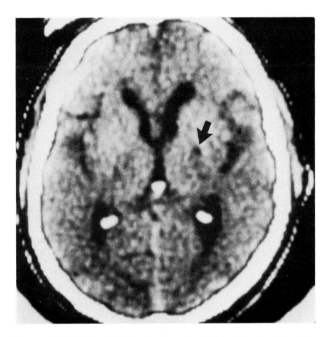

Figure 15-30 Small old anterior choroidal artery territory lacunar infarct hypodensity in region of globus pallidus and knee of internal capsule (arrow).

capsule, and the retrolenticular capsular fibers. Less frequently, lacunar infarcts involve the thalamus. Brainstem lacunar infarcts are commonly observed pathologically, but these as a rule are not delineated on CT, especially in the early stage (Fig. 15-31).

Depending on the size of the occluded lenticulostriate artery, the basal ganglia lacunar infarct may or may not be revealed in the acute phase by CT (Nelson 1980). Those less than 1 cm in size are usually not defined during the first week after the infarct but may become evident after 3 to 4 weeks when cystic encephalomalacic change has developed (Fig. 15-32). Larger lesions are usually demonstrated by 48 hours, appearing as ill-defined oval regions of hypodensity with their longest dimension in the anterior posterior direction (Fig. 15-16). They lie within the confines of the basal ganglia and adjacent internal capsule. Comparison with the tissue density in the contralateral homologous basal ganglia region will aid in appreciating early, minimal, low-density change. Not infrequently the region of decreased attenuation involves only the

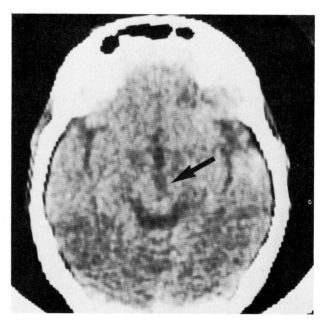

Figure 15-31 Delayed appearance of midbrain lacunar infarct: CT 3 years after acute onset of persistent midbrain symptoms. Initial CT normal. Small hypodensity behind third ventricle in midbrain (arrow). Confirmed at autopsy.

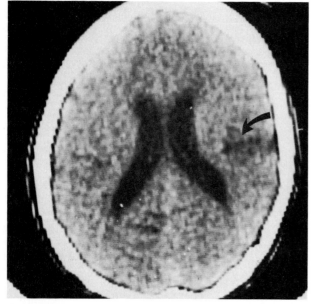

A

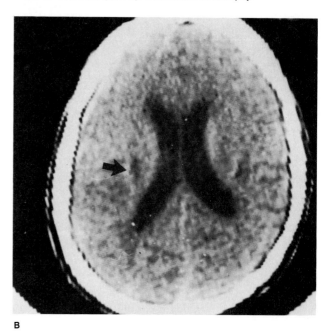

B

Figure 15-32 Delayed appearance of small lacunar infarct. **A.** Three days after onset of symptoms in right hemisphere, CT fails to disclose abnormality, although hypodensity from old infarct is visible in left hemisphere (arrow). **B.** CT at 2 weeks. Small hypodensity appears in superior posterior putamen and periventricular internal capsule (arrow).

most superior portion of the putamen and the white matter adjacent to the outer angle of the lateral ventricle (Fig. 15-32). Slight mass effect and contrast enhancement may develop at the appropriate times, that is, 3 to 5 days for mass effect and 7 to 10 days for enhancement (Fig. 15-14). After 3 to 4 weeks a more sharply defined and lower-density lesion becomes evident. Small lacunes not previously identified may be revealed, confined to a single CT section (Fig. 15-32). The thinner the CT section, the more likely it is that small lesions will be identified.

BINSWANGER'S DISEASE (SUBCORTICAL ARTERIOSCLEROTIC ENCEPHALOPATHY) At times the arteriolosclerotic vasculopathy of hypertension may predominantly involve the long, penetrating transmedullary arterioles which extend from the brain surface into the deep frontal and parietal white matter. The arteries to the basal ganglia are usually also affected. Progressive dementia is the cardinal clinical feature of this peculiar variety of hypertensive vascular disease. There is usually also a history, physical findings, and CT evidence of previous stroke.

The neuropathologic changes in Binswanger's disease consist of diffuse demyelination or focal areas of partial necrosis in the cerebral white matter (or both), mainly in the frontal and occipital lobes. Lacunar infarcts in the basal ganglia are frequently present. The white matter and basal ganglia arterioles are affected by arteriolosclerosis.

On CT, Binswanger's disease demonstrates either diffuse or patchy low-density areas in the white matter of the centrum semiovale and the frontal and occipital regions with prominent involvement of the periventricular area. The changes occur bilaterally but not always in a symmetrical pattern. One or more lacunar infarcts are usually evident in the basal ganglia–internal capsule region or thalamus (Fig. 15-33) (Rosenberg 1979; Zeumer 1980).

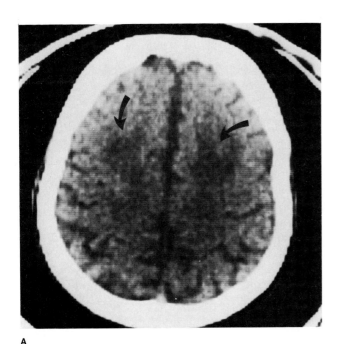

A

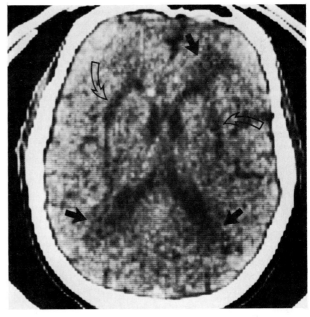

B

Figure 15-33 Binswanger's disease. **A.** Diffuse bilateral patchy white-matter hypodensity (arrows). **B.** Section at level of basal ganglia: large bilateral lacunar infarcts (curved arrows) and periventricular hypodensity adjacent to frontal and occipital horns (arrows).

Arteritis

Cerebral arteritis may involve the large arteries at the base of the brain, the convexity branches, the smaller intracerebral arterioles, or a combination of the three (Sole-Llenas 1978). Many of the disease processes causing arteritis characteristically involve arteries of only one size. Cranial arteritis may be primary or secondary. When primary, the disease process primarily involves the arteries; when secondary, the disease is primarily affecting the meninges or brain parenchyma and involves the arteries secondarily.

With *primary arteritis* the cerebral involvement may be just one of many manifestations of a systemic disorder, such as collagen disease, giant cell arteritis, sarcoidosis, or tertiary syphilis. Occasionally the intracranial arteritis is the sole manifestation at the time of one of these disease processes. Alternatively, primary arteritis may be caused by a disease process which affects mainly the brain arteries, such as granulomatous and chemical arteritis. Cerebral chemical arteritis may be caused by amphetamine and heroin abuse (Rumbaugh 1971), ergotamine, and anovulatory medication. There are undoubtedly other drugs and chemical agents which produce cerebral arteritis. In many cases the exact cause for a primary arteritis cannot be identified.

The CT alterations caused by primary cerebral arteritis are nonspecific and quite varied. Correlation of the CT findings with the clinical history, physical examination, age, and sex of the patient will greatly aid in arriving at the most appropriate diagnosis.

Cerebral arteritis develops with systemic lupus erythematosus (SLE) and occurs mainly in young women, who may manifest psychosis, mental alterations, seizures, or focal neurologic deficits (Johnson 1968; Glaser 1952, 1955; Bilaniuk 1977). Nervous-system involvement in SLE has been reported in 25 to 75 percent of cases (Johnson 1968), but arteritis is not common, being present in from 6 to 13 percent of cases (Ellis 1979). It primarily involves the small cerebral arteries. On CT the most frequent abnormality is enlargement of cortical sulci (Fig. 15-

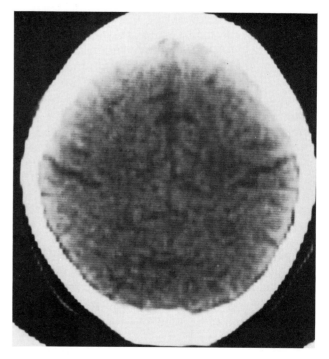

Figure 15-34 Systemic lupus erythematosus. Progressive mental deterioration in 18-year-old female. Enlargement of sulci for age.

34) (Bilaniuk 1977). This change reflects arteritic involvement of the cortical arterioles, resulting in microinfarcts in this region (Johnson 1968). The small arteries supplying the basal ganglia–internal capsule region may also be involved causing either lacunar infarcts or intracerebral hemorrhage (Bilaniuk 1977; Ellis 1979). Arteritic involvement of the large arteries at the base of the brain and the medium-sized arteries in the sylvian fissures and over the convexity on occasion may cause more typical cerebral hemispheric infarcts (Trevor 1972).

Granulomatous arteritis predominantly involves the small leptomeningeal and penetrating arteries and veins of less than 200 μm in diameter to the white matter. Occasionally the larger cerebral arteries are affected (Cravioto 1959; Nurick 1972; Rosenblum 1972). The CT manifestation of this involvement is a diffuse edematous-like, bilateral, white-matter low-density pattern (Fig. 15-35) (Faer 1977). Contrast enhancement is generally not seen with white-matter involvement (Faer 1977). There may

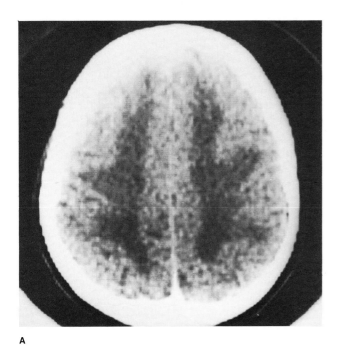

A

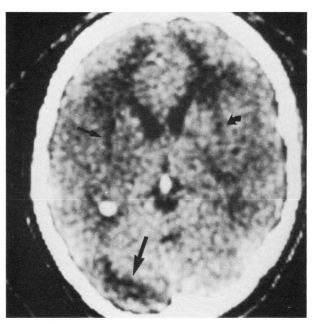

B

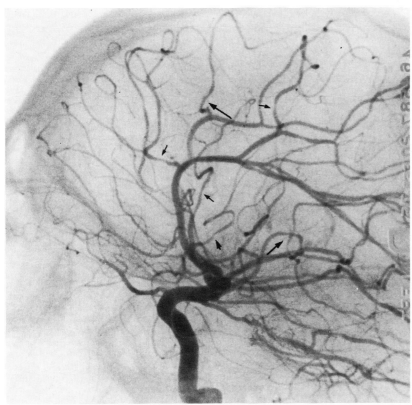

C

Figure 15-35 Granulomatous arteritis in 38-year-old male (biopsy confirmation). **A.** Diffuse bilateral white-matter hypodensity. **B.** Diffuse bilateral anterior frontal white-matter hypodensity. Focal infarct hypodensities at left posterior putamen (curved arrow), right anterior putamen (small arrow), and right occipital region (large arrow). **C.** Lateral carotid angiogram: multiple focal regions of peripheral arterial branch narrowing (arrows).

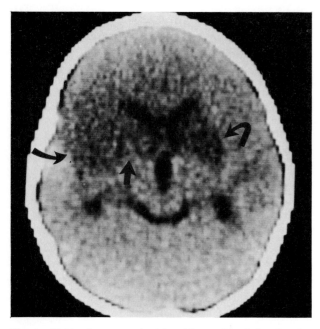

Figure 15-36 Acute meningitis with arteritis: infarction hypodensity in bilateral basal ganglia and right middle cerebral artery territory anteriorly (arrows).

also be focal low-density regions of the cortex and white matter representing more typical infarcts and reflecting arteritic involvement of large and medium-sized branches (Fig. 15-35). Contrast enhancement and mass effect develop with lesions in this location (Valvanis 1979).

In many cases of primary arteritis there is bilateral involvement, with multiple areas of infarction similar to those seen with emboli. Angiography is usually required to substantiate the diagnosis and will demonstrate multiple segmental regions of irregular narrowing in the secondary and tertiary peripheral branches of the main cerebral arteries (Fig. 15-35).

Secondary cerebral arteritis is caused by central nervous system inflammatory disease. Although the diagnosis can usually be readily established clinically and by cerebral spinal fluid examination, occasionally the appropriate clinical manifestations are not apparent and only the manifestations caused by the arteritis are evident. In these instances the CT may reveal alterations which will suggest the correct diagnosis. This situation may occur with the more

indolent types of meningitis such as tuberculous and fungal.

Secondary arteritis, besides revealing CT alterations of ischemic disease, frequently reveals other abnormalities related to the subarachnoid inflammatory disease which are suggestive of this diagnosis. CECT may show enhancement of the subarachnoid spaces around the basal cisterns, in the sylvian fissure, over the convexity, or in a combination of these locations (Enzmann 1976; Bilaniuk 1978; Chu 1980). Hydrocephalus may develop from obstruction of the subarachnoid pathways, the ventricular outflow at the exit foramina of the fourth ventricle, or the aqueduct of Sylvius by inflammatory exudate and fibrosis (Sole-Llenas 1978).

Purulent meningitis causes a heavy inflammatory exudate which mainly accumulates around the base of the brain. Here it may produce arteritic involvement of the supraclinoid carotid (Leeds 1971), the proximal segments of the anterior and middle cerebral arteries, or the penetrating arteries to the basal ganglia and thalamic region (Cairns 1946). Bilateral or unilateral infarctions may develop in basal

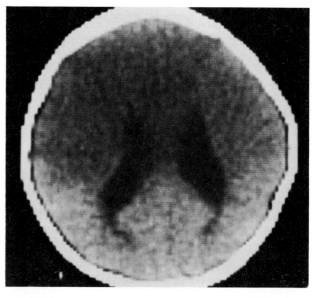

Figure 15-37 *Haemophilus influenzae* meningitis with bilateral large anteriorly located infarctions in anterior and middle cerebral artery territories. Diffuse bilateral hypodensity anteriorly in the brain, more marked on the right side. Moderate hydrocephalus.

ganglia, cerebral hemisphere, or both (Fig. 15-36).

With *Haemophilus influenzae* meningitis the purulent exudate may be around the base but is also located more peripherally over the brain surface, causing arteritis in the insula and convexity arteries (Leeds 1971). This may produce multiple small or large regions of infarction, which are more frequently located anteriorly in the frontal lobes (Fig. 15-37) (Cockrill 1978).

Tuberculous meningitis may involve both the basal and convexity subarachnoid spaces (Fig. 15-38) and can affect the arteries at either or both locations (Dastur 1966; Lehrer 1966; Leeds 1971). Depending on which region is primarily involved, the CT may reveal either a large infarct in one vascular territory or one or more small infarcts in several vascular teritories (Chu 1980). Hydrocephalus may be a prominent feature with tuberculous meningitis (see Chap. 13).

Moyamoya Disease

Moyamoya disease is a condition of unknown etiology resulting in progressive occlusion of the terminal segment of the supraclinoid portion of the internal carotid artery and the proximal portions of the anterior and middle cerebral arteries. The proximal posterior cerebral arteries may also be affected. The disease usually develops in childhood and is most prevalent in the Japanese (Kudo 1968) but has been reported in other races as well (Taveras 1969).

In children the initial manifestations are usually related to cerebral ischemia and include motor and sensory disturbance, involuntary movements, convulsions, headaches, and mental deterioration. In adults the disease usually presents with subarachnoid or intracerebral hemorrhage.

Angiography and pathologic examination reveal tapered partial-to-complete occlusions of the vessels

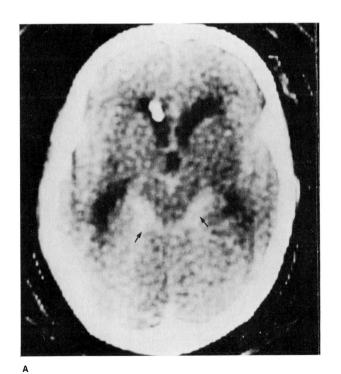
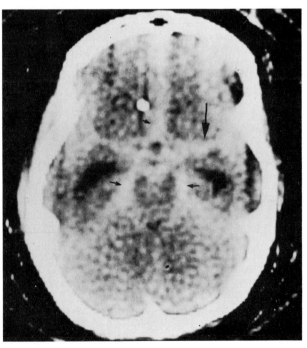

A   B

Figure 15-38 Tuberculous meningitis with clinical brainstem vasculitis. **A** and **B.** CECT: diffuse enhancement throughout basal and sylvian cisterns (arrows). Cisterns isodense on NCCT. Residual hydrocephalus shortly after ventricular shunting.

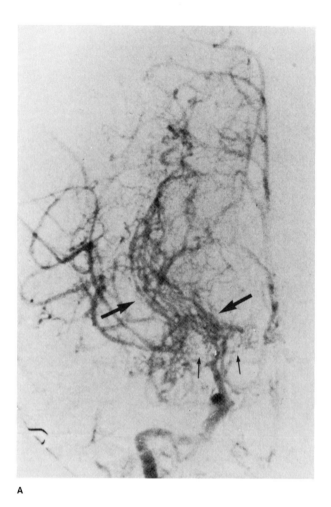

A

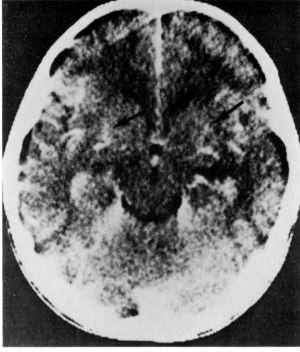

B

Figure 15-39 Moyamoya disease. **A.** Frontal carotid angiogram: tapered occlusion of proximal segments of anterior and middle cerebral arteries (small arrows). Marked dilatation of lenticulostriate arteries representing the moyamoya blush (large arrows). **B.** CECT: prominent curvilinear and punctate vascular-like densities in lenticulostriate artery distribution (arrows). (*From Takahashi M, et al. 1980.*)

about the internal carotid artery bifurcation bilaterally. Marked dilatation develops in the intraparenchymal arteries in the basal ganglia, upper brainstem, and thalamus, which provide collateral circulation to the middle and anterior cerebral arteries distal to their occlusions. This vascular dilatation is the so-called moyamoya blush (Fig. 15-39), *moyamoya* meaning "puff of smoke" in Japanese. The collateral vessels arise from the internal carotid artery proximal to its occlusion and from the anterior choroidal, posterior communicating, and terminal basilar artery bifurcation (Nishimoto 1968; Suzuki 1969; Taveras 1969; Pecker 1973).

The CT scan may reveal nonspecific abnormalities related to focal and diffuse ischemia, such as multiple small areas of parenchymal hypodensity and evidence of cerebral atrophy consisting of dilatation of sulci, interhemispheric and sylvian fissures, and ventricles (Handa 1977). In adults and occasionally in children hemorrhage occurs which may be subarachnoid, basal ganglionic (Fig. 15-40), or intraventricular. The hemorrhage is caused by rupture of a dilated collateral vessel which may develop pseudoaneurysms (Kodama 1978). Takahashi et al. (1980) recently reported a more characteristic abnormality consisting of irregular interrupted or tortuous curvilinear densities in the basal ganglia on CECT. These densities correspond to the location of the most prominent parenchymal collaterals on carotid angiography (Fig. 15-39).

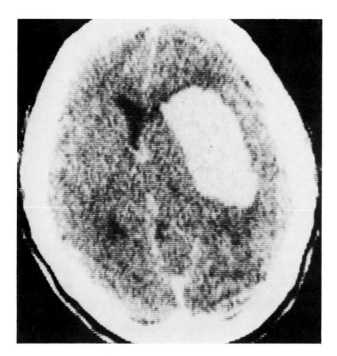

Figure 15-40 Moyamoya disease with large hematoma in basal ganglia on left. (*Courtesy of J. H. Suh, M.D. Severance Hospital, Seoul, Korea.*)

Complicated Migraine

The majority of patients with classical migraine have EEG abnormalities during the attack, usually most marked in the occipital region, and many of these patients develop focal neurologic changes at this time. It is postulated that during the prodromal phase vasospasm develops in some intracranial arteries, resulting in localized cerebral ischemia. This is supported by angiographic and cerebral blood-flow studies, which have shown vasospasm and decreased flow during the attack.

Abnormal CT scans have been noted during and sometimes shortly after the migraine attack in one-third to one-half of the patients (Mathew 1976; Hungerford 1976). The CT reveals focal low-density regions that do not enhance or cause mass effect. They are more commonly located posteriorly in the cerebral hemispheres (Fig. 15-41). The hypodensities will resolve completely on follow-up scans obtained after several weeks if the neurologic deficit clears.

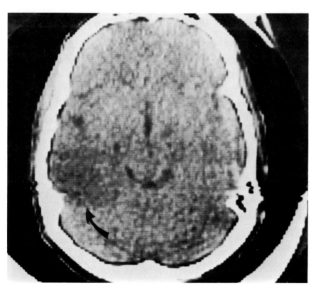

A

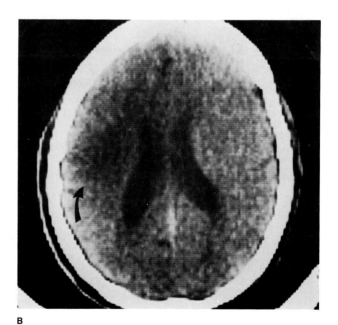

B

Figure 15-41 Complicated migraine: recurrent neurologic deficits associated with headaches. **A.** Diffuse mild hypodensity in right posterior temporal region (arrow). **B.** Diffuse hypodensity in right parietal and posterior frontal region (arrow). Moderate ventricular dilatation.

Brainstem and Cerebellar Infarction

Fewer infarcts are detected by CT in the posterior fossa (Campbell 1978; Kingsley 1980), in part because of inherent computer artifacts in this region from the dense petrous ridges and the occipital bony crest which degrade the images. In addition, significant neurologic deficit may result from very small, critically located infarcts in the brainstem. These small lesions are frequently below the resolution capability of the CT scanner, especially during the acute phase of the infarct. Follow-up scans at 3 months may reveal a higher percentage of infarcts because of the sharper demarcation and greater hypodensity of residual small cystic areas of necrosis (Fig. 15-31). The fourth ventricle and brainstem cisterns may dilate in the chronic phase. In patients with a diffuse ischemic insult, degeneration in the cerebellar cortex may be a prominent abnormality (Brierley 1976). Large brainstem infarctions

are more readily identifiable on CT, usually by 48 hours (Fig. 15-42).

Infarcts in the anterior and inferior portions of the cerebellum may be difficult to define, particularly in the acute phase, because of their proximity to the regions where bone artifacts are maximal. Superior cerebellar infarcts are more readily identified, but care must be taken to distinguish them from infarcts in the adjacent inferior occipital lobe on the opposite side of the tentorium (Fig. 15-42). In this situation, CECT will usually aid in determining the correct location by identifying the enhancing tentorium, especially in coronal views.

With a large cerebellar infarct, severe secondary neurologic deficits may develop from brainstem compression secondary to cerebellar swelling and tonsillar herniation. The infarct edema usually becomes maximum between the third and fifth days. It may be difficult to distinguish between infarction and tumor at this time; the fourth ventricle will be

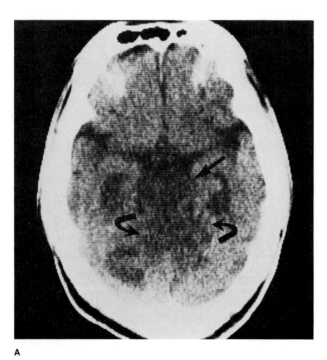

A

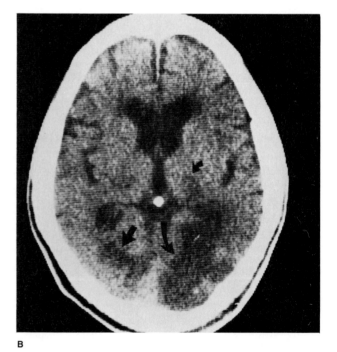

B

Figure 15-42 Basilar occlusion with large infarcts of the brainstem, superior cerebellum, and occipital lobe. **A.** CT through upper brainstem: diffuse hypodensity of midbrain (arrow) and superior cerebellum (curved arrows). **B.** CT through occipital lobes: large posterior cerebral artery territory occipital (large curved arrow) and posterior thalamic hypodensity (small curved arrow) on left with smaller occipital hypodensity on right (straight arrow).

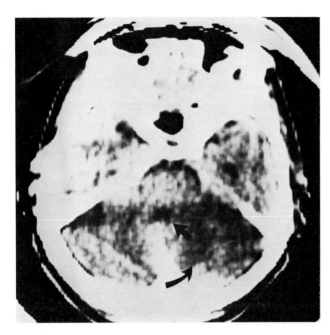

Figure 15-43 Acute cerebellar infarct with mass effect. Left cerebellar hypodensity (curved arrow) with compression and displacement of fourth ventricle (straight arrow).

displaced and the brainstem cisterns compressed in both situations. With infarction, however, the low density tends to remain localized within a vascular distribution and usually does not cross the vermis to the opposite side of the midline (Fig. 15-43). In addition, contrast enhancement is not present at this time with most infarctions but is frequently present with tumor. It is important to carefully evaluate for any early evidence of swelling due to infarction so as to alert the clinicians to the possibility of later severe developments; prognosis might then be favorably affected by early surgical decompression and removal of necrotic cerebellar tissue.

Follow-up CT scans after the first week that show contrast enhancement in the cerebellar folia suggest infarction in one or more branches of the vertebral and basilar arteries. After several months a sharply demarcated low-density region will usually become evident involving the cerebellar surface and extending into the white matter. Focal dilatation of the ipsilateral side of the fourth ventricle may also develop (Fig. 15-44).

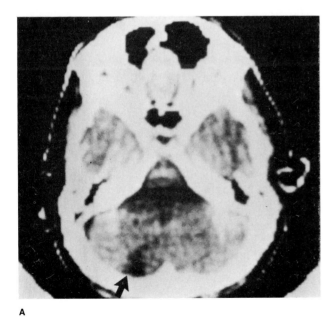

A

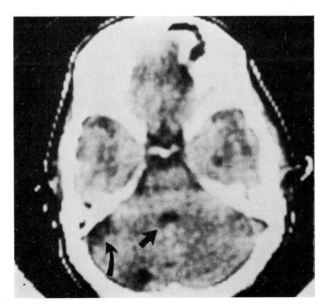

B

Figure 15-44 Old posterior inferior cerebellar artery territory infarct. **A.** Section below fourth ventricle: wedge-shaped marked hypodensity in right posterior inferior cerebellum (arrow). **B.** Higher section through fourth ventricle: decreased size of inferior cerebellar hypodensity. Right posterior lateral cerebellar atrophy (dilated CSF space) (curved arrow). Posterior aspect of fourth ventricle (arrow) shows slight enlargement.

Anoxic Ischemic Encephalopathy and Carbon Monoxide Poisoning

Individuals who suffer acute respiratory insufficiency such as may occur with allergic reaction, primary central respiratory failure, or overdose from central respiratory depressant drugs such as alcohol, narcotics, or barbiturates may develop either acute or delayed onset of brain damage. Carbon monoxide intoxication may cause similar clinical manifestations and brain pathologic alterations (Brucher 1967; Lapresle 1967; Ginsberg 1974, 1979). Anoxia or prolonged hypoxia usually results in hypotension and cardiac failure, adding cerebral ischemic insult to the hypoxemia. Conversely, acute cardiac failure or hypotension may lead to respiratory failure (De Reuck 1978), possibly as a result of brainstem ischemia.

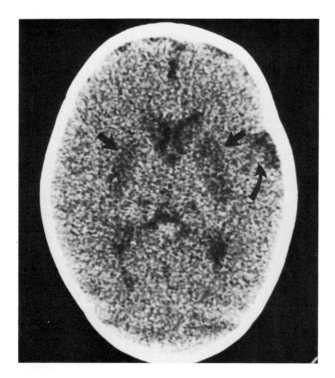

Figure 15-45 Respiratory arrest in 4-month-old child (crib anoxia), at 2 weeks. Hypodensity involving caudate and putamen bilaterally (arrows) and left anterior temporal (curved arrow) and frontal pole regions of the cortex.

Clinically, most patients with anoxic ischemia present with coma (De Reuck 1978; Ginsberg 1979). Some never demonstrate any significant recovery, while others awaken and initially improve, only to have a delayed onset of progressive neurologic deterioration after a period of several weeks (Plum 1962; Ginsberg 1976, 1979). Pathologically the patients with irreversible acute brain injury reveal necrosis, which may affect predominantly either the gray or the white matter. The watershed region, particularly the periventricular white matter, is usually the most severely affected area (Brierley 1976; De Reuck 1978). The deep parts of the basal ganglia, which can also be considered a terminal field of supply, are also commonly involved (De Reuck 1971; Brierley 1976). The pathologic change that develops in those patients with delayed onset of hypoxic ischemic symptoms is progressive demyelination, with or without zones of focal necrosis which is most severe in the periventricular region (Plum 1962; Ginsberg 1976, 1979). Rarely, the neuropathologic alterations are confined to the basal ganglia in patients with the delayed-onset hypoxic ischemic syndrome (Ginsberg 1979).

The CT in patients with unremitting neurologic deficits demonstrates by 24 to 48 hours low-density regions which may be situated in the basal ganglia, the watershed cortex and white matter, or the periventricular white matter (Fig. 15-45). Involved gray matter may be isodense during the acute phase, since reperfusion hyperemia during this period could counterbalance the basic hypoxic ischemic low-density tissue change. On CECT, diffuse enhancement in the watershed cortex may appear, indicating probably hyperemia with blood-brain-barrier abnormality (Fig. 15-46). If the patient survives the acute phase, marked enlargement of the lateral ventricular system and cortical sulci will develop during the next few months, and previously isodense enhancing regions will become hypodense (Fig. 15-47).

In the most severe cases of anoxic ischemic insult, all the cortical, basal ganglia, and white-matter regions of the cerebrum may be involved and reveal diffuse hypodensity after a few days (Fig. 15-48). Initially there is preservation of normal tissue den-

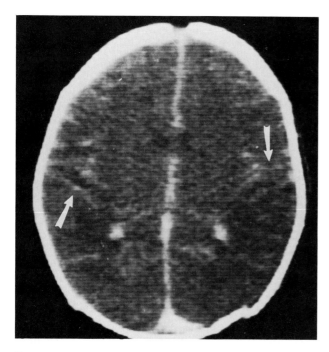

Figure 15-46 CECT: postanoxic cortical enhancement (arrows). Cortical ribbon isodense on NCCT. Diffuse white-matter hypodensity.

sity in the posterior fossa region. The lateral ventricles and basal cisterns are obliterated, reflecting the development of marked brain swelling and increased supratentorial intracranial pressure, which causes further ischemic insult by reducing perfusion pressure. Eventually this vicious circle causes cessation of blood flow in the supratentorial region. The vertebral-basilar circulation to the posterior fossa is similarly affected as the increased intracranial pressure is transmitted transtentorially. A state of cerebral death exists when circulation ceases both supra- and infratentorially. If the patient is kept alive by artificial measures, low density develops in all posterior fossa tissues. Once cerebral death occurs, the large arteries at the base of the brain (in-

Figure 15-47 Chronic post-anoxic-ischemic changes. **A.** Six months after anoxic-ischemic insult: diffuse cortical and ventricular enlargement. CT normal before episode of respiratory arrest. **B.** Another patient (2 years old) several months after smoke-inhalation: hypodensity of globus pallidus bilaterally (arrows), marked cortical and ventricular enlargement.

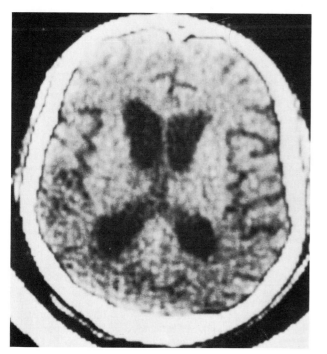

A

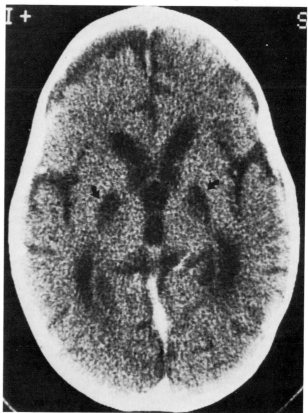

B

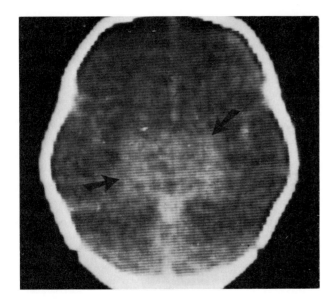

Figure 15-48 Severe anoxic ischemia in neonate: diffuse hypodensity of the cerebrum with normal density of thalamus and posterior basal ganglia (arrows). Isodense cortical bands.

ternal carotid, proximal anterior, and middle cerebral and basilar) and the large cerebral veins and sinuses (vein of Galen, superior sagittal, straight and transverse sinuses) are not visualized on CECT (Rangel 1978; Rappaport 1978). Rapid bolus contrast injection (40 ml in 5 seconds) or large bolus infusion (80 g iodine) more dramatically indicates the lack of vascular contrast filling. Although the CT findings may strongly indicate an absence of cerebral circulation, angiography is still needed for confirmation.

In those patients who manifest the biphasic clinical response to hypoxic ischemic insult with delayed onset of secondary neurologic deterioration, the CT obtained during the first 1 to 2 weeks may be entirely normal. With the onset of neurologic deterioration after a period of 3 to 5 weeks, a mild, diffuse low density will appear in the white matter. Over the next 3 to 4 weeks the hypodensity becomes

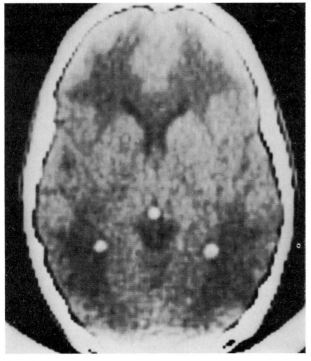

A

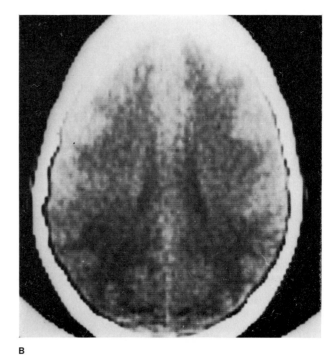

B

Figure 15-49 Delayed-onset clinical deterioration from anoxic ischemic injury. CT normal for several weeks. **A** and **B.** CT 6 weeks after anoxic-ischemic insult from drug abuse. Diffuse hypodensity throughout white matter. Gray-matter regions normal.

progressively more marked (Yagnik 1980). The hypodensity is most severe in the deep white-matter regions but extends in a pseudopod-like manner outward in the white-matter tracks between the involved cortical convolutions (Fig. 15-49).

With acute *carbon monoxide* poisoning (a form of anemic hypoxia due to a reduction in the amount of circulating oxyhemoglobin) the prevalent CT abnormality appears to be bilateral hypodensity in the basal ganglia, most conspicuous in the region of the globus pallidus (Fig. 15-50). This was eventually present in all nine of the patients reported by Kim et al. (1980). It was observed in four of five patients examined during the first week, being present as early as the first day in two. Five of five patients examined after 6 weeks had bilateral basal ganglia involvement. Diffuse bilateral white-matter hypodensity developed in three of the nine patients. Only one of these patients had a relapsing clinical course with delayed onset of neurologic deterioration after recovery from initial coma. All the rest had severe original deficits, which showed little, if any, improvement.

Hypertensive Encephalopathy

Those persons, particularly normotensive ones, who experience a rapid and sustained elevation in blood pressure may develop hypertensive encephalopathy (Ziegler 1965). This is manifested by severe headache, vomiting, convulsions, focal neurologic signs, and drowsiness or coma. Pathologically the brain demonstrates generalized edema, petechial hemorrhages, and patchy vessel-wall necrosis (Yates 1972). These changes are believed to occur because the normal limit of autoregulatory vasoconstriction has been exceeded (Lassen 1972). This breakthrough in the upper limits of autoregulation leads to increased cerebral blood flow and capillary perfusion pressure, and these hemodynamic alterations result in the pathologic abnormalities.

The CT appearance reflects the main pathologic change, diffuse edema. Generalized, well-demarcated, symmetrical hypodensity is present in the cerebral white matter (Kendall 1977), which may be more marked in the upper posterior parts of the cerebral hemispheres (Fig. 15-51) (Rail 1980). Follow-up scans demonstrate resolution of the hypodensity after the blood pressure is reduced for a period of time.

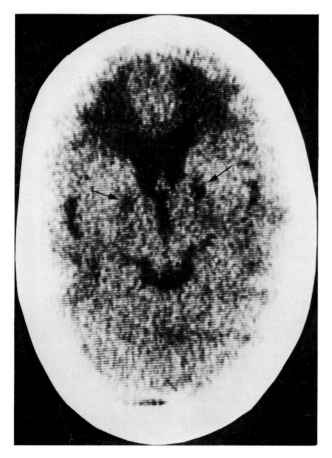

Figure 15-50 Carbon monoxide insult. Bilateral globus pallidus (arrows) and diffuse frontal white-matter hypodensity. (*Courtesy of J. H. Suh, M.D., Yonsei University, Seoul, Korea.*)

Cerebral Venous Thrombosis

Venous thrombosis in the brain may involve the major venous sinuses, superficial cortical veins, or deep venous system, or two or more of these regions may be affected simultaneously. There is a high incidence of grave morbidity and mortality with cerebral sinovenous occlusion (Kalberg 1967).

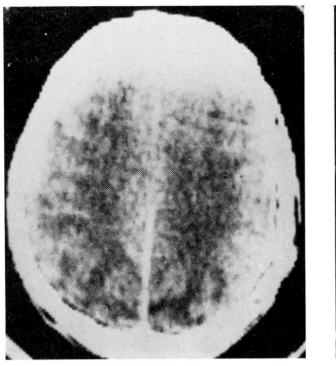 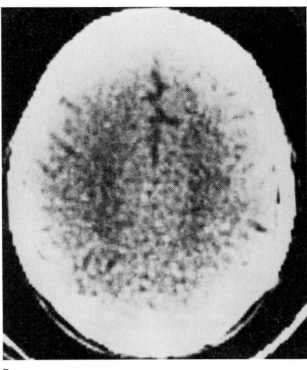

A   **B**

Figure 15-51 Hypertensive encephalopathy.   **A.** CT at time of severe hypertension and symptoms: hypodensity throughout white matter most marked in the upper posterior portions of the cerebral hemispheres.   **B.** CT 2 months after control of hypertension, with mild residual mental function deficits: resolution of white-matter hypodensity, moderate prominence of cortical sulci. (*From Rail DL 1980.*)

To improve survival and reduce debilitating complications, early recognition and institution of appropriate therapy are essential.

The causes of cerebral venous thrombosis fall in two main categories—septic and aseptic. Septic sinovenous occlusion is the result of inflammatory vasculitis, which may be caused either by direct involvement of the cerebral veins from intracranial infections such as meningitis, encephalitis, and subdural and epidural empyema or by intracranial spread of paracranial infections along emissary and communicating veins from inflammatory disease in such areas as the mastoids, paranasal sinuses, face, and scalp (Rao 1981; Eick 1981).

The aseptic causes of venous sinus thrombosis are numerous (Buonanno 1978). They include pregnancy in the prepartum and postpartum periods, use of oral contraceptives, dehydration, rapid di-

uresis, polycythemia vera, sickle cell disease, sickle cell trait, leukemia, thrombocytopenia, disseminated intravascular coagulation, cryofibrinogenemia, malnutrition, acquired and congenital heart disease, head trauma, diabetes mellitus, collagen vascular disease, cerebral arterial occlusion, cerebral and dural arteriovenous malformations, carotid cavernous fistula, compression or invasion by intracranial tumor, and indirect effects of extracranial neoplasms and chronic inflammatory diseases (Merritt 1979). In addition, many cases are idiopathic.

The clinical manifestations are nonspecific and include headache, increased intracranial pressure, stroke, seizures, personality change, hallucinations, decreased mental function, diplopia, blurred vision, and coma (Merritt 1979). Patients with this disorder not infrequently are initially diagnosed as having "functional" problems or benign pseudotumor cerebri. The clinical symptomatology may develop over a relatively long period of time or be fulminant, with rapid progression to coma and death. The mortality rate has been reported to range from 40 percent to as high as 88 percent (Krayenbuhl 1954; Buonanno 1978).

The CT reveals a wide spectrum of abnormalities, which may change over the course of the disease. Some of the CT abnormalities are diagnostic for sinovenous occlusion, while others may be either strongly suggestive or nonspecific. The CT abnormalities may be present singly or in combination. If subsequent scans are obtained, additional abnormalities may be identified. Occasionally, no abnormality is present. Buonanno et al. (1978) reported that only 1 patient out of 11 with sinovenous occlusion had a normal-appearing CT.

A diagnostic CT abnormality which may be present during the first 1 to 2 weeks after the development of sinovenous occlusion is increased density on the NCCT within the region of a dural sinus or a superficial or deep vein (Wendling 1978; Buonanno 1978; Eick 1981). This hyperdensity on CT is due to formation of a recent blood clot and measures betwen 50 and 90 HU. It is best seen when the scan plane is perpendicular to the long axis of the thrombosed sinus or vein. Small thrombosed convexity veins situated immediately adjacent to the calvarium may be obscured by the overlying bony density. Fresh thrombus in the straight sinus region can usually be readily appreciated, since it is sufficiently removed from the skull table. Here it appears as an elongated oval or a bandlike density following the expected course of the straight sinus (Fig. 15-52).

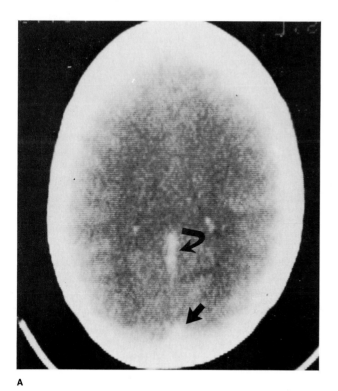

A

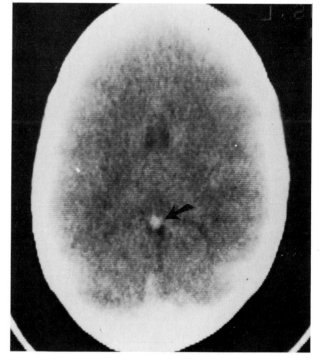

B

Figure 15-52   Venous thrombosis 3 days after onset of symptoms. Dense thrombus in straight sinus, superior sagittal sinus, and vein of Galen; diffuse brain swelling.   **A.** NCCT: band of increased density along course of straight sinus (curved arrow) and posterior aspect of superior sagittal sinus (straight arrow). Diffuse increased hypodensity throughout white matter with compressed lateral ventricles.   **B.** NCCT, section 1 cm below **A:** increased density of vein of Galen (arrow). Diffuse white-matter hypodensity with ventricular compression.

Likewise, recent thrombosis of the vein of Galen, which is situated just anterior and inferior to the beginning of the straight sinus, should be visualized (Fig. 15-52). Care must be taken not to confuse the thrombosed vein of Galen with a partially calcified pineal gland; the latter is located slightly anterior and inferior to the vein of Galen and immediately adjacent to the posterior third ventricle. A fresh thrombus within the superior sagittal sinus may be identified by its density on axial scans if the occlusion is in its posterior vertical portion. In this location the scan plane is relatively perpendicular to the sinus and, because of the large size of the sinus at this location, should not be obscured by the overlying bone (Fig. 15-53). For occlusions more anteriorly situated in the horizontal portion of the superior sagittal sinus, coronal scans made perpendicular to its long axis are necessary. Occasionally the increased density of small thrombosed surface veins is evident if they are not located close to the calvarium—for example, those in sulci or in the sylvian cistern (Fig. 15-53).

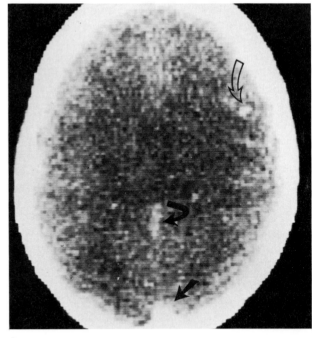

A

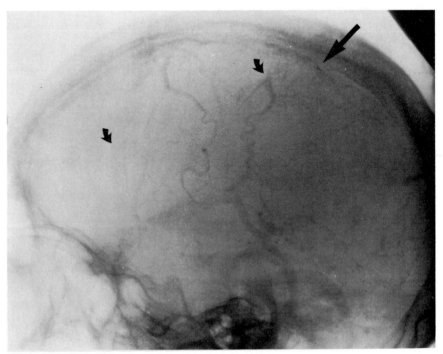

Figure 15-53 Venous thrombosis. Development of dense thrombus in cortical vein. **A.** NCCT: same patient as in Figure 15-52 four days later. Persistent hyperdensity of superior sagittal sinus (straight arrow) and straight sinus (curved arrow). Nodular hyperdensity has appeared near brain surface on left (open arrow). **B.** Lateral carotid angiogram, late venous phase: occlusion of superior sagittal sinus (straight arrow), vein of Galen, and straight sinus (not filled), and cortical veins (curved arrows). Tortuous convexity veins provide collateral drainage inferiorly for the superior aspect of the brain.

B

Another diagnostic CT abnormality of venous sinus occlusion may appear on CECT, usually not becoming evident for at least a week or more after the development of sinus thrombosis, since it follows on the breakdown of the hemoglobin molecules in the clotted blood of the sinus, which then becomes isodense. The superior sagittal sinus, normally demonstrable on CECT as a homogeneous region of increased density, will reveal only enhancement of its outer triangular margin; its central luminal area remains relatively hypodense—the "empty triangle" or "delta" sign (Fig. 15-54) (Buonanno 1978). This appearance represents absence of contrast flow into the sinus (the nonenhanced center) in that region. The enhancing outer triangle represents the normal enhancement of the dural walls of the sinus in combination with the added increased density from the collateral venous channels which develop in the dura (Vines 1971) and

from the neovascularity which is probably appearing in the outer portion of the thrombus secondary to its organization. Both these processes may cause the sinus wall to appear thickened and to encroach on the lumen.

On the standard axial scan the delta sign will be identified mainly in those cases in which the sinus thrombosis involves the posterior third of the superior sagittal sinus, since this is the region where the scan plane is most perpendicular to the sinus. It may be necessary to utilize a high window setting to identify the delta sign, since the thickened enhanced wall of the sinus may obscure the central hypodensity when viewed at normal brain window settings (Fig. 15-55) (Zilkha 1980). On the axial scan the anterior third of the superior sagittal sinus is also perpendicular to the scan plane, and the delta sign may be seen with thrombosis in this location (Rao 1981). It may not be evident, however, because

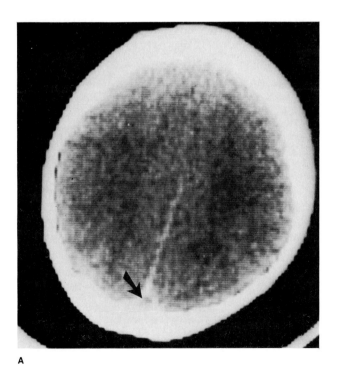

A

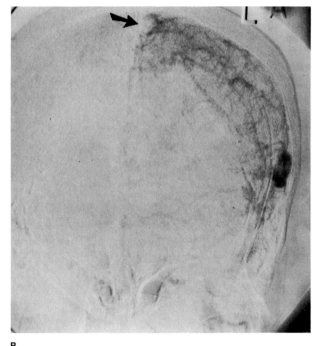

B

Figure 15-54 Venous thrombosis "delta" sign. **A.** CECT: no contrast density in central lumen of posterior aspect of superior sagittal sinus with thick enhancement of its walls (arrow). **B.** Frontal carotid angiogram, venous phase: no contrast filling of superior sagittal sinus (arrow).

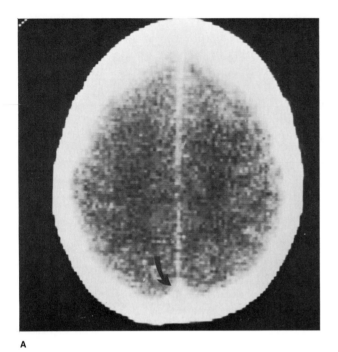

A

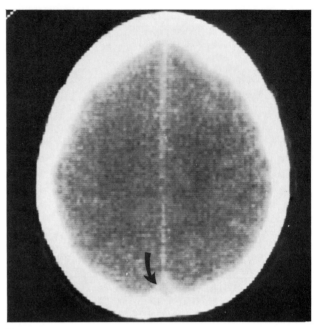

B

Figure 15-55 Wide window setting to identify some cases with "delta" sign. **A.** CECT: at standard window setting "delta" sign is not evident in superior sagittal sinus (arrow). **B.** Same CT section as **A** at wide window setting.

Slightly reduced density of superior sagittal sinus lumen is evident relative to its enhanced walls (arrow). Slight density of lumen related to recent sinus thrombosis.

of the small size of the sinus in this region. To identify the delta sign in occlusion of the middle portion of the superior sagittal sinus, coronal scans are needed for perpendicular sections of this region. Buonanno et al. (1978) observed the delta sign in only 2 of 11 cases (18 percent) of sinovenous occlusion, whereas Rao et al. (1981) identified it in 8 of their 11 patients (72 percent). In addition, Rao observed the delta sign outside the usual location in the superior sagittal sinus in two cases. It was demonstrated as a filling defect in the transverse sinus in one case and in the straight sinus in a second.

Another highly probable pathognomonic finding of venous thrombosis on CECT is visualization of punctate and streaklike hyperdensities within the deep white matter of the brain (Fig. 15-56) (Banna 1979). These have been postulated to represent engorgement and dilatation of transcerebral medullary veins, which serve as collateral channels between the cortical and deep venous systems. Angiograph-

ically, dilated medullary veins may be observed with occlusion of either the deep or the superficial venous systems. (Gabrielsen 1969). To identify these dilated medullary veins on CT, scans with very high spatial resolution are needed.

CT abnormalities similar to those of arterial infarction frequently develop with sinovenous occlusion but usually have characteristics more indicative of venous than of arterial infarction. Since the major cerebral veins generally drain more than one arterial distribution venous infarcts are not always strictly confined, as with arterial infarcts, to the territory of a single artery or to the watershed zone (Fig. 15-57). The involvement, particularly in the white matter, may extend asymmetrically, usually between the three main arterial regions. On NCCT the white matter is hypodense due to congestive edema and necrosis. The pattern of white-matter low density in venous infarcts usually appears different from that in arterial infarcts (Fig. 15-57). In venous in-

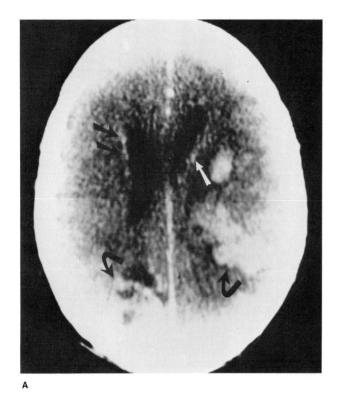

A

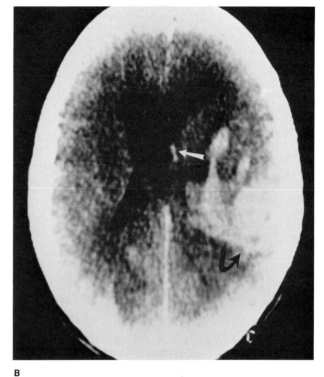

B

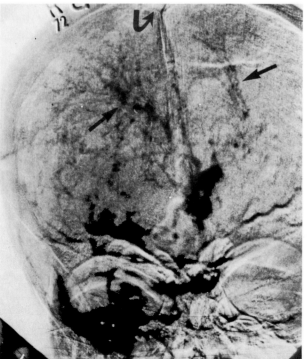

C

Figure 15-56 Venous thrombosis with dilated medullary veins. **A** and **B.** CECT: bilateral hemorrhagic venous infarcts (curved arrows). Multiple punctate periventricular nodular densities (arrows) were not present before enhancement. **C.** Frontal carotid angiogram, venous phase: non-filling of superior sagittal sinus (curved arrow) and superficial veins. Marked dilatation of medullary veins (arrows) draining into deep venous system.

farction the white-matter hypodensity tends to have a rounded, ill-defined border, compared to the more sharply marginated wedge or rectangular shape of an arterial infarct. These differences are probably related to a greater degree of vasogenic edema in venous infarction caused by the high capillary pressure from back-pressure congestion. This factor also results in a greater mass effect on venous infarction for a lesion of comparable size.

With venous infarcts the cortex is usually isodense to slightly hyperdense on NCCT because of congestive dilatation of the capillaries and petechial hemorrhages. On CECT a frequent cortical abnormality is an intense gyral enhancement pattern over and around the region of the venous infarction (Fig.

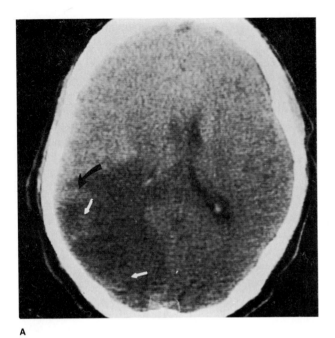

A

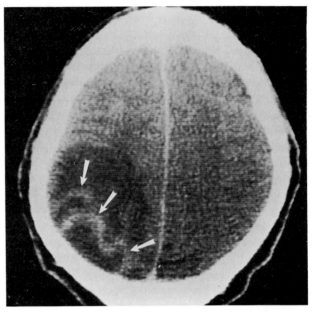

B

Figure 15-57   Venous infarct, mass effect, and enhancement. **A.** NCCT: large hypodensity involving right posterior temporal, parietal, and occipital regions. Hypodensity not confined to an arterial territory. Cortical density within infarct territory, al-

though reduced, is more isodense than the white matter (arrows). Considerable compression of ipsilateral ventricle.   **B.** CECT at higher level: enhancement of cortical ribbon (arrows) centrally in posterior part of infarct.

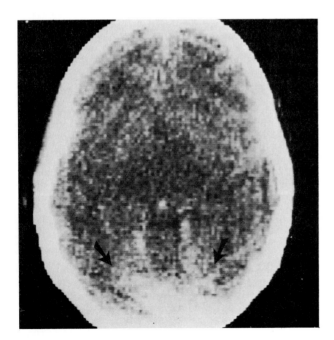

15-57). Prominent gyral enhancement may also occur in the absence of other evidence for venous infarction. The gyral enhancement is caused by capillary engorgement and breakdown of the blood-brain barrier related to high venous back pressure and its associated ischemic effects. Rao et al. (1981) observed gyral enhancement in 7 of 11 patients with venous infarcts. This is a considerably higher frequency than they found on review of the literature, where only 4 of 14 patients having CECT demonstrated gyral enhancement.

Intense enhancement, considerably greater than normal, may develop in the tentorium and falx (Fig. 15-58). This probably reflects enlargement of dural venous collateral channels (Vines 1971) and increased dural capillary pressure, leading to a greater leakage of contrast into the dura. This enhancement has been observed most commonly in the tento-

Figure 15-58   Increased tentorial enhancement (arrow) in venous thrombosis.

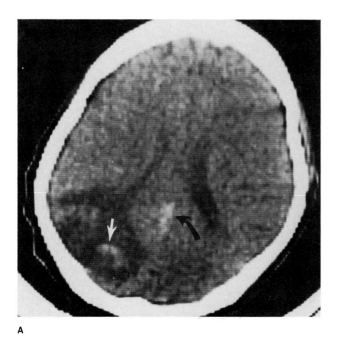 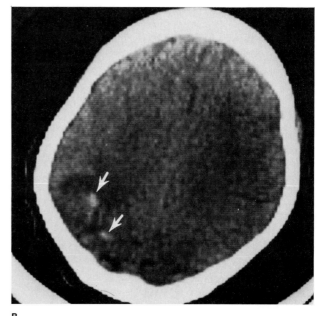

A   **B**

Figure 15-59 Hemorrhagic venous infarct. **A** and **B.** NCCT: hypodensity in posterior parietal occipital territory. Multiple foci of hemorrhage (hyperdensities) (straight arrow) within the isodense cortical ribbon. Hyperdense straight sinus (curved arrow) in **A** due to recent thrombosis.

rium, associated with thrombosis of the straight sinus (Buonanno 1978; Rao 1981).

Hemorrhage is also frequently associated with venous infarcts. The hemorrhage most commonly involves the cortex (Fig. 15-59) but may affect the white matter in the central and deep portions of the infarct (Fig. 15-56). Extensive low density in the white matter when the hemorrhage is first observed is related to the necrosis and edema caused by the venous infarction. The venous-infarction hemorrhage may assume a dense gyral pattern similar in appearance to that of arterial hemorrhagic infarction. Venous hemorrhages tend to be more bulky and less strictly confined to the cortical ribbon. In addition, the white-matter hypodensity and the hemorrhagic region may not be located within the territory of a single major cerebral artery (Fig. 15-59) as with arterial hemorrhagic infarction. At times the venous hemorrhage will be very bulky and extend deeply into the white matter, strongly resembling an arterial intracerebral hematoma. The ve-

nous hemorrhage may, however, reveal changes different from those occurring with an arterial hemispheric hematoma. With venous infarction the hematoma is not so sharply demarcated, and its density may be slightly nonhomogeneous. It is also more superficially located and is surrounded by a greater degree of hypodensity in the white matter, especially in its early stage.

Not infrequently, multiple separate regions of venous infarction may develop. A common pattern seen with multiple venous infarcts is bilateral involvement in the parasagittal high-convexity region of the brain (Fig. 15-60). This may reveal bilateral hypodensities in the anterior cerebral territory, frequently extending beyond the watershed zone into the middle cerebral artery territory. Occasionally multiple venous hemorrhagic infarcts develop in this same distribution.

Nonspecific alterations that may develop with sinovenous thrombosis include small ventricles, mild, diffuse white-matter hypodensity which may

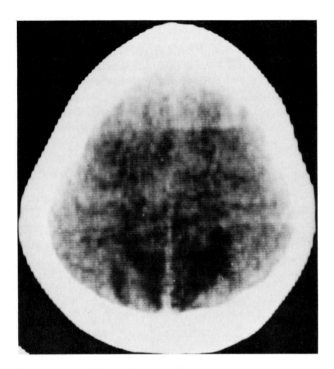

Figure 15-60 Bilateral venous infarction: patchy hypodensities in parasagittal region on both sides.

INTRACEREBRAL HEMORRHAGE

CT is the most accurate and reliable method for diagnosing intracerebral hematoma. The true incidence of this diagnosis has increased since the advent of CT. The density of freshly clotted blood on CT (55 to 95 HU) is significantly greater than that of brain tissue, permitting reliable identification of even very small intracerebral hematomas. Hemorrhages of 1 cm or possibly less in diameter can usually be diagnosed if technically good scans are obtained using collimators 0.8 cm or less in size (Fig. 15-61). Intracerebral hematomas may extend to the brain surface or rupture intraventricularly, resulting in secondary subarachnoid hemorrhage.

Aside from head trauma, the principal cause of intracerebral hematoma is hypertensive vascular disease. Rupture of a berry aneurysm and arteriovenous malformation are less frequent causes.

be unilateral or bilateral, and obliteration of the basal cisterns (Fig. 15-52). These alterations reflect increased intracranial pressure from vasogenic edema caused by the increasing outflow resistance from venous obstruction.

CT may demonstrate nonfilling of a variable segment of the superior sagittal, straight, transverse, or sigmoid sinuses and/or obstruction of superficial convexity or deep veins (Figs. 15-53, 15-54). Thrombi may be identified within occluded or partially obstructed venous sinuses and cerebral veins. Enlargement and frequently corkscrew tortuosity of anastomotic collateral veins (Fig. 15-53) and medullary veins (Fig. 15-56) may be observed. Although the characteristic and highly specific CT findings frequently strongly suggest the diagnosis of sinovenous thrombosis, cerebral angiography is the definitive method for diagnosis and is indicated in questionable cases for confirmation (Krayenbuhl 1954; Gabrielsen 1969, 1981; Vines 1971).

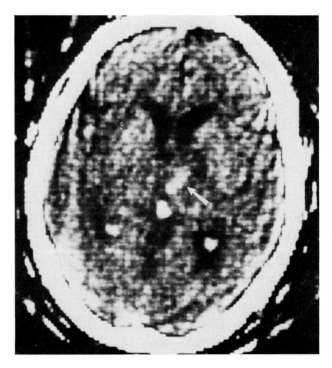

Figure 15-61 Small spontaneous thalamic hematoma (arrow) in hypertensive individual.

Other etiologies include venous thrombosis, amyloid angiopathy, collagen vascular disease, anticoagulation therapy, primary and metastatic brain tumor, and prematurity in the neonate. Although hematomas from various causes may present a similar CT appearance, frequently the correct etiology may be suggested by consideration of the patient's age, the clinical history, and the location of the hematoma. Use of contrast may reveal associated specific enhancement characteristics which will indicate the diagnosis (Weisberg 1979). Hematomas caused by venous infarction have been discussed earlier in this chapter; those associated with trauma, aneurysm, arteriovenous malformation, and tumor are presented in other chapters in this book.

Hypertensive Hematoma

Intracerebral hematomas caused by hypertensive vascular disease tend to occur in older patients, usually those in their seventh decade. These hematomas are most commonly situated in the basal ganglia and internal capsule region. They predominantly involve the lateral portion of the putamen but also occur in the head of the caudate nucleus and the thalamus, brainstem, and cerebellum. They occasionally develop in the deep cerebral white matter in the parietal and posterior temporal occipital area (Cole 1967). Small hematomas may present clinically as a vasoocclusive stroke (Kinkel 1976). CT is then needed for appropriate diagnosis and management.

Larger basal ganglia–capsular hematomas not infrequently rupture into the lateral ventricle. Since the advent of CT, intraventricular rupture has been recognized as being much more common than previously believed. Small amounts of intraventricular bleeding do not significantly increase mortality. With large intraventricular rupture the prognosis becomes very grave (Fig. 15-62) (Weisberg 1979). Once it becomes intraventricular, a hemorrhage from any region can spread throughout the entire ventricular system and into the subarachnoid space.

Intracerebral hemorrhage frequently extends away from its site of origin into adjacent regions

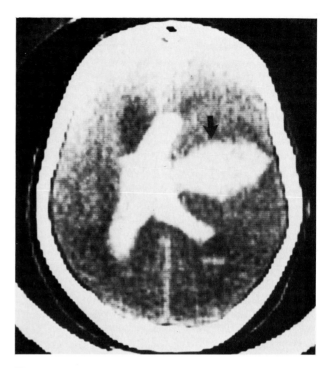

Figure 15-62 Large hematoma of superior ganglion–internal capsule (arrow) with extensive intraventricular rupture.

along white-matter tracts (Fig. 15-63). Occasionally, the degree of spread may be so great that determining the primary site of hemorrhage is difficult. Basal ganglia–capsular hemorrhage may extend superiorly into the deep frontoparietal white matter via the internal capsule or inferiorly into the temporal lobe via the external capsule. Intraventricular rupture into the body of the lateral ventricle is frequent from this location. Thalamic hematomas may dissect inferiorly into the brainstem, laterally into the posterior limb of the internal capsule, or medially into the third ventricle. Superior extension into the lateral ventricle is not usual, probably because of the intervening subarachnoid space of the velum interpositum. Brainstem hematomas may extend superiorly into the thalamus or posteriorly either into the cerebellum through the cerebellar peduncles or directly into the fourth ventricle. Conversely, cerebellar hematomas can dissect anteriorly into the pons. Large cerebellar hematomas cause significant

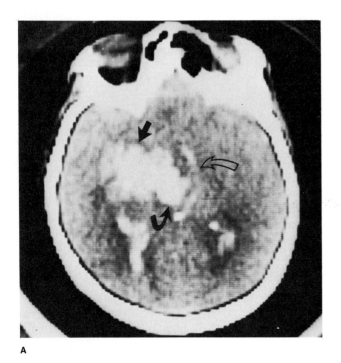

A

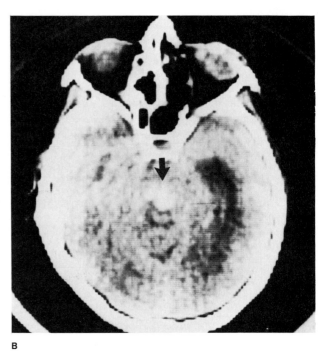

B

Figure 15-63 Spread of thalamic hematoma. **A.** Thalamic hematoma (curved arrow). Large lateral dissection into region of basal ganglia–internal capsule (straight arrow). Medial rupture into displaced third ventricle (open arrow) with spread to occipital horns of lateral ventricle. **B.** Inferior dissection of hematoma into brainstem (arrow).

brainstem compression and tonsillar herniation and frequently require urgent surgical evacuation.

Hypertensive hematoma is believed by many to be caused by rupture of microaneurysms on the penetrating arteries. These aneurysms were first described by Charcot and Bouchard (1868) and are frequently referred to by their names. Recent elegant microradiographic and histopathologic studies have reconfirmed their presence, their strong association with hypertension, and their prevalence at the usual sites of intracerebral hemorrhage, being most frequent in the basal ganglia–internal capsule region (Russell 1963; Cole 1967). They result from hyalin degeneration in the walls of the penetrating arteries, with loss of elastic fibers and smooth muscle in the intima and media. These microaneurysms are most often located at points of branching and are either fusiform or saccular dilatations ranging in size from 50 to 1000 μm (Kido 1978). They may occasionally be demonstrated with high-detail-mag-

nification angiography and angiotomography (Goldberg 1973).

A fresh hematoma on NCCT appears as a homogeneously dense (55 to 90 HU), well-defined lesion with a rounded to oval configuration. The hemorrhage separates brain tissue rather than intermixing with it. A thin, well-defined low-density zone surrounding the hematoma can be observed as early as a few hours after the hemorrhage (Fig. 15-64A). This early hypodense rim is probably caused by the clotting of the liquid hemorrhage with extrusion of the low-density plasma at the periphery of the hematoma. After 3 to 4 days, additional low density appears around the hematoma, spreading peripherally in the white matter. This is caused by compression ischemic necrosis of surrounding tissue and the development of edema related to clot lysis, with breakdown of the blood-brain barrier (Fig. 15-64B) (Stehbens 1972; Grubb 1974; Laster 1978). Hematomas produce ventricular compression

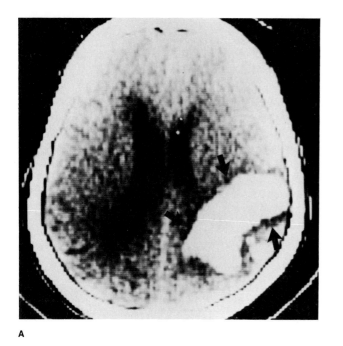

A

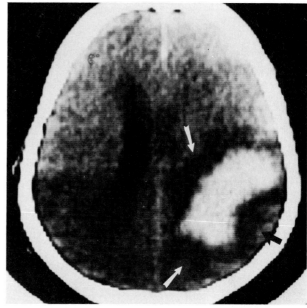

B

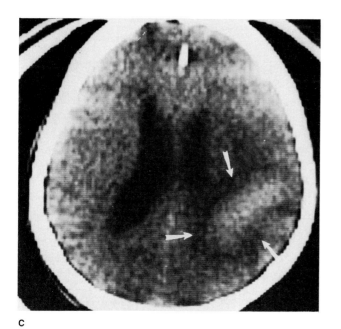

C

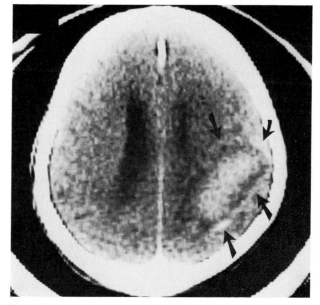

D

Figure 15-64 Evolution of CT alterations of large parietal-occipital hypertensive hematoma. **A.** CT at day 1: large hyperdense parietal-occipital hematoma with ventricular compression. Thin rim of hypodensity around hematoma (arrows). **B.** NCCT at day 9: slight reduction in size of hematoma. Increased size of surrounding hypodensity (edema) which extends beyond the initial hematoma margins (arrows). More marked ventricular compression than at day 1. **C.** NCCT at day 38: hematoma density considerably reduced, especially peripherally, resulting in apparent decreased size. Surrounding hypodensity extends only to location of original hematoma margin (arrows). **D.** CECT at same time as **C:** faint rim of enhancement at outer margin of surrounding hypodensity (arrows). (*Continued on p. 644.*)

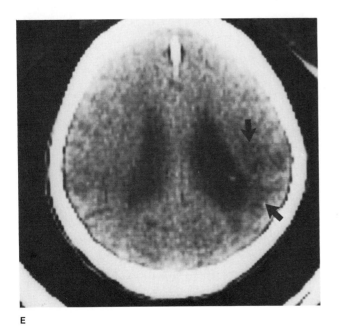

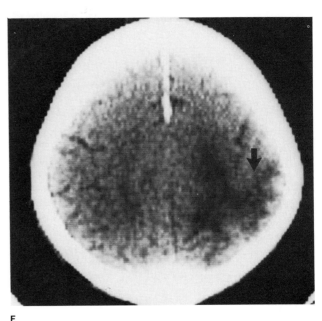

E

F

Figure 15-64 (Cont.)   **E** and **F**. CT at 6 months: focal dilatation of lateral ventricle and irregular parenchymal hypodensity (arrows) in the region of the previous hematoma.

and, when large, considerable midline shift and brain herniation. Mass effect may increase during the third to seventh days from the development of edema. Steroid treatment, especially in nontraumatic hematomas, will usually control edema formation and therefore eliminate or considerably reduce the secondary increased mass effect both clinically and on CT.

A hematoma which is nonhomogeneously dense should lead the physician to consider hemorrhage occurring with tumor, inflammation, contusion, or arterial and venous infarction. In these situations the hemorrhage usually develops within the abnormal and necrotic tissue and, depending on the etiology, may appear either as a poorly marginated and patchy region of increased density, a nonhomogenous region of hyperdensity centrally located in an area of hypodensity, or a complete or incomplete irregular ring of increased density around a low-density or isodense center with surrounding edema. CECT will frequently reveal abnormal enhancement associated with hemorrhages not caused

by hypertensive vascular disease which will aid in their differentiation.

Dolinskas et al. (1977a) reported that hematomas show a decreasing peak density averaging 0.7 ± 0.31 EMI units per day (these values would be approximately double in Hounsfield units). Small hematomas tended to lose their density faster than the larger ones: hematomas of 2 cm or less reached isodensity on or before the nineteenth day after the bleeding, while larger hematomas frequently took 4 to 6 weeks to become isodense. The decreasing density of a hematoma is due to breakdown and absorption of the hemoglobin molecule. Hematomas lose their peripheral density rapidly and therefore show a progressive decrease in apparent size (Fig. 15-64C). Dolinskas et al. (1977a) found a reduction in the visualized size of the hematoma averaging 0.65 ± 0.32 mm per day. Small hematomas showed this size reduction sooner than large ones. Although the visualized portion of the hematoma becomes smaller on CT, the actual size of the clot is not changing significantly at this time; it is merely

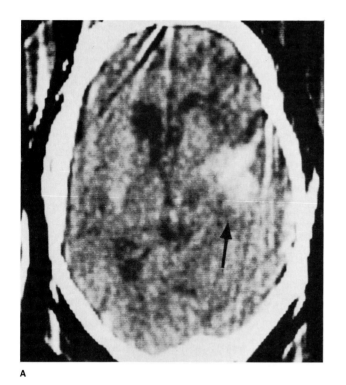

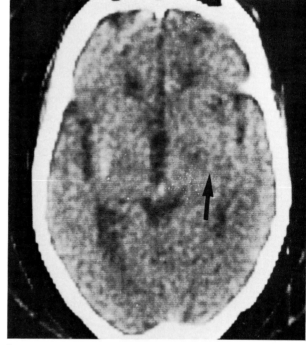

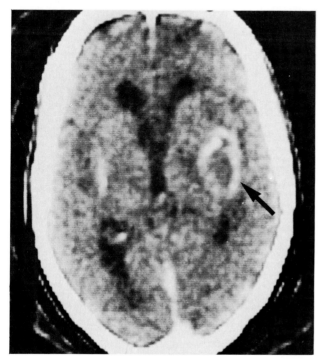

Figure 15-65 Lateral ganglionic hypertensive hematoma: evolution to isodensity and ring enhancement.   **A.** NCCT: hyperdensity of fresh hematoma in lateral putamen (arrow) with compression of frontal horn and third ventricle. Calcific density in opposite putamen.   **B.** NCCT at 14 days: hematoma isodense (arrow). Unchanged hyperdensity in opposite putamen.   **C.** CECT at same time as **B:** ring enhancement (arrow) around isodense hematoma site. Mild residual compression of frontal horn and third ventricle.

becoming isodense, and this is reflected in a delay in the reduction of its mass effect. Mass effect may be prominent for as long as 4 weeks with a large hematoma. These authors also noted that the earliest visualized decrease in mass effect for hematomas of all sizes averaged 16.7 days after the bleeding. Smaller hematomas lost their mass effect faster than the larger ones. In addition it was found that mass effect did not increase unless an operation was performed or the hematoma was secondary to trauma.

Over the next 2 to 3 months the density of a hematoma becomes progressively lower. After passing through the isodense stage (Fig. 15-65) the hematoma becomes hypodense (Dolinskas 1977a; Laster 1978). At its end stage, which may vary between 3 and 6 months, depending on the initial size, a well-defined low-density region, which may be considerably smaller than the original lesion, is present at the site of the original hematoma. With small hematomas a slitlike cystic area may be the residual change. Atrophic dilatation of the adjacent portion of the ventricular system occurs, as well as sulcal enlargement (Fig. 15-64E, F). Rarely calcification develops at the hematoma site. The residual low density and the focal atrophic changes are pathologically related to the formation of a cystic encephalomalacic cavity containing a yellowish, high-protein fluid with vascular trabeculations. This region is surrounded by a variable degree of gliosis (Stehbens 1972).

Contrast enhancement usually develops around the periphery of a hematoma after about 7 to 9 days (Zimmerman 1977; Laster 1978). The appearance of contrast enhancement corresponds to the time at which radionuclide studies become positive (Dolinskas 1977b). Pathologically there is ingrowth of capillary neovascularity at the margin of the hematoma by the end of the first week (Sugitani 1973; Zimmerman 1977). These newly formed capillaries, as in infarctions, have an abnormal blood-brain barrier which results in extravasation of contrast material around the hematoma (Molinari 1967; Di Chiro 1974).

The contrast enhancement appears as a ringlike density situated near the inner margin of the surrounding low-density zone and separated from the hematoma density by a thin isodense or hypodense zone (Fig. 15-64D) (Dolinskas 1977b; Laster 1978). At the time when the hematoma is passing through its isodense stage, NCCT may show little abnormality except for possibly a slight residual mass effect. However, the ring contrast enhancement on CECT persists through the isodense period and into the first few months of the hypodense state (Fig. 15-65C). The surrounding edema is clearing during the third to fourth weeks, and the ring enhancement then appears to surround an isodense or hypodense core, with normal surrounding brain tissue and no mass effect (Zimmerman 1977). The en-

hancing capsule becomes more intense and thicker over the next 4 to 6 weeks before beginning to fade. Pathologically at this stage there is a well-developed glial vascular capsule (Stehbens 1972; Laster 1978) which may be identified angiographically (Leeds 1973). The diameter of the enhancing ring decreases during the final hypodense stage as the gliotic capsule constricts around the absorbed hematoma. The CT appearance of the enhancing ring may easily be confused with that of a tumor or abscess. The lack of enhancement of the central region when the hematoma is isodense and the lack of surrounding edema and mass effect, particularly during the hypodense phase, tend to strongly favor a diagnosis of an evolving hematoma. In addition, with hemorrhagic tumors the enhancing rim is usually present on the initial scan during the first day, and it is thicker and irregular in shape (Gildersleve 1977).

Amyloid Angiopathy

Amyloid angiopathy is an infrequent cause of non-hypertensive massive spontaneous intracerebral hemorrhage in older persons. Over the age of 70, more than 40 percent of brains surveyed in one autopsy series demonstrated the presence of amyloid in the cerebral parenchymal blood vessels. Between the ages of 60 and 70 only about 12 percent of brains demonstrated amyloid change in the blood vessels. The disease affects only the arterioles of the cortex. This vascular disease has not been found in the white matter, basal ganglia, brainstem, or cerebellum. The cortical arterioles are most frequently involved in the parietal region (Vinters 1981).

The patients commonly have dementia, and pathologically Alzheimer's plaques may be found in association with the vascular lesions. The angiopathy, however, is often present in the absence of Alzheimer's changes or clinical dementia. The amyloid change is probably not related to a specific disease entity but rather is due to age-related change in the blood vessels.

Pathologically the hemorrhage associated with amyloid angiopathy primarily involves the cortex, with spread into the adjacent portion of the brain

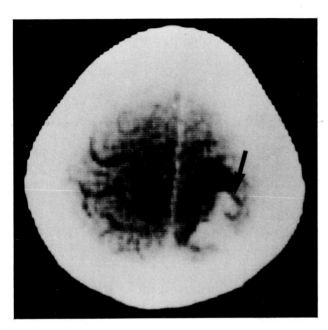

Figure 15-66 Superficial brain hemorrhage (arrow) in elderly individual with dementia suggesting amyloid angiopathy with hemorrhage.

(Fig. 15-66). This is in contrast to the usual deep location of hypertensive hemorrhages, which only on occasion extend to the brain surface. As might be expected from its superficial origin, subarachnoid hemorrhage is commonly associated with the amyloid vasculopathy hemorrhage.

Hemorrhage in Premature Neonates

Intracerebral hemorrhage develops in 40 to 70 percent of neonates weighing less than 1500 g (Burstein 1979; Lee 1979). The hemorrhage is mild in about 25 percent. Intraventricular hemorrhage of varying degree develops in over 75 percent of such cases (Albright 1981). The hemorrhage is clinically unsuspected in the majority of these infants. Burstein et al. (1979) reported that 68 percent of surviving premature infants had unsuspected hemorrhage found on CT.

These neonatal hemorrhages originate in the germinal matrix, a loose meshwork of highly vas-

cular tissue with little supporting stroma which contains primitive nerve cells (DeReuck 1977) and is located beneath the ependyma lining the lateral wall of the lateral ventricle. The germinal matrix is largest in the region of the head of the caudate nucleus. Its size is greatest between the twenty-fourth and thirty-second week of gestation, after which involution occurs. It is the source of nerve cells which migrate to the surface cortex during fetal development (Friede 1976). The exact cause of germinal-matrix hemorrhage is uncertain, but cerebral hypoxia related to neonatal respiratory distress, which is frequently associated with cardiac and vasomotor instability, is thought to predispose to this hemorrhage (Lou 1980). The hemorrhage usually develops during the first 4 days of life and is frequently not present at birth (Lee 1979).

The hemorrhages may range in degree from mild to very severe. They may be localized in one or several regions of the germinal matrix. The head of the caudate nucleus adjacent to the frontal horn is the site most frequently involved (Fig. 15-67) with hemorrhages, which may also originate from the region of the body and trigone of the lateral ventricle (Fig. 15-68) (Lee 1979). Varying degrees of intraventricular rupture occur in the majority of cases, being mild in about 25 percent (Fig. 15-68). Large brain hemorrhage or ventricular hemorrhage (Fig. 15-69) develops in about 25 percent of the cases and carries a grave prognosis (Burstein 1979).

Small intraventricular hemorrhages clear by 7 to 9 days; large ones take up to 2 weeks (Albright 1981), and parenchymal hemorrhages may take up to 3 weeks to resolve (Fig. 15-68). The last frequently lead to porencephalic ventricular dilatation. Intraventricular hemorrhage results in hydrocephalus about one-third of the time (Fig. 15-69). Burstein et al. (1979) reported that small intraventricular hemorrhages did not cause hydrocephalus, whereas 90 percent of large ones did. In contrast, Albright and Fellows (1981) observed that the size of the intraventricular hemorrhage did not correlate well with the subsequent development of hydrocephalus. In their series hydrocephalus was closely related to the ventricular size at the time of the initial hemorrhage; the larger the initial size of the ventricles, the greater

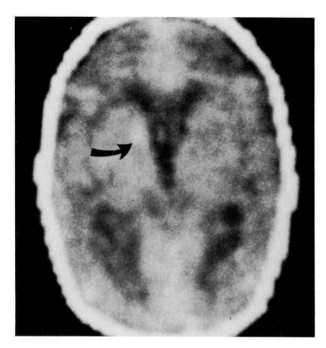

Figure 15-67   Premature neonate with small subependymal germinal matrix hemorrhage, head of caudate nucleus (arrow). Increased hypodensity of periventricular white matter in anterior frontal and posterior temporal regions.

was the probability for development of progressive hydrocephalus requiring shunting. Symptomatic hydrocephalus usually becomes evident between the first and the third week after birth.

Periventricular Leukomalacia

Periventricular hypodensity greater than would be expected with prematurity alone (Robinson 1966) has been observed in about 95 percent of premature neonates with intracerebral hemorrhage (Fig. 15-70) (Albright 1981). Serial CT scans on these infants have shown worsening of the periventricular hypodensity in 54 percent on scans obtained during the following several weeks. The areas of white-matter hypodensity become larger, with a progressively lower attenuation value. Subsequently, atrophic mild to severe ventricular and sulcal dilatation develops, depending on the maximum severity of periventricular hypodensity (Volpe 1966). The parenchymal hypodensity becomes less evident with the ventricular enlargement, although there

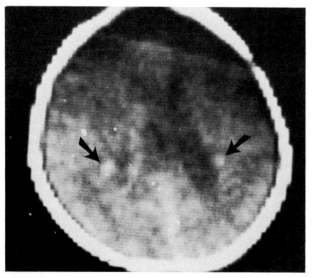

A

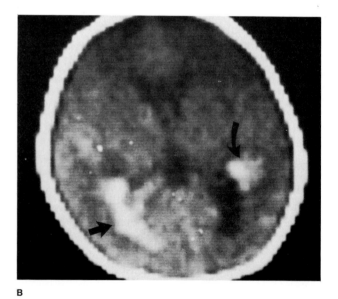

B

Figure 15-68   Multiple germinal matrix hemorrhages with parenchymal and small interventricular extension.   **A.** Bilateral subependymal hemorrhages in the atrial region of the lateral ventricles (arrows).   **B.** Parenchymal extension into left posterior temporal region (curved arrow); small ventricular rupture into right occipital horn (straight arrow).

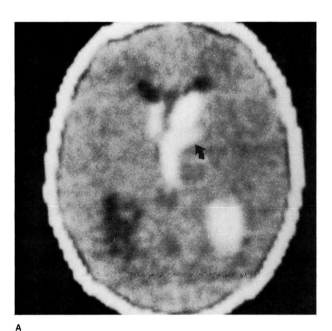

A

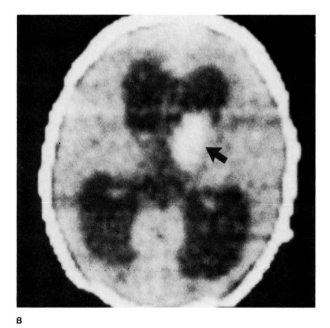

B

Figure 15-69 Large intraventricular rupture of germinal matrix hemorrhage with development of hydrocephalus. **A.** Extensive hemorrhage filling left lateral and third ventricles with small extension into right frontal horn. Site of hemorrhage appears to be subependymal in the posterior portion of cau-

date nucleus head (arrow). **B.** Two weeks after **A:** Marked hydrocephalus has developed. Residual localized hematoma remains against the lateral wall at the posterior aspect of left frontal horn.

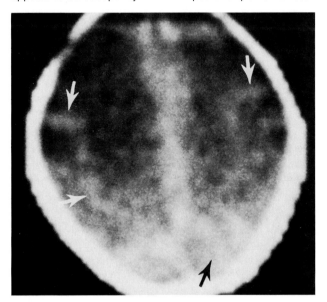

Figure 15-70 Periventricular leukomalacia in premature infant with small germinal matrix hemorrhage—same patient as in Figure 15-67. Marked white-matter hypodensity which accentuates cortical gray-matter density (arrows).

may be some persistence of hypodensity in the white matter. Pathologic studies have shown leukomalacia and white-matter coagulation necrosis, indicating that an anoxic ischemic insult to the brain is the most probable cause (de Reuck 1972). The hypodensity involves the frontal white matter alone in 45 percent, the frontal and parietal-occipital white matter together in 33 percent, the parietal-occipital white matter alone in eight percent, and the white matter diffusely in 15 percent of cases (Albright 1981). Its bilateral distribution in the white matter is frequently asymmetric.

Abnormal and progressive periventricular low density also develops in premature infants who have respiratory distress without intracerebral hemorrhage (Di Chiro 1978); a majority of these premature neonates develop this hypodensity (Albright 1981). Its distribution is similar to that seen in those infants with germinal-matrix hemorrhage. Caution must be exercised when calling periventricular hypodensity abnormal during the first 1 to 2 weeks post partum in premature infants, in whom the white matter is normally less dense than that of full-term infants because of less developed myelinization (Estrada 1980). In order to accurately evaluate these infants for possible periventricular leukomalacia, follow-up scans should be obtained in 4 to 6 weeks. The ultimate prognosis for surviving premature infants, both those with and those without intracerebral hemorrhage, appears most closely related to the degree and persistence of periventricular hypodensity and its subsequent atrophic consequences.

Bibliography

ADAMS RD, VANDER EECKEN HM: Vascular diseases of brain. *Ann Rev Med* **4:**213, 1953.

ADAMS RD and SIDMAN RL: *Introduction to Neuropathology.* New York, McGraw-Hill Book Company, 1968.

ALBRIGHT L, FELLOWS R: Sequential CT scanning after neonatal intracerebral hemorrhage. *Am J Neuroradiol* **2:**133–137, 1981.

ALCALA H, GADO M, TORACK RM: The effect of size, histologic elements, and water content on the visualization of cerebral infarcts. *Arch Neurol* **35:**1–7, 1978.

ANDERSON DC, COSS DT, JACOBSON RL, MEYER MW: Tissue pertechnetate and iodinated contrast material in ischemic stroke. *Stroke* **11:**617–622, 1980.

BAKER HL JR, CAMPBELL JK, HOUSER OW et al: Early experience with the EMI scanner for study of the brain. *Radiology* **116:**327–333, 1975.

BANNA, M, GROVES JT: Deep vascular congestion in dural venous thrombosis on computed tomography. *J Comput Assist Tomogr* **3:**539–541, 1979.

BILANIUK LT, PATEL S, ZIMMERMAN RA: Computed tomography of systemic lupus erythematosus. *Radiology* **124:**119–121, 1977.

BILANIUK LT, ZIMMERMAN RA, BROWN L, YOO HJ, GOLDBERG HI: Computed tomography in meningitis. *Neuroradiology* **16:**13–14, 1978.

BLAHD WH: *Nuclear Medicine.* New York, McGraw-Hill Book Company, 1971, pp 262–267.

BRADAC GM, OBERSON R: CT and angiography in cases with occlusive disease of supratentorial cerebral vessels. *Neuroradiology* **19:**193–200, 1980.

BRIERLEY JB: Cerebral hypoxia, in Blackwood W, Corsellis JAN (eds): *Greenfield's Neuropathology.* London, Edward Arnold Ltd., 1976, pp 43–85.

BRUCHER JM: Neuropathological problems posed by carbon-monoxide poisoning and anoxia. *Prog Brain Res* **24:**75–100, 1967.

BUELL V, KAZNER E, RATH M, STEINHOFF H, KLEINHANS E, LANKSCH W: Sensitivity of computed tomography and serial scintigraphy in cerebrovascular disease. *Radiology* **131:**393, 1979.

BUONANNO FS, MOODY DM, BALL MR, LASTER DW: Computed cranial tomographic findings in cerebral sinovenous occlusion. *J Comput Assist Tomogr* **2:**281–290, 1978.

BURSTEIN J, PAPILE LA, BURSTEIN R: Intraventricular hemorrhage and hydrocephalus in premature newborns: A prospective study with CT. *Am J Roentgenol* **132:**631–535, 1979.

CAIRNS H, RUSSELL DS: Cerebral arteritis and phlebitis in pneumococcal meningitis. *J Pathol Bacteriol* **58:**649–665, 1946.

CAMPBELL JK, HOUSER OW, STEVENS JC, WAHNER HW, BAKER HL, FOLGER WN: Computed tomography and radionuclide imaging in the evaluation of ischemic stroke. *Radiology* **126**:695–702, 1978.

CHARCOT JD, BOUCHARD C: Nouvelles recherches sur la pathogénie de l'hémorrhagie cérébrale. *Arch Physiol Norm Path (Paris)* **1**:110–127, 1868.

CHIU LC, CHRISTIE JH, SCHAPIRO RL: Nuclide imaging and computed tomography in cerebral vascular disease. *Semin Nucl Med* **7**:175–195, 1977.

CHU NS: Tuberculous meningitis: Computerized tomographic manifestations. *Arch Neurol* **37**:458–460, 1980.

COLE FM, YATES PO: The occurrence and significance of intracerebral microaneurysms. *J Pathol Bacteriol* **93**:393–411, 1967.

COCKRILL HH JR, DREISBACH J, LOWE B, YAMAUCHI T: Computed tomography in leptomeningeal infections. *Am J Roentgenol* **130**:511–515, 1978.

CRAVIOTO H, FEIGIN, I: Noninfectious granulomatous angiitis with a predilection for the nervous system. *Neurology* **9**:599–609, 1959.

CRONQVIST S, BRISMAR J, KJELLIN K, SODERSTROM CE: Computer assisted axial tomography in cerebrovascular lesions. *Radiology* **118**:498, 1976.

CRONQVIST S, LAROCHE F: Transient hyperaemia in focal cerebral vascular lesions studied by angiography and regional cerebral blood flow measurements. *Br J Radiol* **40**:270–274, 1967.

CRONQVIST S: Regional cerebral blood flow and angiography in apoplexy. *Acta Radiol [Diagn] (Stockholm)* **7**:521–534, 1968.

DASTER DK, UDANI PM: The pathology and pathogenesis of tuberculous encephalopathy. *Acta Neuropathol (Berl)* **6**:311–326, 1966.

DAVIS KR, ACKERMAN RH, KISTLER JP, MOHR JP: Computed tomography of cerebral infarction: Hemorrhagic, contrast enhancement, and time of appearance. *Comput Tomogr* **1**:71–86, 1977.

DAVIS KR, TAVERAS JM, NEW PFJ, SCHNUR JA, ROBERSON GH: Cerebral infarction diagnosis by computerized tomography: Analysis and evaluation of findings. *Am J Roentgenol* **124**:643–660, 1975.

DENNY-BROWN D: Recurrent cerebrovascular episodes. *Arch Neurol* **2**:194–210, 1960.

DE REUCK J: Arterial vascularisation and angioarchitecture of the nucleus caudatus in human brain. *Eur Neurol* **5**:130–136, 1971*a*.

DE REUCK JL, VANDER EECKEN HM: Periventricular leukomalacia in adults. *Arch Neurol* **35**:517–521, 1978.

DE REUCK J, CHATTA AS, RICHARDSON EP: Pathogenesis and evolution of periventricular leukomalacia in infancy. *Arch Neurol* **27**:229–236, 1972.

DE REUCK JL: The significance of the arterial angioarchitecture in perinatal cerebral damage. *Acta Neurol Belg* **77**:65–94, 1977.

DE REUCK J: The human periventricular arterial blood supply and the anatomy of cerebral infarctions. *Eur Neurol* **5**:321–334, 1971*b*.

DI CHIRO G, ARIMITSU T, PELLOCK JM, LANDES RD: Periventricular leukomalacia related to neonatal anoxia: Recognition by computed tomography. *J Comput Assist Tomogr* **2**:352–355, 1978.

DI CHIRO G, TIMINS EL, JONES AE, JOHNSTON GS, HAMMOCK MK, SWANN SJ: Radionuclide scanning and microangiography of evolving and completed brain infarction: A correlative study in monkeys. *Neurology* **24**:418–423, 1974.

DOLINSKAS CA, BILANIUK LT, ZIMMERMAN RA, KUHL DE: Computed tomography of intracerebral hematomas. I. Transmission CT observations on hematoma resolution. *Am J Roentgenol* **129**:681–688, 1977*a*.

DOLINSKAS CA, BILANIUK LT, ZIMMERMAN RA, KUHL DE, ALAVI A: Computed tomography of intracerebral hematomas: II. Radionuclide and transmission CT studies of the perihematoma region. *Am J Roentgenol* **129**:689–692, 1977b.

DUDLEY AW JR, LUNZER S, HEYMAN A: Localization of radioisotope (chlormerodrin He-203) in experimental cerebral infarction. *Stroke* **1**:143–148, 1970.

EICK JJ, MILLER KD, BELL KA, TUTTON RH: Computed tomography of deep cerebral venous thrombosis in children. *Radiology* **140**:399–402, 1981.

EISENBERG H, MORRISON JT, SULLIVAN P, FOOTE FM: Cerebrovascular accidents. *JAMA* **189**:883–888, 1964.

ELLIS GG, VERITY MA: Central nervous system involvement in systemic lupus erythematosus: A review of neuropathologic findings in 57 cases, 1955-1977. *Semin Arthritis Rheum* **8**:212–221, 1979.

ENZMANN DR, NORMAN D, MANI J, NEWTON H: Computed tomography of granulomatous basal arachnoiditis. *Radiology* **120**:341–344, 1976.

ESTRADA M, GAMMA TE, DYKEN PR: Periventricular low attenuations: A normal finding in computerized tomographic scans of neonates? *Arch Neurol* **37**:754–756, 1980.

FAER MJ, MEAD JH, LYNCH RD: Cerebral granulomatous angiitis: Case report and literature review. *Am J Roentgenol* **129**:463–467, 1977.

FERRIS EJ, SHAPIRO JH, SIMEONE FA: Arteriovenous shunting in cerebrovascular occlusive disease. *Am J Roentgenol Radium Ther Nucl Med* **98**:631–636, 1966.

FISHER CM, ADAMS RD: Observations on brain embolism with special reference to the mechanism of hemorrhagic infarction. *J Neuropathol Exp Neurol* **10**:92–94, 1951.

FISHER CM, CURRY HB: Pure motor hemiplegia of vascular origin. *Arch Neurol* **13**:30–44, 1965.

FISHER CM: Capsular infarcts: The underlying vascular lesion. *Arch Neurol* **36**:65–73, 1979.

FISHMAN RA: Brain edema. *N Engl J Med* **293**:706–711, 1975.

FRIEDE RL: *Developmental Neuropathology*. New York, Springer, 1976, pp 1–37.

GABRIELSEN TO, HEINZ ER: Spontaneous aseptic thrombosis of the superior sagittal sinus and cerebral veins. *Am J Roentgenol Radium Ther Nucl Med* **107**:579–588, 1969.

GABRIELSEN TO, SEEGER JF, KNAKE JE, STILWILL EW: Radiology of cerebral vein occlusion without dural sinus occlusion. *Radiology* **140**:403–408, 1981.

GADO MH, PHELPS ME, COLEMAN RE: An extravascular component of contrast enhancement in cranial computed tomography. *Radiology* **117**:595–597, 1975.

GILDERSLEVE N, KOO AH, MCCONALD CJ: Metastatic tumor presenting as intracerebral hemorrhage. *Radiology* **124**:109–112, 1977.

GINSBERG MD, MYERS RE, MCDONAGH BF: Experimental carbon-monoxide encephalopathy in the primate: II. Clinical aspects, neuropathology, and physiological correlation. *Arch Neurol* **30**:209–216, 1974.

GINSBERG MD, HEDLEY-WHYTE TE, RICHARDSON EP JR: Hypoxic ischemic leukoencephalopathy in man. *Arch Neurol* **33**:5–14, 1976.

GINSBERG MD: Delayed neurological deterioration following hypoxia, in Fahn S et al (eds), *Advances in Neurology*. New York, Raven Press, 1979, pp 21–47.

GLASER GH: Lesions of CNS in disseminated lupus erythematosus. *Arch Neurol Psychiatr* **67**:745–753, 1952.

GLASER GH: Neurologic manifestion in collagen diseases. *Neurology* **5**:751–766, 1955.

GOLDBERG HI: Clinical cerebral microangiography—magnification angiography and angiotomography, in Hilal S (ed), *Symposium on Small Vessel Angiography*. St. Louis, C.V. Mosby Company, 1973, pp 219–237.

GRUBB RL, COXE WS: Central nervous system trauma: Cranial, in Eliasson SG, Prensky AL, Hardin WB (eds), *Neurological Pathophysiology*. New York, Oxford University Press, 1974, pp 292–309.

HANDA J, HANDA H, NAKANO Y, OKUNO T: Computed tomography in moyamoya: Analysis of 16 cases. *Comput Axial Tomogr* **1**:165–174, 1977.

HAYMAN LA, EVANS RA, BASTION FO, HINCK VC: Delayed high dose contrast CT; Identifying patients at risk of massive hemorrhagic infarction. *Am J Neuroradiol* **2**:139–147, 1981.

HAYMAN LA, SAKAI F, MEYER JS, ARMSTRONG D, HINCK VC: Iodine-enhanced CT patterns after cerebral arterial embolization in baboons. *Am J Neuroradiol* **1**:233–238, 1980.

HEINZ ER, DUBOIS P, OSBORNE D et al: Dynamic computed tomography study of the brain. *J Comput Assist Tomogr* **3**:641–649, 1979.

HOEDT-RASMUSSEN K, SKINHOJ E, PAULSON O et al: Regional cerebral blood flow in acute apoplexy: The "luxury perfusion syndrome" of brain tissue. *Arch Neurol* **17**:271–281, 1967.

HUNGERFORD GD, DUBOULAY GH: CT in patients with severe migraine. *Neurol Neurosurg Psychiatr* **39**:990, 1976.

INOUE Y, TAKEMOTA K, MIYAMOTO T, YOSHIKAWA N, TANIGUCHI S, SAIWAI S, NISHIMURA Y, KOMATSU T: Sequential computed tomography scans in acute cerebral infarction. *Radiology* **135**:655–662, 1980.

IRINO T, MINAMI T, TANEDA M, HARA K: Brain edema and angiographical hyperemia in postrecanalized cerebral infarction. *Acta Neurol Scand* [Suppl] **64**:134–135, 1977a.

IRINO T, TANEDA M, MINAMI T: Angiographic manifestations in postrecanalized cerebral infarction. *Neurology* **17**:471–475, 1977b.

ITO U, OHNO K, TOMITA H, INABA Y: Cerebral changes during recirculation following temporary ischemia in mongolian gerbils, with special reference to blood brain barrier change, in Schmiedek P (ed), *Microsurgery for Stroke: Third Symposium.* New York, Springer, 1976, pp 29–38.

JOHNSON RT, RICHARDSON EP: The neurological manifestations of systemic lupus erythematosus: A clinical pathological study of 24 cases and review of literature. *Medicine* **47**:337–367, 1968.

JORGENSEN L, TORBIK A: Ischaemic cerebrovascular diseases in an autopsy series: II. Prevalency, location, pathogenesis and clinical course of cerebral infarcts. *J Neurol Sci* **9**:285–320, 1969.

KASSIK AE, NILSSON L, SIESJO BK: Acid-base and lactate-pyruvate changes in brain and CSF in asphyxia and stagnant hypoxia. *Scand J Clin Lab Invest* 22 (suppl 102) **3**:6, 1968.

KALBAG RM, WOOLF AL: *Cerebral Venous Thrombosis*, with Special Reference to Primary Aseptic Thrombosis. London, Oxford University Press, 1967, p. 237.

KAMIJYO Y, GARCIA JH, COOPER J: Temporary regional cerebral ischemia in the cat. *J Neuropathol Exp Neurol* **36**:338–350, 1977.

KENDALL BE, CLAVERIA LE, QUIROGA W: CAT in leukodystrophy and neuronal degeneration, in du Boulay GH, Moseley IF (eds): *Computerized Axial Tomography in Medical Practice.* New York, Springer-Verlag, 1977.

KIDO DK, GOMEZ DG, SANTOS-BUCH CA, CASTON TV, POTTS DG: Microradiographic study of cerebral and ocular aneurysms in hypertensive rabbits. *Neuroradiology* **15**:21–26, 1978.

KIM KS, WEINBERG PE, SUH JH, HO SU: Acute carbon monoxide poisoning: Computed tomography of the brain. *Am J Neuroradiol* **1**:399–402, 1980.

KINDT GW, YOUMANS JR, ALBRAND O: Factors influencing the autoregulation of cerebral blood flow during hypotension and hypertension. *J Neurosurg* **26**:299–305, 1967.

KINGSLEY DPE, WRADUE E, DUBOULAY EPGH: Evaluation of computed tomography in vascular lesions of the vertebrobasilar territory. *J Neurol Neurosurg Psychiatr* **43**:193–197, 1980.

KINKEL WR, JACOBS L: Computerized axial transverse tomography in cerebrovascular disease. *Neurology* **26**:924–930, 1976.

KLATZO J: Pathophysiological aspects of brain edema, in Reulen HJ, Schurmann K (eds): *Steroids and Brain Edema.* New York, Springer-Verlag, 1972, pp 1–8.

KODAMA N, SUZUKI J: Moyamoya disease associated with aneurysm. *J Neurosurg* **58:**565–569, 1978.

KOHLMEYER K, GRASER C: Comparative studies of computed tomography and measurements of regional cerebral blood flow in stroke patients. *Neuroradiology* **16:**233–237, 1978.

KRAYENBUHL H: Cerebral venous thrombosis: The diagnostic value of cerebral angiography. *Schweiz Arch Neurol Psychiatr* **74:**261–287, 1954.

KUDO T: Spontaneous occlusion of the circle of Willis: A disease apparently confined to Japanese. *Neurology* **18:**485–496, 1968.

KURTZKE JF: Epidemiology of cerebrovascular disease, in *Cerebrovascular Survey Report.* National Institute of Neurological and Communicative Disorders and Stroke and National Heart and Lung Institute, Joint Council Subcommittee on Cerebrovascular Disease, 1980, pp 135–176.

LADURNER G, SAGER WD, ILIFF LD, LECHNER H: A correlation of clinical findings and CT in ischaemic cerebrovascular disease. *Eur Neurol* **18:**281–288, 1979.

LAPRESLE J, FARDEAU M: The central nervous system and carbonmonoxide poisoning: II. Anatomical study of brain lesions following intoxication with carbonmonoxide (22 cases). *Prog Brain Res* **24:**31–75, 1967.

LASSEN NA: The luxury-perfusion syndrome and its possible relation to acute metabolic acidosis localized within the brain. *Lancet* **2:**1113–1115, 1966.

LASSEN NA, AGNOLI A: The upper limit of autoregulation of cerebral blood flow in the pathogenesis of hypertensive encephalopathy. *Scand J Clin Lab Invest* **30:**113–115, 1972.

LASTER DW, MOODY DM, BALL MR: Resolving intracerebral hematoma: Alteration of the "ring sign" with steroids. *Am J Roentgenol* **130:**935–939, 1978.

LAURENT JP, MOLINARI GF, OAKLEY JC: Primate model of cerebral hematoma. *J Neuropathol Exp Neurol* **35:**560–568, 1976.

LEE KF, CHAMBERS RA, DIAMOND C, PARK CH, THOMPSON NL, SCHNAPF D, PRIPSTEIN S: Evaluation of cerebral infarction by computed tomography with special emphasis on microinfarction. *Neuroradiology* **16:**156–158, 1978.

LEE BCP, GRASSI AE, SCHECHNER S, AULD PAM: Neonatal intraventricular hemorrhage: A serial computed tomography study. *J Comput Assist Tomogr* **3:**483–490, 1979.

LEEDS NE, GOLDBERG HI: Angiographic manifestations in cerebral inflammatory disease. *Radiology* **98:**595–604, 1971.

LEEDS NE, GOLDBERG HI: Abnormal vascular patterns in benign intracranial lesions: Pseudotumors of the brain. *Am J Roentgenol* **118:**567–575, 1973.

LEHRER H: The angiographic triad in tuberculous meningitis. *Radiology* **87:**829–835, 1966.

LEWIS SE, HICKEY DC, PARKEY RW: Radionuclide brain imaging: Its role and relation to CT scanning. *Comput Tomogr* **2:**155–172, 1978.

LHERMITTE F, GAUTIER JC, DEROUSNE C: Nature of occlusion of the middle cerebral artery. *Neurology* **20:**82, 1970.

LOU HC: Perinatal hypoxic-ischemic brain damage and intraventricular hemorrhage: A pathogenic model. *Arch Neurol* **37:**585–587, 1980.

MANELFE C, CLANET M, GIGUAD M, BONAFE A, GUIRAUD B, RASCOL A: Internal capsule: Normal anatomy and ischemic changes demonstrated by computed tomography. *Am J Neuroradiol* **2:**149–155, 1981.

MASDEU JC, BERHOOZ A-K, RUBINA, FA: Evaluation of recent cerebral infarction by computerized tomography. *Arch Neurol* **34:**417–421, 1977.

MATHEW NT, MEYERS JS: Abnormal CT scans in migraine. *Headache* **16:**272, 1976.

MATSUMOTO N, WHISNANT JP, KURLAND LT, OKAZAKI H: Natural history of stroke in Rochester, Minn., 1955 through 1969: An extension of a previous study, 1945 through 1954. *Stroke* **4:**20–29, 1973.

MCCALL AJ, FLETCHER PJH: Pathology, in Kutchinson EC, Ackason EJ, (eds), *Strokes: Natural History, Pathology and Surgical Treatment.* Philadelphia, WB Saunders Company, 1975, pp 36–105.

MERRITT HH: *A Textbook of Neurology,* 6th ed. Philadelphia, Lea & Febiger, 1979, pp 40–45.

MOHR JP, FISHER CM, ADAMS RD: Cerebrovascular diseases, in Isselbacher KJ, Adams RD, Braunwald E, Petersdorf RG, Wilson JD (eds) *Harrison's Principles of Internal Medicine,* 9th ed. McGraw-Hill Book Company, 1980, pp 1911–1942.

MOLINARI GF, PIRCHER F, HEYMAN A: Serial brain scanning using technetium 99m in patients with cerebral infarction. *Neurology* **17**:627, 1967.

MYER JS, DENNY-BROWN D: The cerebral collateral circulation: I. Factors influencing collateral blood flow. *Neurology* **7**:447–458, 1957.

NELSON RF, PULLICINO P, KENDALL BE, MARSHALL J: Computed tomography in patients presenting with lacunar syndromes. *Stroke* **11**:256–261, 1980.

NISHIMOTO A, TAKEUCHI S: Abnormal cerebrovascular network related to the internal carotid arteries. *J Neurosurg* **29**:255–260, 1968.

NORMAN D, AXEL L, BERNINGER WH, EDWARD MS, CANN C, REDINGTON RW, COX L: Dynamic computed tomography of the brain: Techniques, data analysis, and applications. *Am J Neuroradiol* **2**:1–12, 1981.

NORTON GA, KISHORE PRS, LIN J: CT contrast enhancement in cerebral infarction. *Am J Roentgenol* **131**:881–885, 1978.

NURICK S, BLACKWOOD W, MAIR WGP: Giant cell granulomatous angiitis of the central nervous system. *Brain* **95**:133–142, 1972.

O'BRIEN MD, JORDAN MM, WALTZ AG: Ischemic cerebral edema and the blood-brain barrier: Distribution of pertechnetate, albumin, sodium, and antipyrine in brains of cats after occlusion of the middle cerebral artery. *Arch Neurol* **30**:461–465, 1974.

OLSSON Y, CROWELL RM, KLATZO I: The blood brain barrier to protein tracers in focal cerebral ischemia and infarction caused by occlusion of the middle cerebral artery. *Acta Neuropathol* **18**:89–102, 1971.

PAULSON OB, LASSEN NA, SKINHOJ E: Regional cerebral blood flow in apoplexy without arterial occlusion. *Neurology* **20**:125–138, 1970.

PECKER J, SIMON J, GUY G, HERRY JF: Nishimoto's disease: Significance of its angiographic appearances. *Neuroradiology* **5**:223–230, 1973.

PERRONE P, CANDELISE L, SCOTTI G, DE GRANDI C, SCIALFA G: CT evaluation in patients with transient ischemic attack: Correlation between clinical and angiographic findings. *Eur Neurol* **18**:217–221, 1979.

PITTS FW, HASKIN ME, RIGGS HE, GROFF RA: Tumor-strain in cerebrovascular disease. *J Neurosurg* **21**:298–300, 1964.

PLUM F, POSNER JB, HAIN RF: Delayed neurological deterioration after anoxia. *Arch Intern Med* **110**:18–25, 1962.

PRINEAS J, MARSHALL J: Hypertension and cerebral infarction. *Br Med J* **1**:14–17, 1966.

PULLICINO P, KENDALL BE: Contrast enhancement in ischaemic lesions: I. Relationship to prognosis. *Neuroradiology* **19**:235–239, 1980.

RAIL DL, PERKIN GD: Computerized tomographic appearance of hypertensive encephalopathy. *Arch Neurol* **37**:310–311, 1980.

RANGEL RA: Computerized axial tomography in brain death. *Stroke* **9**:597–598, 1978.

RAO KCVG, KNIPP HC, WAGNER EJ: Computed tomographic findings in cerebral sinus and venous thrombosis. *Radiology* **140**:391–398, 1981.

RAPPAPORT ZH, BRINKER RA, ROVIT RL: Evaluation of brain death with contrast enhanced computerized cranial tomography. *Neurosurgery* **2**:230–232, 1978.

Report to the President: A National Program to Conquer Heart Disease, Cancer and Stroke. Washington, President's Commission on Heart Disease, Cancer and Stroke, 1964, 1965.

ROBINSON MA, TIZARD MA: The cerebral nervous system in the newborn. *Br Med Bull* **22**:49–55, 1966.

ROMANUL FCA, ABRAMOWICZ A: Changes in brain and pial vessels in arterial border zones. *Arch Neurol* **11**:40–65, 1964.

ROSENBLUM WI, HADFIELD MG: Granulomatous angiitis of the nervous system in cases of herpes zoster and lymphosarcoma. *Neurology* **22**:348–354, 1972.

ROSENBERG GA, KORNFELD M, STOVRING J, BICKNELL JM: Subcortical arteriosclerotic encephalopathy (Binswanger): Computerized tomography. *Neurology* **29**:1102–1106, 1979.

RUFF RL, TALMAN WT, PETITO F: Transient ischemic attacks associated with hypotension in hypertensive patients with carotid artery stenosis. *Stroke* **12**:353–355, 1981.

RUMBAUGH CL, BERGERON RT, FANG HCH, MCCORMICK R: Cerebral angiographic changes in drug abuse patients. *Radiology* **101**:335–344, 1971.

RUSSELL RWR: Observations on intracerebral aneurysms. *Brain* **86**:425–442, 1963.

SOIN JS, BURDINE JA: Acute cerebral vascular accident associated with hyperfusion. *Radiology* **118**:109–112, 1976.

SOLE-LLENAS J, PONS-TORTELLA E: Cerebral angiitis. *Neuroradiology* **15**:1–11, 1978.

STEHBENS WE: *Pathology of the Cerebral Blood Vessels.* St. Louis, C.V. Mosby Company, 1972, pp 291–323.

SUGITANI Y, NAKAMA M, YAMAGUCHI Y, IMAIZUMI M, NAKADA T, ABE H: Neovascularization and increased uptake of ^{99}m Tc in experimentally produced cerebral hematoma. *J Nucl Med* **14**:912–916, 1973.

SUZUKI J, TAKAKU A: Cerebrovascular "moyamoya" disease: Disease showing abnormal net-like vessels in base of brain. *Arch Neurol* **20**:88–299, 1969.

TABOADA D, ALONSO A, OLAGUE R, MULAS F, ANDREW V: Radiological diagnosis of periventricular and subcortical leukomalacia. *Neuroradiology* **20**:33–41, 1980.

TAKAHASHI M, SAITO Y, KONNO K: Intraventricular hemorrhage in childhood moyamoya disease. *J Comput Assist Tomogr* **4**:117–120, 1980.

TAVERAS JM: Multiple progressive intracranial arterial occlusion: A syndrome of children and young adults. *Am J Roentgenol Radium Ther Nucl Med* **106**:235–268, 1969.

TREVOR RP, SONDHEINER FK, FESSEL WJ et al: Angiographic demonstrations of major cerebral vessel occlusion in systemic lupus erythematosus. *Neuroradiology* **4**:202–207, 1972.

VALAVANIS A, FRIEDE R, SCHUBIGER O, HAYEK J: Cerebral granulomatous angiitis simulating brain tumor. *J Comput Assist Tomgr* **3**:536–538, 1979.

VALK J: *Computed Tomography and Cerebral Infarction.* New York, Raven Press, 1980, p. 56.

VINES FS, DAVIS DO: Clinical-radiological correlation in cerebral venous occlusive disease. *Radiology* **98**:9–22, 1971.

VINTERS HV, GILBERT JJ: Amyloid angiopathy: Its incidence and complications in the aging brain. *Stroke* **12**:118, 1981.

VOLPE JJ: Perinatal hypoxic ischemia brain injury. *Pediatr Clin North Am* **23**:383–397, 1976.

WEISBERG LA: Computerized tomography in intracranial hemorrhage. *Arch Neurol* **36**:422–426, 1979.

WEISBERG LA: Computerized tomographic enhancement patterns in cerebral infarction. *Arch Neurol* **37**:21, 1980.

WENDLING LR: Intracranial venous sinus thrombosis: Diagnosis suggested by computed tomography. *Am J Roentgenol* **130**:978–980, 1978.

WHISNANT JP, FITZGIBBONS JP, KURLAND LT, SAYRE GP: Natural history of stroke in Rochester, Minnesota, 1945 through 1954. *Stroke* **2**:11–21, 1971.

WING SD, NORMAN D, POLLOCK JA, NEWTON TH: Contrast enhancement of cerebral infarcts in computed tomography. *Radiology* **121**:89–92, 1976.

WOOD MW, WAKIM KG, SAYRE, GP, MILLIKAN CH, WHISNANT JP: Relationship between anticoagulants and hemorrhagic cerebral infarction in experimental animals. *Arch Neurol Psychiatr* **79**:390–396, 1958.

YAGNIK P, GONZALEZ C.: White matter involvement in anoxic encephalopathy in adults. *J Comput Assist Tomogr* **4**:788–790, 1980.

YAMAGUCHI T, WALTZ AG, OKAZAKI H: Hyperemia and ischemia in experimental cerebral infarction: Correlation of histopathology and regional blood flow. *Neurology* **21**:565–578, 1971.

YARNELL PR, EARNEST MP, SANDERS B, BURDICK D: The "hot stroke" and transient vascular occlusions. *Stroke* **6**:517–520, 1975.

YOCK DH JR, MARSHALL WH JR: Recent ischemic brain infarcts at computed tomography: Appearances pre- and postcontrast infusion. *Radiology* **117**:599–608, 1975.

YOCK DH JR: CT demonstration of cerebral emboli. *J Comput Assist Tomogr* **5**:190–196, 1981.

ZEUMER H, SCHONSKY B, STRUM KW: Predominant white matter involvement in subcortical arteriosclerotic encephalopathy (Binswanger disease). *J Comput Assist Tomogr* **4**:14–19, 1980.

ZILKHA A, DAIZ AS: Computed tomography in the diagnosis of superior sagittal sinus thrombosis. *J Comput Assist Tomogr* **4**:124–126, 1980.

ZIMMERMAN RD, LEEDS NE, NAIDICH TP: Ring blush with intracerebral hematoma. *Radiology* **122**:707–711, 1977.

ZIEGLER DK, ZOSA A, ZILELI T: Hypertensive encephalopathy. *Arch Neurol* **12**:472–478, 1965.

WHITE MATTER DISEASE OF THE BRAIN*

Richard E. Fernandez

Pulla R. S. Kishore

There are many diseases that affect the white matter of the brain, ranging from intracerebral hemorrhage to tuberous sclerosis (Garrick 1979). In this chapter, we deal with those diseases listed in Table 16-1 which are considered to involve primarily the white matter. It should be kept in mind, however, that any such classification by its very nature must be somewhat arbitrary. This group can be further subdivided into those which are considered to be the result of breakdown of normal myelin, termed *myelinoclastic*, and those diseases involving either the formation of abnormal myelin or abnormal myelin maintenance, termed *dysmyelinating diseases*. The discussion of white matter disease is somewhat hampered by the numerous clinical entities which have been described in the literature prior to the present century and which have been subsequently classified and reclassified. The current discussion thus deals with the most common of these diseases which the practicing clinician may encounter.

With the advent of computed tomography (CT), there is a whole new method of investigating white matter disease. Where a diagnosis was previously made solely on clinical impression with or without biopsy proof, there is now a noninvasive method for evaluating these diseases. Computed tomography also offers a noninvasive method of following the progression and extent of the pathologic processes. While some of these entities are sufficiently common to have been fully evaluated in the litera-

* The authors express their appreciation to Dr. N. R. Ghatak for reviewing the manuscript.

Table 16-1 White Matter Disease of the Brain

Myelinoclastic diseases

  Multiple sclerosis

  Progressive multifocal leukoencephalopathy

  Disseminated necrotizing leukoencephalopathy

  Acute disseminated encephalomyelitis

  Schilder's disease

Dysmyelinating diseases

  Metachromatic leukodystrophy

  Spongy degeneration (Canavan's disease)

  Globoid cell leukodystrophy (Krabbe's disease)

  Alexander's disease

  Pelizaeus-Merzbacher disease

  Cockayne's syndrome

  Adrenoleukodystrophy

ture, others are exceedingly rare, and full comprehension of their pathologic pattern as demonstrated by CT continues to evolve. It should also be remembered when reading the pathological descriptions in this chapter that the pathologist frequently sees an end-stage process while CT will demonstrate the disease as it is evolving.

MYELINOCLASTIC DISEASES

These entities are acquired diseases having inflammatory characteristics. To this group of demyelinating diseases could also be added secondary demyelination of any etiology such as intoxication, anoxia, deficiency syndromes, cerebral infarct, brain abscess, and cerebral tumors, either primary or metastatic (Heinz 1979; Rubinstein 1978).

Multiple Sclerosis

Multiple sclerosis is a disease of unknown etiology affecting the central nervous system with primary involvement of the central white matter. The peak incidence is between 20 and 40 years of age, with no sex or race predilection. The clinical course is widely variable, with multiple relapses and remissions. The lesions themselves consist of localized areas of myelin breakdown and appear to expand by focal diffusion in the white matter by an as of yet unknown process. Pathologically, the lesions commonly progress to glial scarring (Schumacher 1965).

Computed tomography can play an important role in the diagnosis of multiple sclerosis by revealing characteristic findings. Computed tomography also helps to exclude other entities such as extraaxial tumors around the tentorium and foramen magnum which have been known to cause neurological findings simulating those of multiple sclerosis (Lausberg 1974). The appearance of white matter disease in multiple sclerosis will depend on whether the patient is in remission or in relapse.

Old inactive disease will characteristically show multiple, rather well defined areas of decreased attenuation situated in the deep white matter and periventricular regions (Cala 1978; Lane 1978) (Fig. 16-1). The plaques of multiple sclerosis may also occur in other white matter areas, including the cerebellum and spinal cord; however, these lesions are more difficult to visualize, as CT resolution is more difficult in this area. The size of the demyelinating plaques may vary in size up to several centimeters in diameter (Lane 1978), with the majority much smaller. The multiplicity and asymmetric appearance of the demyelinating plaques in multiple sclerosis is an important clue in making the diagnosis. Also, relative absence of surrounding edema is a usual finding and helps to differentiate from metastatic disease (Fig. 16-1).

In the acute phase, the evolving plaques may show enhancement on CECT (Fig. 16-1). The CT appearance is often that of a mixture of nonenhancing focal areas of decreased density representing old areas of demyelination, intermixed with enhancing regions, representing active foci. Enhancement patterns have been described as homogeneous, diffuse, peripheral, edge, ring, and central (Marano 1980; Weisberg 1981). Thus the pattern is nonspecific and may not help in suggesting the diagnosis. The enhancement may occur in a lesion seen as a low-density area on noncontrast computed tomog-

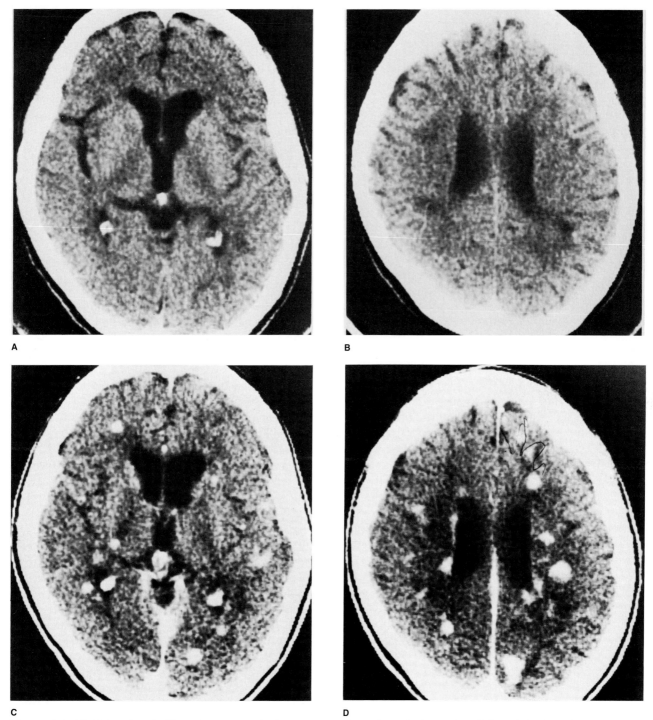

A

B

C

D

Figure 16-1 Multiple sclerosis. These images are of a 31-year-old female with a long history of known multiple sclerosis. **A** and **B.** NCCT images reveal diffuse central and cortical atrophy of both hemispheres. There are multiple areas of hypodensity in the white matter. **C** and **D.** CECT images disclose multiple contrast-enhancing plaques in the white matter, particularly in the periventricular region. A few of the hypodense areas do not show contrast enhancement, indicating old plaques. Dramatic improvement in clinical condition and almost complete disappearance of the multiple sclerosis plaques were noted after steroid therapy. Left frontal artifact is present.

raphy (NCCT) or it may occur in an isodense area of brain (Aita 1978; Lebow 1978). These areas of enhancement in isodense brain may not show enhancement on follow-up studies or may develop into focal low-density lesions (Aita 1978). Demyelinating plaques with decreased attenuation may also enhance so that they appear isodense on CECT and may not be detected if only CECT is performed (Sears 1978). Mass effect in association with active multiple sclerosis has been reported (Van der Velden 1979; Weisberg 1981). This mass effect may be confusing and lead to misinterpretation. Contrast enhancement may also be visualized only with delayed scans (Morariu 1980). Contrast enhancement in a lesion has also been reported 12 hours prior to its clinical recurrence (Sears 1978). Following steroid therapy a previously enhancing lesion may show a lesser degree of enhancement or no enhancement at all (Sears 1978; Weisberg 1981). This finding gives credence to the theory that the mode of enhancement is related to alteration in the blood-brain barrier, which is lessened by the administration of corticosteroids (Sears 1978). It should also be noted, however, that contrast enhancement has been noted in an enlarging lesion that was demonstrated to be nonenhancing prior to the initiation of steroid treatment and in the face of clinical improvement (Marano 1980).

In the face of long-standing disease, atrophy of the cerebral hemispheres (Fig. 16-1) and the cerebellum, especially the vermis, is common (Cala 1978). Low-density areas of the optic nerves have been reported; however, the small size of the optic nerves along with the problem of volume averaging makes this finding tenuous, and these areas may actually represent artifacts, at least in part (Cala 1978). The identification of demyelination of multiple sclerosis in the spinal cord has also been reported (Coin 1979).

Previous reports have noted a poor correlation between specific foci of disease and clinical findings (Cala 1978; Reisner 1980). These studies, however, were not carried out during the active stage of the disease, and contrast enhancement was not consistently employed. As we have already noted, an active focus of multiple sclerosis may appear isodense on non-contrast-enhanced CT and then enhance following contrast administration. These areas may thus, at least in part, be responsible for the low radiologic-clinical correlation. Further investigation in this area during acute bouts of multiple sclerosis with new acute neurological findings is needed to evaluate this specific area. These same reports also noted a significant number of clinically silent low-density plaques in the cerebral hemisphere, especially in a periventricular location (Cala 1978; Reisner 1980).

Progressive Multifocal Leukoencephalopathy

Progressive multifocal leukoencephalopathy (PML) is a progressive disease of the central nervous system showing white matter involvement as a constant feature. The disease occurs usually in immunosuppressed patients. The majority of these patients either have leukemia or lymphoma. It has also been reported in renal transplant recipients and in patients with tuberculosis, sarcoidosis, and macroglobulinemia (Carroll 1977; Lyon 1971; McCormick 1976). Only rarely was PML reported in patients with no known cause for immunosuppression (Richardson 1974). Papovavirus (JC, SV 40) has been isolated from the lesions of progressive multifocal leukoencephalopathy (Peters 1980). The usual clinical course is one of progression to coma, leading to death usually in 3 to 6 months after the onset of symptoms (Carroll 1977). The final diagnosis of progressive multifocal leukoencephalopathy depends on biopsy or postmortem examination (Peters 1980). Drug therapy has had varied success.

Pathological examination in PML demonstrates multifocal areas of demyelination with relative sparing of neurons. The mechanism for demyelination is considered by some to be a result of the death of oligodendroglia, the cells responsible for the sheath formation (Carroll 1977). The demyelinating lesions of PML appear to have a predilection for the subcortical white matter. Atrophy is a late occurrence in the disease.

Computed tomography plays an important role in the diagnosis of progressive multifocal leukoencephalopathy by suggesting the diagnosis as well as selecting sites for biopsy by revealing the characteristic low-density foci in the subcortical white matter (Carroll 1977). The lesions are sharply marginated with a scalloped outer border (Fig. 16-2). There appears to be a predilection for the parieto-occipital region (Bosch 1976; Carroll 1977). Follow-up examinations may show progressive enlargement of the demyelinating areas (Carroll 1977). Al-

though rare, mass effect may be present (Cunningham 1977), as may contrast enhancement (Heinz 1979).

Disseminated Necrotizing Leukoencephalopathy

Disseminated necrotizing leukoencephalopathy is a disease affecting patients who have been treated

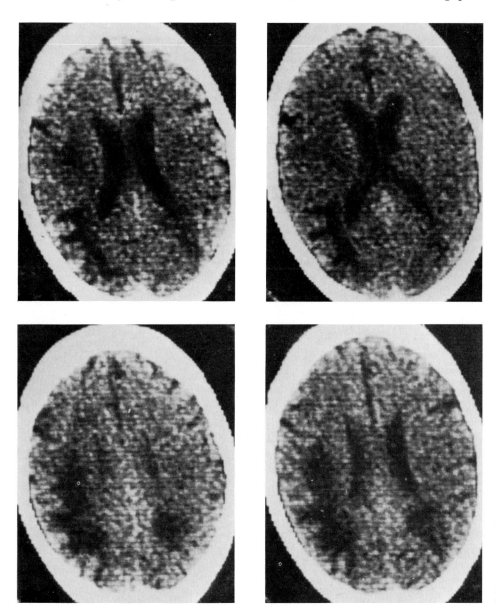

Figure 16-2 Progressive multifocal leukoencephalopathy. NCCTs of a 68-year-old man with history of chronic lymphocytic leukemia reveal low-density zones (10–12 HU) in both hemispheres. Note the characteristic well-marginated medial aspect and scalloped outer border at junction of gray and white matter. No contrast enhancement was noted. (*Reproduced by permission from Carroll et al., 1977.*)

with methotrexate, usually intrathecally for the pre-vention or treatment of meningeal leukemia or lym-phoma as well as for the treatment of solid tumors (Allen 1978). In patients with leukemia or lym-phoma who have been treated with systemic anti-tumor drugs, the central nervous system serves as a reservoir for tumor cells which are protected from the systemic drugs by the blood-brain barrier. To prevent relapse in these patients, radiation therapy and intrathecal administration of antitumor drugs have been undertaken (Aur 1972; Rubinstein 1975). Diffuse necrotizing leukoencephalopathy may occur following administration of systemic methotrexate without craniospinal irradiation (Allen 1978). The disease usually is clinically manifest as confusion, somnolence, spasticity, seizures, ataxia, and de-mentia and may lead to coma and death (Kay 1972; McIntosh 1973; Price 1975; De Vivo 1977).

Pathology of disseminated necrotizing leukoen-cephalopathy reveals multiple foci of coagulative necrosis of the white matter in a random manner which appears to extend by confluence and dissem-inates in the cerebral white matter (Rubinstein 1975, 1978). With progression of the disease, the demye-lination may appear extensive and symmetrical (Rubinstein 1975). In the later phase of the disease, dystrophic calcification may occur in the basal gan-glia or gray-white matter margin (Peylan-Ramu 1977).

Computed tomography can play an important role in necrotizing leukoencephalopathy because there has been some indication that the effects of this process may be partially reversible on discon-tinuation of the methotrexate therapy (Allen 1978; Pizzo 1976). Computed tomography in necrotizing leukoencephalopathy is to be distinguished from other changes seen in these patients such as dila-tation of ventricular and subarachnoid spaces. These changes may be a result of cranial irradiation rather than those of necrotizing leukoencephalopa-thy (Peylan-Ramu 1978).

Computed tomography of necrotizing leukoen-cephalopathy demonstrates areas of decreased at-tenuation in the centrum semiovale and periven-tricular areas (Fig. 16-3) (Allen 1978; Peylan-Ramu

1977). On CECT there may be enhancement of the low-density lesions (Lane 1978). Mass effect may also be seen. When methotrexate is introduced via a reservoir in the ventricular system, necrotizing leukoencephalopathy may then be seen as a focal process at the tube tip, with edema and the ap-pearance of a mass which may enhance following contrast administration and which may be confused with an abscess or other process (Bjorgen 1977). The intracerebral calcifications of necrotizing leukoen-cephalopathy have been demonstrated by CT (Mueller 1976; Peylan-Ramu 1977, 1978).

Acute Disseminated Encephalomyelitis

Acute disseminated encephalomyelitis is usually an explosive although sometimes subacute widespread central nervous system inflammatory condition which severely affects the white matter, leading to a marked neurologic impairment. The clinical out-come is varied, and the disease may be fatal, com-pletely reversible, or may give permanent neurolog-ical disability (Schumacher 1965). There is no age or sex predilection. It is usually monophasic; however, a few recurrent cases have been reported (Poser 1978). The disease can be divided into four types on the basis of etiology (Oppenheimer 1976): (1) post-infectious (measles, vaccinia, or varicella); (2) spon-taneous or during the course of a nonspecific respi-ratory infection; (3) allergic (postvaccination); and (4) fulminating (nearly always fatal and character-ized by multiple punctate intracerebral hemor-rhages). An immune complex etiology has been pro-posed for acute disseminated encephalomyelitis (Reik 1980).

Pathologically, the lesions may be indistinguish-able from those of multiple sclerosis while others may show a more typical pattern of perivascular extraadventitial demyelinization with microglial re-action following the course of the cerebral veins. The foci are not limited to the white matter of the cerebrum but are frequently seen in the cerebral cortex, cerebellum, basal ganglia, brainstem, and spinal cord as well (Oppenheimer 1976; Reik 1980;

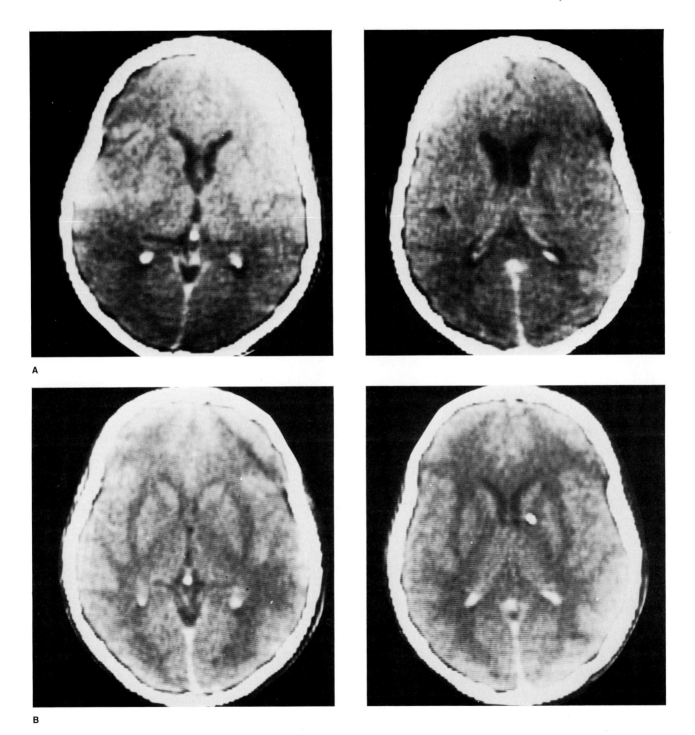

Figure 16-3 Disseminated necrotizing leukoencephalopathy. **A.** Initial CT of a patient on intrathecal methotrexate therapy reveals no gross abnormality. **B.** CT images on the same patient performed 3 months later reveal diffuse low-density zones in both hemispheres.

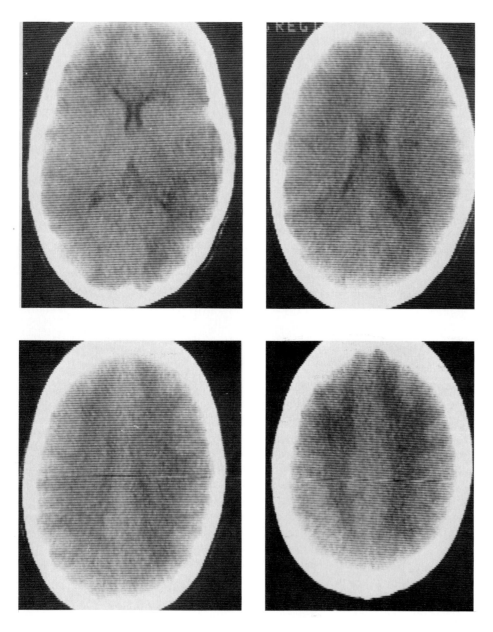

Figure 16-4 Acute disseminated encephalomyelitis. 18-year-old woman with bilateral hemispheric dysfunction and altered mental status. CT images reveal diffuse low-density zones in both hemispheres. Cerebrospinal fluid revealed markedly elevated gamma globulins with elevated rubella titers (1024:1).

Schumacher 1965). Edema is a major component of the acute phase of the disease.

CT in acute disseminated encephalomyelitis would show cerebral edema in the acute phase. In the chronic stage CT would show variable amounts of white and gray matter loss with atrophy, depending on the severity and extent of involvement (Fig. 16-4).

It should be mentioned when considering acute disseminated encephalomyelitis that there is another clinical entity known as *subacute sclerosing panencephalitis* which has been linked to the measles virus. Subacute sclerosing panencephalitis, unlike acute disseminated encephalomyelitis, is a progressive disease showing at least two phases with the second phase characterized by periodic involuntary movements which may consist of jerking of the face, fingers, or limbs and may include torsion spasms of the trunk (Adams 1976). The CT appearance of subacute sclerosing panencephalitis has been described as showing no abnormality, cerebral atrophy either focal or diffuse, and low density areas of the basal ganglia as well as the white and gray matter (Duda 1980).

Schilder's Disease

"Schilder's disease" is an eponymic term which previously received some attention but has lost most of its meaning. It has been advocated that the cases described under this term be reclassified as examples of a variant of multiple sclerosis, adrenoleukodystrophy, or demyelination accompanying subacute viral encephalitis or as other variants of familial leukodystrophies (Rubinstein 1978). The advocates of Schilder's disease believe that it can be differentiated from multiple sclerosis, and report a larger size of the lesions and an absence of separate lesions in the brainstem and spinal cord (Schumacher 1965). The pathological changes are described as massive degeneration of the central and subcortical white matter of the cerebrum which appear to begin in one focus and then spread by contiguity (Schumacher 1965). Computed tomography of Schilder's disease in most cases will show a pattern resembling either multiple sclerosis or adrenoleukodystrophy (Fig. 16-5).

DYSMYELINATING DISEASES

Dysmyelination was originally introduced to differentiate conditions in which normally formed myelin is destroyed (e.g., multiple sclerosis) from a group of diseases in which there appears to be abnormal myelin formation or maintenance (Poser 1957). The dysmyelinating diseases can be subdivided into those which are considered primarily white matter disease and those which, either additionally or primarily, affect gray matter, which would include Niemann-Pick disease, Gaucher's disease, and Tay-Sachs disease (Malone 1976; Poser 1978). Only those diseases that affect white matter primarily are discussed in this chapter.

This group of dysmyelinating diseases is made up largely of the leukodystrophies. These diseases are inherited diseases showing either autosomal recessive, autosomal dominant or sex-linked recessive modes of inheritance. Specific enzyme deficiencies have been shown in two of the leukodystrophies, namely, globoid cell leukodystrophy and metachromatic leukodystrophy (Rubinstein 1978). While most authors feel that the pathological changes in leukodystrophy are secondary to a specific enzyme deficiency, this hypothesis has been questioned by others (Poser 1978). With the exception of metachromatic leukodystrophy and globoid cell leukodystrophy, the leukodystrophies do not affect the peripheral nervous system (Malone 1976).

Metachromatic Leukodystrophy

Metachromatic leukodystrophy is a progressive autosomal recessive disorder which derives its name from the marked staining of metachromatic lipids. It may occur from the perinatal period (Feigin 1954) to advanced life. The oldest reported case is a man who became symptomatic for the first time at the age of 62 (Bosch 1978). The majority of the cases, however, present around the second year of life and become progressively worse with death by the third or fourth year. Occasional prolonged survival for several years has been reported (Malone 1976). The classic case is believed to have three clinical stages. The child is initially normal and then develops decreased truncal control, intellectual decline, and decreased responsiveness to the environment (Malone 1976). There is subsequent decline to an essentially unresponsive state with spasticity and "twitchlike" movements. In the late-onset type, there is a slower progression. The late juvenile and adult forms show dementia as a prominent feature, which may be the result of accumulation of sulfatides in neurons (Rubinstein 1978).

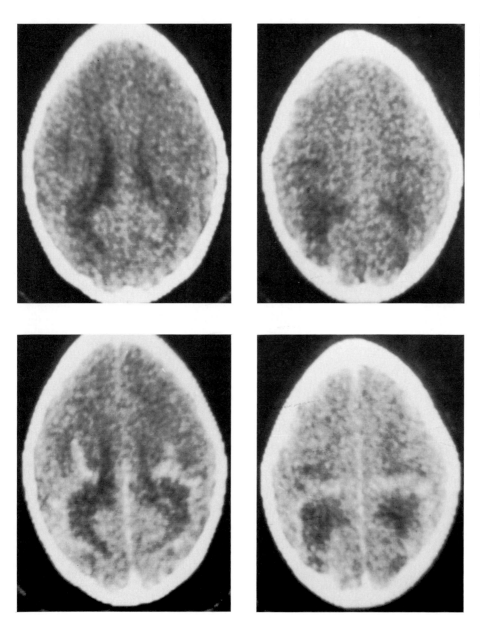

Figure 16-5 Schilder's disease. Noncontrast CT (*left*) and CECT (*right*) of a 6-year-old boy reveal periventricular hypodense zones that enhance markedly. These findings are consistent with adrenoleukodystrophic form of Schilder's disease.

Enzyme deficiencies of aryl sulfatase A or multiple sulfatases have been found in metachromatic leukodystrophy, and definitive diagnosis may be established by an absence of aryl sulfatase in the urine and serum (Crome 1976; Malone 1976).

Pathological examination in metachromatic leukodystrophy demonstrates diffuse widespread foci of disease in the centrum semiovale, cerebellum, and brainstem. In the late infantile form the brain is often noted to be larger and heavier than normal. Peripheral nerves demonstrate mild demyelination. Demyelination in the central nervous system is often intensified around vascular structures (Crome 1976).

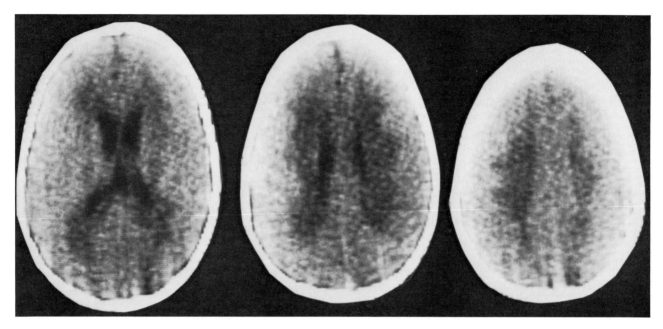

Figure 16-6   Metachromatic leukodystrophy. CT images of a 33-month-old girl reveal hypodense zones in the white matter without conforming to either lobar or vascular distribution. (*Reproduced by permission from Buonanno et al., 1978.*)

The role of CT in metachromatic leukodystrophy is to exclude other etiologies for the clinical findings. The definitive diagnostic test as already noted is the demonstration of an aryl sulfatase A deficiency in the urine or serum. CT findings typically consist of diffuse symmetrical decrease in attenuation in the centrum semiovale (Fig. 16-6). Contrast enhancement or mass effect has not been reported (Buonanno 1978; Robertson 1977). Minimal ventricular dilatation suggesting atrophy has been described. A single case of late adult-onset type in which CT demonstrated normal attenuation of white matter has been described (Bosch 1978). Atrophy probably reflecting the patient's age was noted in this case.

Spongy Degeneration (Canavan's Disease)

Spongy degeneration is a disease of infancy demonstrating megalencephaly, blindness, initial hypotonia followed by spasticity, and progressive psychomotor deterioration with onset between the second and ninth months of life (Adornato 1972;

Crome 1976). Deafness has sometimes been noted. The disease is apparently transmitted as an autosomal recessive. Some authors feel that this leukodystrophy should no longer be considered as a single entity and that it actually represents a rather nonspecific manifestation of a large and diverse group of metabolic disturbances (Poser 1978).

Pathologically, there is considerable variation in the extent and location of the demyelination. Most severely affected is the centrum semiovale, where there is little evidence of myelin (Crome 1976; Poser 1978). Megalencephaly has been noted (Boltshauser 1976; Lane 1978). With the exception of Alexander's disease, spongy degeneration is the only degenerative neurologic syndrome in this age group which demonstrates megalencephaly.

Spongy degeneration is diagnosed by brain biopsy. Computed tomography assists in this diagnosis by demonstrating a marked decrease in the attenuation of the entire white matter in a symmetric fashion throughout both hemispheres (Fig. 16-7). Contrast enhancement is not reported.

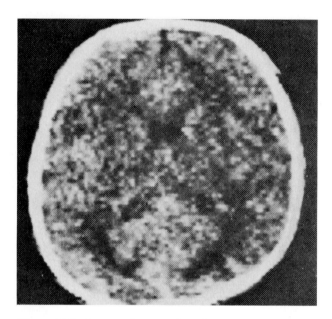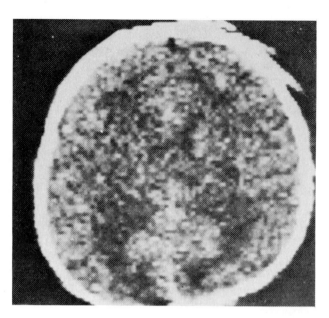

Figure 16-7   Spongy degeneration (Canavan's disease). CT images in a patient with spongy degeneration confirmed by brain biopsy reveal extensive areas of low attenuation in both hemispheres. (*Reproduced by permission from Boltshauser and Isler, 1976.*)

Globoid Cell Leukodystrophy (Krabbe's Disease)

Globoid cell leukodystrophy is an autosomal recessive disorder causing progressive neurologic impairment. The disease receives its name from characteristic large multinucleated histiocytes (Crome 1976). The disease usually presents in the first year of life. Although late forms of the disease are known, globoid cell leukodystrophy occurs almost exclusively as an acute early infantile disorder. A subacute type with clinical similarities to metachromatic leukodystrophy is also known to occur. Two striking clinical features consisting of rapid spontaneous nystagmus and poikilothermia (sudden decrease and elevation of temperature) associated with globoid cell leukodystrophy should help to distinguish the two (Crome 1976; Malone 1976). The labile temperatures may cause confusion with sepsis. A specific enzyme deficiency of galactoside-β-galactosidase has been identified (Malone 1976; Suzuki 1970).

On pathological inspection the brain demonstrates widespread foci of disease in the centrum semiovale, cerebellum, and brainstem. There is severe or total lack of myelin in the white matter.

Sufficient data have not yet been accumulated for computed tomographic characterization. In the only biopsy-proven report of globoid cell leukodystrophy published thus far, CT demonstrated diffuse cerebral atrophy without detectable white matter abnormality (Lane 1978). This is in agreement with the authors' experience (Fig. 16-8).

Alexander's Disease

Alexander's disease is a rare condition which is usually clinically manifest during the first year of life and shows gradual enlargement of the head, with progressive retardation, convulsions, and spasticity. All cases reported thus far have been sporadic (Crome 1976). A case occurring in an adult has been reported (Seil 1968).

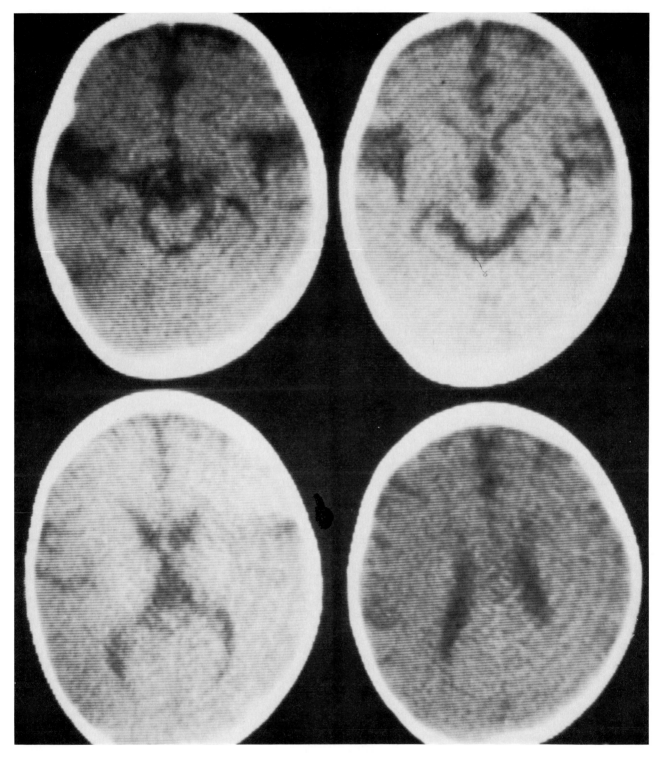

Figure 16-8 Globoid cell leukodystrophy (Krabbe's disease). CT images in a 6-month-old child with biopsy-proven Krabbe's disease show evidence of enlarged subarachnoid spaces including sylvian fissures and lateral ventricles consistent with atrophy.

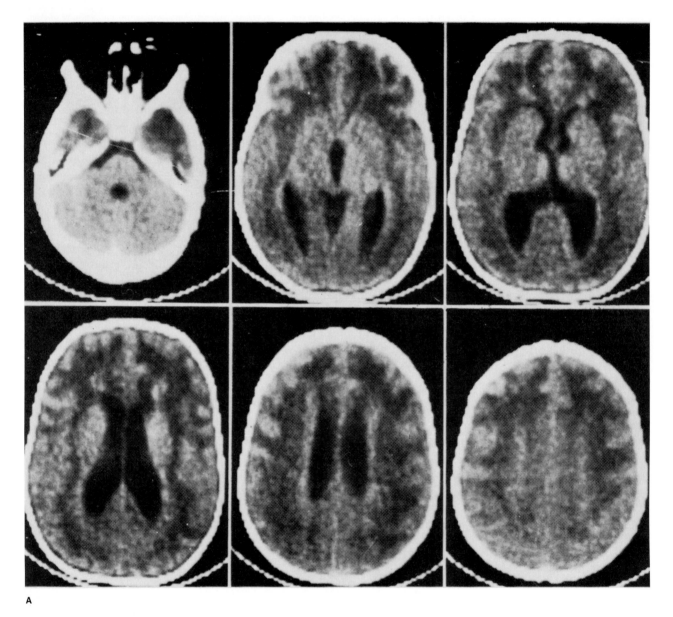

A

Figure 16-9 Alexander's disease. NCCT (**A**) and CECT (**B**) images reveal symmetrical low attenuation in deep white matter with more extensive changes in the frontal regions. Marked enhancement is seen in the caudate nuclei, anterior columns of fornices, and periventricular brain substance. (*Reproduced by permission from Holland and Kendall, 1980.*)

On histologic examination of the brain, there is little stainable myelin. The characteristic feature of Alexander's disease is the presence of large numbers of Rosenthal bodies in a perivascular distribution (Holland 1980).

Computed tomography in Alexander's disease has been reported to show decreased attenuation of the cerebral white matter with relative sparing of subependymal regions. The findings are predominantly in the frontal lobes, and there may be dila-

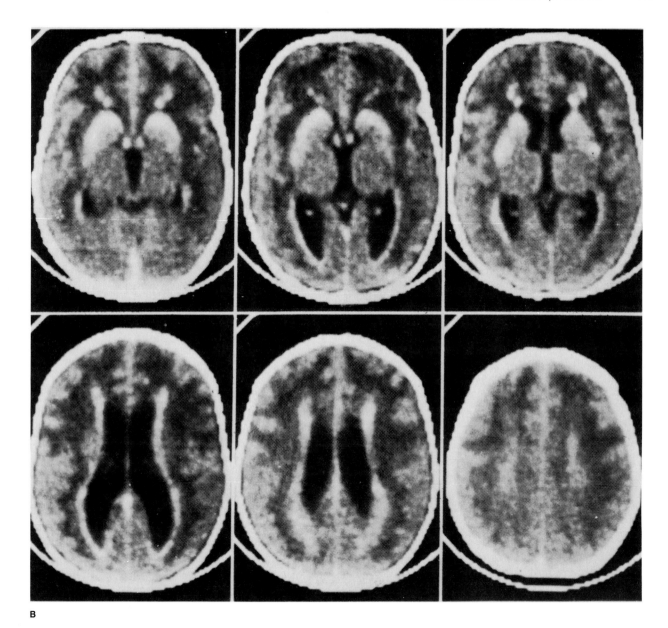

B

tation of the lateral ventricles (Boltshauser 1978; Holland 1980). Apparent marked contrast enhancement of the caudate nuclei, anterior columns of the fornices, and periventricular areas were reported in a case where the white matter low density abutted these structures (Fig. 16-9) (Holland 1980). Megalencephaly, characteristic of this disease, may be evident on CT (see the section on spongy degenera-

tion). While CT may show rather characteristic findings of megalencephaly and decreased white matter attenuation most pronounced in the frontal lobes, the diagnosis of Alexander's disease, as of now, still rests with brain biopsy. Needless to say, CT is extremely useful in making the diagnosis and as a guide to biopsy.

Pelizaeus-Merzbacher Disease

Pelizaeus-Merzbacher disease is a disease of the central white matter showing a very slow progression. There are apparently two types of this disease. One is a sex-linked recessive form presenting in early infancy. The second type appears later in childhood and seems to be transmitted by a dominant mode of inheritance and may present in later adulthood (Crome 1976; Malone 1976).

Pathological descriptions indicate a diffuse and symmetrical demyelination of the cerebral and cerebellar white matter as well as the brainstem and spinal cord with conspicuous residual "islands" of preserved or partially demyelinated fibers, which are considered the characteristic pathological finding of Pelizaeus-Merzbacher disease (Crome 1976; Malone 1976).

Computed tomography in a case of Pelizaeus-Merzbacher disease of long-standing duration and severe clinical involvement did not demonstrate any gross abnormality (Heinz 1979).

Cockayne's Syndrome

Cockayne's syndrome is an autosomal recessive disorder in which there is dwarfism, cachexia, thickened cranium, retinal pigmentation, and associated mental retardation. Cataracts, optic atrophy, deafness, broad hands and feet, flexion contractures, and dermal photosensitivity may also be associated to varying degrees. The patient starts out as a normal infant but by the second year begins to show retarded growth. At the same time, motor skills deteriorate, with loss of speech, and the patient reverts to infantile behavior (Alton 1972; Cockayne 1936; Moossy 1967).

On pathological examination there is marked reduction in the cerebral white matter, atrophy, and resultant enlarged ventricles. There may also be cerebellar atrophy. The demyelination is patchy in all areas of the white matter. There may be mineralization of the basal ganglia and the cerebral and cerebellar cortex. The patchy demyelination tends to preserve "islands" similar to those found in Pelizaeus-Merzbacher disease, and some people have advocated classifying Cockayne's syndrome as a form of Pelizaeus-Merzbacher disease (Jellinger 1969; Moossy 1967).

CT features of Cockayne's syndrome include microcephaly, calcification of the basal ganglia and dentate nuclei, and evidence of cerebral atrophy (Vermess 1976).

Cockayne's syndrome should be distinguished from Kearns-Sayre syndrome (oculocraniosomatic disease), which is a clinical triad of progressive external ophthalmoplegia, atypical pigmentary degeneration of the retina, and heart block. Microcephaly may also be present. CT in these patients has demonstrated decreased attenuation of the white matter, basal ganglia, thalami, and cerebral hemispheres (Seigel 1979). Plain radiographic findings of Cockayne's syndrome including the plain skull findings have been described (Alton 1972).

Adrenoleukodystrophy

Adrenoleukodystrophy is a sex-linked recessive disorder showing adrenal atrophy and cerebral demyelination. The disease occurs predominantly in males between the ages of 3 and 12 years. Adult cases have also been reported. Clinically the patients demonstrate abnormal behavior as well as disturbances of vision and gait. There may be asymmetry of clinical findings early in the disease. Adrenal insufficiency may not be apparent. The disease is progressive without remission. The diagnosis rests on adrenal biopsy findings. Brain biopsy at times may be misleading (Powell 1975; Schaumburg 1975). Steroid therapy appears to be ineffective in altering the course of the neurologic disease (Schaumburg 1975).

Pathological inspection reveals demyelination of the subcortical white matter in the posterior cerebrum. The disease tends to be most severe in the parietal, occipital, and posterior temporal lobes. In the posterior cerebrum the disease is symmetric; however, when the frontal lobes are involved, it may be asymmetric. The disease appears to take a caudorostral direction of progression. The disease tends to extend across the splenium of the corpus callosum and be contiguous with the opposite hemisphere. Schaumburg et al. (1975) have identified three histologic zones. The first two zones contain macrophages and appear to be active areas of myelin destruction. The first two zones are most prominent along the frontal edge of the lesion. The third appears to be an inactive area of glial fibrosis. Dystrophic deposits of calcium may be identified.

Computed tomography demonstrates a striking correlation to the gross and microscopic findings in adrenoleukodystrophy. Early in the disease there is bilateral symmetric decreased attenuation to the posterior cerebral white matter. There may be edge enhancement at the periphery of the lesion following contrast administration. Patients undergoing corticosteroid treatment may show decreased contrast enhancement (Eiben 1977). It is interesting to note that the maximal area of contrast enhancement along the anterior margin of the lesion corresponds to the histologic zones of active demyelination as described by Schaumburg. This correlation was de-

scribed previously, and the zones of enhancement were considered to represent either Schaumburg's zone 1 (Quisling 1979) or Schaumburg's zones 1 and 2 (Greenberg 1977). The disease shows contiguity on CT across the splenium of the corpus callosum without involving the remainder of the corpus callosum. CT demonstrates progression in a caudorostral direction. The anterior edge of the lesion will show the most significant contrast enhancement and has been described as "serpiginous" (Lane 1978). As the disease progresses, there may be a decrease in the degree of contrast enhancement. With involvement of the frontal lobes, the low-attenuation areas may become asymmetric. The disease eventually progresses to involve the cerebellum as well as the frontal lobes and there is extensive generalized cerebral atrophy (Greenberg 1977; Quisling 1979). The white matter may become so low in attenuation that it may appear indistinguishable from the conspicuously enlarged ventricles (Eiben 1977). Two cases of adrenoleukodystrophy are illustrated in Figure 16-10.

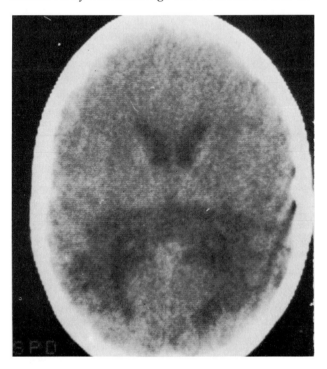
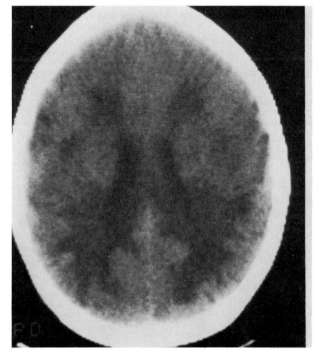
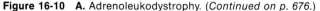

Figure 16-10 **A.** Adrenoleukodystrophy. (*Continued on p. 676.*)

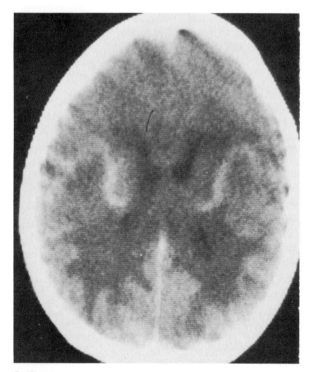

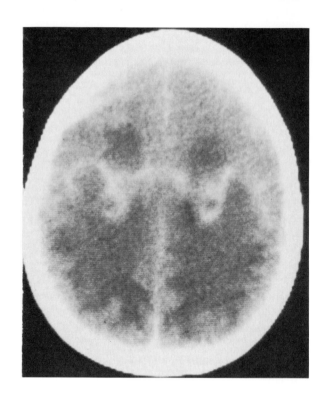

B (Cont.)

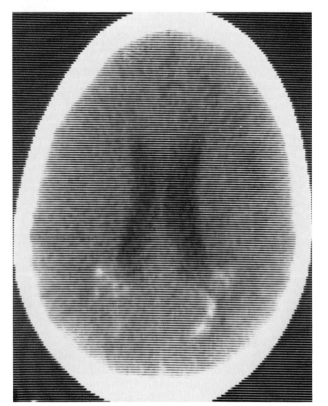

C

Figure 16-10 (Cont.)   **A.** CT images of a 10-year-old boy with a 2-year history of loss of visual acuity and mental deterioration. NCCT (*p. 675*) shows areas of decreased attenuation in both hemispheres in the periventricular area posteriorly; CECT (**B**) reveals peripheral enhancement of these low-density zones.   **C.** CT image of a 1-year-old boy with known adrenoleukodystrophy shows areas of high density with Hounsfield numbers in the range of calcium in the previously demonstrated areas of low density. Dystrophic calcification in this area was confirmed at autopsy (see text).

Bibliography

ADAMS JH, Virus diseases of the venous system, in Blackwood W, Corsellis JAN, (eds): *Greenfield's Neuropathology,* Chicago, Year Book Medical Publishers, 1976, pp 312–314.

ADORNATO BT, O'BRIEN JS, LAMPERT PW, ROE TF, NEOSTEIN HB: Cerebral spongy degeneration of infancy: A biochemical and ultrastructural study of affected twins. *Neurology* **22:**202–210, 1972.

AITA JF, BENNETT DR, ANDERSON RE, ZITER F: Cranial CT appearance of acute multiple sclerosis. *Neurology* **28:**251–255, 1978.

ALLEN JC, THALER HT, DECK F, ROTTENBERG DA: Leukoencephalopathy following high dose intravenous methotrexate chemotherapy: Quantitative assessment of white matter attenuation using computed tomography. *Neuroradiology* **16:**44–47, 1978.

ALTON DJ, MCDONALD P, REILLY BJ: Cockayne's syndrome: A report of three cases. *Radiology* **102:**403–406, 1972.

AUR RJA, SIMONE JV, HUSTU HO, VERZOSA MS: A comparative study of central nervous system irradiation and intensive chemotherapy early in remission of childhood acute lymphocytic leukemia. *Cancer* **29:**381–391, 1972.

BJORGEN JE, GOLD LHA: Computed tomographic appearance of methotrexate-inducing necrotizing leukoencephalopathy. *Radiology* **122:**377–378, 1977.

BOLTSHAUSER E, ISLER W: Computerized axial tomography in spongy degeneration. *Lancet* **1:**1123, 1976.

BOLTSHAUSER E, SPEISS H, ISLER W: Computed tomography in neurodegenerative disorders in childhood. *Neuroradiology* **16:**41–43, 1978.

BOSCH EP, HART MN: Late adult-onset metachromatic leukodystrophy. *Arch Neurol* **35:**475–477, 1978.

BOSCH EP, CANCILLA PA, CORNELL SH: Computerized tomography in progressive multifocal leukoencephalopathy. *Arch Neurol* **33:**216, 1976.

BUONANNO FS, BALL MR, LASTER DW, MOODY DM, MCLEAN WT: Computed tomography in late-infantile metachromatic leukodystrophy. *Ann Neurol* **4:**43–46, 1978.

CALA LA, MASTAGLIA FL, BLACK JL: Computerized tomography of brain and optic nerve in multiple sclerosis. *J Neurol* **36:**411–426, 1978.

CARROLL BA, LANE B, NORMAN D, ENZMANN D: Diagnosis of progressive multifocal leukoencephalopathy by computed tomography. *Radiology* **122:**137–141, 1977.

COCKAYNE EA: Dwarfism with retinal atrophy and deafness. *Arch Dis Childh* **11:**1–8, 1936.

COIN CG, HUCKS-FOLLISS A: Cervical computed tomography in multiple sclerosis with spinal cord involvement. *J Comput Assist Tomogr* **3:**421–422, 1979.

CROME L, STERN J: Inborn lysosomal enzyme deficiencies, in Blackwood W, Corsellis JAN (eds): *Greenfield's Neuropathology,* Chicago, Year Book Medical Publishers, 1976, pp 541–557.

CUNNINGHAM ME, KISHORE PRS, RENGACHARY SS, PRESKORN S: Progressive multifocal leukoencephalopathy presenting as focal mass lesion in the brain. *Surg Neurol* **8:**448–450, 1977.

DE VIVO DC, MALAS D, NELSON JS, LAND VJ: Leukoencephalopathy in childhood leukemia. *Neurology* **27:**609–613, 1977.

DUDA EE, HUTTENLOCHER PR, PATRONAS NT: CT of subacute sclerosing panencephalitis. *Am J Neuroradiol* **1:**35–38, 1980.

EIBEN RM, DI CHIRO G: Computer assisted tomography in adrenoleukodystrophy. *J Comput Assist Tomogr* **1:**308–314, 1977.

FEIGIN I: Diffuse cerebral sclerosis (metachromatic leukoencephalopathy). *Am J Pathol* **30:**715, 1954.

GARRICK R, GOMEZ MR, HOUSER OW: Demyelination of the brain in tuberous sclerosis: Computed tomography evidence. *Mayo Clin Proc* **54**:685–689, 1979.

GREENBERG HS, HALVERSON D, LANE B: CT scanning and diagnosis of adrenoleukodystrophy. *Neurology* **27**:884–886, 1977.

HEINZ ER, DRAYER BP, HAENGGELI CA, PAINTER MJ, CROMRINE P: Computed tomography in white-matter disease. *Radiology* **130**:371–378, 1979.

HOLLAND IM, KENDALL BE: Computed tomography in Alexander's disease. *Neuroradiology* **20**:103–106, 1980.

JELLINGER K, SEIFELBERGER F: Pelizaeus-Merzbacher disease: Transitional form between classical and co-natal (Seitelberger) type. *Acta Neuropath (Berlin)* **14**:108–117, 1969.

KAY HEM et al: Encephalopathy in acute leukemia associated with methotrexate therapy. *Arch Dis Childh* **47**:344–354, 1972.

LANE B, CARROLL BA, PEDLEY TA: Computerized cranial tomography in cerebral diseases of white matter. *Neurology* **28**:534–544, 1978.

LAUSBERG G et al: Misdiagnosis—cerebral form of multiple sclerosis, in Klug W, Brock M, Klinger M, Spoerri O (eds): *Advances in Neurosurgery, No. 2*, Berlin, Springer-Verlag, 1974, pp 169–182.

LEBOW S, ANDERSON DC, MASTRI A, LARSON D: Acute multiple sclerosis with contrast-enhancing plaques. *Arch Neurol* **35**:435–439, 1978.

LYON LW, MCCORMICK WF, SCHOCHET SS: Progressive multifocal leukoencephalopathy. *Arch Intern Med* **128**:420–426, 1971.

MALONE MJ: The cerebral lipidoses. *Pediatr Clin North Am* **23**:303–326, 1976.

MALONE MJ, SZOKE MC, LOONEY GL: Globoid leukodystrophy: Clinical and enzymatic studies. *Arch Neurol* **32**:606–612, 1975.

MARANO GD, GOODWIN GA, KO JP: Atypical contrast enhancement in computerized tomography of demyelinating disease. *Arch Neurol* **37**:523–524, 1980.

MCCORMICK WF, SCHOCHET SS, SARLES HE, CALVERLEY JR: Progressive multifocal leukoencephalopathy in renal transplant recipients. *Arch Intern Med* **136**:829–834, 1976.

MCINTOSH S, ASPNES GT: Encephalopathy following CNS prophylaxis in childhood lymphoblastic leukemia. *Pediatrics* **52**:612–615, 1973.

MOOSSY J: The neuropathology of Cockayne's syndrome. *Exper Neurol* **26**:654–660, 1967.

MORARIU MA, WILKINS DE, PATEL S: Multiple sclerosis and serial computerized tomography: Delayed contrast enhancement of acute and early lesions. *Arch Neurol* **37**:189–190, 1980.

MUELLER S, BELL W, SEIBERT J: Cerebral calcifications associated with intrathecal methotrexate therapy in acute lymphocytic leukemia. *J Pediatr* **88**:650–653, 1976.

OPPENHEIMER DR: Demyelinating diseases, in Blackwood W, Corsellis JAN (eds): *Greenfield's Neuropathology*, Chicago, Year Book Medical Publishers, 1976, pp 487–495.

PETERS ACB, VERSTEEG J, BOTS GTAM, BOOGERD W, VIELVOYE GT: Progressive multifocal leukoencephalopathy: Immunofluorescent demonstration of Simian virus 40 antigen in CSF cells and response to cyturabine therapy. *Arch Neurol* **37**:497–501, 1980.

PEYLAN-RAMU N, POPLACK DG, BLEI L, HERDT TR, VERMESS M, DI CHIRO G: Computer assisted tomography in methotrexate encephalopathy. *J Comput Assist Tomogr* **1**:216–221, 1977.

PEYLAN-RAMU N, POPLACK DG, PIZZO PH, ADORNATO BT, DI CHIRO G: Abnormal CT scans of the brain in asymptomatic children with acute lymphocytic leukemia after prophylactic treatment of the central nervous system with radiation and intrathecal chemotherapy. *New Engl J Med* **298**:815–818, 1978.

PIZZO PA, BLEYER WA, POPLACK DG, LEVENTHAL BG: Reversible dementia temporarily associated with intraventricular therapy with methotrexate in a child with acute myelogenous leukemia. *J Pediatr* **88:**131–133, 1976.

POSER C: Leukodystrophy as an example of dysmyelinating disease. *Proceedings of the Third International Congress on Neuropathology, Brussels,* Editions *Acta Medica Belgica,* 1957, pp 106–111.

POSER C: Dysmyelination revisited. *Arch Neurol* **35:**401–408, 1978.

POSER C, ROMAN G, EMERY S III: Recurrent disseminated vasculomyelinopathy. *Arch Neurol* **35:**166–170, 1978.

POWELL H, TINDALL R, SCHULTZ P, PAA D, O'BRIEN J, LAMPERT P: Adrenoleukodystrophy: Electron microscopic findings. *Arch Neurol* **32:**250–260, 1975.

PRICE RA, JAMIESON PA: The central nervous system in childhood leukemia: II. Subacute leukoencephalopathy. *Cancer* **35:**306–318, 1975.

QUISLING RG, ANDRIOLA MR: Computed tomographic evaluation of the early phase of adrenoleukodystrophy. *Neuroradiology* **17:**285–288, 1979.

REIK L: Disseminated vasculomyelinopathy an immune complex disease. *Ann Neurol* **7:**291–296, 1980.

REISNER T, MAIDA E: Computerized tomography in multiple sclerosis. *Arch Neurol* **37:**475–477, 1980.

RICHARDSON EP: Our evolving understanding of progressive multifocal leukoencephalopathy. *Ann NY Acad Sci* **230:**358–364, 1974.

ROBERTSON WC, GOMEZ RC, REESE DF, OKAZAKI H: Computerized tomography in demyelinating disease of the young. *Neurology* **27:**838–842, 1977.

RUBINSTEIN LJ: Pathology of white matter disease of the brain. Keynote Lecture, 16 Annual Meeting, American Society of Neuroradiology, New Orleans, LA, 1978.

RUBINSTEIN LJ, HERMAN MM, LONG TF, WILBUR JR: Disseminated necrotizing leukoencephalopathy: A complication of treated central nervous system leukemia and lymphoma. *Cancer* **35:**291–305, 1975.

SCHAUMBURG HH, POWERS JM, RAINE CS, SUZUKI K, RICHARDSON EP: Adrenoleukodystrophy: A clinical and pathological study of 17 cases. *Arch Neurol* **32:**577–591, 1975.

SCHUMACHER GA: The demyelinating diseases, in Baker AB (ed): *Clinical Neurology,* New York, Harper and Row, 1965, pp 1226–1284.

SEARS ES, TINDALL RSA, ZARNOW H: Active multiple sclerosis. Enhanced computerized tomographic imaging of lesions and the effect of corticosteroids. *Arch Neurol* **35:**426–434, 1978.

SEIGEL RS, SEEGER JF, GABRIELSON TO, ALLEN RJ: Computed tomography in oculocraniosomatic disease (Kearns-Sayre syndrome). *Radiology* **130:**159–164, 1979.

SEIL FJ, SCHOCHET SS, EARLE KM: Alexander's disease in an adult: Report of a case. *Arch Neurol* **19:**494–502, 1968.

SUZUKI K, SUZUKI Y: Globoid leukodystrophy (Krabbe disease) deficiency of galactocerebroside-beta-galactosidase. *Proc Natl Acad Sci (USA)* **66:**302–308, 1970.

VAN DER VELDEN M, BOTS GTAM, ENDTZ L: Cranial CT in multiple sclerosis showing a mass effect. *Surg Neurol* **12:**307–310, 1979.

VERMESS M: Computer assisted tomography in Cockayne's syndrome (abstracted). Paper presented at the International Symposium on Computer Assisted Tomography in Non-tumoral Diseases of the Brain, Spinal Cord and Eye. NIH, Bethesda, MD, 1976.

WEISBERG L: Contrast enhancement visualized by computerized tomography in acute multiple sclerosis. *J Comput Assist Tomogr* **5:**293–300, 1981.

17

PITFALLS AND LIMITATIONS OF CT IN NEURODIAGNOSIS

Seungho Howard Lee

Stephen A. Kieffer

Jaime H. Montoya

Despite initial skepticism in some quarters, the value and efficacy of computed tomography of the brain was quickly established. CT has emerged as the primary diagnostic screening modality for the *detection* of intracranial pathology. Accuracy of *localization* of structural abnormalities of the brain by CT often exceeds that which can be obtained by cerebral angiography or other invasive diagnostic procedure. Frequently CT can also provide information permitting *characterization* of the nature of the disease process.

Accumulated experience with CT scanning of the head indicates that even this remarkable diagnostic tool has its limitations. However, the limitations of CT are probably fewer in number and less in severity than those associated with any other neurological diagnostic modality.

TECHNICAL

Motion artifacts have been a severe problem for the radiologist from the earliest 4 1/2-minute translate-rotate scanners up to the present fourth-generation stationary detector array units capable of scanning times of 2 seconds or less (Ter-Pogossian 1977). The severity of motion artifacts depends on the extent of displacement of the object being scanned. They are most prominent in regions of sharp gradients of x-ray attenuation. The artifacts due to intracranial metallic foreign bodies (e.g., vascular clips, shunt catheters, bullet fragments) (Fig. 17-1) are particularly aggravated by motion. While the much shorter scan time of the newer CT units has reduced the likelihood of patient movement during scanning,

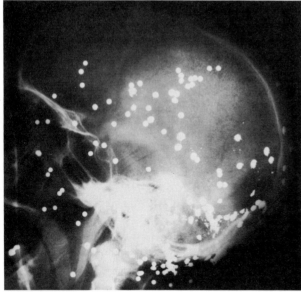

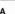

A

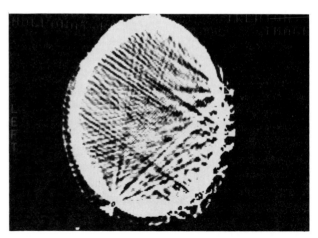

B

Figure 17-1 Metallic artifacts. **A.** Lateral view of skull demonstrates numerous metallic pellets overlying the cranial vault and face. **B.** CT image demonstrates multiple linear artifacts emanating from the metallic pellets in the scalp. Intracranial anatomy cannot be recognized.

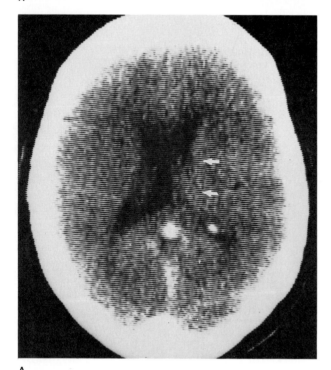

A

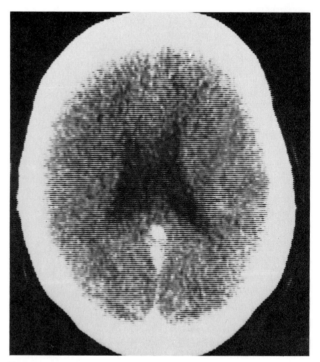

B

Figure 17-2 Tilting of head simulating a thalamic mass. **A.** Initial CT image suggests the presence of a mass in the body of the left lateral ventricle in a 52-year-old female (arrows). CT images at lower levels demonstrated asymmetry of structures at the skull base, indicating that the patient's head was tilted within the gantry. **B.** Following repositioning of the patient's head, a repeat CT image at the same level as in **A** shows no evidence of a mass in the left lateral ventricle.

the severity of such artifacts, when they occur, has not been significantly altered.

Meticulous care in patient positioning is essential for successful and reliable CT scanning. Even slight degrees of *tilting of the head* can result in factitious abnormalities, notably apparent shifts of midline structures. An apparent mass in the floor of the body of one lateral ventricle may be simulated by the normal thalamus if the plane of section is slightly tilted (Fig. 17-2).

Despite considerable improvement in resolution, even the newer scanners have not solved the problems resulting from *beam hardening* due to absorption of "softer" incident radiation by areas of thick, dense bone (Brooks 1976). This is a particular prob-

lem in the posterior cranial fossa, where a narrow transverse hypodense stripe (the Hounsfield artifact) is frequently observed extending between the two petrous pyramids and obscuring definition of the pons and aqueduct (Fig. 17-3).

Small lesions with a diameter less than or approximating the thickness of the scan slice may not be accurately represented on the CT image. If the volume of the lesion does not occupy the entire thickness of the slice, the attenuation coefficient on the CT image will reflect averaging of the x-ray attenuation of the lesion and the surrounding normal tissue (*volume averaging*) (Dohrmann 1978). Volume averaging is also a problem at the margins of larger lesions. Reduction in scan slice thickness and in size of matrix pixels diminishes the impact of volume averaging on CT scan accuracy.

Failure to identify the fourth ventricle should not be lightly disregarded, particularly when the lateral and third ventricles are mildly enlarged. A mass lesion in or adjacent to the brainstem or cerebellum compressing the fourth ventricle could easily be overlooked (Gado 1977). Repeat scans in alternate planes or thinner section studies will usually demonstrate the elusive ventricle.

Proper *window and center settings* are important in elucidating subtle tissue-density differences (Fig. 17-4). Dense peripheral intracranial lesions may blend with the overlying calvarium and be overlooked. At conventional window and center settings, a thin bandlike acute subdural hematoma which does not produce a significant shift of midline structures could be missed. To precisely define such peripheral densities, a relatively high center setting (60 or 70 HU) and a wider window (200 to 400 HU) should be employed (Fig. 17-5).

NORMAL VARIATIONS

A thorough understanding of the normal gross anatomy of the brain on CT studies and an awareness of common normal anatomic variations will reduce the likelihood of false positive diagnoses and thus obviate the need for invasive studies.

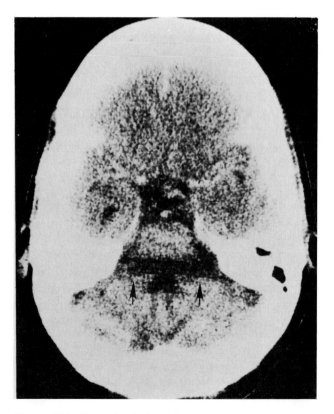

Figure 17-3 Beam-hardening (Hounsfield) artifact. A narrow transverse hypodense stripe extends between the two petrous pyramids (arrows) and obscures definition of the posterior aspect of the pons and the middle cerebellar peduncles.

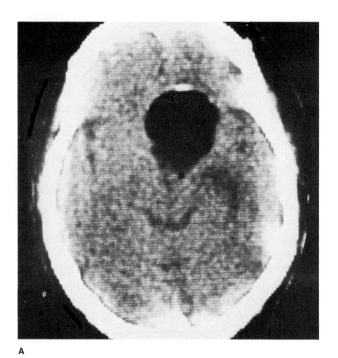

A

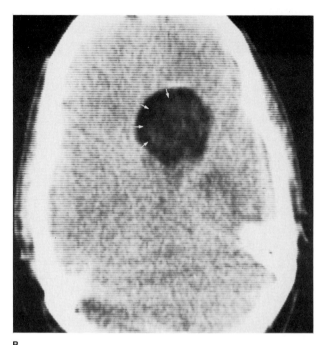

B

Figure 17-4 Dermoid cyst: importance of varying center and window settings. **A.** On the initial CT image obtained with a low center level and a narrow window (usual settings for head CT studies), a round, fatty tumor with a partially calcified wall was considered to be a lipoma. **B.** A repeat CT image with a slightly higher center level and a much wider window demonstrates soft-tissue mass within the cyst (arrows). At surgery, a hair ball was found inside a dermoid cyst.

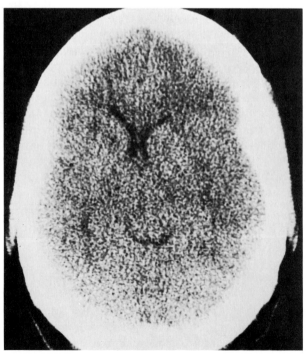

A

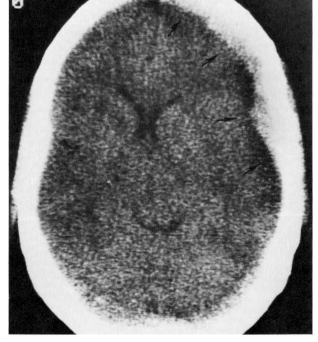

B

The *jugular tubercles* are rounded bony elevations arising from the inner surface of the occipital bone adjacent to the anterolateral margins of the foramen magnum on each side. The tubercles vary widely in size and shape and are often asymmetric. Axial CT sections through the posterior fossa often demonstrate one or both jugular tubercles as rounded densities located medial and just inferior to the internal auditory meatus. These densities can be confused with extraaxial mass lesions in the cerebellopontine angle (Fig. 17-6). Careful review of adjacent consecutive axial CT images in this region, repetition of axial scanning with reduced scan slice thickness, and obtaining scans in alternate planes (e.g., coronal) will usually clarify the situation.

The right *jugular foramen* is larger than the left in 50 to 70 percent of persons; this disparity is related to the size of the corresponding transverse and sigmoid sinuses. One jugular bulb may be hypoplastic while the opposite bulb is markedly enlarged, mimicking a tumor in the jugular foramen (Fig. 17-7).

A *large cisterna magna* may simulate a cystic lesion in the posterior cranial fossa (Leo 1979). The size of the cisterna magna varies widely in the normal population. It may normally extend up to the level of the internal occipital protuberance, and rarely it may protrude farther upward through a defect in the tentorium (Liliequist 1960). The adjacent occipital bone may be thinned. The absence of compression of the fourth ventricle usually permits a definitive diagnosis of an enlarged cisterna magna (Adam 1978) (Fig. 17-8).

The *inferior vermis* of the cerebellum occasionally appears quite dense on NCCT in normal persons. On CECT, the normal vermis often exhibits homo-

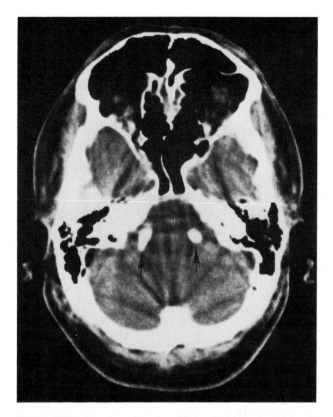

Figure 17-6 Jugular tubercles. Bilateral oblong bony densities are identified within the posterior fossa medial and inferior to the internal auditory meatus (arrows). A clear separation from the adjacent petrous temporal bones, with intervening normal brain tissue or subarachnoid cisterns, is an important finding in differentiating a jugular tubercle from a possible meningioma or other hyperdense or calcified tumor in this region.

geneous opacification, appearing as a triangular or elliptical homogeneous density extending on axial CT images from the posterior margin of the fourth ventricle to the cisterna magna (Kramer 1977). The increased density and prominent contrast enhancement may reflect the high concentration of cortical tissue surrounded by CSF spaces (Fig. 17-9). Differentiation from neoplasm or other pathologic condition is based on the lack of deformity or displacement of the adjacent fourth ventricle.

Physiological calcification of the basal ganglia is occasionally recognized on CT studies of the brain (Fig. 17-10). The calcification is typically located in the globus pallidus, is usually but not always bilat-

---

◀**Figure 17-5** Acute subdural hematoma: importance of varying center and window settings. **A.** A 55-year-old man was found somnolent and unresponsive following head trauma. CT image at usual center and window settings demonstrates a shift of the septum pellucidum to the right of the midline but no evident intracerebral mass to account for the shift. **B.** The same image as in **A** is viewed with a higher center level and a wider window. A crescentic band of increased density (acute subdural hematoma) is identified along the lateral margin of the left frontal and temporal lobes (arrows).

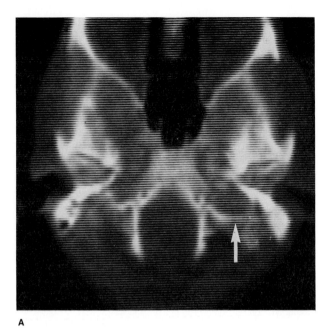

A

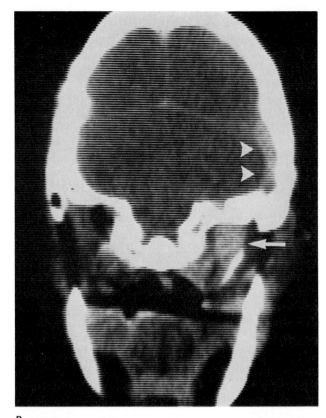

B

Figure 17-7 Large left jugular foramen. **A.** Axial CT image at the level of the foramen magnum shows the left jugular foramen (arrow) to be larger than its companion on the right. Note that the cortical margin of the foramen is intact. **B.** Coronal CECT demonstrates a large ipsilateral transverse sinus (arrowheads) and jugular bulb (arrow).

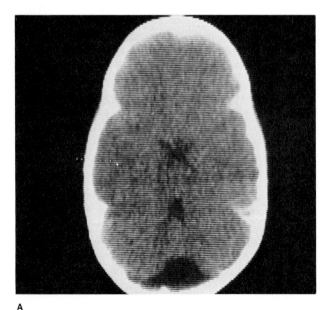

A

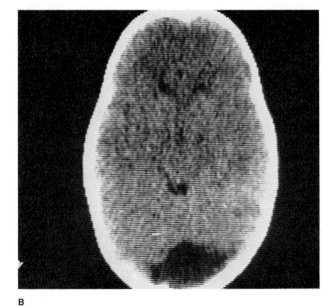

B

Figure 17-8 Large cisterna magna. Axial CT images demonstrate a sharply marginated triangular hypodensity between the posterior margin of the cerebellum and the inner table of the occipital bone, with superior extension. Note that the fourth ventricle is normal in size, shape, and position.

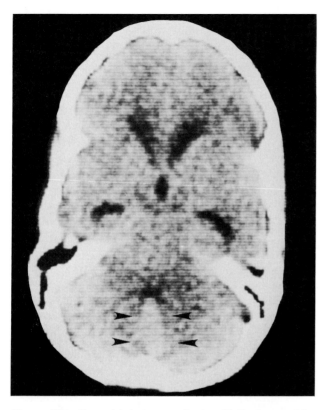

Figure 17-9 Normal inferior vermis. An elliptical area of increased density extends posteriorly in the midline from the fourth ventricle toward the internal occipital crest (arrows) on this CECT image. Note that the fourth ventricle has a normal triangular shape and is not displaced or compressed.

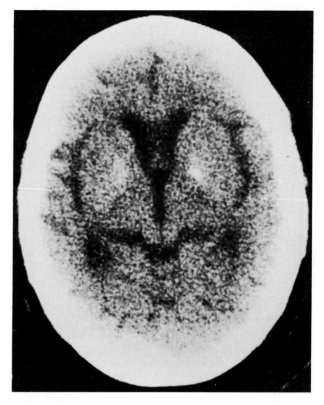

Figure 17-10 Basal ganglia calcification. On this NCCT image of a 42-year-old male, calcifications are noted in the region of the globus pallidus bilaterally.

eral, and almost always occurs in persons above age 40 (Cohen 1980). Demonstration of basal ganglia calcification in a patient under age 40 should prompt a search for associated pathologic conditions (e.g., hypoparathyroidism, pseudohypoparathyroidism). Children with Down's syndrome may show early calcification of the basal ganglia.

Physiological calcification of the choroid plexuses in the bodies of the lateral ventricles (Fig. 17-11) is 5 to 15 times more commonly detected on CT studies, as compared with plain skull radiographs. Demonstration of calcification in the choroid plexus of the temporal horn or third ventricle suggests the presence of neurofibromatosis (Modic 1980).

Asymmetry of the frontal or occipital horns of the lateral ventricles is a common normal developmental variant (LeMay 1978). Coarctation of ependymal surfaces during fetal development may produce interruption or obliteration (either unilateral or bilateral) of these portions of the ventricular system (Fig. 17-12A). The lack of ventricular compression or displacement or of any focal parenchymal abnormality differentiates this normal variation from compression due to a mass lesion.

Other cerebral asymmetries may be demonstrated by CT (LeMay 1978). The left occipital pole is frequently wider and protrudes farther posteriorly than the right occipital pole; thus the calcified choroid plexus glomus of the left lateral ventricle often

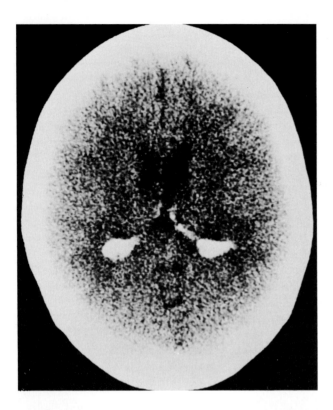

Figure 17-11 Physiological calcification of the choroid plexuses. Bilateral calcifications of the choroid plexus of the lateral ventricles are identified on this NCCT image. In this patient, calcification is heaviest in the glomera but also extends anteriorly to the region of the foramen of Monro.

Figure 17-12 Asymmetry of the lateral ventricles. The left lateral ventricle is larger than its companion on the right in this right-handed person with normal mentation and function. The left frontal horn projects farther anteriorly than the right frontal horn. The sharp lateral angle of the right frontal horn suggests coaptation of its ependymal surfaces.

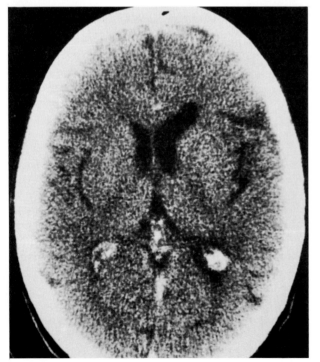

A

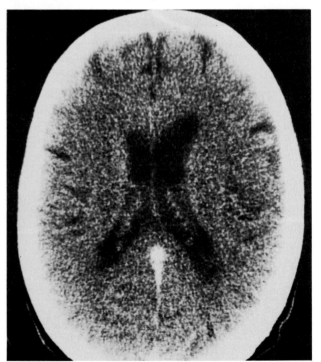

B

is located slightly posterior to the right glomus. The right frontal pole often protrudes slightly more anteriorly than the left, and the right frontal horn is frequently smaller than its companion on the left (Fig. 17-12B). These asymmetries are more common in right-handed persons; hemispheric asymmetry is less common and less striking in left-handed persons. The pineal gland often lies slightly to the left of the midline in normal persons.

Contrast enhancement of the *choroid plexus of the temporal horn* produces a crescentic density on the medial aspect of the temporal horn. In combination with the diverging bandlike blush of the adjacent contrast-enhanced tentorium, this forms an incomplete ringlike density which can simulate the CECT appearance of a medial temporal lobe tumor (Naidich 1977) but is usually bilateral and symmetrical

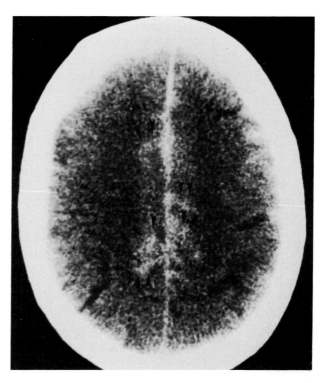

Figure 17-14 Subarachnoid hemorrhage in the interhemispheric fissure extending into the paramedian sulci. NCCT of a middle-aged man with a ruptured aneurysm shows a midline increased density in the interhemispheric fissure (subarachnoid hemorrhage) and its extension into the contiguous paramedian cortical sulci (arrowheads). The CT diagnosis of subarachnoid hemorrhage can be confirmed by the presence of free blood in the cortical sulci and other subarachnoid cisterns.

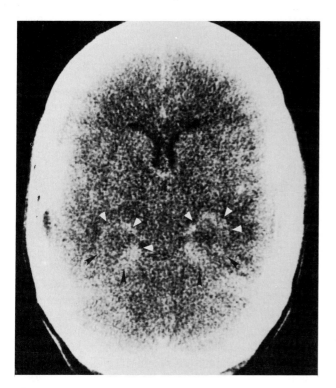

Figure 17-13 Incomplete density ring in medial temporal region. Bilateral symmetrical curvilinear contrast enhancement in the posteromedial temporal regions is due to a combination of the choroid plexuses of the temporal horns (arrowheads) and the anterolateral margins of the tentorium.

and is not associated with any mass effect (Fig. 17-13).

The *falx cerebri* is commonly visualized as a long, thin band of slightly increased density in the region of the interhemispheric fissure in normal persons on NCCT (false falx sign) (Osborn 1980). This finding must be differentiated from the appearance of subarachnoid hemorrhage in the interhemispheric fissure (Dolinskas 1978)—the falx sign—which appears as a midline band of increased density extending into the paramedian cerebral sulci (Fig. 17-14) and is confirmatory of the presence of extracerebral blood (Osborn 1980).

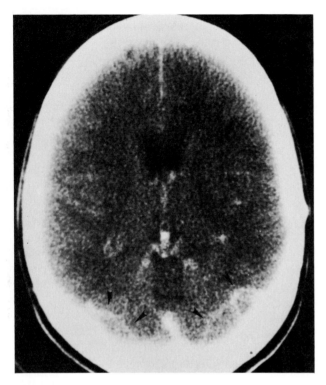

Figure 17-15 Prominent dural veins in the tentorium cerebelli. CECT shows multiple curvilinear densities (arrows) at the upper level of tentorial surfaces mimicking vascular malformation or an infarct of unusual appearance. These are normal dural veins frequently found in the normal pediatric age group.

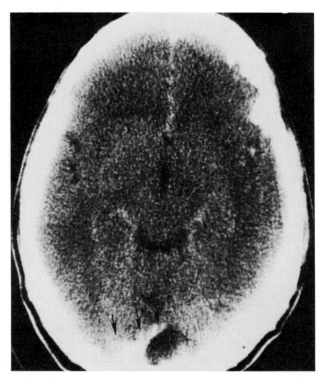

Figure 17-16 Torcular Herophili: normal variant. A thick, bandlike, contrast-enhancing structure to the right of the midline (arrow) represents the opacified confluence of the dural venous sinuses, displaced from the midline by a superior extension of a large cisterna magna. Also note temporal "rings."

Occasionally, prominent *dural veins* in the tentorial leaves present as multiple curvilinear densities on CECT, mimicking a bizarre appearance of a tumor or arteriovenous malformation (Fig. 17-15). These are more frequently observed in infants and children than in adults.

The *torcular Herophili* typically appears triangular on normal CECT studies and is located in close approximation to the occipital bone in the midline (Naidich 1977). However, variations in the location and configuration of this confluence of the dural venous sinuses are common. It may appear round or elongated and may lie as much as a centimeter anterior to the occipital bone or to one side of the midline (Fig. 17-16).

LOCALIZATION

It is the accepted convention in CT scanning of the skull and brain to angle the gantry (and therefore the plane of CT section) slightly craniocaudad (about 10° to 15° with respect to the canthomeatal line) in order to include the volume of the brain in the smallest number of scans. Thus, "axial" CT images of the brain are really modified transaxial sections, and the anatomy visualized on these images differs considerably from true horizontal sections. Accurate surgical localization of intracranial lesions demonstrated on axial CT scans is often difficult, particularly when the lesion is small and situated superiorly in the high convexity; the absence of cal-varial landmarks on the CT image and the angled plane of section contribute to this difficulty (Fig. 17-17). Solutions to this problem include the use of radiopaque external marking devices (Lee 1980) or the digital radiographic imaging mode available in many of the newer CT scanning units.

Differentiation of extra- from intracerebral masses on axial CT images is a frequent problem. Many extracerebral masses invaginate the underlying brain and thus simulate intracerebral lesions on CT. Notorious in this regard are meningiomas, cranial nerve neuromas, and large arterial aneurysms. Factors which may aid in establishing a lesion as extracerebral include demonstration of adjacent

bone destruction, widening of adjacent subarachnoid spaces and cisterns, and continuity of the lesion with the falx or tentorium (Miller 1978). Rescanning in a modified coronal plane may also be helpful. Extracerebral masses displacing and compressing the adjacent brain produce inward buckling of the underlying white matter, while intracerebral tumors tend to stretch the adjacent white matter (George 1980). However, if the CT findings do not permit clear differentiation of extra- from intracerebral mass, angiography may be of value.

Mass lesions in the region of the tentorial incisura may be supratentorial or infratentorial (that is, either above or below the tentorium). A clear understanding of normal tentorial anatomy on axial CT scans is invaluable in making this differentiation (Naidich 1977). The authors have found that images in the modified coronal plane are frequently of great help in this situation (Fig. 17-18).

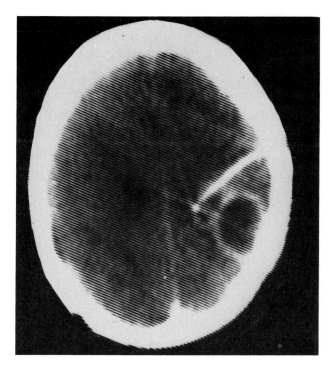

Figure 17-17 Parietal convexity abscesses. CT image obtained in the modified transaxial plane (angled craniocaudad approximately 15° with respect to the canthomeatal line) following surgery demonstrates an opaque cannula entering a daughter abscess. The position of the cannula is anterior to the major abscess cavity. Surgical localization of high-convexity masses may be difficult because of the absence of anatomic landmarks and the angulation of the plane of the CT image.

NONSPECIFICITY

Not long after the advent of CT scanning as a clinical modality, it was realized that intravenous injection of iodinated contrast media aided considerably in the discrimination of the various causes of intracranial masses. However, in the case of low-density lesions, cerebral edema is often a major contributor to both the apparent size and the low density of the mass. Edematous tissue does not exhibit contrast enhancement, but neither do many low-grade gliomas (Tans 1978). It is important to recognize that many infarcts provoke significant local edema and thus appear as space-occupying masses with ventricular compression and shift of midline structures (Davis 1975). Thus it may be very difficult to differentiate a cerebral infarct from a low-grade glioma on CT (Handa 1978); both lesions may appear as low-density masses without contrast enhancement. Clinical signs and history may be misleading, and often only follow-up CT studies a few weeks later will clarify the situation (Fig. 17-19).

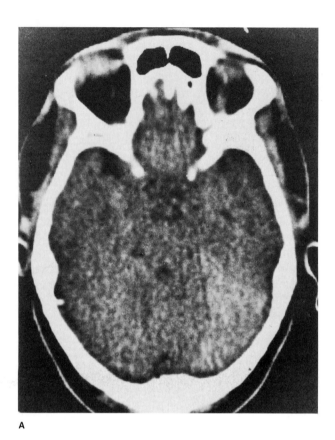

A

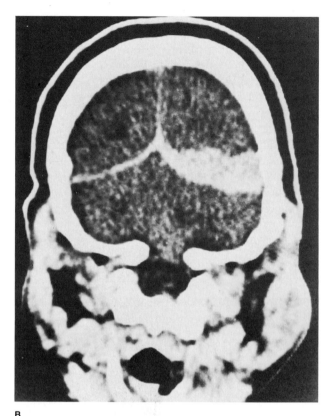

B

Figure 17-18 Tentorial en plaque meningioma. **A.** Trans-axial CECT image demonstrates a large, well-marginated tri-angular area of increased density on the left posteriorly. On this image, it is not possible to be certain whether the lesion lies above the tentorium or in the posterior fossa. **B.** Coronal

CECT image shows a homogeneous contrast-enhancing mass which appears continuous with the superior aspect of the tentorium. Surgery confirmed the presence of an en plaque meningioma attached to the tentorium and growing into the supratentorial compartment.

However, many infarcts exhibit contrast en-hancement, usually between 1 and 4 weeks after the acute ischemic episode (Wing 1976). This often appears as a gyral pattern of opacification in the area of infarction. This gyral enhancement pattern is also nonspecific; its persistence beyond 4 weeks postictus should suggest the possibility of an in-flammatory or neoplastic process in the meninges and adjacent cerebral parenchyma (Fig. 17-20).

Round, well-marginated, hypodense (5 to 15 HU) lesions strongly suggest fluid-filled cysts. How-ever, these are not always found, and both solid and microcystic masses may have a similar appear-ance (Latchaw 1977) (Fig. 17-21).

Figure 17-20 Tuberculous meningoencephalitis simulating cerebral infarction. **A.** CECT image obtained 4 days after the sudden onset of ataxia, dysarthria, and right hemiparesis in a 45-year-old female. Note contrast enhancement of several gyri in the left frontoparietal convexity, with underlying white mat-ter edema. The CT and clinical findings were interpreted as being compatible with a diagnosis of cerebral infarction. **B.** A follow-up CECT study 5 weeks later demonstrates persistent gyral enhancement with significant increase in white matter edema. The patient's clinical condition had not improved. Sur-gical exploration revealed extensive meningoencephalitis; his-tologic examination confirmed a diagnosis of tuberculosis. ▶

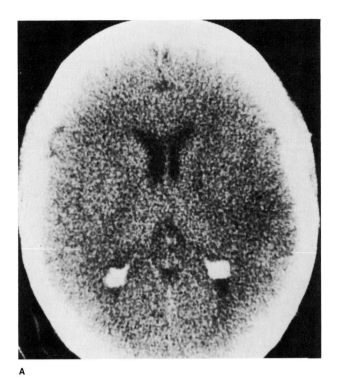

A

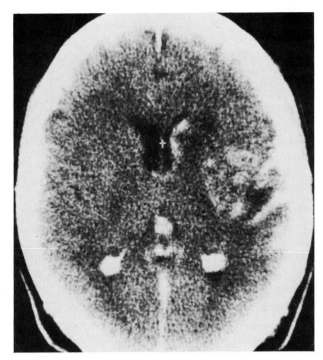

B

Figure 17-19 Evolution of recent infarction and CT distinction from low-grade glioma. **A.** CT within 2 days after ictus demonstrates a poorly defined area of hypodensity in the left temporoparietal lobe. No contrast enhancement was noted in the area, but mild mass effect was present on the same side. **B.** CECT, a week later, demonstrates extensive enhancement in the same area with no apparent shift of the midline or localized mass effect. A focal area of infarction in the head of the caudate nucleus on the left side is also visible. This rapid evolution of the contrast-enhancement pattern, which is gyral in configuration, and relative absence of mass effect are rather characteristic of a recent infarction rather than a low-grade glioma.

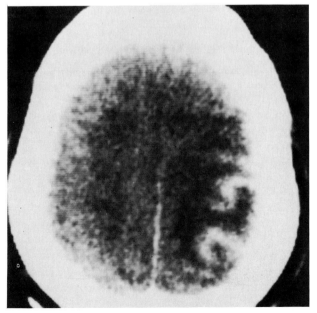

A

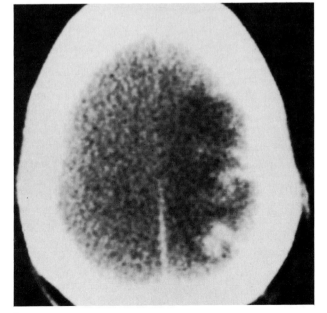

B

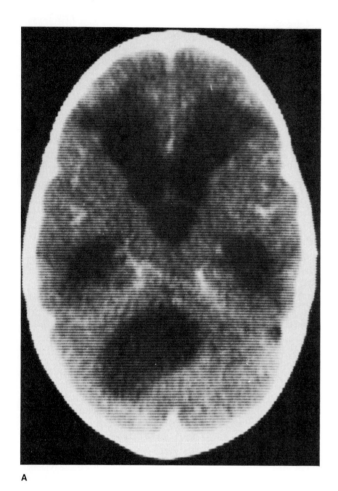

A

B

Figure 17-21 Microcystic astrocytoma of the cerebellum. NCCT **(A)** and CECT **(B)** images demonstrate a cystic-appearing hypodense (12 HU) mass in the right cerebellar hemisphere extending across the midline, with contrast enhancement of the margin of the "cyst." Exploration revealed a well-encapsulated solid mass. Histologic examination showed the lesion to be composed of a myriad of microcysts, probably accounting for the low attenuation values. The tumor has compressed and obstructed the fourth ventricle. Note the markedly distended third and lateral ventricles, with periventricular hypodensity (interstitial edema) in both frontal regions.

Intracerebral masses exhibiting significantly increased density on NCCT may represent tumor or hemorrhage. Glioma, metastatic carcinoma, and meningioma may all exhibit increased density on NCCT and may be difficult to differentiate from intracerebral hematoma. Hemorrhage within a tumor may further complicate this problem. Enhancement of the periphery of the dense mass following intravenous injection of contrast medium is seen in many of these tumors (Russell 1980). When a dense mass on NCCT fails to show contrast enhancement, serial studies may be necessary for differentiation of tumor from hematoma. One should be able to observe a significant decline in CT numbers of a hematoma within 10 to 14 days, as the packed red blood cells lyse and hemoglobin is broken down and absorbed (Davis K. 1977). Omission of serial follow-up studies in dense lesions presumed to be hematomas may prove tragic for the patient (Fig. 17-22).

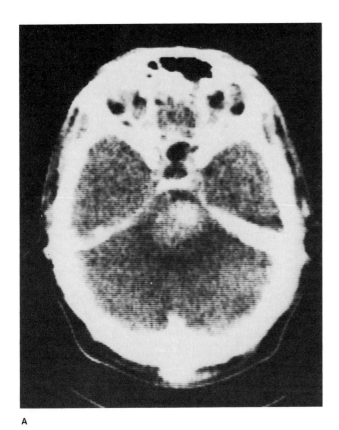

A

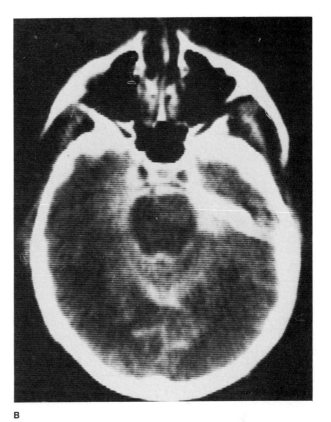

B

Figure 17-22 Hyperdense lesion in pons. **A.** NCCT image obtained following the sudden onset of left hemiparesis in a 58-year-old male. A rounded, hyperdense lesion is noted in the left side of the pons, extending across the midline and posteriorly. In view of the patient's history, a diagnosis of pontine hematoma was suggested. However, serial CT studies over the ensuing 8 weeks showed no change in the size or density of the mass. **B.** Metrizimide CT cisternogram obtained 8 weeks after **A** shows asymmetry, with bulging of the left anterolateral margin of the pons. The hyperdense lesion is still evident on this high center–wide window image. The patient subsequently died, and autopsy confirmed a diagnosis of pontine glioma.

In the immediate postoperative period following resection of a space-occupying mass, the appearance in the former tumor site of a well-defined area of slightly increased density (40 to 50 HU) may suggest hemorrhage and lead to reoperation. The density of such masses is significantly less than an acute hematoma (usually in the range of 60 to 80 HU). This postoperative abnormality is due to Oxycel or Gelfoam strips laid in the tumor bed which become soaked with blood and tissue fluids (Fig. 17-23).

A *ring pattern* of peripheral rimlike contrast enhancement of a hypodense mass was originally presumed to be characteristic of a malignant neoplasm (glioblastoma or metastasis) with central coagulative necrosis. It was quickly realized that intracerebral abscess often presented the same appearance on CT (Davis D. 1977; Whelan 1980). Some meningiomas contain foci of necrosis or cystic degeneration, which may produce a ring pattern on CECT (Russell 1980). A wide margin of low density surrounding the opacified ring and due to cerebral edema may be seen in all these lesions. However, serial follow-up studies in other disease processes have demonstrated that the ring sign is even less specific. In the process of resolution of an intracerebral hematoma (Zimmerman 1977) or a cerebral infarct (Wing 1976;

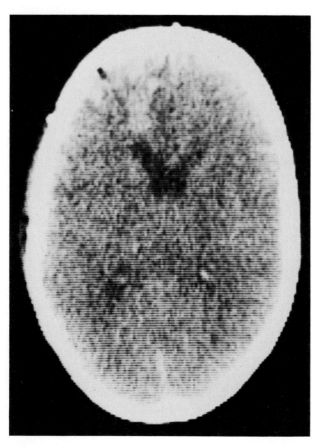

Figure 17-23 Surgical packing simulating postoperative hemorrhage. NCCT image demonstrates an irregularly marginated, slightly hyperdense (43 HU) lesion in the right anterior frontal region. There is no evident compression or displacement of the adjacent right frontal horn. The image was obtained 5 hours following the excision of a meningioma in the same location. Hemorrhage into the former tumor site was questioned, although the density of the lesion is less than what might be expected in an acute hematoma. Reexploration demonstrated no hematoma or other mass, only blood and serum-soaked strips of surgical packing.

Yock 1975), a ring of contrast enhancement may develop around the periphery of the resolving mass. Gliosis and neovascularity, typical components of the repair process, probably account for this pattern (Fig. 17-24).

It is well recognized that intracranial meningiomas frequently have the same density as adjacent normal brain and cannot be differentiated on CT studies without contrast injection (Davis D. 1977). However, this pattern is also nonspecific. Extraaxial neuroma, carcinomatous metastasis, and intracerebral histiocytic lymphoma (Brant-Zawadzki 1978) may also be of the same density as the surrounding brain and may be defined only after contrast medium is administered intravenously. A subacute subdural hematoma (10 to 20 days after the acute bleeding) may also be indistinguishable from adjacent brain, due to partial resorption of protein from the hematoma; restudy after intravenous contrast injection may demonstrate marginal membrane formation (Davis K. 1977) or displaced surface veins on the inner aspect of the hematoma (Kim 1978). In all these lesions, the plain CT study usually gives some indication of a space-occupying mass, for example, compression or shift of portions of the ventricular system, which should alert the radiologist to the necessity for repeat study with intravenous contrast (Fig. 17-25).

COEXISTENCE OF TWO LESIONS

The presence of a dominant abnormality may mask recognition of a coexisting second disease process. Dominance may be on the basis of size, location, or attenuation coefficient. The second lesion is often, but not always, causally related to the dominant abnormality. A relatively thin subdural hematoma may not completely explain a large contralateral shift of midline structures; the intervening brain may be edematous and may exhibit small scattered areas of hemorrhage, indicating the presence of cerebral contusion (Zimmerman 1978). When the CT pattern of the dominant lesion does not unequivocally fit the clinical findings, a careful search should be made for a second abnormality (Fig. 17-26).

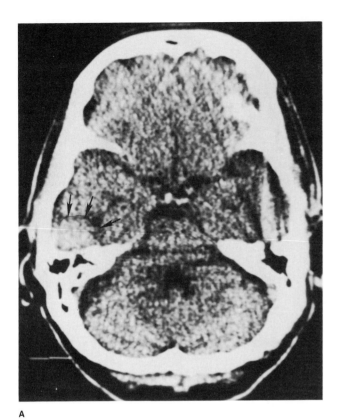

A

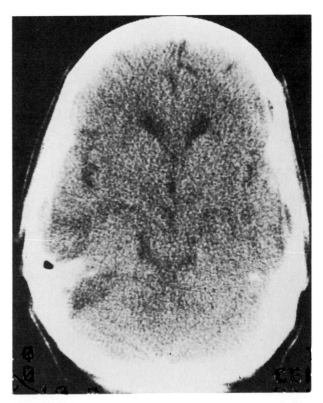

B

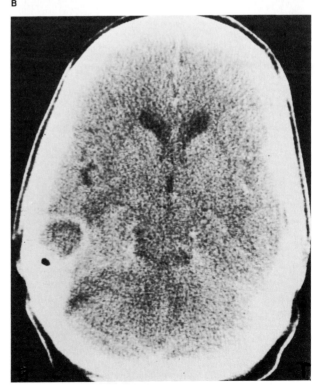

C

Figure 17-24 Ringlike contrast enhancement: intracerebral hematoma. **A.** NCCT image obtained shortly after patient fell out of a moving vehicle, striking the right side of his head on the pavement. A slightly hyperdense round mass is identified in the right temporal lobe laterally and inferiorly (arrows). A very thin peripheral hypodense rim around the anteromedial margin of the mass probably represents edema. **B.** Ten days later, an NCCT image shows significant diminution in size and density of the temporal lobe mass, consistent with a diagnosis of resolving intracerebral hematoma. The peripheral hypodense rim is now much wider (edema? gliosis?). **C.** CECT immediately following **B** shows smooth, uniform contrast enhancement of the peripheral hypodense rim due to gliosis and neovascularity (repair reaction).

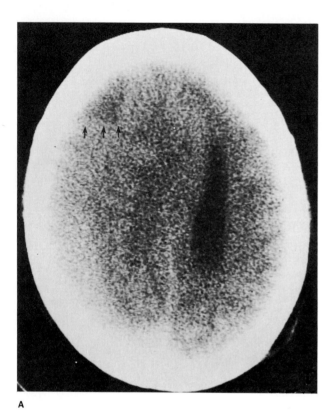

A

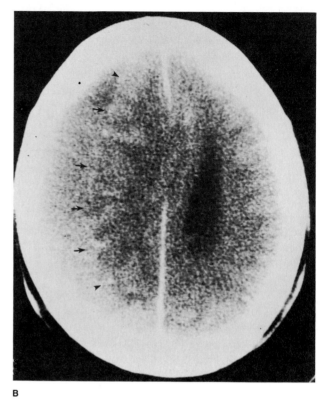

B

Figure 17-25 Isodense subacute subdural hematoma. **A.** NCCT image in a 60-year-old man who presented with low-grade fever, recent personality change, and disorientation. Cerebral abscess was suspected clinically. There is compression of the right lateral ventricle, and the gyral pattern of the right frontoparietal cortex is displaced inward from the skull margin, separated by a thick homogeneous band which is virtually isodense with the cortex. A fluid level near the anterior margin of the band (arrow) probably represents a fluid level within the subdural hematoma. **B.** CECT image accentuates the interface between hematoma and cortex by demonstrating opacified veins on the convexity of the right hemisphere (arrows).

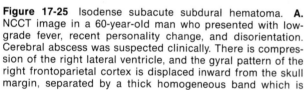

Figure 17-26 Coexistence of two lesions. **A.** Posteroanterior view of the skull in a 12-year-old male with a 2-week history of increasingly severe headache and vomiting who was found to have papilledema and a dilated left pupil. Since infancy, he had been known to have asymmetry of the cranial vault. Note the outward bulging of the left hemicranium with elevation of the left sphenoid ridge, suggesting a long-standing mass in the left middle cranial fossa. **B.** CECT image demonstrates compression of the left frontal horn, with displacement across the midline to the right. There is a large, sharply marginated, hypodense mass in the left middle fossa. The radiological diagnosis was arachnoid cyst in the anterior portion of the left middle fossa, but the surgeon attending the patient felt that this diagnosis did not explain the recent clinical deterioration. **C.** CECT image at a higher level displays the thin superior extension of the hypodense mass. Note also a minimally hyperdense band (arrow) adjacent to the left frontal bone anterior to the hypodense mass. **D.** CECT image at level of centrum semiovale demonstrates the considerable thickness of the peripheral homogeneous band (arrows), which is isodense with the adjacent cortex. Surgical exploration confirmed the presence of both an arachnoid cyst of the left middle fossa and a large subacute subdural hematoma over the left frontal and parietal convexities. ▶

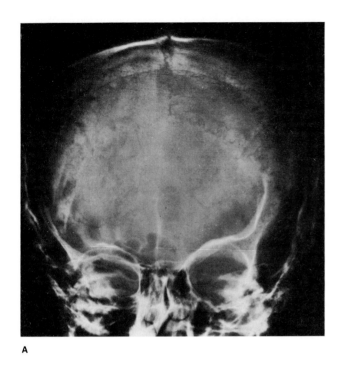

A

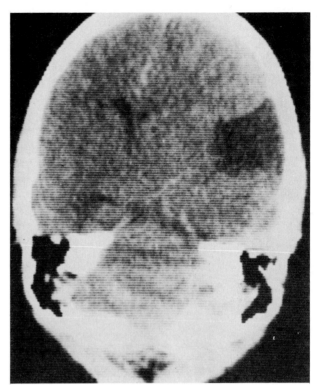

B

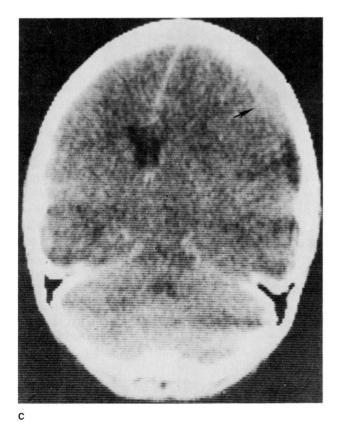

C

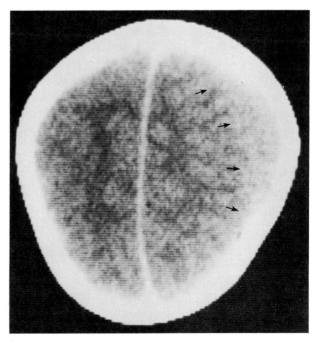

D

Bibliography

ADAM R, GREENBERG JO: The large cisterna magna. Neurosurgery 48(2): 109–192, 1978.

BRANT-ZAWADZKI M, ENZMANN DR: Computed tomographic brain scanning in patients with lymphoma. *Radiology* **129**:67–71, 1978.

BROOKS RA, DICHIRO G: Beam hardening in x-ray reconstructive tomography. *Phys Med Biol* **21**:390–398, 1976.

COHEN CR, DUCHESNEAU P, WEINSTEIN MA: Calcification of the basal ganglia as visualized by CT. *Radiology* **134**:97–99, 1980.

DAVIS DO: CT in the diagnosis of supratentorial tumors. *Semin Roentgenol* **12**:97–108, 1977.

DAVIS KR, TAVERAS JM, NEW PFJ, SCHNUR JA, ROBERSON GH: Cerebral infarction diagnosed by computerized tomography analysis and evaluation of findings. *Am J Roentgenol* **124**:643–660, 1975.

DAVIS KR et al: Computed tomography in head trauma. *Semin Roentgenol* **12**:53–62, 1977.

DOHRMANN GJ, GEEHR RB, ROBINSON F: Small hemorrhages vs. small calcifications in brain tumors: Difficulty in differentiation by CT. *Surg Neurol* **10**:309–312, 1978.

DOLINSKAS CA, ZIMMERMAN RA, BILANIUK LT: A sign of subarachnoid bleeding on cranial computed tomograms of pediatric head trauma patients. *Radiology* **126**:409–411, 1978.

GADO M, HEUTE I, MIKHAEL M: Computerized tomography of infratentorial tumors. *Semin Roentgenol* **12**:109–120, 1977.

GEORGE AE, RUSSELL EJ, KRICHEFF II: White matter buckling: CT sign of extra-axial intracranial mass. *Am J Neuroradiol* **1**:425–430, 1980.

HANDA J, NAKANO Y, HANDA H: Computed tomography in the differential diagnosis of low-density intracranial lesions. *Surg Neurol* **10**:179–185, 1978.

KIM KS, HEMMATI M, WEINBERG PE: Computed tomography in isodense subdural hematoma. *Radiology* **128**:71–72, 1978.

KRAMER RA: Vermian pseudotumor: A potential pitfall of CT brain scanning with contrast enhancement. *Neuroradiology* **13**:229–230, 1977.

LATCHAW RE et al: The monospecificity of absorption coefficients in the differentiation of solid tumors and cystic lesions. *Radiology* **125**:141–144, 1977.

LEE SH, VILLAFANA T: Localization of vertex lesions on cranial computed tomography. *Radiology* **134**:539–540, 1980.

LEMAY M, KIDO D: Asymmetries of the cerebral hemispheres on CT. *J Comput Assist Tomogr* **2**:471–476, 1978.

LEO JS, PINTO RS, HULVAT GF, EPSTEIN F, KRICHEFF II: Computed tomography of arachnoid cysts. *Radiology* **130**:675–680, 1979.

LILIEQUIST B, TOVI D, SCHISANO G: Developmental defects of the tentorium and cisterna magna. *Acta Psychiatr Neurol Scand* **35**:223–234, 1960.

MILLER EM, NEWTON TH: Extra-axial posterior fossa lesions simulating intra-axial lesions on CT. *Radiology* **127**:675–679, 1978.

MODIC MT et al: Calcification of the choroid plexus visualized by computed tomography. *Radiology* **135**:369–372, 1980.

NAIDICH TP et al: The normal contrast-enhanced computed axial tomogram of the brain. *J Comput Assist Tomogr* **1**:16–29, 1977.

NORMAN D et al: Quantitative aspects of computed tomography of the blood and cerebrospinal fluid. *Radiology* **123**:335–338, 1977.

OSBORN AG, ANDERSON RE, WING SD: The false falx sign. *Radiology* **134:**421–425, 1980.

RUSSELL EJ et al: Atypical computed tomographic features of intracranial meningioma. *Radiology* **135:**673–682, 1980.

TANS J, DE JONGH IE: Computed tomography of supratentorial astrocytoma. *Clin Neurol Neurosurg* **80:**156–168, 1978.

TER-POGOSSIAN MM: Computerized cranial tomography: Equipment and physics. *Semin Roentgenol* **12:**13–25, 1977.

WHELAN MA, HILAL SK: CT as a guide in the diagnosis and follow-up of brain abscesses. *Radiology* **135:**663–671, 1980.

WING SD et al: Contrast enhancement of cerebral infarcts in computed tomography. *Radiology* **121:**89–92, 1976.

YOCK DH, MARSHALL WH: Recent ischemic brain infarcts at computed tomography: Appearance pre- and post-contrast infusion. *Radiology* **117:**599–608, 1975.

ZIMMERMAN RA et al: Cranial computed tomography in diagnosis and management of acute head trauma. *Am J Roentgenol* **131:**27–34, 1978.

ZIMMERMAN RD, LEEDS NE, NAIDICH TP: Ring blush associated with intracerebral hematoma. *Radiology* **122:**707–711, 1977.

EPILOGUE: FUTURE EXPECTATIONS

Norman E. Chase

Irvin I. Kricheff

Projections of the future of CT should be divided into short- and long-range. Short-range, as defined in this chapter, means under 3 years, in the authors' projections, and long-range on the order of 10 years. Unfortunately, in our projections we cannot allow for the influence that changes in the economy of the industrialized world or modifications in government regulations in the major industrialized nations may have on the speed of development of new technologies.

First, it should be realized that at the time of publication of this book, there are virtually no CT scanners manufactured that cannot be recommended for clinical application. There are differences in quality and convenience features among them, but all the commonly distributed CT scanners are adequate for reasonably good anatomic diagnosis within the limits of the technique.

It is probable that within the next 1 to 3 years, all the major manufacturers will offer true scan times per slice of under 3 seconds, with density and spatial resolution equal or superior to that available in the best of the current scanners (Margulis 1980). Most of these modifications probably will be retrofittable on the earlier-model scanners that do not now offer that convenience. Standard slice reconstruction time should be under 20 seconds for all the new major manufactured scanners. Reconstruction times under 20 seconds are generally not essential in clinical practice, but rapid-sequence (dynamic) CT scanning will have use in studying intracranial physiologic events (Norman 1981).

Most of the currently available scanners offer spatial resolution of 1 millimeter or less. Some offer fractional-millimeter spatial resolution on high-contrast objects such as bone. It is probable that within the next 1 to 3 years, fractional-millimeter spatial resolution will be available on all units, particularly for high-contrast objects. The universal availability of fractional-millimeter spatial resolution on bony structures should have the side effect of virtually eliminating the market for complex motion tomography equipment.

It is highly unlikely that there will be massive improvement in spatial or density resolution over the next few years. The cost involved in such improvements would probably not be offset by the small amount of additional clinical information that could be obtained with the improvements. The continuing decrease in cost and size of computation equipment probably will permit better utilization of data acquired during scanning and will cause a reduction in artifacts on the final image and somewhat increased reliability of the information.

Marked improvements in scanner software are constantly being made, so it is reasonable to expect that multiplanar reconstructions will be available as a standard feature, and that some types of three-dimensional reconstruction will also be made available. Most will be the pseudo-three-dimensional reconstructions of computer graphics. In addition, some manufacturers may be able to offer holographic reconstructions.

Since all these three-dimensional reconstructions take advantage only of high-contrast difference structures, their usefulness will be rather limited. However, they may be of value in tumor mapping, stereotactic procedures, and teaching detailed normal and abnormal anatomy.

Genuine breakthroughs in CT will require major innovations, such as scanners that are capable of scanning a mass as a whole, rather than in individual slices, and scanners that can complete a scan in less than 50 milliseconds. It is doubtful that such scanners will be available in less than 5 to 10 years, but they will be necessary for such developments as visualization of the heart and its major vessels,

and a number of the other organs in the trunk (Ritman 1980). It is probable that within a decade, the combination of CT and a variation of digital radiography will eliminate virtually all invasive diagnostic procedures of the central nervous system.

CT will be improved for use in stereotactic surgery, since the spatial orientation available with CT is vastly superior to that available by any other means. Integration of scanners and stereotactic probes is possible and, indeed, has been accomplished in a number of universities.

It is possible that in the not too distant future, many intracranial lesions that have been considered inoperable will become approachable by some stereotactic surgical techniques. Certainly we stand to learn a great deal about the electrophysiology of the brain from the accurate placement of probes by the use of modifications of CT.

An unfortunate accompaniment of these changes and of the reduction in the number of manufacturers that can be expected, as well as of the uncertainties of the marketplace caused at least partially by the uncertainties of government regulation, will be an increase in the cost of scanners. It is probable that were market forces allowed to operate freely, the real cost of scanners in constant dollars would be significantly reduced, but such a free market has not been in effect and probably will not be. The standard scanner will certainly be a million dollars or more in constant 1980 dollars.

CT will influence the development of digital radiography, which should offer alternatives to virtually all our film techniques.

What about other techniques that may be related to CT, such as nuclear magnetic resonance (NMR) (James 1981) and positron emission tomography (PET) (Phelps 1980)?

First, the authors would like to suggest that there is no likelihood that these techniques can replace CT and the use of x-ray sources as anatomic imaging systems. If all that NMR can provide is another imaging system, we predict that it will remain inferior to CT. However, if NMR can be used primarily as a nonimaging system for information presently obtained in vitro that could be obtained in vivo, such as the determination of concentrations of metabolites in organs and organ systems, it may have great potential.

PET is potentially inferior as an anatomic imaging device even to NMR. However, PET too is a technique that may offer information not obtainable by means of CT or other x-ray diagnostic modalities. If current investigational work with PET proves to be consistently reproducible, and if cyclotrons can be made smaller, more reliable, and cheaper, PET could become a valuable diagnostic tool in areas such as the diagnosis of mental disorders and the evaluation of cardiac metabolism.

We live in a time of rapidly advancing technology, the medical science fiction of today becoming the accepted technique of tomorrow. As radiologists, we are among the first of our profession to be exposed to innovations. Thus we bear a responsibility to our patients and our peers to constantly stay abreast of new methods in order to apply to our patients only the most rewarding examinations.

Bibliography

JAMES AE JR, PARTIAN CL: Proceedings of the nuclear magnetic resonance (NMR) imaging symposium. *J Comput Assist Tomogr* **5**(2):285–305, April 1981.

MARGULIS A et al: Desirable properties of computed tomography scanners (Opin). *Radiology* **134**:261, 1980.

NORMAN D et al: Dynamic computed tomography of the brain: Techniques, data analysis and applications. *Am J Roentgenol Radium Ther Nucl Med* **136**:759–770, April 1981.

PHELPS ME: Emission computed tomography. *Semin Nucl Med* **7**:568, 1980.

RITMAN E et al: Physics and technical considerations in the design of the DSR: High temporal resolution volume scanners. *Am J Roentgenol Radium Ther Nucl Med* **134**:369, 1980.

Index

Page numbers in *italic* indicate illustrations and tables.